CLINICAL COMPANION
to MEDICAL-SURGICAL NURSING

CLINICAL COMPANION

to MEDICAL-SURGICAL NURSING

Shannon Ruff Dirksen, RN, PhD
Assistant Professor, College of Nursing,
University of New Mexico,
Albuquerque, New Mexico

Sharon Mantik Lewis, RN, PhD, FAAN
Professor, College of Nursing,
Research Associate Professor, Department of Pathology,
University of New Mexico,
Albuquerque, New Mexico

Idolia Cox Collier, RNCS, DNSc
Professor Emeritus, College of Nursing,
University of New Mexico,
Albuquerque, New Mexico

with 32 illustrations

Mosby

St. Louis Baltimore Boston Carlsbad Chicago Naples New York
Philadelphia Portland London Madrid Mexico City Singapore
Sydney Tokyo Toronto Wiesbaden

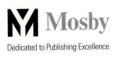

M Mosby

Dedicated to Publishing Excellence

A Times Mirror Company

Vice President and Publisher *Nancy Coon*
Editor *Robin Carter*
Developmental Editor *Jeanne Allison*
Project Manager *Dana Peick*
Production Editor *Dottie Martin*
Designer *Amy Buxton*
Manufacturing Supervisor *Linda Ierardi*

Printed in the United States of America
Editing, production, and composition by Top Graphics
Printing/binding by R.R. Donnelley & Sons Company

Mosby–Year Book, Inc.
11830 Westline Industrial Drive
St. Louis, Missouri 63146

Library of Congress Cataloging-in-Publication Data

Dirksen, Shannon Ruff.
    Clinical companion to Medical-surgical nursing / Shannon Ruff Dirksen, Sharon Mantik Lewis, Idolia Cox Collier.
        p.   cm.
    Companion v. to: Medical-surgical nursing / [edited by] Sharon Mantik Lewis, Idolia Cox Collier, Margaret M. Heitkemper. 4th ed. c1996.
    Includes index.
    ISBN 0-8151-5420-8
    1. Nursing—Handbooks, manuals, etc.   2. Surgical nursing—Handbooks, manuals, etc.   I. Lewis, Sharon Mantik.   II. Collier, Idolia Cox.   III. Medical-surgical nursing.   IV. Title.
    [DNLM: 1. Perioperative Nursing—handbooks.   2. Nursing Care—handbooks.   3. Nursing Assessment.   WY 49 D599c 1996]
RT41.M488   1996 Suppl.
    610.73—dc20
    DNLM/DLC
    for Library of Congress
                                                    95-26642
                                                        CIP

97 98 99 00 / 9 8 7 6 5 4 3 2

PREFACE

The *Clinical Companion* for Lewis, Collier, and Heitkemper's *Medical-Surgical Nursing: Assessment and Management of Clinical Problems,* fourth edition, was developed as a condensed reference of essential information for approximately 225 medical-surgical diseases, disorders, and clinically related subjects. This pocket-sized book provides nurses and nursing students easy access to concise and important information needed when caring for patients with a variety of clinical problems in diverse settings. The *Clinical Companion* can be used independently as a reference or in conjunction with *Medical-Surgical Nursing: Assessment and Management of Clinical Problems.*

The book is divided into three parts. Part One presents commonly encountered medical-surgical disorders arranged alphabetically and organized in a standard format. The disorders are extensively cross-referenced to *Medical-Surgical Nursing,* fourth edition, for the reader who desires more detailed information. Part Two includes brief explanations of common medical-surgical treatments and procedures, such as dialysis, traction, and chemotherapy. Part Three contains reference material related to information frequently used in clinical practice, for example, blood and urine laboratory values, ECG monitoring, and breath sounds. This part also discusses health care resources available on the Internet. An index of disorder and procedure names and their synonyms is provided for easy location of information.

We are especially grateful to our persevering typist, Christa Cooper. We also appreciate the patience and understanding of our families.

We hope that the *Clinical Companion* will become an invaluable reference and resource in helping nurses meet the challenges of caring for patients and their families during states of altered health and well-being.

Shannon Ruff Dirksen
Sharon Mantik Lewis
Idolia Cox Collier

CONTENTS

PART TWO

TREATMENTS AND PROCEDURES

PART THREE

REFERENCE APPENDIX

PART ONE

DISORDERS

ABDOMINAL PAIN, ACUTE

Definition/Description

Causes of acute abdominal pain are varied (Table 1). Although sometimes called "surgical" abdomen, acute abdominal pain does not always necessitate surgery. Many disorders must be ruled out before a diagnosis is confirmed.

Clinical Manifestations

Pain is the most important symptom of acute abdominal pain. A patient may also complain of abdominal tenderness, vomiting, diarrhea, constipation, flatulence, fatigue, and an increase in abdominal girth.

Diagnostic Studies

- Diagnosis begins with a complete health history and physical examination. Physical examination should include both a rectal and a pelvic examination.
- Complete blood count (CBC), urinalysis, abdominal x-ray examination, and an ECG are done initially.
- A pregnancy test should be performed on a woman of childbearing age who has acute abdominal pain.

Therapeutic Management

The goal of management is to identify and treat the cause. A differential diagnosis needs to be made because many causes of abdominal pain do not require surgery (see Table 1).

- In addition to being a therapeutic measure, surgery can be diagnostic. Operative exploration is usually done after careful examination of the patient, and it is justified when "look and see" is better than "wait and see."
- An *exploratory laparotomy* in which an opening is made through the abdominal wall into the peritoneal cavity is done to determine the cause of an acute abdomen. If the cause of acute abdomen can be surgically removed (e.g., inflamed appendix) or surgically repaired (e.g., ruptured abdominal aneurysm), then surgery is considered definitive therapy.

Nursing Management After Laparotomy
Goals

The patient will have a satisfactory level of pain control, relief of nausea and vomiting, normal bowel sounds within 72 hours, absence of fever, and lungs clear to auscultation.

Table 1	**Causes of Acute Abdomen**
Abdominal penetrating trauma	Pancreatitis
Acute ischemic bowel	Pelvic inflammatory disease
Appendicitis	Peptic ulcer
Bowel obstruction with perforation or necrosis	Perforated GI malignancy
Cholecystitis	Peritonitis
Crohn's disease	Ruptured abdominal aneurysm
Diverticulitis with peritonitis	Ruptured ectopic pregnancy
Foreign body perforation	Ruptured ovarian cyst
Gastritis	Ulcerative colitis

See the nursing care plan for the patient after laparotomy in Lewis/Collier/Heitkemper, *Medical-Surgical Nursing,* edition 4, p. 1218.

Nursing Diagnoses

- Pain related to surgical incision and inadequate pain control measures
- Nausea and vomiting related to decreased GI motility, GI distention, and narcotics
- Ineffective airway clearance related to effects of anesthesia, sedation, pain, immobility, and location of incision
- Constipation related to immobility, pain, medication, and decreased motility

Nursing Interventions

General care for the patient involves management of fluid and electrolyte imbalances, pain, and anxiety. Preoperative preparation of a patient with an acute abdomen includes a CBC count, typing and crossmatching of blood, and clotting studies. Catheterization, preparation of abdominal skin, and passage of a nasogastric (NG) tube may be done in the emergency department or operating room (OR).

Increased use of laparoscopic procedures has reduced the risk of postoperative complications related to wound care and altered GI motility. These procedures generally result in shorter hospital stays. A general nursing care plan for the postoperative patient is presented in Lewis/Collier/Heitkemper, *Medical-Surgical Nursing,* edition 4, p. 396. A nursing care plan for the patient after laparotomy is presented in Lewis/Collier/Heitkemper, *Medical-Surgical Nursing,* edition 4, p. 1218.

- If an NG tube is present, it is connected to suction as ordered. The purpose of this tube is to empty the stomach of secretions and gas to prevent gastric dilatation. The NG tube is checked frequently for patency because it may become obstructed with mucus, sediment, or old blood. An order is usually written to irrigate the tube with 20 to 30 ml of normal saline solution if needed. Repositioning the tube may facilitate drainage. Mouth care and nasal care are essential.

- Parenteral fluids are administered to provide the patient with fluids and electrolytes until bowel sounds return. Occasionally, ice chips may be ordered because they relieve a dry mouth.

- Although nausea and vomiting are not uncommon after abdominal surgery, these problems are often self-limiting. Observation is important in determining the cause. Antiemetics such as promethazine (Phenergan), prochlorperazine (Compazine), or trimethobenzamide (Tigan) may be ordered.

- Abdominal distention and gas pains are also common after a laparotomy; they are due to swallowed air and impaired peristalsis resulting from immobility, manipulation of abdominal contents during surgery, and side effects of anesthesia. The resulting pain can be so uncomfortable that medications to stimulate peristalsis, such as bethanechol (Urecholine) or neostigmine methylsulfate (Prostigmin), may be given. A rectal tube or moist heat on the abdomen may be effective in relieving distention. The physician should be informed of abdominal distention and rigidity. As intestinal activity increases, distention and gas pains gradually decrease.

- Emotional support from the nursing staff is important. Honest, clear, concise explanations of all procedures in language the patient and family can understand will assist in allaying anxiety.

Patient Teaching

Patient teaching for discharge begins when the patient returns from the OR. Instructions to the patient and family should include any modifications in activity, care of the incision, diet, and drug therapy.

- Small, frequent meals that are high in calories should be taken initially, with a gradual increase in food intake as tolerated.

- Normal activities should be resumed gradually with planned rest periods.

- The patient should be aware of possible complications after surgery and should notify the physician immediately if vomiting, pain, weight loss, incisional drainage, or changes in bowel function occur.

ACHALASIA

Definition/Description
In achalasia (cardiospasm), peristalsis of the lower two thirds (smooth muscle) of the esophagus is absent. Lower esophageal sphincter (LES) pressure is increased, along with incomplete relaxation of the LES. Achalasia affects all ages and both genders, and the disease has a chronic course.

Pathophysiology
This condition results in dilatation of the lower esophagus. Obstruction of the esophagus at or near the diaphragm also occurs with food and fluid accumulating in the lower esophagus. The altered peristalsis is a result of impairment of the autonomic nervous system innervating the esophagus.

Clinical Manifestations
- Dysphagia (difficulty in swallowing) is the most common symptom and occurs more frequently with liquids.
- Substernal chest pain (similar to the pain of angina) occurs during or immediately after a meal.
- Halitosis (bad breath) and the inability to erucate (belch) are other symptoms.
- Another common symptom is regurgitation of sour-tasting food and liquids, especially when the patient is in a horizontal position.
- Weight loss is typical.

Therapeutic and Nursing Management
Symptomatic treatment consists of eating a semisoft bland diet, eating slowly, drinking fluid with meals, and sleeping with the head elevated. More definitive treatment consists of dilatation, surgery, and the use of drugs directed at relieving the stasis caused by increased LES pressure, nonrelaxing LES, and aperistaltic esophagus.
  - Esophageal dilatation (bougienage) is an effective treatment measure for many patients. Pneumatic dilatation of the LES with a balloon-tipped dilator passed orally is usually used. The forceful dilatation does not restore normal esophageal motility but does provide for emptying of the esophagus into the stomach.
  - Surgical intervention, such as an esophagomyotomy, may become necessary. In this procedure the muscle fibers that enclose the narrowed area of the esophagus are divided.
  - Classes of drugs used include anticholinergics, calcium channel antagonists (nifedipine is one of the most effective), and long-acting nitrates.

ACUTE RESPIRATORY DISTRESS SYNDROME

Definition/Description

Acute respiratory distress syndrome (ARDS) is a sudden, progressive disorder consisting of pulmonary edema of noncardiac origin, severe dyspnea, hypoxemia refractory to supplemental O_2, reduced lung compliance, and diffuse pulmonary infiltrates. ARDS is either a cause or a consequence of the systemic inflammatory response syndrome (SIRS), which occurs as a response to a severe insult. SIRS is characterized by widespread inflammation or clinical responses to inflammation occurring in a patient with a variety of insults. When SIRS is the result of infection, the term *sepsis* is used.

- ARDS itself may initiate SIRS, or it may be one of the earliest manifestations of the multiple organ dysfunction syndrome (MODS), which develops as a consequence of SIRS. MODS results from progressive failure of several interdependent organ systems following a significant insult, such as trauma, burns, or infection.
- Risk factors for the development of SIRS or MODS include delayed resuscitation, persistent infection, shock (especially septic shock), multiple trauma with massive tissue injury, bowel infarction, diabetes mellitus, and cancer. Many clinical disorders cause either direct lung injury (e.g., pneumonia, gastric aspiration) or indirect lung injury caused by mediators produced by SIRS.

Pathophysiology

Initial insult to the lungs occurs in the patient who may have a variety of clinical disorders as previously mentioned. The common abnormal finding is diffuse alveolar-capillary membrane damage with subsequent leakage of fluid from the vascular space into the interstitium and alveoli.

The exact cause for damage to the alveolar-capillary membrane is not known; however, many cellular and humoral mediators are thought to be involved. Release of these inflammatory mediators results in structural damage to lungs, increased vascular permeability, development of microemboli of platelets and fibrin within the pulmonary vasculature, vasoconstriction leading to increased vascular resistance, and bronchoconstriction.

Pathophysiologic changes in ARDS are divided into three phases: injury or exudative, reparative or proliferative, and fibrotic.

- *Injury* or *exudative phase* occurs approximately 1 to 7 days (usually 24 to 48 hours) after initial direct lung injury. An influx of neutrophils, which adhere to the pulmonary microcirculation, causes alveolar-capillary injury. Because of this disruption in normal alveolar-capillary membrane, fluid accumulates (proteinaceous pulmonary edema). As alveoli collapse and fill with fluid, increased shunting of blood occurs, and alveolar hypoventilation, decreased cardiac output, and decreased tissue perfusion develop.
- *Reparative* or *proliferative phase* begins 1 to 2 weeks after initial lung injury. During this phase there is an influx of granulocytes, monocytes, and lymphocytes. The injured lung has an immense regenerative capacity after acute lung injury.
- *Fibrotic phase* occurs approximately 2 to 3 weeks after initial lung injury. This phase is also called the *chronic* or *late phase* of ARDS. By this time, the lung is completely remodeled by sparsely collagenous and fibrous tissues. There is diffuse scarring and fibrosis, resulting in decreased lung compliance and decreased surface area for gas exchange. Pulmonary hypertension results from fibrosis.

Progression of ARDS varies among patients for unknown reasons. Some persons survive the acute phase of lung injury; pulmonary edema resolves, and the patient completely recovers in a few days. Others progress to the fibrotic (late or chronic) phase requiring long-term mechanical ventilation, with a poor chance of survival.

Clinical Manifestations

At the time of initial injury and for several hours to 1 to 2 days afterward, the patient may not experience respiratory symptoms.

- *Initial presentation* of ARDS is often insidious. The patient may exhibit dyspnea, cough, and restlessness. Chest auscultation may be normal or reveal fine, scattered crackles. Arterial blood gas (ABG) analysis demonstrates mild hypoxemia and respiratory alkalosis. Chest x-ray may be normal or exhibit evidence of minimal scattered interstitial infiltrates. Edema may not manifest until there is a 30% increase in lung fluid content.
- *As ARDS progresses,* symptoms develop that are related to increased fluid accumulation in the lungs and decreased lung compliance. Respiratory discomfort becomes evident as the work of breathing increases. Noisy tachypneic respirations, and intercostal retractions may be present. Tachycardia, diaphoresis, changes in sensorium with decreased mentation, cyanosis, and pallor may be present. Chest auscultation usually reveals scattered to diffuse crackles and rhonchi.

Complications of ARDS are summarized in Table 2. A major cause of death in ARDS is MODS, often accompanied by sepsis. Organs most commonly involved are the kidneys, liver, and heart; systems most often involved are the central nervous system, hematologic system, and GI system.

Diagnostic Studies

- Pulmonary function tests reveal decreased compliance and decreased lung volumes, particularly functional residual capacity (FRC).
- Chest x-ray demonstrates diffuse and extensive bilateral interstitial and alveolar infiltrates. Chest x-ray is often termed *white out* or *white lung* because consolidation and coalescing infiltrates pervade the lungs, leaving few recognizable air spaces. Pleural effusions may also be present.
- Diagnosis of ARDS is confirmed if pulmonary capillary wedge pressure is within normal limits. Typically, pulmonary artery pressures increase in heart failure.

Table 2	Complications Associated with Acute Respiratory Distress Syndrome

Infection Nosocomial pneumonia Catheter-related infection Sepsis (bacteremia)	**Renal Complications** **Cardiac Complications** Decreased cardiac output Dysrhythmias
Respiratory Complications Pulmonary emboli Pulmonary barotrauma (e.g., pneumothorax, pneumomediastinum, subcutaneous emphysema) O_2 toxicity Pulmonary fibrosis	**Hematologic Complications** Anemia Thrombocytopenia Disseminated intravascular coagulation **CNS Complications**
GI Complications Stress ulceration and hemorrhage Ileus	**Endotracheal Intubation Complications** Laryngeal ulceration Tracheal ulceration Tracheal stenosis

CNS, Central nervous system.

- Progressive arterial hypoxemia, despite an increased fraction of inspired oxygen (FIO_2) by mask, cannula, or endotracheal tube, is a *hallmark* of ARDS. This development is called *refractory hypoxemia.*
- ABG values may demonstrate a normal partial pressure of carbon dioxide in arterial blood ($PaCO_2$) despite severe dyspnea and hypoxemia.
- As ARDS continues to the fibrotic phase, it is associated with profound respiratory distress requiring endotracheal intubation and assisted ventilation.
- Severe hypoxemia, hypercapnia, and metabolic acidosis with symptoms of target organ or tissue hypoxia may ensue if prompt therapy is not instituted.

Therapeutic and Nursing Management

Therapeutic and nursing management of ARDS and acute respiratory failure are strongly interdependent and are presented in Tables 3 and 4.

Prevention of ARDS. Observation of the respiratory status of a patient at risk for ARDS is especially important. Judicious fluid administration and monitoring of fluid status by intake and output records, weights, clinical manifestations of increased fluid in the lung (e.g., crackles, deteriorating ABGs, increased work of breathing), and body fluid accumulation (e.g., jugular venous distention; sacral or peripheral edema; splenomegaly) are important. Expeditious treatment of the initial disorder (e.g., prompt treatment with antibiotics or surgery to remove the source of infection in sepsis and maintenance of BP and renal blood flow in shock) is necessary and may prevent further deterioration of the patient and the development of ARDS.

Treatment of underlying disorder. Sepsis is often an initiating mechanism of ARDS. Prompt culture of exudates, secretions, and blood and surgical debridement (if indicated) of an infected area are necessary. Antibiotic therapy should be instituted as soon as possible.

- If severe arterial hypotension and shock are initiating factors, restoration of adequate BP is essential. Frequently, overzealous administration of fluids in the attempt to restore BP leads to circulatory overload and pulmonary edema.

Maintenance of adequate oxygenation
- Endotracheal intubation with subsequent mechanical ventilation is almost always required (see Intubation, Endotracheal, p. 657, and Mechanical Ventilation, p. 662).
- When adequate oxygenation is not achieved by conventional mechanical ventilation and when PaO_2 remains <60 mm Hg with an FIO_2 of >0.5 to 0.6, use of positive expiratory end pressure (PEEP) is indicated.

Table 3	Principles of Therapeutic Management of Acute Respiratory Distress Syndrome

- Identify and treat underlying condition
- Establish an airway (usually endotracheal tube)
- Institute mechanical ventilation
    Volume-cycled ventilator
    PEEP
- Maintain oxygenation
    O_2 administration
    Packed RBCs
- Increase cardiac output and maintain blood pressure
    Dolbutamine
    Dopamine
- Monitor oxygenation and cardiac output
    Arterial line
    Pulmonary artery catheter
    Oximetry
- Maintain fluid balance
    Colloids, crystalloids
    Diuretics
- Treat infections

PEEP, positive end expiratory pressure; *RBCs*, red blood cells.

Maintenance of cardiac output and hemoglobin concentration. Continuous hemodynamic monitoring of the patient with ARDS who is receiving ventilator and PEEP therapy is required. An arterial line should be inserted to obtain continuous recording of BP and to make it easier to obtain frequent ABG measurements. Cardiac output can be assessed by the thermodilution port of the pulmonary artery catheter.

Maintenance of fluid balance. Leaky capillaries increase fluid in the lungs and cause pulmonary edema. However, the patient may be volume depleted and prone to hypotension and decreased cardiac output from mechanical ventilation and PEEP.

- Pulmonary capillary wedge pressure (which indicates fluid status of the left side of the heart) is kept as low as possible without impairing cardiac output. The patient is usually placed on mild fluid restriction and diuretics are used as necessary. Strict intake and output and daily weights are done. Electrolytes and fluid status are monitored.

Table 4	Therapeutic and Nursing Management: Acute Respiratory Failure

Maintenance of Adequate Oxygenation
O_2 administration to keep PaO_2 >60 mm Hg
Maintenance of adequate hemoglobin concentration
Maintenance of adequate cardiac output
Prevention and assessment of tissue hypoxia
Measures to decrease stress and anxiety and promote comfort

Improvement of Alveolar Ventilation
- Maintenance of patent airway
  Effective coughing
  Suctioning
  Positioning
- Measures to assist in liquefaction and movement of secretions
  Humidification
  Adequate hydration
  Chest physiotherapy (if indicated)
  Bland aerosols and ultrasonic nebulization
- Relief of bronchospasm
  Bronchodilators
  Aerosolized bronchodilators
  Corticosteroids (when indicated)
- Reduction of pulmonary congestion
  Diuretics
- Ventilatory assistance
  Continuous positive pressure breathing
  Noninvasive positive pressure ventilation

Treatment of Underlying Cause of Failure

Continuous Monitoring and Evaluation of Treatment

PaO$_2$, Partial pressure of oxygen in arterial blood.

Goals

The patient with ARDS will have a PaO_2 within limits of normal for age, oxygen saturation in blood (as measured by arterial blood gas analysis) (SaO_2) >90%, a patent airway, and clear lungs on auscultation.

Nursing Diagnoses/Collaborative Problems
- Ineffective breathing pattern related to neuromuscular impairment, anxiety, respiratory muscle fatigue, and expiratory obstruction to airflow
- Ineffective airway clearance related to accumulation of secretions, decreased level of consciousness, presence of an artifi-

cial airway, thoracic and/or abdominal neuromuscular dysfunction, and pain

- Dyspnea related to increased airway resistance, airtrapping or hyperinflation, decreased lung compliance, and decreased chest wall compliance
- Anxiety related to dyspnea, intubation, severity of illness, loss of personal control, and uncertain outcome
- Risk for fluid volume excess related to increases in peripheral or pulmonary fluid secondary to heart failure or acute respiratory distress
- Potential complication: hypercapnia related to alveolar hypoventilation and $\dot{V}/\dot{Q}$ mismatch
- Potential complication: hypoxemia related to alveolar hypoventilation, intrapulmonary shunting, and $\dot{V}/\dot{Q}$ mismatch

Patient Teaching

Teaching slow pursed-lip breathing techniques can help the patient feel some sense of control over breathing. Fear of suffocation or death is not uncommon.

- Providing reassurance, spending time with the patient, and ensuring that help can be received immediately (e.g., call light is readily available) may help to decrease the patient's anxiety level. Anxiety may also be reduced through instruction and use of progressive relaxation, guided imagery, and meditation.
- It is helpful to explain to the patient any possible sensations that may be encountered with each new experience (e.g., suctioning, drawing ABGs) so that coping strategies can be purposefully selected.

ADDISON'S DISEASE

Definition/Description

Addison's disease is a hypofunction of the adrenal cortex or adrenocortical insufficiency in which all three classes of adrenal steroids (glucocorticoids, mineralocorticoids, and androgens) are reduced. In North America the most common cause of primary Addison's disease (which is a rare condition) is autoimmune; adrenal tissue is destroyed by antibodies against the patient's own adrenal cortex. Less common causes include hemorrhage, infarction, fungal infections (e.g., histoplasmosis), acquired immunodeficiency syndrome (AIDS), and metastatic cancer. Iatrogenic Addison's disease may be due to anticoagulant therapy (causing adrenal hemorrhage), antineoplastic chemotherapy, ketoconazole therapy for AIDS, or bilateral adrenalectomy.

Clinical Manifestations

Primary manifestations are progressive weakness, fatigue, weight loss, and anorexia. Skin hyperpigmentation, a striking feature, is seen primarily in sun-exposed areas of the body, at pressure points, over joints, and in creases, especially palmar creases.

- Other frequent manifestations are hypotension, hyponatremia, hyperkalemia, nausea and vomiting, and diarrhea.
- The most dangerous feature is hypotension, which may cause shock, especially during stress. Circulatory collapse from this cause is unresponsive to the usual treatment (vasopressors and fluid replacement) and requires glucocorticoid administration.

A patient with adrenocortical insufficiency is at risk for *acute adrenal insufficiency (Addisonian crisis)*, which is a life-threatening emergency caused by insufficient adrenocortical hormones or a sudden sharp decrease in these hormones.

- This crisis may occur during stress (e.g., from infection, surgery, trauma, or psychologic distress), sudden cessation of adrenocortical hormone replacement therapy (often done by a patient who lacks knowledge regarding replacement therapy), adrenal surgery, or sudden pituitary gland destruction (pituitary apoplexy).

Diagnostic Studies

- Plasma cortisol levels are subnormal or fail to rise over basal levels with an adrenocorticotropic hormone (ACTH) stimulation test. Free cortisol urine levels are decreased.
- Serum electrolytes show hyperkalemia, hypochloremia, and hyponatremia.
- CT scan and MRI are used to localize tumors or identify adrenal enlargement.

Therapeutic Management

Treatment is focused on the management of the underlying cause when possible. Regardless of etiology, the mainstay of treatment is replacement therapy with glucocorticoids. A patient who takes medications consistently can have a normal life expectancy.

- Hydrocortisone, the most commonly used form of replacement therapy, also has mineralocorticoid properties.
- When any illness or stress occurs, whether mild or acute, glucocorticoid dosage must be increased to prevent adrenal crisis. The patient should take two to three times the usual dose and notify the physician.
- If vomiting or diarrhea occurs, as may happen with the flu, the physician must be notified immediately because electrolyte replacement may be necessary. In addition, these symptoms may be early indicators of crisis.

A

Management of Addisonian crisis requires immediate glucocorticoid replacement therapy. Treatment must be vigorous and directed toward shock management. IV administration of hydrocortisone 100 mg every 6 hours, sodium, fluids, and dextrose (for hypoglycemia) are necessary for 24 hours or until BP returns to normal.

Nursing Management

Goals

The patient with Addison's disease will manage self-care activities, experience relief of symptoms, learn to adjust the medication dosage to life situations, avoid acute adrenocortical insufficiency, and actively participate in the long-term therapeutic plan.

Nursing Diagnoses

- Activity intolerance related to weakness and hypotension
- Self-care deficit related to weakness, lack of interest, depression
- Self-esteem disturbances related to inability to perform usual activities, loss of hair, skin hyperpigmentation
- Altered health maintenance related to lack of knowledge of management of lifelong hormone replacement therapy

Nursing Interventions

When the patient with Addison's disease is hospitalized, whether for diagnosis, an acute crisis, or some other health problem, frequent nursing assessment is necessary.

- Vital signs and signs of fluid volume deficit and electrolyte imbalance should be assessed every 30 minutes to 4 hours for the first 24 hours, depending on the patient's instability.
- Nursing interventions include daily weights, diligent steroid administration, protection against exposure to infection (reverse isolation), and complete assistance with daily hygiene.
- The patient should be protected from noise, light, and environmental temperature extremes. (The patient cannot cope with these stresses because corticosteroids cannot be produced.)

If hospitalization is due to an adrenal crisis, a patient usually responds by the second day and can start oral corticosteroid replacement.

- Because discharge frequently occurs before the usual maintenance dose of corticosteroids is reached, the patient should be instructed on the importance of keeping scheduled follow-up appointments.

Patient Teaching

Because of the serious nature of the disease and the need for lifelong replacement therapy, a well-organized and carefully presented teaching plan is important to the health of the patient. The major areas that must be included in the teaching plan are the following:

1. Names, dosages, and actions of drugs
2. Symptoms of overdosage and underdosage
3. Conditions requiring increased medication (e.g., trauma, surgery, emotional crisis)
4. Course of action to take relative to changes in need for medication
5. Prevention of infection and need for prompt and vigorous treatment of existing infections
6. Need for lifelong replacement therapy and medical supervision
7. Need for medical-alert identification device

Patients who can control or manage the degree of stress they experience can maintain a better hormone balance than those who cannot. The nurse should help the patient develop effective coping skills and techniques for handling stress or make appropriate referrals.

- The patient should have an emergency kit nearby at all times. The kit should consist of 100 mg of intramuscular (IM) hydrocortisone, syringes, and instructions for use.
- The patient and significant others should be instructed on how to give an IM injection if replacement therapy cannot be taken orally. The patient should verbalize instructions, practice IM injections with saline, and have written instructions as to when to alter the dosage.

ALLERGIC DISORDERS

Definition/Description

Although an alteration in the immune system may be manifested in many ways, allergies or type I hypersensitivity reactions are the most frequently seen alterations (see Hypersensitivity Reactions, p. 314).

Diagnostic Studies

A complete blood count (CBC) with a white blood cell (WBC) differential is required with an eosinophil count. Eosinophil count is elevated with type I hypersensitivity reactions involving IgE immunoglobulins. Serum IgE level is also elevated in type I hypersensitivity reactions and serves as a diagnostic indicator of atopic (allergic) diseases.

- Radioallergosorbent test (RAST) is an in vitro diagnostic test for IgE antibodies to a specific allergen.

- If asthma is suspected, pulmonary function tests for vital capacity, forced expiratory volume, and maximum midexpiratory flow rates are helpful.
- Skin testing is used to confirm specific sensitivity in patients with atopic disease after the health history has suggested possible allergens for testing.

Therapeutic and Nursing Management

After an allergic disorder is diagnosed, therapeutic treatment attempts the following: (1) reducing exposure to offending allergens, (2) treating symptoms, and (3) desensitizing the person through immunotherapy. All health care workers must be prepared for the rare but life-threatening anaphylactic reaction that requires immediate medical and nursing interventions. It is important that all of a patient's allergies are listed on the chart, nursing care plan, and medication record.

Anaphylaxis. Anaphylactic reactions occur suddenly in hypersensitive patients after exposure to the offending allergen. They may occur after parenteral injection of drugs (especially antibiotics) and insect stings.

- The cardinal principle in therapeutic management is *speed* in the following: (1) recognition of signs and symptoms of an anaphylactic reaction, (2) maintenance of a patent airway, (3) prevention of allergen spread by using a tourniquet, (4) administration of drugs, and (5) treatment for shock.
- Mild symptoms such as pruritus and urticaria can be controlled by administration of epinephrine given subcutaneously every 20 minutes according to the physician's orders or hospital emergency drug protocol. An IV infusion should be initiated to provide a route for administration of epinephrine, volume expanders, and vasopressor agents such as dopamine if intractable hypotension occurs.
- O_2 given through a nasal catheter or intermittent positive pressure breathing of O_2 with isoproterenol (Isuprel) may be helpful. Endotracheal intubation or a tracheostomy is necessary for O_2 delivery if progressive hypoxia exists.
- Other agents are used, including an antihistamine such as diphenhydramine (Benadryl) for urticaria and angioedema and aminophylline IV for bronchospasm.
- Hypovolemic shock may occur because of intravascular fluid loss into the interstitial spaces. Unless shock is treated early, the body will no longer be able to compensate, and irreversible tissue damage will occur, leading to death (see Shock, p. 521).

Chronic allergies. Most allergic reactions are chronic and are characterized by remissions and exacerbations of symptoms. Treatment focuses on identification and control of allergens, relief of symptoms through pharmacologic interventions, and hyposensitization of the patient to the offending allergen.

- The nurse plays an important role in helping the patient make lifestyle adjustments so that there is minimal exposure to offending allergens. The nurse must reinforce that, even with drug therapy and immunotherapy, the patient will never be totally desensitized or completely free of symptoms.

The major categories of drugs used for symptomatic relief of chronic allergic disorders include the following:

1. Antihistamines (e.g., Benadryl)
2. Sympathomimetic-decongestant drugs (e.g., epinephrine)
3. Corticosteroids (e.g., Vancenase inhaler)
4. Antipruritic drugs (e.g., Temaril)
5. Antiinflammatory agents (e.g., cromolyn [Intal])

Many of these drugs may be obtained over the counter and are often misused by patients. (See Table 10-13 in Lewis/Collier/Heitkemper, *Medical-Surgical Nursing,* edition 4, p. 223.)

Patient Teaching

- Of primary importance is the need to identify the offending allergen; sometimes this is done through skin testing. In the case of food allergies, an elimination diet is a useful strategy. If an allergic reaction occurs, all food eaten should be eliminated and gradually reintroduced one at a time until the offending food is detected.
- Many allergic reactions, especially asthma and urticaria, may be aggravated by fatigue and emotional stress. The nurse can be instrumental in initiating a stress management program with the patient.
- Control of allergic symptoms may require environmental control, including changing occupations, moving to a different climate, or giving up a pet. In the case of airborne allergens, sleeping in an air-conditioned room, damp dusting daily, and wearing a mask outdoors may be helpful.
- If the allergen is a drug, the patient should be instructed to avoid the drug. The patient also has the responsibility to make drug intolerance well known to all health care providers. The patient should wear a medical-alert bracelet listing the particular drug allergy and have the drug listed on all medical and dental records.
- For a patient allergic to insect stings, commercial bee-sting kits containing preinjectable epinephrine and a tourniquet are available. The nurse has the responsibility to instruct the patient about applying the tourniquet and self-injecting subcutaneous

epinephrine. This patient also should wear a medical-alert bracelet and carry a bee-sting kit along whenever going outdoors.

Alzheimer's Disease

Definition/Description

Alzheimer's disease is a type of dementia characterized by progressive deterioration in memory and other aspects of cognition. The term *dementia of the Alzheimer type (DAT)* is used to identify this type of dementia, regardless of age. DAT is increasingly recognized as a major health problem in the United States, particularly for persons more than 65 years of age.

Pathophysiology

Although no single cause for DAT has been found, there are several etiologic hypotheses, including disordered immune function, viral infection, and genetic factors.

- Cellular changes associated with DAT include neurofibrillary tangles and β-amyloid plaques in the cerebral cortex and hippocampus. There is also an excessive loss of cholinergic neurons, particularly in regions essential for memory and cognition.
- Genes on chromosome 21 (site of abnormality for patients with Down syndrome) have been linked to a predisposition to DAT. In the familial form of DAT, age of onset is younger (50 to 60 years) and severity of dementia is greater than in nonfamilial cases.

Clinical Manifestations

- An initial sign is subtle deterioration in memory. Inevitably this progresses to more profound memory loss that interferes with the patient's ability to function. Recent events and new information cannot be recalled. Personal hygiene deteriorates as does the ability to maintain attention.
- Later in the disease, long-term memory fails, and a patient loses the ability to recognize family members. Eventually the ability to communicate and to perform activities of daily living is lost.
- Progression of deterioration, which eventually leads to death, varies but can last as long as 20 years.
- DAT must be distinguished from depression, a clinically similar condition, because depression is potentially reversible and often responds to appropriate treatment. A careful assessment can distinguish the two clinical conditions (Table 5).

Table 5	Differentiation of Depression and Alzheimer's-Type Dementia	
	Depression	**Dementia**
Onset	Abrupt (weeks)	Insidious
Psychiatric history	Previous depression common	Usually no history
Mental status	Pervasive dysphoria	Flattening of affect
	Normal or impaired cognition	Impaired cognition
	Variable performance	Stable performance
	Variable memory disturbance	Memory deteriorates
Sleep disturbance	Initial and early-morning insomnia	Frequent awakenings
Somatic complaints	Often multiple	Often none
Self-image	Poor	Normal
Suicidal ideation	Present	Absent
Treatment	High effectiveness of antidepressants	Very limited usefulness of antidepressants
Weight loss	Yes, with appetite disturbance	No

Diagnostic Studies

Diagnosis of DAT is one of exclusion. When all other possible conditions that can cause mental impairment have been ruled out and manifestations of dementia persist, the diagnosis of DAT can be made.

- A CT scan or MRI may show brain atrophy and enlarged ventricles in later stages of disease, although this finding occurs in other diseases and in normal persons.
- Neuropsychologic testing can help document the degree of cognitive dysfunction in early stages.
- Definitive diagnosis of DAT can be made only at autopsy when the presence of neurofibrillary tangles is observed.

Therapeutic Management

Pharmacologic agents are used to control undesirable symptoms that the patient may exhibit. These may include tricyclic antidepressants, antipsychotics, benzodiazepines, and neuroleptic medications. The drug tacrine, an acetylcholinesterase inhibitor, may delay deterioration in cognitive function. Its long-term efficacy remains to be determined. It is important for the nurse to be aware that this type of drug does not alter the course of the disease.

Nursing Management

Goals

The patient with Alzheimer's disease will maintain functional ability for as long as possible, be maintained in a safe environment with a minimum of injuries, and have personal care needs met.

See the nursing care plan for the patient with Alzheimer's disease in Lewis/Collier/Heitkemper, *Medical-Surgical Nursing,* edition 4, p. 1785.

Nursing Diagnoses

- Altered thought processes related to effects of dementia
- Total self-care deficit related to memory deficit and inability to distinguish appropriate from inappropriate patterns of dressing, grooming, eating, and toileting
- Ineffective individual coping related to depression in response to diagnosis
- Sleep pattern disturbance related to physical discomfort, excessive napping secondary to inability to initiate activities, lack of physical activity
- Risk for injury related to impaired judgment, muscle weakness, sensory or perceptual alteration
- Risk for ineffective management of therapeutic regimen related to decreasing level of cognitive functioning and memory
- Risk for violence related to sensory overload, lack of appropriate coping mechanisms, and unfamiliar environment

Nursing Interventions

Although there is no current effective treatment for DAT, there is a need for ongoing monitoring of both the patient and the patient's caregiver. An important nursing responsibility is to work collaboratively with the patient's physician to manage symptoms effectively as they change with time.

- The nurse is often responsible for teaching the caregiver to perform essential tasks for the patient. To aid in identifying caregiver problems, a nursing care plan for the caregiver of the patient with Alzheimer's disease is presented in Lewis/Collier/Heitkemper, *Medical-Surgical Nursing,* edition 4, p. 1787. Adult day care is one of the options available to caregivers. Common goals of all day-care programs are to provide respite for family and protective services for the patient.
- The nursing care needs of the patient change as the disease progresses, emphasizing the need for regular assessment, monitoring, and support. Regardless of the setting, the severity of symptoms and amount of care required intensify with time.

- A patient with DAT is subject to acute and other chronic illnesses. The inability of the patient to communicate health symptoms and problems places responsibility for assessment and diagnosis on caregivers and health professionals. Hospitalization of the patient can be a traumatic event for both the patient and caregiver and can precipitate a crisis.

AMYOTROPHIC LATERAL SCLEROSIS

Amyotrophic lateral sclerosis (ALS), a rare progressive neurologic disease, results from a loss of motor neurons. This disease became known as Lou Gehrig's disease when the famous baseball player was stricken with it in the early 1940s. The onset is between the ages of 40 and 70 years, and twice as many men as women are affected.

- For unknown reasons, motor neurons in the brain stem and spinal cord gradually degenerate in ALS. Consequently, electrical and chemical messages originating in the brain never reach the muscles to activate them.
- Primary symptoms are weakness of upper extremities, dysarthria, and dysphagia. Muscle wasting and fasciculations result from denervation of muscles and lack of use.
- Death usually results from respiratory infection secondary to compromised respiratory function.
- There is no cure or treatment for ALS. This illness is devastating because the patient remains cognitively intact while wasting away.
- The challenge of nursing care is to support the patient's cognitive and emotional functions by facilitating communication, providing diversional activities such as reading and human companionship, and helping the person and family with anticipatory grieving related to loss of motor function and ultimate death.

ANEMIA

Definition/Description
Anemia is a reduction below normal in the number of erythrocytes, the quantity of hemoglobin (Hb), and/or the volume of packed red cells (hematocrit). This disorder can be caused by rapid blood loss, impaired production of erythrocytes, and/or increased destruction of erythrocytes.

Table 6	**Etiologic Classification of Anemia**

Decreased Erythrocyte Production
- Decreased hemoglobin synthesis
  Iron deficiency
  Thalassemias (decreased globin synthesis)
  Sideroblastic anemia (decreased porphyrin)
- Defective DNA synthesis
  Vitamin B_{12} deficiency
  Folic acid deficiency
- Decreased number of erythrocyte precursors
  Aplastic anemia
  Anemia of leukemia and myelodysplasia
  Chronic diseases or disorders

Blood Loss
- Acute
  Trauma
  Blood vessel rupture
- Chronic
  Gastritis
  Menstrual flow
  Hemorrhoids

Increased Erythrocyte Destruction*
- Intrinsic
  Abnormal hemoglobin (HbS–sickle-cell anemia)
  Enzyme deficiency (G6PD)
  Membrane abnormalities (paroxysmal nocturnal
    hemoglobinuria)
- Extrinsic
  Physical trauma (prosthetic heart valves, extracorporeal
    circulation)
  Antibodies (isoimmune and autoimmune)
  Infectious agents and toxins (malaria)

*Hemolytic anemias.

- Because erythrocytes transport O_2, erythrocyte disorders can lead to tissue hypoxia. This hypoxia accounts for many of the clinical manifestations of anemia.
- Anemia is not a specific disease; it is a manifestation of a pathologic process. Anemia is identified and classified by laboratory evaluation.

- Anemia can result from primary hematologic problems or can develop as a secondary consequence of defects in other body systems.

The different types of anemia can be classified according to either etiology or morphology.

- Etiologic classification is related to the clinical conditions causing anemia, such as decreased erythrocyte production, blood loss, or increased erythrocyte destruction (Table 6).
- Morphologic classification is based on the descriptive and objective laboratory information about erythrocyte size and color.

Although the morphologic system is the most accurate means of classifying anemia, it is easier to discuss patient care by focusing on the etiologic problem. Table 7 relates morphologic classifications to various etiologies.

Clinical Manifestations

Manifestations of anemia are primarily caused by the body's response to tissue hypoxia. The intensity of the manifestations varies depending on the severity of anemia and the presence of coexisting diseases. Severity of anemia may be determined by Hb levels.

- *Mild* states of anemia (Hb 10 to 14 g/dl [100 to 140 g/L]) may exist without causing symptoms. If symptoms develop, they are usually caused by the underlying disease or a compensatory response to heavy exercise. These symptoms include palpitations, dyspnea, and diaphoresis.

Table 7	Relationship of Morphologic Classification and Etiologies of Anemia

Morphology	Etiology
Normocytic, normochromic	Acute blood loss, hemolysis, chronic renal disease, chronic disease, cancers, sideroblastic anemia, refractory anemia, diseases of endocrine dysfunction, megaloblastic anemia, pregnancy
Macrocytic, normochromic	Vitamin B_{12} deficiency, folic acid deficiency, liver disease (including effects of alcohol abuse), postsplenectomy
Microcytic, hypochromic	Iron-deficiency anemia, thalassemia, lead poisoning

Table 8   Clinical Manifestations of Anemia

Body system	Severity of anemia			
	Mild (Hb 10-14 g/dl [100-140 g/L])	Moderate (Hb 6-10 g/dl [60-100 g/L])	Severe (Hb <6 g/dl [<60 g/L])	
Integument	None	None	Pallor, jaundice,* pruritus*	
Eyes	None	None	Icteric conjunctiva and sclera,* retinal hemorrhage, blurred vision	
Mouth	None	None	Glossitis, smooth tongue	
Cardiovascular	Palpitations	Increased palpitations	Tachycardia, increased pulse pressure, systolic murmurs, intermittent claudication, angina, CHF, MI	
Pulmonary	Exertional dyspnea	Dyspnea	Tachypnea, orthopnea, dyspnea at rest	
Neurologic	None	None	Headache, vertigo, irritability, depression, impaired thought processes	
Gastrointestinal	None	None	Anorexia, hepatomegaly, splenomegaly	
Musculoskeletal	None	None	Bone pain	
General	None	Fatigue	Sensitivity to cold, weight loss, lethargy	

CHF, Congestive heart failure; *Hb*, hemoglobin; *MI*, myocardial infarction.
*Caused by hemolysis.

- In cases of *moderate* anemia (Hb 6 to 10 g/dl [60 to 100 g/L]), cardiopulmonary symptoms may be increased and can be present with rest as well as activity.
- Patients with *severe* anemia (Hb <6 g/dl [<60 g/L]) display many clinical manifestations that involve multiple body systems (Table 8).

Nursing Management
Goals
The patient with anemia will be able to participate in activities of daily living (ADLs), experience no fatigue with activity, have a nutritional intake containing essential nutrients for erythropoiesis, and understand and follow the therapeutic regimen. See the nursing care plan for the patient with anemia in Lewis/Collier/Heitkemper, *Medical-Surgical Nursing,* edition 4, p. 779.

Nursing Diagnoses
- Impaired physical mobility related to fatigue and weakness
- Activity intolerance related to decreased hemoglobin and imbalance between oxygen supply and demand
- Anxiety related to inability to care for self and lack of knowledge of cause of weakness and prognosis
- Altered health maintenance related to lack of knowledge about lifestyle adjustments, appropriate nutrition, medication regimen
- Self-care deficit: partial to total related to weakness and fatigue

Nursing Interventions
The numerous causes of anemia necessitate different nursing interventions specific to patient needs. General components of care for all patients with anemia may include:
- Dietary and lifestyle changes that may reverse some anemias and return patients to their former state of health.
- Acute interventions such as blood transfusions, pharmacologic management (e.g., erythropoietin, vitamin replacements), and O_2 therapy. Correcting the etiology of the anemia is the ultimate goal of therapy.
- Chronic management that may require long-term transfusion therapy or erythropoeitin injections.

Specific types of anemia are listed under separate headings.

ANEMIA, APLASTIC

Definition/Description
One of the most severe forms of anemia related to reduced erythrocyte production is a group of disorders termed aplastic or hy-

poplastic anemias. These anemias are life-threatening stem cell disorders, characterized by hypoplastic fatty bone marrow, that result in pancytopenia. Aplastic anemia is somewhat of a misnomer because in most cases all marrow elements—erythrocytes, leukocytes, and platelets—are quantitatively decreased.

Pathophysiology

There are various etiologic classifications for aplastic anemia, but they can be divided into two major groups: congenital or acquired (Table 9).

- Congenital aplastic anemia is caused by chromosomal alterations.
- Acquired aplastic anemia is a result of exposure to ionizing radiation, chemical agents (e.g., benzene, insecticides, alcohol), viral and bacterial infections (e.g., hepatitis, miliary tuberculosis), and prescribed medications (e.g., analgesics, anticonvulsants, antimicrobials).

Clinical Manifestations

Aplastic anemia usually develops insidiously. Clinically, the patient may have symptoms caused by suppression of any or all bone marrow elements.

- General manifestations of anemia such as fatigue and dyspnea, as well as cardiovascular and cerebral responses, may be seen (see Table 8, p. 25).
- The patient with granulocytopenia is susceptible to infection and generally has a fever.
- Thrombocytopenia is manifested by a predisposition to bleed (e.g., petechiae, ecchymoses, epistaxis).

Table 9	Causes of Aplastic Anemia

Congenital
Fanconi syndrome
Familial aplastic anemia

Acquired
Radiation
Chemical agents and toxins
Drugs
Viral and bacterial infections
Pregnancy
Idiopathic

Diagnostic Studies

Diagnosis is confirmed by laboratory studies.

- All marrow elements are affected: hemoglobin (Hb), white blood cell (WBC), and platelet values are often decreased (Table 10).
- Reticulocyte count is low and bleeding time is prolonged.
- Serum iron and total iron-binding capacity (TIBC) are elevated as initial signs of erythroid suppression.
- Bone marrow examination may be done for any anemic state. Findings are especially important in aplastic anemia because the marrow is hypocellular with increased yellow marrow (fat content), a finding referred to as a *dry tap*.

Therapeutic and Nursing Management

Management of aplastic anemia is based on identifying and removing the causative agent (when possible) and providing supportive care until the pancytopenia reverses.

Nursing interventions appropriate for the patient with pancytopenia from aplastic anemia are presented in the nursing care plans for the patient with thrombocytopenia and the patient with neutropenia. (See Lewis/Collier/Heitkemper, *Medical-Surgical Nursing,* edition 4, p. 798 and p. 809, respectively.) Nursing actions are directed at preventing complications from infection and hemorrhage.

- Prognosis of untreated aplastic anemia is poor (approximately 75% fatal). However, advances in medical management, including bone marrow transplantation and/or immunosuppressive therapy with antithymocyte globulin (ATG) and cyclosporine, have improved outcomes significantly. ATG is a horse serum containing polyclonal antibodies against human T cells. Rationale for this therapy is that aplastic anemia is an immune-mediated disease.
- Treatment of choice for adults less than 45 years of age who have a human leukocyte antigen (HLA)–matched sibling donor is allogeneic bone marrow transplantation. Best results occur in a younger patient who has not had previous transfusions. Prior transfusions increase the risk of graft rejection.
- For the older adult or the patient without HLA-matched siblings, the treatment of choice is immunosuppression with ATG and/or cyclosporine. Response to this therapy may only be partial, but usually transfusions can be avoided.

Table 10 Laboratory Study Findings in Anemias

	Iron deficiency	Thalassemia major	Vitamin B$_{12}$ deficiency	Folic acid deficiency	Aplastic anemia	Sickle cell anemia
Hb/Hct	↓	↓	↓	↓	↓	↓
MCV	↓	N	↑	↑	N	N
MCH	↓	N	N or slight ↓	N or slight ↓	N	N
MCHC	↓	N	↑	N	N	N
Retic	N or ↓	↑	N	N	↓	↑
Serum iron	↓	↑	N	N	±N	N to ↑
TIBC	↑	↑	N	N	±N	N to ↓
Bilirubin	N to ↓	↑	↑	N	N	↑
Platelets	N or ↑	—	↓	↓	↓	—
Other findings	—	—	↓ Vitamin B$_{12}$, positive Schilling's test	↓ Folate	↓ WBC	See note below

Hb, Hemoglobin; *Hct*, hematocrit; *MCH*, mean corpuscular hemoglobin; *MCHC*, mean corpuscular hemoglobin concentration; *MCV*, mean corpuscular volume; *N*, normal; *TIBC*, total iron-binding capacity; *WBC*, white blood cell.
NOTE: See Table 28-11 in Lewis/Collier/Heitkemper, *Medical-Surgical Nursing*, edition 4, p. 791.

ANEMIA, FOLIC ACID DEFICIENCY

Folic acid is required for DNA synthesis leading to red blood cell (RBC) formation and maturation. Four common causes of folic acid deficiency are:

1. Poor nutrition, especially a lack of leafy green vegetables, liver, citrus fruits, yeast, dried beans, nuts, and grains
2. Malabsorption syndromes, particularly small bowel disorders
3. Drugs that impede absorption and use of folic acid (e.g., methotrexate, oral contraceptives) and anticonvulsants (e.g., phenobarbital, diphenylhydantoin)
4. Alcohol abuse and anorexia

Clinical manifestations of folic acid deficiency are similar to those of vitamin B_{12} deficiency. The disease develops insidiously, and the patient's symptoms may be attributed to other coexisting problems such as cirrhosis or esophageal varices.

- GI disturbances include dyspepsia and a smooth, beefy red tongue.
- Absence of neurologic problems is an important diagnostic finding; this lack of neurologic involvement differentiates folic acid deficiency from vitamin B_{12} deficiency.

Diagnostic findings for folic acid deficiency are presented in Table 10 (p. 29). In addition, serum folate level is low, serum vitamin B_{12} level is normal, and gastric analysis is positive for hydrochloric acid.

Treatment for folic acid deficiency is by replacement therapy with the usual dose of 1 mg/day by mouth. In malabsorption states, up to 5 mg/day may be required. Duration of treatment depends on the reason for deficiency. The patient should be encouraged to eat foods containing large amounts of folic acid.

ANEMIA, IRON-DEFICIENCY

Definition/Description

Iron-deficiency anemia is one of the most common chronic hematologic disorders found in North America, occurring in 10% to 30% of the population. Regardless of economics or geography, iron-deficiency anemia is most common in infants, children, women who are premenopausal or pregnant, and older adults.

Pathophysiology

Iron deficiency may develop from inadequate dietary intake, malabsorption, or blood loss. Iron is obtained from dietary intake in which only 5% to 10% of all ingested iron is absorbed in the duodenum. This amount of dietary iron is adequate to meet the needs of men and older women, but it may be inadequate for those individuals who have higher iron needs (e.g., children, pregnant women).

Malabsorption of iron may occur after certain types of GI surgery and in malabsorption syndromes. Surgical procedures such as Billroth I or II often involve removal of or bypass of the duodenum. Malabsorption syndromes commonly involve disease of the duodenum, where iron is normally absorbed.

Blood loss is a major cause of iron deficiency in adults. The main sources of chronic blood loss are from the GI and genitourinary (GU) systems.

- GI bleeding is often not apparent and therefore may exist for a considerable time before the problem is identified. Loss of 50 to 75 ml of blood from the upper GI tract is required to cause stools to appear as *melena*. The black color of melena results from iron in red blood cells (RBCs).
- Common causes of adult GI blood loss are peptic ulcer, esophagitis, diverticuli, hemorrhoids, neoplasia, and gastritis. GU blood loss occurs primarily from menstrual bleeding. The average monthly menstrual blood loss is about 45 ml, which causes a loss of about 22 mg of iron.
- Pregnancy contributes to iron deficiency because of iron diversion to the fetus for erythropoiesis, blood loss at delivery, and lactation.

Clinical Manifestations

In the early course of iron-deficiency anemia, the patient may be free of symptoms. As the disease becomes chronic, any of the general manifestations of anemia may develop (see Table 8, p. 25). In addition, specific clinical symptoms may occur related to iron-deficiency anemia.

- Pallor is the most common finding and *glossitis* (inflammation of tongue) is the second most common; another finding is *cheilitis* (inflammation of lips).
- In addition, the patient may report headache, paresthesias, and a burning sensation of the tongue, all of which are caused by lack of iron in tissues.

Diagnostic Studies

Laboratory abnormalities characteristic of iron-deficiency anemia are presented in Table 10 (p. 29). Other diagnostic studies are done to determine the cause of iron deficiency. For example, endoscopy and colonoscopy may be used to detect GI bleeding.

Therapeutic Management

The main management goal in iron-deficiency anemia is to treat the underlying cause of reduced intake (e.g., malnutrition, alcoholism) or malabsorption of iron. Efforts are directed toward replacing iron, which may be done through increasing iron intake.

- The patient should be taught which foods are good sources of iron. If nutrition is adequate, increasing iron intake by dietary means may not be reasonable because it is difficult for nutritional intake to exceed 7 mg of iron per 1000 kcal without dietary supplement use. Consequently, oral parenteral iron supplements are used.
- If iron deficiency results from significant acute blood loss, transfusion of packed RBCs may be required. (See Blood Transfusion Therapy, p. 620.)

Nursing Management

It is important to recognize groups of individuals who are at increased risk for development of iron-deficiency anemia, including infants, teenage girls, premenopausal and pregnant women, persons from low socioeconomic backgrounds, older adults, and individuals experiencing blood loss. Dietary teaching, with an emphasis on foods high in iron, is important for these groups. Supplemental iron is especially important for pregnant women. Appropriate nursing measures are presented in the nursing care plan for the patient with anemia in Lewis/Collier/Heitkemper, *Medical-Surgical Nursing,* edition 4, p. 779.

Patient Teaching

- If anemia is present, it is important to discuss with the patient the need for diagnostic studies to identify the cause. The hemoglobin (Hb) level and RBC count should be reassessed to evaluate the response to therapy.
- Compliance with dietary and drug therapy needs to be emphasized. To replenish the body's iron stores, the patient should take iron therapy for 2 to 3 months after the Hb level returns to normal. An older adult patient may require lifelong iron supplementation.

ANEMIA, SICKLE CELL

Definition/Description

Sickle cell anemia is a genetic disorder characterized by the production of abnormal hemoglobin (Hb), anemia, and acute and chronic tissue damage from vascular blockage by abnormal red blood cells (RBCs). In sickle cell anemia, abnormal Hb (hemoglobin S [HbS]), instead of normal hemoglobin A (HbA), is produced. The disease affects more than 50,000 Americans and is predominant in African-Americans, occurring in an estimated prevalence of 1 in 375 live births. It can also affect persons of Mediterranean, Caribbean, South and Central American, Arabian, or East Indian ancestry. It is an incurable type of anemia that is often fatal by middle age.

Pathophysiology

Sickle cell anemia is an autosomal recessive genetic disorder in which the person is homozygous for HbS.

- Some persons may have sickle cell trait, a mild condition that may be asymptomatic. A person with *sickle cell trait* is heterozygous, with approximately one fourth of the hemoglobin in the abnormal S form and three fourths in the normal A form.
- The mutation that causes HbS to develop involves one amino acid. One valine amino acid is substituted for a glutamic acid; this substitution leads to an abnormal linking reaction that causes development of deformed crescent-shaped cells when O_2 tension is lowered.

When hypoxia occurs in a patient with sickle cell disease, HbS assumes various crescent or sickle shapes. Erythrostasis develops when sickled red cells are trapped in small blood vessels. Erythrostasis causes further O_2 deprivation, which potentiates more sickling. The increased concentration of sickled cells makes the circulation more sluggish, thus exerting a profound effect on all major organs. The abnormal hemoglobin shape is recognized by the body, and the cell is hemolyzed.

- Initially the sickling is reversible on reoxygenation but eventually becomes irreversible, with cells being hemolyzed. *Sickle cell crises* (exacerbations of sickling) develop if a patient becomes extremely hypoxic.

Precipitating factors include conditions that cause hypoxia or deoxygenation of RBCs, including viral or bacterial infections, high altitudes, emotional or physical stress, surgery, and blood loss.

- Crises can also be precipitated by elevated blood viscosity, which may result from dehydration due to vomiting, diarrhea, or diaphoresis. Sometimes the crisis occurs spontaneously with no apparent precipitating event.

Clinical Manifestations

Infants do not manifest symptoms until 10 to 12 weeks of age, at which time most of the fetal hemoglobin (HbF) has been replaced by HbS.

- Affected children manifest a general impairment of growth and development and a failure to thrive. Puberty is delayed, but considerable growth occurs in late adolescence.
- Most patients with sickle cell anemia are in reasonably good health most of the time.

The frequency of sickle cell crisis varies. Crises may occur frequently and then may not recur for months or years. The attack may last for 4 to 6 days.

- These attacks may appear suddenly and affect various parts of the body, especially the chest, abdomen, bones, and joints. Organs that have a high need for O_2 are the most immediately affected and form the basis for many of the complications of sickle cell disease, including an enlarged heart, pulmonary infarctions, seizures with impaired consciousness, and ultimately shock. Additional chronic manifestations include hepatomegaly, osteoporosis, joint aching, and chronic leg ulcers.
- Pain may occur spontaneously or may be precipitated by infection and cold intolerance. The pain usually begins in the extremities and lasts 4 to 6 days. Aplastic crises occur when a stressor significantly decreases erythropoiesis.
- The patient with sickle cell disease is particularly prone to infection due to impairment of the spleen to phagocytize foreign substances. Pneumonia is the most common infection and often is of pneumococcal origin. Infections need to be treated vigorously with antibiotics.

Diagnostic Studies

- Hb level usually ranges from 5 to 11 g/dl (50 to 110 g/L) with a mean RBC survival time of 10 to 15 days.
- Characteristic clinical findings of hemolysis (jaundice, elevated serum bilirubin levels) are noted with abnormal laboratory test results summarized in Table 10 (see p. 29).
- Skeletal x-rays may demonstrate bone and joint deformities and flattening.
- MRI may reveal a stroke due to blocked cerebral vessels from sickled cells.

Therapeutic Management

Therapeutic care is essentially supportive because there is no specific treatment.

- Therapy is directed toward alleviating symptoms from complications of the disease. For example, chronic leg ulcers may be treated with bed rest, antibiotics, warm saline soaks, debridement, and dressings.
- Sickle cell crises may require hospitalization. O$_2$ is administered to alter hypoxia and control sickling. Rest is instituted to reduce metabolic requirements, and fluids and electrolytes are given to reduce blood viscosity and maintain renal function.
- Analgesics are used to treat pain.
- Transfusion therapy is indicated when an aplastic crisis occurs. They have little, if any, role in treatment between crises.
- Because these patients have an increased need for folic acid, it is important they obtain daily supplements. Iron therapy is generally not indicated.

Nursing Management

- Because of the hereditary nature of sickle cell disease, genetic counseling is the only form of prevention. For genetic counseling to be effective, screening must be done to detect persons who have sickle cell trait.
- Basic care for the patient with sickle cell anemia is discussed in the nursing care plan for the patient with anemia in Lewis/Collier/Heitkemper, *Medical-Surgical Nursing,* edition 4, p. 779. Long-term care for the patient is based mainly on patient education. Patient and family must understand the basis of the disease and the reasons for supportive care.
- The patient must be taught ways to avoid crises, which include taking steps to reduce the chance of developing hypoxia, such as avoiding high altitudes, and seeking medical attention quickly to counteract problems such as upper respiratory tract infections.
- Education on pain control is also needed since the pain during a crisis may be severe and often requires considerable analgesia.

ANEMIA, VITAMIN B$_{12}$ DEFICIENCY

Definition/Description

There are many conditions in which vitamin B$_{12}$ deficiency anemia can occur. Normally a protein known as intrinsic factor (IF) is secreted by the parietal cells of the gastric mucosa. IF is required for vitamin B$_{12}$ (extrinsic factor) absorption. Therefore if intrinsic factor is not secreted, vitamin B_{12} cannot be absorbed. (Vitamin B_{12} is normally absorbed in the distal ileum.)

- In *pernicious anemia,* gastric secretion of intrinsic factor is defective. Pernicious anemia is only one cause of vitamin B_{12} deficiency, and the term should be used only to describe situations in which the gastric mucosa is clearly not secreting IF.

Pathophysiology

Vitamin B_{12} deficiency can occur in a patient who has a total gastrectomy or small bowel resection involving the ileum. This deficiency results from loss of IF-secreting gastric mucosal surface or impaired absorption of vitamin B_{12} in the distal ileum. Pernicious anemia is an autoimmune disease of insidious onset that generally begins in middle age. In this condition IF secretion fails because of gastric mucosal atrophy, which probably results from destruction of parietal cells. Pernicious anemia occurs frequently in persons of Northern European ancestry (particularly Scandinavians) and African-Americans. In African-Americans the disease tends to begin at an early age, has a high frequency in women, and is often severe.

Clinical Manifestations

Manifestations of anemia related to vitamin B_{12} deficiency develop because of tissue hypoxia (see Table 8, p. 25).

- GI manifestations include a sore tongue, anorexia, nausea, vomiting, and abdominal pain.
- Neuromuscular manifestations include weakness, paresthesias of feet and hands, reduced vibratory and position sense, ataxia, muscle weakness, and impaired thought processes ranging from confusion to dementia.
- Because vitamin B_{12} deficiency–related anemia has an insidious onset, it may take several months for these manifestations to develop.

Diagnostic Studies

- Laboratory data reflective of vitamin B_{12} deficiency anemia are presented in Table 10 (see p. 29). Erythrocytes appear large (macrocytic) and have abnormal shapes. This structure contributes to erythrocyte destruction because the cell membrane is very fragile.
- Serum vitamin B_{12} levels will be reduced.
- Gastric analysis may determine the cause of vitamin B_{12} deficiency.
- Schilling's test is diagnostic of pernicious anemia and assesses parietal cell function and absorption of vitamin B_{12} when IF is given parenterally.

Therapeutic Management

Regardless of how much vitamin B_{12} is ingested, the patient is not able to absorb it if IF is lacking or if there is impaired ileum absorption. Therefore dietary management is not used for vitamin B_{12} replacement.

- Parenteral administration of vitamin B_{12} (cyanocobalamin or hydroxocobalamin) is the treatment of choice. A typical treatment schedule consists of 1000 µg cobalamin IM daily for 2 weeks, then weekly until the hematocrit (Hct) is normal, then monthly for life. Hematologic manifestations can be completely reversed with supplemental vitamin B_{12}. However, most long-standing (>3 months) neuromuscular complications will not be reversed by this therapy.

Nursing Management

- Patients who have a positive family history of pernicious anemia should be evaluated for symptoms. Although disease development cannot be prevented, early detection and treatment can lead to reversal of symptoms.
- Nursing interventions for the patient with anemia are appropriate for the patient with vitamin B_{12} deficiency (see Anemia, p. 22). In addition to these measures, the patient should be protected from burns and trauma because of diminished sensation to heat and pain.
- Ongoing care is primarily related to ensuring patient compliance in returning for monthly vitamin B_{12} injections. There must also be careful follow-up to assess for neurologic difficulties that were not fully corrected by adequate vitamin B_{12} replacement therapy. Because the potential for gastric carcinoma is increased in pernicious anemia, patients should have frequent and careful evaluation for this problem.

ANEURYSM

Definition/Description

An aneurysm is an outpouching or dilatation of the arterial wall, commonly involving the aorta. Most aneurysms are found in the abdominal aorta below the level of the renal arteries. The aortic wall weakens and dilates with turbulent blood flow. The growth rate of aneurysms is unpredictable, but the larger the aneurysm, the greater the risk of rupture.

Pathophysiology

- Although the cause is unknown, there are several risk factors associated with development of aneurysms, including hypertension, smoking, and atherosclerosis. A common cause of aortic aneurysm is atherosclerosis with plaques composed of lipids, cholesterol, fibrin, and other debris deposited beneath the intima or lining of the artery. This plaque formation causes degenerative changes in the media (middle layer of arterial wall), leading to loss of elasticity, weakening, and eventual dilatation of the aorta.

- Other less common causes of aneurysm formation include trauma, acute or chronic infections (e.g., tuberculosis, syphilis), and anastomotic disruptions.

Aneurysms are generally divided into two basic classifications, *true* and *false*.

  - A true aneurysm is one in which the wall of the artery forms the aneurysm, with at least one vessel layer still intact. True aneurysms can be further subdivided into fusiform and saccular dilatations. A *fusiform aneurysm* is circumferential and relatively uniform in shape; whereas a *saccular aneurysm* is pouchlike and has a narrow neck connecting the bulge to one side of the arterial wall.

  - A false aneurysm, or *pseudoaneurysm,* is not an aneurysm but a disruption of all layers of the arterial wall resulting in leakage of blood that is contained or tamponaded by surrounding structures. False aneurysms may result from trauma, infection, or disruption of an arterial suture line after surgery.

Clinical Manifestations

- Thoracic aneurysms are usually asymptomatic. When manifestations are present, they are varied, with deep, diffuse chest pain the most common sign.
- Aneurysms in the ascending aorta and aortic arch can produce hoarseness as a result of pressure on the recurrent laryngeal nerve. Pressure on the esophagus can cause dysphagia. If the aneurysm presses on the superior vena cava, it can cause distended neck veins and edema of the head and arms. Pressure on pulmonary structures can lead to coughing, dyspnea, and airway obstruction.
- Abdominal aneurysms are usually asymptomatic and are often detected on routine physical examination or coincidentally when the patient is being examined for an unrelated problem (e.g., abdominal x-ray). On examination a pulsatile mass in the periumbilical area slightly to the left of midline may be detected. Bruits (murmurlike sounds resulting from turbulent blood flow) may be audible when a stethoscope is placed over the aneurysm.
- Symptoms of an abdominal aortic aneurysm may mimic pain associated with any abdominal or back disorder. Symptoms may result from compression of nearby anatomic structures (e.g., back pain caused by lumbar nerve compression).

- Occasionally aneurysms, even small ones, spontaneously embolize plaque and thrombi. This can cause "blue toe syndrome" in which patchy mottling of the feet and toes occurs in the presence of pedal pulses.

  Complications can be catastrophic. The most common complication is rupture. If rupture occurs posteriorly into retroperitoneal space, bleeding may be tamponaded by surrounding structures, preventing exsanguination. In this case the patient has severe back pain and may or may not have back or flank ecchymosis (Turner's sign).

  - If the rupture occurs anteriorly into the abdominal cavity, death from massive hemorrhage is likely. If the patient does reach the hospital, presenting signs are manifestations of shock such as tachycardia, hypotension, pale clammy skin, decreased urine output, and altered sensorium.
  - Paraplegia is a rare but devastating possible complication. If blood supply to the spinal cord is severely compromised as a result of rupture, prolonged hypotension, or prolonged clamping time during surgery, permanent paralysis may develop. This complication would most likely occur with a thoracic aneurysm.

Diagnostic Studies

- Chest x-ray demonstrates mediastinal silhouette and abnormal widening of the thoracic aorta.
- Echocardiography may show aortic insufficiency related to aortic dilatation.
- ECG is done to rule out myocardial infarction.
- CT scan determines anteroposterior and cross-sectional diameter of aneurysm. MRI is used to diagnose and assess aneurysm severity.
- Aortography is performed if arterial occlusive disease is suspected or if the aneurysm extends above the renal arteries.

Therapeutic Management

The management goal is to prevent rupture of the aneurysm. Therefore early detection and prompt treatment of the patient are imperative. Once an aneurysm is suspected, studies are performed to determine its exact size and location.

Generally, if coexisting problems are not severe, surgery is the treatment of choice, with the type of surgery depending on the location of the aneurysm.

- Surgery to repair a fusiform aneurysm is known as *endoaneurysmorrhaphy*. If the iliac arteries are also aneurysmal, the entire diseased segment is replaced with a bifurcation graft.
- If the aneurysm has ruptured, the treatment of choice is immediate surgical intervention. Even with prompt care, the mortal-

ity rate is high (about 50%) after rupture and increases with the age of the patient.

Nursing Management After Surgery

Goals

The patient with an aneurysm will have normal tissue perfusion, intact motor and neurologic function, and no complications related to surgical repair.

Nursing Diagnoses/Collaborative Problems

- Risk for infection related to presence of a prosthetic vascular graft and invasive lines
- Risk for altered peripheral tissue perfusion related to bypass graft occlusion
- Risk for sensory and perceptual alteration related to electrolyte imbalance, cerebral hypoxia, altered sensory input
- Potential complication: hypovolemia secondary to hemorrhage, extravascular fluid redistribution, prolonged diuresis
- Potential complication: altered renal perfusion related to renal artery embolism, prolonged hypotension, prolonged aortic cross-clamping intraoperatively
- Potential complication: cardiac dysrhythmia related to hypothermia, electrolyte imbalance, coexisting coronary artery disease
- Potential complication: paralytic ileus secondary to bowel manipulation, pain medication, immobility

Nursing Interventions

Special attention should be given to patients with a strong familial history of aneurysm or any evidence of other cardiovascular disease. Trauma victims should be urged to seek medical attention even in the absence of symptoms.

- Patients should be encouraged to reduce risk factors known to be associated with this disease process, including controlling hypertension, cessation of smoking, and following a diet low in fat and cholesterol.
- The patient who does not undergo surgical repair should be urged to receive regular routine physical examinations and should be reminded that any symptom, no matter how minor, must be investigated if it persists.
- The nursing role during the preoperative period should include patient teaching, providing support to patient and family, and carefully assessing all body systems. It is imperative that problems be identified early and proper intervention instituted.
- In the postoperative period adequate respiratory function, fluid and electrolyte balance, and pain control need to be maintained; the nurse needs to monitor graft patency, pulmonary status, renal perfusion, and circulation. The nurse can also assist in pre-

venting ventricular dysrhythmias, infections, and neurologic complications. Care of the patient after aneurysm repair is described in Lewis/Collier/Heitkemper, *Medical-Surgical Nursing,* edition 4, pp. 1040-1043.

Patient Teaching

- The patient may be apprehensive about returning home after major surgery involving the aorta. Encourage the patient to express any concerns and reassure the patient that normal activities can be gradually resumed. Fatigue, poor appetite, and irregular bowel habits are to be expected. Heavy lifting should be avoided for at least 4 to 6 weeks following surgery.
- Observation of incisions for signs and symptoms of infection should be encouraged. Any redness, increased pain, fever >100° F (>37.8° C), or drainage from incisions should be reported to the physician.
- Sexual dysfunction in male patients is not uncommon after aneurysm repair surgery. This effect may occur because the internal hypogastric artery is disrupted, leading to altered blood flow to the penis.
- The patient should be taught to observe for changes in extremity color or warmth and how to palpate peripheral pulses and assess for changes in their quality.
- The patient who has received a synthetic graft should be aware that prophylactic antibiotics may be required before future invasive procedures.

ANGINA PECTORIS

Definition/Description

Angina pectoris is literally translated as pain *(angina)* in the chest *(pectoris).* Myocardial ischemia is expressed symptomatically as angina. More specifically, angina pectoris is transient chest pain due to myocardial ischemia. It usually lasts for only a short time (3 to 5 minutes) and commonly subsides when the precipitating factor (usually exertion) is relieved. Typical exertional angina should not persist longer than 20 minutes after rest and/or administration of nitroglycerin.

Pathophysiology

Myocardial ischemia develops when the demand for myocardial oxygen exceeds the ability of the coronary arteries to supply it. The primary reason for insufficient flow is narrowing of the coronary arteries by atherosclerosis. If myocardial O_2 needs are not met, coronary blood flow is increased through vasodilatation and increased rate of flow.

- In the person with coronary artery disease (CAD), the coronary arteries are unable to dilate to meet increased metabolic needs because they are already chronically dilated beyond the obstructed area. In addition, the diseased heart has difficulty increasing the rate of blood flow, creating an O_2 deficit.
- Up to 90% of ischemia is asymptomatic, referred to as *silent ischemia*. Ischemia with pain (angina) or without pain has the same prognosis. Diabetes mellitus and hypertension are associated with an increased prevalence of silent ischemia.
- On the cellular level, the myocardium becomes cyanotic within the first 10 seconds of coronary occlusion, and ECG changes appear. With total occlusion of coronary arteries, contractility ceases after several minutes, depriving myocardial cells of glucose for aerobic metabolism. Myocardial nerve fibers are irritated by increased lactic acid and transmit a pain message to cardiac nerves and upper thoracic posterior roots (the reason for referred cardiac pain to left shoulder and arm). Under ischemic conditions, cardiac cells are viable for about 20 minutes.
- With restoration of blood flow, aerobic metabolism resumes and contractility is restored. Cellular repair begins.
- Extracardiac factors may precipitate myocardial ischemia and anginal pain, including physical exertion, strong emotions, consumption of a heavy meal (especially if physical exertion occurs afterward), hot or cold temperature extremes, cigarette smoking, sexual activity, stimulants (e.g., cocaine or caffeine), and circadian rhythm patterns. (CAD manifestations are noted more frequently in early morning on awakening.)

Types of Angina

Stable angina (classic angina) refers to chest pain occurring intermittently over a long time with the same pattern of onset, duration, and intensity of symptoms. Stable angina is usually exercise induced. Pain at rest is unusual.

- An ECG usually reveals ST-segment depression, indicating subendocardial ischemia. Discomfort may be mild or severe and disabling but is usually infrequent.
- Stable angina can be controlled with medications on an outpatient basis. Because stable angina is often predictable, medications can be timed to provide peak effects during the time of day when angina is likely to occur.

Unstable angina (progressive, crescendo, or *preinfarction angina)* is different from stable angina in that it is unpredictable. Patients with stable angina may develop unstable angina, which can be the first clinical manifestation of CAD (see Coronary Artery Disease, p. 154).

- Unstable angina is associated with deterioration of a once stable atherosclerotic plaque. This unstable lesion is at increased risk of complete thrombosis of the lumen with progression to myocardial infarction (MI). This is why these patients require immediate hospitalization with ECG monitoring and bed rest.
- Aspirin and systemic anticoagulation are the treatments of choice for unstable angina. Since it is also believed that unstable angina may include a spasm component, calcium channel blockers are also administered.

Prinzmetal's angina (variant angina) often occurs at rest, usually in response to spasm of a major coronary artery. It is a rare form of angina and may occur in the absence of atherosclerotic disease.

- Factors that may precipitate coronary artery spasm include increased myocardial O_2 demand and increased levels of a variety of substances such as histamine, angiotensin, epinephrine, norepinephrine, and prostaglandins.
- When spasm occurs, the patient experiences pain and marked, transient ST-segment elevation. The pain may occur during rapid eye movement (REM) sleep when myocardial O_2 consumption increases. It may be relieved by some form of exercise, or it may disappear spontaneously.

Nocturnal angina occurs only at night but not necessarily when the person is in a recumbent position or sleeping. *Angina decubitus* is chest pain that occurs only while the person is lying down and is usually relieved by standing or sitting.

Clinical Manifestations

The most common initial symptom of angina is chest pain or discomfort. The exact cause of pain is unknown, but neurogenic pain at the site of ischemia is most likely.

- On direct questioning, some patients may deny feeling pain but will refer to a vague sensation, pressure, or ache in the chest. It is an unpleasant feeling, often described as a constrictive, squeezing, heavy, choking, or suffocating sensation.
- Many persons complain of severe indigestion or burning. Although discomfort is usually felt substernally, the sensation may occur in the neck or radiate to various locations, including the jaw, shoulders, and down the arms.
- Associated symptoms may include shortness of breath, cold sweat, weakness, or paresthesias of arm(s). Relief of classic angina pectoris is usually obtained with rest or cessation of activity. Prinzmetal's angina differs from stable or unstable angina in that it is longer in duration and may wake people from sleep. See Table 31-9 in Lewis/Collier/Heitkemper, *Med-*

ical-Surgical Nursing, edition 4, p. 901, for a comparison of the pain of angina pectoris and that of MI.

Diagnostic Studies

- Chest x-ray to detect cardiac enlargement, cardiac calcifications, and/or pulmonary congestion
- ECG to compare to earlier tracing when possible
- Serum enzyme levels to rule out MI
- Serum lipid levels to screen for positive risk factors
- Exercise stress tests to examine ST-segment changes with stable angina
- Nuclear imaging studies to determine myocardial perfusion
- Angiography studies for visualization of coronary arteries to determine extent of disease
- Echocardiography with exercise for diagnosing coronary artery stenosis

Therapeutic Management

The most common initial therapeutic intervention for angina is the use of nitrate therapy to enhance coronary blood flow. Emergency care of the patient with chest pain is presented in Table 31-11 in Lewis/Collier/Heitkemper, *Medical-Surgical Nursing,* edition 4, p. 903. Treatment of coronary artery disease (CAD) may include *percutaneous transluminal coronary angioplasty (PTCA), stent placement, atherectomy,* and *laser angioplasty.*

   Percutaneous transluminal coronary angioplasty. In a catheterization laboratory a catheter equipped with a balloon tip is inserted into the appropriate coronary artery. When the lesion is located, the catheter is passed through and just past the lesion, the balloon is inflated, and the atherosclerotic plaque is compressed, resulting in vessel dilatation.

- Advantages of PTCA are that (1) it provides an alternative to surgical intervention, (2) it is performed with local anesthesia, (3) it eliminates recovery from thoracotomy required for bypass surgery and its complications, (4) the patient is ambulatory 24 hours after procedure, (5) the length of hospital stay is approximately 1 to 3 days compared with 5- to 7-day stay of someone having open heart surgery with a coronary artery bypass graft (CABG), thus reducing hospital costs, and (6) there is rapid return to work (approximately 1 week after PTCA) instead of a 1- to 8-week convalescence after CABG.
- Today PTCA is more frequently performed than CABG. Reduction of lesion size by >20% occurs in 91% of patients.
- The most serious complication of PTCA is dissection of the dilated artery where an intimal lesion is pushed farther up or down the intimal lining instead of being compressed. If damage

is extensive, the coronary artery could rupture, causing cardiac tamponade, a fall in cardiac output (CO), and possible death.

- Risk of restenosis after PTCA is about 30% in the first 3 to 6 months. Restenosis occurs more commonly in smokers, patients with diabetes, and patients with hypercholesteremia.

Stent placement. Stents are used to treat abrupt or threatened abrupt closure following PTCA. Stents are expandable meshlike structures designed to maintain vessel patency by compressing arterial walls and resisting vasoconstriction. Because stents are thrombogenic, patients must undergo anticoagulation for at least 3 months.

- Primary complications from stent placement are hemorrhage and vascular injury. Less common complications are stent thrombosis, acute MI, need for emergency CABG, stent embolization, and coronary spasm. The possibility of dysrhythmias is always present.

Atherectomy. With atherectomy the plaque is shaved off with a type of rotational blade. Atherectomy decreases the incidence of abrupt closure as compared to PTCA. However, it is limited to use in proximal and middle portions of a vessel. It is superior to PTCA for lesions located in branches or attachment sites of a bypass graft, but it carries the same risk for thrombosis and restenosis rate as conventional PTCA.

Laser angioplasty. A catheter is introduced through a peripheral artery into the diseased coronary artery. A small laser on the tip of the catheter vaporizes the plaqued areas of artery, thereby facilitating blood flow. A disadvantage of this procedure is that the technique needs refinement so that the proper laser strength for a given thickness of atherosclerotic plaque will be known.

Coronary artery bypass graft (CABG) surgery. Generally, CABG is recommended if the patient has (1) significant left main coronary artery obstruction, (2) triple-vessel disease, or (3) two-vessel disease unresponsive to medical therapy. Bypass surgery is usually recommended for the person with unstable angina who demonstrates a poor response to therapy, requiring repeat angioplasty. (See Coronary Artery Bypass Graft Surgery, p. 642.)

Pharmacologic Management

- *Antiplatelet aggregation therapy* is the first line of pharmacologic intervention in the treatment of angina. Aspirin is the drug of choice. Dipyridamole (Persantine) is also used as an antiplatelet-aggregation agent.
- *Nitrates,* which are commonly classified as vasodilators, are the next step in treatment of angina. These drugs produce their principal effects by dilating peripheral blood vessels, coronary arteries, and collateral vessels. Nitroglycerin can be used pro-

phylactically before undertaking an activity that the patient knows may precipitate an anginal attack.

- β-*blocking agents* available for the prophylaxis of angina include propranolol (Inderal) and metoprolol (Lopressor). These drugs produce a direct decrease in myocardial contractility, heart rate, systemic vascular resistance (SVR), and BP, all of which reduce myocardial O_2 demand.
- *Calcium-blocking agents* such as nifedipine (Procardia), verapamil (Calan, Isoptin), and diltiazem (Cardizem) are the next step in management of angina. Primary effects of calcium channel blockers are (1) systemic vasodilatation with decreased SVR, (2) decreased myocardial contractility, and (3) coronary vasodilatation.

Nursing Management
Goals
The patient with angina will experience pain relief, have reduced anxiety, have adequate knowledge of the problem and prescribed treatment, and modify risk factors.

Nursing Diagnoses
- Pain (chest pain or discomfort) related to ischemic myocardium
- Anxiety related to diagnosis, pain and limited activity tolerance, uncertainties about future, diagnostic tests, pending surgery
- Decreased cardiac output related to myocardial ischemia affecting contractility
- Activity intolerance related to myocardial ischemia

Nursing Interventions
The main nursing objectives for the patient with angina are pain assessment, evaluation of treatment, and reinforcement of appropriate therapy. Because chest pain can be caused by many factors other than ischemia (e.g., pericarditis, valvular disease, MI), it is important to have a clear understanding of the patient's chest pain.

- The nurse needs to elicit a history of anginal pain. It is important to determine whether breathing in or out or changing positions makes the patient's chest pain better or worse. Anginal pain does not vary with body position or respirations. In contrast, the pain of pericarditis does.
- It should be ascertained whether pain is deep or superficial, mild or intense, diffuse or localized. Cardiac pain is usually described as deep and intense, but occasionally it may be characterized as a dull ache.
- The nurse should instruct the patient to quantify each pain experience by rating the pain on a scale from 1 to 10, with 10 being excruciating pain and 1 being barely noticeable. By doing this, the nurse can assess the effectiveness of treatment during

a pain experience and discriminate between subsequent pain experiences.

- If a nurse is present during an anginal attack, the following measures should be instituted: (1) administration of O_2, (2) determination of vital signs, (3) 12-lead ECG, (4) prompt pain relief with nitrate or narcotic analgesic, (5) physical assessment of chest, and (6) comfortable positioning of patient. Supportive and realistic assurance and a calm, soothing manner help to reduce patient anxiety.

Patient Teaching

- The patient needs to be reassured that a long, productive life is possible, even with angina. Prevention of angina is preferable to treatment. The patient needs to be educated regarding CAD and angina, precipitating factors, risk factors, and medications.
- Patient teaching can be handled in a variety of ways. One-to-one contact between nurse and patient is often the most effective procedure. Time spent in providing daily care is often an ideal teaching period. Teaching tools, such as pamphlets, films at the bedside, a heart model, and especially written information, are important components of patient and family education.
- The patient needs to be assisted in identifying factors that precipitate angina and given instruction on how to avoid or control these factors.
- The patient needs to be assisted in identifying personal risk factors in CAD. Once these risk factors are known, various methods of decreasing them should be discussed.
- Educating the patient and family about diets that are low in sodium and saturated fat may be appropriate. Maintaining ideal body weight is most important in controlling angina since weight above this level increases myocardial workload and may cause pain. Eating large meals also contributes to angina, and patients may need to eat several small meals in place of three moderate to large meals each day.
- Adhering to a regular individualized exercise program that conditions the heart rather than overstressing it is important. The nurse should consult with a physician or a physical therapist in instructing the patient regarding an exercise program.
- Counseling should be provided to assess the psychologic adjustment of the patient and family to the diagnosis of CAD and resulting angina pectoris. Many patients feel a threat to their identity and self-esteem.

ANKYLOSING SPONDYLITIS

Definition/Description

Anklyosing spondylitis (AS) is a chronic inflammatory disease that primarily affects sacroiliac joints, apophyseal and costovertebral joints of the spine, and adjacent soft tissues. Approximately 90% of Caucasian patients with AS are positive for HLA-B27. The disease typically appears in adolescence or young adulthood. There appears to be a definite familial tendency, and the disease is unusual in African-Americans.

Pathophysiology

The cause of AS is unknown. Genetic predisposition appears to play an important role in disease pathogenesis, but the precise mechanisms are unknown. Environmental factors and infectious agents are also suspected. Inflammation in joints and adjacent tissue causes the formation of granulation tissue, eroding vertebral margins and resulting in spondylitis. Calcification tends to follow the inflammation process, leading to bony ankylosis.

Clinical Manifestations

- The patient typically has lower back pain, stiffness, and limitation of motion that is worse during the night and in the morning but improves with mild activity.
- General constitutional features such as fever, fatigue, anorexia, and weight loss are rarely present. Other symptoms depend on the stage of disease and may include peripheral arthritis of the shoulders, hips, and knees and occasional ocular inflammation (iritis).
- Advancing kyphosis leads to a bent-over posture, and compensating hip-flexion contractures may occur. There is pronounced impairment of neck motion in all directions.
- Extraskeletal involvement may include iritis, aortic valvular regurgitation, and apical pulmonary fibrosis.

Diagnostic Studies

When abnormalities are present, they include sacroiliac joints that show pseudowidening of joint space and later obliteration with ankylosis.

- New bone formation (syndesmophytes) may be spotty or generalized (classic "bamboo spine").
- Erythrocyte sedimentation rate (ESR), alkaline phosphatase, and creatine kinase levels are usually elevated.
- Tissue typing is positive for HLA-B27 in the majority of patients.

Therapeutic Management

Prevention of AS is not possible. However, families with diagnosed HLA-B27–positive rheumatic diseases should be alert to signs of lower back pain and arthritis symptoms.

Therapeutic management is aimed at maintaining maximal skeletal mobility. Proper posture is important in all activities. Although drugs do not halt the progression of the disease, drugs such as phenylbutazone and indomethacin can provide pain relief, which makes proper posture easier. Surgery to correct extreme flexion deformities may be performed in certain cases. A total hip replacement is done for patients with crippling hip ankylosis.

Nursing Management

Nursing responsibilities include education about the nature of the disease and principles of therapy. A home management program consists of local heat and exercise and proper use of medications.

- Pain should be managed by appropriate medication, heat, massage, and gentle exercise. Application of moist heat should be followed by range-of-motion (ROM) exercises and daily chest expansion and deep-breathing exercises.
- Excessive physical exertion during periods of active inflammation should be discouraged.
- Proper positioning at rest is essential. The mattress should be firm, and the use of pillows must be avoided. The patient should sleep on the back and avoid positions that encourage flexion deformity.
- Postural training emphasizes avoiding forward flexion (e.g., leaning over a desk), heavy lifting, and prolonged walking, standing, or sitting. Sports that facilitate natural stretching, such as swimming and racquet games, should be encouraged.
- Family counseling and vocational rehabilitation are important.

ANORECTAL ABSCESS

Definition/Description

Anorectal abscesses are undrained collections of perianal pus that are due to perirectal infections in patients who have compromised local circulation or active inflammatory disease.

- The most common causative organisms are *Escherichia coli,* staphylococci, and streptococci. Clinical manifestations include local pain and swelling, foul-smelling drainage, tenderness, and elevated temperature. Sepsis can occur as a complication.

- Surgical treatment consists of abscess drainage. If packing is used, it should be impregnated with petroleum jelly and the area should be allowed to heal by granulation. The packing is changed every day, and moist, hot compresses are applied to the area. Care must be taken to avoid soiling the dressing during urination or defecation. A low-residue diet is given. The patient may leave the hospital with the area open.
- Discharge teaching should include wound care, the importance of sitz baths, thorough cleaning after bowel movements, and follow-up visits to the physician.

ANOREXIA NERVOSA

Definition/Description
Anorexia nervosa is a specific psychiatric disorder characterized by refusal to maintain body weight to >85% of that expected for age and height.

- Two subgroups of anorexia nervosa are the *bulimic* type and the *restrictive* type, depending on whether or not there are cycles of binging and purging. This condition is found predominantly in adolescent girls.
- Once anorexia nervosa has developed, the person will go to almost any extreme to hide eating behavior from parents or peers. Eating habits are severely disturbed. If purging is present, it is often accomplished by self-induced vomiting, use of cathartics, or enemas.
- If the eating pattern is permitted to continue for a prolonged time, body wasting and signs of severe malnutrition become evident. Restricted intake occurs even in the presence of hunger.

Clinical Manifestations
- Common physical signs and symptoms of anorexia nervosa include amenorrhea, bradycardia, orthostatic hypotension, cold intolerance, breast atrophy, lanugo (soft, downlike hair normally associated with a fetus), dry skin, hair loss, severe constipation, and edema with altered fluid balance.
- Chronic anorexia nervosa places the patient at risk for serious complications affecting multiple systems such as the cardiovascular, musculoskeletal, GI, and endocrine systems.
- Life-threatening cardiac complications include hypotension, bradycardia, and malignant dysrhythmias.

Therapeutic Management

Multidisciplinary treatment must involve a combination of improved nutrition and supportive and psychiatric care. Hospitalization may be necessary if there are severe physical complications that cannot be managed in an outpatient therapy program.

- Nutritional replenishment must be closely supervised, not merely for the few pounds the person can rapidly gain but for consistent and ongoing gains. The use of tube or parenteral feedings may be necessary. Improved nutrition, however, is not a cure for anorexia nervosa.
- The underlying psychologic problem must be addressed by identification of the disturbed patterns of individual and family interactions and followed by individual and family counseling.

AORTIC DISSECTION

Definition/Description

Aortic dissection is a longitudinal splitting of the medial layer of the artery by a column of blood, occurring most commonly in the thoracic aorta.

Pathophysiology

Aortic dissection results from a small tear in the intimal lining of the artery, allowing blood to "track" between intima and media and creating a false lumen of blood flow.

- As the heart contracts, each systolic pulsation causes increased pressure, which further increases dissection. As the dissection extends proximally or distally, it may occlude major branches of the aorta, cutting off blood supply to the brain, abdominal organs, spinal cord, and extremities.
- The exact cause is uncertain. Cystic medial necrosis (destruction of medial layer elastic fibers) may be the leading cause. Most people with dissection problems have hypertension. Persons with Marfan syndrome (a connective tissue disease) have a high incidence of dissection. Pregnancy also promotes vascular stress as a result of increased blood volume. Areas that seem to undergo the greatest amount of stress and are thus most prone to dissection are the ascending aorta, aortic arch, and descending aorta beyond the origin of the left subclavian artery.

Clinical Manifestations and Complications

The patient with aortic dissection usually has sudden, severe pain in the back, chest, or abdomen. The pain is described as "tearing" or "ripping" and may mimic that of myocardial infarction (MI). As the dissection progresses, pain may be located both above and below the diaphragm. Dyspnea may also be present.

- If the arch of the aorta is involved, the patient may exhibit neurologic deficiencies, including altered level of consciousness, dizziness, and weakened or absent carotid and temporal pulses.
- An ascending aortic dissection usually produces some degree of aortic valvular insufficiency, and a murmur is audible on auscultation.
- When either subclavian artery is involved, pulse quality and BP readings may vary between the left and right arms.
- As the dissection progresses down the aorta, the abdominal organs and lower extremities may begin to demonstrate evidence of altered tissue perfusion and ischemia.
- A severe complication of dissection of the ascending aortic arch is *cardiac tamponade,* which occurs when blood escapes from the dissection into the pericardial sac. Clinical manifestations include narrowed pulse pressure, distended neck veins, muffled heart sounds, and pulsus paradoxus.
- Because the aorta is weakened by medial dissection, it may rupture. Hemorrhage may occur into the mediastinal, pleural, or abdominal cavities.
- Dissection can lead to occlusion of the arterial supply to many vital organs, including the spinal cord, kidneys, and abdominal structures. Ischemia of the spinal cord produces symptoms varying from weakness to paralysis in lower extremities and decreased pain sensation. Renal ischemia is manifested by low urinary output. Signs of abdominal ischemia include abdominal pain, decreased bowel sounds, and altered bowel elimination.

Diagnostic Studies
- ECG to rule out MI
- Chest x-ray to determine widening of mediastinal silhouette
- CT scan to assess presence and severity of dissection
- Echocardiogram to assess for left ventricular hypertrophy
- Aortography to determine extent of dissection

Therapeutic Management
The goal of therapy for aortic dissection without complications is to lower BP and myocardial contractility so that pulsatile forces within the aorta are diminished. Use of trimethaphan (Arfonad) and nitroprusside (Nipride) IV rapidly reduces BP. IV β-blockers, such as propranolol (Inderal), or α-blockers and β-blockers, such as labetalol (Normodyne), may also be used. Propranolol is used to decrease the force of myocardial contractility.

- The patient without complications can be conservatively treated for a long time. Supportive treatment is directed toward pain relief, blood transfusion (if required), and management of heart failure (if indicated).
- If dissection involves the ascending aorta, surgery is indicated. Surgery is also indicated when drug therapy is ineffective or when complications of aortic dissection (e.g., heart failure, leaking dissection, occlusion of artery) are present. Surgery is delayed for as long as possible to allow time for edema in the area of dissection to resolve, to permit clotting of blood in the false lumen, and to allow the healing process to begin.
- Surgery for aortic dissection involves resection of the aortic segment containing the intimal tear and replacement with synthetic graft material.

Nursing Management

Interventions and nursing care related to an aortic dissection include keeping the patient in bed in a semi-Fowler's position and maintaining a quiet environment. These measures assist in keeping systolic BP at the lowest possible level. Narcotics and tranquilizers should be administered as ordered. Pain and anxiety must be managed because they increase BP.

- Continuous IV administration of antihypertensive agents requires close nursing supervision. A cardiac monitoring device is used and an intraarterial pressure line is usually inserted. Changes in the quality of peripheral pulses and signs of increasing pain, restlessness, and anxiety need to be monitored. A widening pulse pressure may indicate increasing aortic valvular insufficiency. If blood vessels branching off the aortic arch are involved, decreased cerebral blood flow may alter sensorium and level of consciousness.
- Postoperative care after correction of the dissection is similar to after aortic aneurysm repair (see Lewis/Collier/Heitkemper, *Medical-Surgical Nursing,* edition 4, p. 1041).

Patient Teaching

- The therapeutic regimen includes antihypertensive drugs, which are usually taken orally. The patient needs to understand that these drugs must be taken to control BP. Propranolol can be taken orally to continue to decrease myocardial contractility.
- Instruct the patient to return to the health care facility immediately if pain returns or other symptoms progress.

APPENDICITIS

Definition/Description
Appendicitis is an inflammation of the appendix, a narrow blind pouch that extends from the inferior part of the cecum.

Pathophysiology
The most common causes of appendicitis are obstruction of the lumen by a *fecalith* (accumulated feces), foreign bodies, intramural thickening due to lymphoid hyperplasia, or tumor of the cecum or appendix. Obstruction results in distention, venous engorgement, and accumulation of mucus and bacteria.

Clinical Manifestations
Appendicitis typically begins with periumbilical pain, followed by anorexia, nausea, and vomiting. The pain is persistent and continuous, eventually shifting to the right lower quadrant and localizing at McBurney's point (located halfway between umbilicus and right iliac crest). Coughing aggravates the pain.

- Further assessment of the patient reveals localized and rebound tenderness with muscle guarding. The patient usually prefers to lie still, often with the right leg flexed. Low-grade fever may or may not be present. Rovsing's sign may be elicited by palpation of the left lower quadrant, causing pain to be felt in the right lower quadrant.
- Complications of acute appendicitis are perforation, peritonitis, and abscess.

Diagnostic Studies
- Palpation of the abdomen usually reveals tenderness and muscle guarding.
- WBC count indicates leukocytosis.
- Urinalysis is done to rule out genitourinary conditions that mimic manifestations of appendicitis.

Therapeutic Management
Treatment of appendicitis is immediate surgical removal *(appendectomy)* if the inflammation is localized. If the appendix has ruptured and there is evidence of peritonitis or an abscess, conservative treatment, consisting of antibiotic therapy and administration of parenteral fluids, may be used to prevent sepsis and dehydration for 6 to 8 hours before an appendectomy is performed.

Nursing Management

The patient with abdominal pain is encouraged to see a physician and to avoid self-treatment, particularly the use of laxatives and enemas. Increased peristalsis from these procedures may cause perforation.

- Until the patient is seen by the physician, nothing should be taken by mouth (NPO) to ensure that the stomach will be empty if surgery is needed.
- An ice bag may be applied to the right lower quadrant to decrease the flow of blood to the area and impede the inflammatory process. Heat is *never* used because it may cause the appendix to rupture.
- Surgery is usually performed as soon as a diagnosis is made.

Postoperative nursing management is similar to postoperative care of the patient after laparotomy (see pp. 3-5). In addition, the patient should be observed for evidence of peritonitis. Ambulation begins the day of surgery or the first postoperative day. Diet is advanced as tolerated.

- The patient is usually discharged on the first or second postoperative day, and normal activities are resumed 2 to 3 weeks after surgery.

ARTERIOSPASTIC DISEASE (RAYNAUD'S PHENOMENON)

Definition/Description

Arteriospastic disease is an episodic vasospastic disorder of small cutaneous arteries, most frequently involving the fingers and toes. The condition occurs primarily in young women, and the exact etiology is not known. It is seen frequently in association with collagen diseases such as rheumatoid arthritis, scleroderma, and systemic lupus erythematosus. Other contributing factors include occupation-related trauma and pressure to the fingertips as noted in typists, pianists, and those who use hand-held vibrating equipment. Exposure to heavy metals may also be a contributing etiologic factor.

Clinical Manifestations

- The disorder is characterized by three color changes (white, red, and blue). Initially, a vasoconstrictive effect produces pallor (white), followed by cyanosis (bluish-purple). These changes are subsequently followed by rubor (redness) or hyperemia. Because Raynaud's phenomenon is a vasospastic disorder of small blood vessels, wrist pulses are never lost.

- Symptoms are usually precipitated by exposure to cold, emotional upset, caffeine, and tobacco use.
- The patient usually describes cold and numbness in the vasoconstrictive phase and throbbing, aching pain; tingling; and swelling in the hyperemic phase. This type of episode usually lasts only minutes but in severe cases may persist for several hours.
- Complications include punctate (small hole) lesions of the fingertips and superficial gangrenous ulcers in the advanced stages.

Therapeutic and Nursing Management

If symptoms persist for several years in the absence of an associated underlying disorder, the diagnosis of primary Raynaud's disease may be made. It is of diagnostic importance to search for an underlying disease so that appropriate treatment can be instituted. Otherwise, treatment is generally not required because the symptoms are self-limiting.

Treatment of symptoms with calcium channel blockers has been encouraging. Oral vasodilators have been used with variable success. Sympathectomy is considered only in advanced cases.

Patient Teaching

Patient education should be directed toward reassurance that no serious underlying disorder is present and that prevention of recurrent episodes is possible.

- Loose, warm clothing should be worn as protection from cold, including gloves when a refrigerator or freezer is used or when cold objects are being handled.
- Temperature extremes should be avoided. Moving to a warmer climate is not necessarily beneficial because symptoms may still occur during cooler weather and in an air-conditioned environment.
- The patient should stop smoking, avoid caffeine, and develop techniques to cope with anxiety-producing situations. Immersion of hands in warm water often decreases the spasm.

ASTHMA

Definition/Description

Asthma is a lung disease characterized by airway obstruction, inflammation, and increased responsiveness to a variety of stimuli.

Pathophysiology

The most common etiologic factor is nonspecific hyperirritability or hyperresponsiveness of the tracheobronchial tree. The airway hyperresponsiveness seen in asthma is caused by bronchoconstriction in response to physical, chemical, or pharmacologic agents.

Prominent features of asthma are a reduction in airway diameter and an increase in airway resistance related to mucosal inflammation, constriction of bronchial smooth muscles, and excess production of mucus.

Asthma occurs when an allergen cross-links with IgE receptors on mast cells that become activated, resulting in the release of such substances as histamine, bradykinin, and prostaglandins. A similar process can occur in a susceptible patient after exercise.

- These mediators cause an intense inflammatory reaction that consists of bronchial smooth muscle constriction, increased vasodilatation and permeability, and epithelial damage. The effects are bronchospasm, increased mucous secretion, edema, and increased amounts of tenacious sputum.
- This *immediate response* peaks within 30 to 60 minutes of exposure to the trigger (allergen) and subsides in another 30 to 90 minutes. The patient has wheezing, chest tightness, and dyspnea. *Triggers* of asthma attacks include (1) certain allergens such as dust, pollen, and animal danders, (2) respiratory infections (especially viral infections), (3) exercise and cold, dry air, and (4) drugs and food additives such as indomethacin and yellow dye no. 5 (tartrazine).
- The *delayed* or *late-phase reaction* begins 2 to 8 hours after exposure to an allergen and may last for several hours or days or months. This reaction heightens airway reactivity, which in turn worsens the symptoms of future asthma attacks.

Clinical Manifestations

- Asthma attacks may have an abrupt or gradual onset and may last a few minutes to several hours. Between attacks a person may be asymptomatic with normal pulmonary function.
- Characteristic manifestations are wheezing, cough, dyspnea, a feeling of suffocation, and chest tightness.
- Additional signs include restlessness, increased anxiety, increased pulse and BP, and increased respiratory rate with the use of accessory muscles immediately after a meal.
- As asthma progresses, the patient may wheeze during inspiration and expiration. Severely diminished breath sounds are an ominous sign, indicating severe obstruction and impending respiratory failure.

Table 11 presents a correlation between arterial blood gases (ABGs) and clinical manifestations during an acute asthmatic attack.

Table 11		Arterial Blood Gas Results Correlated with Clinical Manifestations During an Acute Asthmatic Attack		

Time frame	pH	PaCO₂	PaO₂	Clinical manifestations
Early in attack	↑	↓	↓	Use of all accessory muscles of ventilation to overcome increased airway resistance
				Increased heart rate, diaphoresis, chest tightness, cough, wheezing
Progressive attack	N	N	↓	Tiring of patient and difficulty with increased work of breathing
Prolonged attack, status asthmaticus	↓	↑	↓	Exhaustion, diminished breath sounds, intubation and mechanical ventilation necessary

N, Normal; $PaCO_2$, partial pressure of arterial CO_2; PaO_2, partial pressure of arterial O_2.

Complications

Status asthmaticus is a severe, life-threatening complication of asthma that may be refractory to usual treatment.

- Causes of status asthmaticus include viral illnesses, ingestion of aspirin or other nonsteroidal antiinflammatory drugs (NSAIDs), emotional stress, increases in allergen exposure, abrupt discontinuation of drug therapy (especially corticosteroids and theophylline), and abuse of aerosol medication. The patient usually reports a history of poorly controlled asthma progressing over days or weeks.
- Clinical manifestations are similar to those of asthma, but they are more severe and prolonged.
- Complications include pneumothorax, pneumomediastinum, acute cor pulmonale, and respiratory muscle fatigue leading to respiratory arrest.
- Death from status asthmaticus is the result of respiratory arrest or cardiac failure.

Diagnostic Studies

- Pulmonary function tests, including bronchodilator therapy response, are used to diagnose asthma and give an objective measurement of airflow obstruction.
- Sputum specimen (Gram stain and culture), if indicated, is used to rule out bacterial infection.
- Chest x-ray during an attack shows hyperinflation.
- Arterial blood gases (ABGs) with mild attack indicate respiratory alkalosis and normal arterial oxygen partial pressure (PaO_2). Hypercapnia and respiratory acidosis indicate severe disease.
- Allergy testing may indicate the specific allergen causing the attack.

Therapeutic Management

- Prevention management includes teaching the patient who has persistent airflow obstruction and frequent attacks of asthma to avoid triggers of acute attacks and to premedicate before exercising.
- The patient with mild to moderate asthma should use inhaled β_2-adrenergic agents or cromolyn (Intal) before exercising or when anticipating exposure to allergens.
- For moderate to severe asthma, inhaled corticosteroids, oral sustained-release theophylline drugs, inhaled cromolyn, and inhaled ipratropium (Atrovent) can be used to prevent or alleviate symptoms.
- Some persons require continuous oral corticosteroids, which should be maintained at as low a dosage as possible and administered on alternate days (if possible) to reduce systemic side effects.

For a listing of drugs used in the treatment of asthma and COPD, see Table 25-4 in Lewis/Collier/Heitkemper, *Medical-Surgical Nursing,* edition 4, p. 692.

Nursing Management
Goals
The patient with asthma will have normal breath sounds, normal or baseline pulmonary function, increased energy, decreased incidence of asthma attacks, and adequate knowledge to participate in and carry out a treatment plan.

See the nursing care plan for the patient with asthma in Lewis/Collier/Heitkemper, *Medical-Surgical Nursing,* edition 4, p. 702.

Nursing Diagnoses
- Ineffective airway clearance related to bronchospasm, ineffective cough, tenacious secretions, fatigue
- Activity intolerance related to fatigue secondary to increased work of breathing and inadequate oxygenation
- Sleep pattern disturbance related to dyspnea, anxiety, frequent assessments and treatments, side effects of some medications
- Anxiety related to difficulty breathing, perceived or actual loss of control, fear of suffocation
- Risk for respiratory infection related to decreased pulmonary function and ineffective airway clearance
- Ineffective management of therapeutic regimen related to lack of knowledge about management of bronchospasms, medications, proper rest and activity, adequate hydration, signs and symptoms of respiratory infection, and factors that may precipitate an asthma attack

Nursing Interventions
During an acute attack of asthma, it is important to monitor the patient's respiratory and cardiovascular systems. This includes auscultating lung sounds; taking pulse rate, respiratory rate, and BP; and monitoring ABGs, pulse oximetry, and peak expiratory flow rates.
- The patient's work of breathing (i.e., use of accessory muscles, degree of fatigue) and response to therapy should be evaluated. If the patient's condition deteriorates, the physician needs to be notified immediately to initiate prompt medical intervention.
- Nursing interventions include administering O_2, bronchodilators, chest physical therapy, and medications.
- A calm, quiet, reassuring attitude may help the patient relax. The patient should be positioned comfortably (usually sitting) to maximize chest expansion. Staying with the patient and being available provide additional comfort. Encouraging slow breathing with pursed lips can be helpful.

A

Patient Teaching

The nursing role in preventing asthma attacks or decreasing their severity focuses on teaching the patient and family.

- The patient should be taught to avoid known personal triggers for asthma (e.g., cigarette smoke, pet dander) and irritants (e.g., cold air, aspirin, foods, cats). If cold air cannot be avoided, dressing properly with a scarf or mask helps reduce the risk of an asthma attack. Aspirin and NSAIDs (e.g., indomethacin) should be avoided if they are known to precipitate an attack. Many OTC drugs contain aspirin, and the patient should be instructed to read labels carefully.

- β-adrenergic blocking agents (e.g., propranolol) should not be used because they inhibit bronchodilatation.

- The patient with asthma needs to learn about medications that may be recommended and to develop self-management strategies. Some patients may benefit from keeping a diary to record medication use, presence of wheezing or coughing, drug side effects, and activity level. This information will be valuable in helping the health care provider adjust the medication.

- The patient needs to be instructed to recognize triggers of acute exacerbation so that it will be possible to medicate early, continue medication according to individually predetermined protocols until symptoms improve, or seek emergency care at a predetermined place.

- It is most helpful for the physician or nurse to write a detailed individual protocol about how to adjust the medications once the early warning signs of an acute exacerbation occur.

- Relaxation therapies (e.g., yoga, meditation relaxation techniques, and breathing techniques) may be of value in helping the patient relax the respiratory muscles and decrease the respiratory rate.

- The patient should be taught to maintain a fluid intake of 2 to 3 L/day. Good nutrition and avoidance of overeating are other important measures. Physical exercise (e.g., swimming, walking, stationary cycling) within the patient's limit of tolerance is also beneficial.

- A plan should be developed with the patient and significant other that defines what can be done to help the patient during an asthma attack. The significant other needs to know where the patient's inhalers, oral medication, and emergency phone numbers are located. The significant other can also be instructed on how to decrease patient anxiety if an asthma attack occurs.

- Counseling may be indicated to help the patient and family resolve personal, family, social, and occupational problems that have resulted from asthma.

BELL'S PALSY

Definition/Description

Bell's palsy (peripheral facial paralysis, acute benign cranial polyneuritis) is a disorder characterized by a disruption of motor branches of the facial nerve (CN VII) on one side of the face in the absence of any other disease such as a stroke.

- Cause is still unknown, but current theories suggest that the herpes simplex virus may cause inflammation and demyelination of the nerve. Onset of Bell's palsy is often accompanied by an outbreak of herpes vesicles in or around the ear.
- Bell's palsy is considered benign with full recovery after 3 to 4 months in about 85% of patients, especially if treatment is instituted immediately. Failure to show spontaneous recovery after 6 months indicates that the problem is probably not Bell's palsy.

Clinical Manifestations

Paralysis of motor branches of the facial nerve typically results in flaccidity of the affected side of the face, with drooping of the mouth accompanied by drooling. Inability to close the bottom eyelid, with upward movement of the eyeball when closure is attempted, is also evident.

- A widened palpebral fissure (opening between the eyelids), flattening of nasolabial fold, unilateral loss of taste, and inability to smile, frown, or whistle are also common.
- Decreased muscle movement may alter chewing ability, and some patients may experience a loss of tearing or excessive tearing.
- Pain may be present behind the ear on the affected side, especially before the onset of paralysis.

Complications can include psychologic withdrawal because of changes in appearance, malnutrition and dehydration, mucous membrane trauma, muscle stretching, and facial spasms and contractures.

Diagnosis of Bell's palsy and its prognosis are indicated by observation of the typical pattern of onset and signs and testing of percutaneous nerve excitability.

Therapeutic Management

- Corticosteroids, especially prednisone, are started immediately, and the best results are obtained if corticosteroids are initiated before paralysis is complete. Corticosteroids should be tapered off over a 2-week period, when the patient improves to the point that they are no longer necessary. Usually corticosteroid treatment decreases the edema and pain, but mild analgesics can be used if necessary.

- Other methods of treatment include moist heat, gentle massage, and electric stimulation of the nerve. Stimulation may maintain muscle tone and prevent atrophy. Care is primarily focused on relief of symptoms and prevention of complications.

Nursing Management
Goals
The patient with Bell's palsy will be pain free or have pain controlled, maintain adequate nutritional status, not experience injury to the eye, return to normal or previous perception of body image, and be optimistic about disease outcome.

Nursing Diagnoses
- Pain related to the inflammation of CN VII (facial nerve)
- Altered nutrition: less than body requirements related to inability to chew secondary to muscle weakness
- Risk for trauma to eye (corneal abrasion) related to inability to blink
- Body image disturbance related to change in facial appearance secondary to facial muscle weakness

Nursing Interventions
- Mild analgesics can relieve pain. Hot wet packs can be used to reduce the discomfort of herpetic lesions and relieve pain.
- The face should be protected from cold and drafts because trigeminal hyperesthesia may accompany the syndrome.
- Maintenance of good nutrition is important. The patient should be taught to chew on opposite (functional) side of mouth to avoid trapping food and to improve taste. Thorough oral hygiene must be carried out after each meal to prevent development of parotitis, caries, and periodontal disease from accumulated residual food.
- Dark glasses may be worn for protective and cosmetic reasons. Artificial tears (methylcellulose) should be instilled frequently during the day to prevent drying of the cornea. Ointment and an impermeable eye shield can be used at night to retain moisture. In some patients taping the lids closed at night may be necessary.
- A facial sling may be helpful to support affected muscles, improve lip alignment, and facilitate eating. Vigorous facial massage can break down tissues, but gentle upward massage has psychologic benefits. When function begins to return, active facial exercises are performed several times a day.
- The change in physical appearance can be devastating; the patient needs to be reassured that a stroke did not occur and that chances for a full recovery are good. The patient's need for privacy should be respected, especially during meals. Enlisting support from family and friends is important.

BENIGN PROSTATIC HYPERPLASIA

Definition/Description

Benign prostatic hyperplasia (BPH) refers to new growth of epithelial and especially stromal elements within the prostate gland and is the most common problem of the adult male reproductive system.

- This problem occurs in about 50% of men over the age of 50 and 75% of men over age 70. BPH is most likely to develop in the innermost part of the prostate, whereas cancer is most likely to develop in the outer part of the prostate.
- Prostatic hyperplasia does not predispose a patient to the development of prostate cancer.

Pathophysiology

BPH begins with enlargement of the glandular tissue. Although the cause is not completely understood, it is thought that the increased number of cells results from endocrine changes associated with aging.

- Excessive accumulation of dihydroxytestosterone (the principal intraprostatic androgen), stimulation of estrogen, and local growth hormone action are proposed causes. Other factors under investigation include diet, race, and lifestyle.

Clinical Manifestations

The patient seeks assistance for relief of symptoms related to urinary obstruction.

- Early symptoms can be minimal because compensatory hypertrophy of the bladder can compensate for resistance to urine flow.
- With increasing blockage, *obstructive symptoms* of BPH develop, including diminution in caliber and force of urinary stream, hesitancy in initiating voiding, dribbling at end of urination, and a feeling of incomplete bladder emptying because of urinary retention. *Irritative symptoms,* including nocturia, dysuria, and urgency, can develop from inflammatory, infectious, or neoplastic causes.

The patient is at increased risk for urinary tract infection because of failure of the bladder to empty completely as a result of partial or complete obstruction of the proximal urethra.

- Residual urine provides a favorable environment for bacterial growth, and calculi may develop as a result of alkalinization of residual urine. Breakage of tiny overstretched blood vessels in the bladder may produce hematuria.
- More serious complications resulting from urinary retention are abnormally distended ureters (hydroureters), destruction of kidney

parenchyma from back pressure of urine (hydronephrosis), and pyelonephritis. These complications can lead to renal failure.

Diagnostic Studies

- Physical examination including digital rectal examination for prostate enlargement
- Urinalysis with culture to determine infection or inflammation
- Serum creatinine and blood urea nitrogen (BUN) to assess renal involvement with long-standing BPH
- Prostate specific antigen (PSA), if indicated
- Urodynamic flow studies
- Transrectal ultrasound
- Cystoscopy (for surgical candidates)

Therapeutic Management

The goals of management are to restore bladder drainage, relieve patient symptoms, and prevent or treat complications of BPH. Although these goals may be temporarily accomplished by catheterization, it does not resolve the underlying problem of prostatic enlargement. The treatment of asymptomatic BPH is referred to as "watchful waiting." T here are numerous treatment options for symptomatic BPH.

Pharmacologic options. Drugs are used to cause regression of hyperplastic tissue through hormonal manipulation, such as suppression or relaxation of smooth muscle fibers of the prostate by androgens.

- Finasteride (Proscar) blocks the conversion of testosterone to the metabolite dihydroxytestosterone and is of benefit to men with a predominance of glandular hyperplasia.
- α-Adrenergic receptor blockers cause smooth muscle relaxation, which ultimately facilitates urinary flow through the prostatic urethra. Three selective α-adrenergic blockers, prazosin (Minipress), doxazosin (Cardura), and terazosin (Hytrin), are currently being used.

Nonsurgical invasive options. If BPH becomes symptomatic, nonsurgical invasive options may be tried before surgery. These options include heat, a prostatic balloon device, laser ablation, and stents or coils.

- Localized application of *heat* is used in an attempt to reduce the size of prostatic tissue. One technique to achieve a desired temperature of 109.4° F (43° C) or greater involves intracavitary placement in the urethra of a radiating microwave antenna that emits heat. This procedure results in a significant increase in urine flow rate, decrease in postvoid residual urine capacity, and decrease in frequency of nocturia. Mild side effects include occasional problems of bladder spasm, hematuria, dysuria, and retention.

- A *prostatic balloon device* dilates the urethra by stretching, fracturing, or compressing the gland to enlarge the passage and allow for the free flow of urine. If the procedure is successful, an indwelling catheter is left in place for the first 24 hours to monitor urinary output and the degree of hematuria. Complications have been rare, and short-term results are encouraging.

- Laser ablation using a *transurethral ultrasound-guided laser-induced prostatectomy (TULIP)* is another treatment approach.

- *Stents* (stainless steel) or *coils* (titanium) placed in the prostatic urethra hold back the walls of the prostate to allow unobstructed flow of urine. In the majority of cases the stents become completely covered by epithelium, thus reducing the risk of encrustation and infection. The procedure is used most often for men who have medical contraindications to anesthesia and surgery because only local anesthesia is required for this procedure.

Advantages and disadvantages of the various nonsurgical invasive treatment options are compared in Table 52-3 in Lewis/Collier/Heitkemper, *Medical-Surgical Nursing,* edition 4, p. 1630.

Surgical invasive options. Surgery is indicated when there is a decrease in urine flow of a magnitude sufficient to cause discomfort, persistent residual urine, acute urinary retention because of obstruction with no reversible precipitating cause, and/or hydronephrosis.

- Treatment of symptomatic BPH primarily involves resection of the prostate. The selection of a surgical approach to remove adenomatous tissue depends on size and position of the prostatic enlargement, degree of debility, and reproductive outlook of the patient.

- Major postoperative complications of surgery are hemorrhage, infection, bladder spasm, and erectile problems.

The *transurethral resection (TUR* or *TURP)* approach is the most common route for partial removal of the prostate. A large three-way indwelling catheter with a 30 ml balloon containing sterile water is usually inserted into the bladder after the procedure to provide hemostasis and facilitate urinary drainage. The bladder is irrigated, either continuously or intermittently, for at least 24 hours to prevent obstruction from mucous threads and blood clots.

- TUR is often the surgery of choice for the debilitated patient or for the patient with moderate prostatic enlargement. Advantages of TUR are that it does not involve an external incision and is less likely to result in erectile dysfunction or long-term incontinence. A disadvantage is that it does not completely remove all prostatic tissue, leaving the potential for recurrence of hyperplasia.

A *transurethral incision of the prostate (TUIP)* can be done in high-risk patients, those with mild obstruction, or in younger patients. Transurethral slits or incisions are made into the prostatic tissue to relieve bladder neck obstruction. This method is usually used to treat intravesical obstruction related to BPH.

- The patient is discharged with an indwelling catheter for the first 24 hours to monitor urinary output and hematuria. For the advantages and disadvantages of this procedure, see Table 52-3 in Lewis/Collier/Heitkemper, *Medical-Surgical Nursing,* edition 4, p. 1630.

Nursing Management
Because primary treatment for BPH is surgical resection of hyperplastic tissue, nursing care focuses on preoperative and postoperative care of the patient having prostatic surgery.

Goals
The patient having prostatic surgery will have restoration of urinary drainage, treatment of any urinary tract infection, and understanding of the upcoming surgery with implications for sexual functioning. Overall postoperative goals are that the patient will have no complications, complete bladder emptying, restoration of urinary control, and satisfying sexual expression.

See the nursing care plan for the patient undergoing transurethral resection in Lewis/Collier/Heitkemper, *Medical-Surgical Nursing,* edition 4, p. 1633.

Nursing Diagnoses/Collaborative Problems
- Acute pain: bladder spasms related to irrigations and clots, presence of catheter, and surgical procedure
- Fear related to actual or potential sexual dysfunction, possible diagnosis of cancer, and lack of knowledge regarding surgical procedure and postoperative care
- Risk for urinary infection related to indwelling catheter, environmental pathogens, and urinary stasis
- Urge incontinence related to poor sphincter control
- Potential complication: hemorrhage related to surgical procedure

Nursing Interventions
Because the cause of BPH is poorly understood, the focus of health promotion is early detection and treatment. The American Cancer Society recommends a yearly medical history and digital rectal examination for men over age 40 in an effort to provide early detection of prostate problems. After age 50 and when symptoms of prostatic hyperplasia become evident, further diagnostic screening may be necessary.

- Some men find that ingestion of alcohol and caffeine tends to increase prostatic symptoms because of the diuretic effect that increases bladder distention. Compounds found in common cough and cold remedies such as pseudoephedrine (in Sudafed) and phenylephrine (in Allerest nasal or Coricidin nasal) often worsen symptoms of BPH.
- Patients with obstructive symptoms should be advised to urinate when they first feel the urge in order to minimize urinary stasis and acute urinary retention. Fluid intake should be maintained at a normal level to avoid dehydration or fluid overload.

Preoperative care. Urinary drainage must be restored before surgery; a urethral catheter such as a Coudé catheter may be needed.

- Any infection of the urinary tract must be treated before surgery. Restoring drainage, encouraging high fluid intake, and providing a diet high in acid ash–producing foods are helpful.
- The patient is usually concerned about the impact of impending surgery on his sexual functioning. The nurse should provide an opportunity for the patient to express his concerns.

Postoperative care. The plan of care should be adjusted to the type of surgery, reasons for surgery, and patient response to surgery. Discharge planning and home care issues are important aspects of postprostatectomy care.

- After prostatectomy the bladder may be continuously irrigated with sterile normal saline solution to remove clotted blood from the bladder and to ensure drainage of urine. Some form of irrigation (continuous or intermittent) may be used for 24 hours or until no clots are noted draining from the bladder.
- Blood clots are normal for the first 24 to 36 hours. However, large amounts of bright-red blood in the urine can indicate hemorrhage.
- Activities that increase abdominal pressure, such as sitting or walking for prolonged periods and straining to have a bowel movement, should be avoided.
- Bladder spasms are a complication after transurethral and suprapubic prostatectomy. They occur as a result of irritation of the bladder mucosa from insertion of a resectoscope, the presence of a catheter, or clots leading to obstruction of the catheter. The patient should be instructed not to attempt to urinate around the catheter because this increases the likelihood of spasm. If bladder spasms develop, the catheter should be checked for clots. If present, the clots should be removed by irrigation so urine can flow freely. Belladonna and opium suppositories, along with relaxation techniques, are used to relieve pain and decrease spasm.

- Sphincter tone may be poor immediately after surgery, resulting in incontinence or dribbling. Sphincter tone can be strengthened by having the patient practice Kegel exercises (pelvic floor muscle technique). Continence can improve for up to 12 months. If continence has not been achieved by that time, the patient may be referred to a continence clinic. A variety of methods, including biofeedback, have been used to achieve positive results. The patient can also use a penile clamp, condom catheter, or incontinence briefs to avoid embarrassment from leakage.

- The patient should be observed for signs of postoperative infection. If an external wound is present, the area should be observed for redness, heat, swelling, and purulent drainage. Special care must be taken if a perineal incision is present because of the proximity of the anus. Rectal procedures, such as rectal temperatures and enemas (except insertion of belladonna and opium suppositories), should be avoided because they may initiate bleeding.

- The catheter should be connected to a closed drainage system secured to the inner thigh and should not be disconnected unless it is being removed, changed, or irrigated. Secretions that accumulate around the meatus should be cleansed daily with soap and water.

- Dietary intervention is important to prevent the patient from straining during bowel movements. Straining increases intraabdominal pressure, which can lead to bleeding at the operative site. A diet high in fiber facilitates passage of stool.

Patient Teaching

After prostatic surgery the patient may be concerned about erectile dysfunction. Physiologic impotence may occur when nerves are cut or damaged during surgery. The patient often experiences anxiety over the loss of sex role, self-esteem, and quality of sexual interaction with his sexual partner.

- Sexual counseling and treatment options may be necessary if erectile dysfunction becomes a chronic or permanent problem.

- Many men experience retrograde ejaculation because of trauma to the internal sphincter. Semen is discharged into the bladder at orgasm and may produce cloudy urine when the patient urinates after orgasm. The nurse should discuss these changes with the patient and his partner and allow them to ask questions and express their concerns.

BLADDER CANCER

Definition/Description

Bladder cancer accounts for nearly 1 in every 20 cancers diagnosed in the United States. The most frequent malignant tumor of the urinary tract is transitional cell carcinoma of the bladder. Cancer of the bladder is most common between the ages of 60 and 70 years and is at least three times as common in men as in women.

Risk factors for bladder cancer include cigarette smoking, exposure to dyes used in the rubber and cable industries, and chronic abuse of phenacetin-containing analgesics. Individuals with chronic, recurrent nephrolithiasis and recurrent upper urinary tract infections also have an increased incidence of bladder cancer.

Clinical Manifestations

- Gross painless hematuria is the most common clinical finding in 75% of patients. Bladder irritability with dysuria, frequent urination, and intermittent bleeding may also be noted.
- When cancer is suspected, urine specimens for cytology can be obtained to determine the presence of neoplastic or atypical cells.

Bladder cancer can be classified as superficial, invasive, or metastatic. Superficial carcinomas are seen in patients with carcinoma in situ, mucosal involvement, and submucosal involvement. The patient with invasive disease has cancer progression into the muscle and/or surrounding fat.

- Bladder tumors are staged using the Jewett-Strong-Marshall system or the TNM system (Table 12). The Jewett-Strong-Marshall system broadly classifies bladder cancer as superficial, invasive, or metastatic disease. Pathologic grading systems are also used to classify malignant potential of tumor cells, indicating a scale from well-differentiated to anaplastic categories. Low-stage, low-grade bladder cancers are most responsive to treatment.

Therapeutic and Nursing Management

Surgical interventions may include one of the following procedures:

- *Endoscopic resection and fulguration* (electrocautery) is used for diagnosis and treatment of superficial lesions with a low recurrence rate. This procedure is also used to control bleeding in patients who are poor operative risks or who have advanced tumors.
- *Laser photocoagulation* can be repeated a number of times for recurrence. The advantages of laser include bloodless destruction of the lesion, minimal risk of perforation, and lack of need for a urinary catheter.

Table 12	TNM Classification System

Primary Tumor (T)

T_0	No evidence of primary tumor
T_{is}	Carcinoma in situ
T_{1-4}	Ascending degrees of increase in tumor size and involvement

Regional Lymph Nodes (N)

N_0	No evidence of disease in lymph nodes
N_{1-4}	Ascending degrees of nodal involvement
N_x	Regional lymph nodes unable to be assessed clinically

Distant Metastases (M)

M_0	No evidence of distant metastases
M_{1-4}	Ascending degrees of metastatic involvement of host, including distant nodes

- *Open-loop resection* (snaring of polyp-type lesions) *and/or fulguration* is used to control bleeding, large superficial tumors, and multiple lesions. Treatment of large lesions entails *segmental resection* of the bladder.

Postoperative management of the patient who has had one of these three surgical procedures includes instructions to drink large amounts of fluid each day, measurement of intake and output, avoidance of alcoholic beverages, use of analgesics and stool softeners (if necessary), and sitz baths to promote muscle relaxation and reduce urinary retention.

- The nurse should also help the patient and family cope with fears about cancer, surgery, and sexuality and should emphasize the importance of regular follow-up care. Frequent routine cystoscopies are required.

When the tumor is invasive or involves the trigone (area where ureters insert into bladder) and the patient otherwise has a good life expectancy and no demonstrated metastases beyond pelvic area, a *total cystectomy* with urinary diversion is the treatment of choice.

- *Radiation therapy* is used with cystectomy or as the primary therapy when the cancer is inoperable or when surgery is refused (see Radiation Therapy, p. 675).
- *Chemotherapy* with local instillation of thiotepa is of some use in the treatment of superficial recurring lesions. It is instilled directly into the patient's bladder and retained for about 2 hours; position of the patient may be changed every 15 minutes for maximum contact with all areas of bladder. Other in-

travesical chemotherapeutic agents include doxorubicin (Adri-amycin), mitomycin (Mutamycin), and bacille-Calmette-Guérin (BCG). BCG is the drug of choice for carcinoma in situ of the bladder.

It is important for the nurse to encourage the patient to increase daily fluid intake and to quit smoking, assess the patient for secondary urinary infection, and stress the need for routine urology follow-up. The patient may have fears or concerns about sexual activity or bladder function; these issues will need to be addressed.

BONE CANCER

Definition/Description

Primary malignant bone neoplasms are rare in adults and account for <1% of all deaths attributed to cancer. They are characterized by their rapid metastasis and bone destruction. Primary neoplasms occur most frequently during childhood through young adulthood.

Types of bone cancers include osteogenic sarcoma, osteoclastoma, Ewing's sarcoma, and multiple myeloma (see Multiple Myeloma, p. 387).

Osteogenic Sarcoma (Osteosarcoma)

Osteogenic sarcoma is a primary neoplasm of bone that is extremely malignant and is characterized by rapid growth and metastasis. It usually occurs in the metaphyseal region of long bones of the extremities, particularly in regions of the distal femur, proximal tibia, and proximal humerus. Osteogenic sarcoma has its highest incidence in 10- to 25-year-old males. Early metastasis to the lungs is responsible for a poor prognosis and a survival rate of 15% to 20%.

Clinical manifestations. Manifestations are usually associated with a past health history of minor injury and gradual onset of pain and swelling. The injury does not cause the neoplasm but rather serves to bring the preexisting condition to medical attention.

- The neoplasm grows rapidly and produces a noticeable increase in size of the general region, which can restrict joint motion.

Diagnosis. The diagnosis is confirmed from biopsied tissue specimens, elevation of serum alkaline phosphatase and calcium levels, and x-ray findings.

Treatment. Management may include amputation (see p. 617). Radiation and chemotherapy may be used before surgery to decrease tumor size or tissue involvement. Limb-salvage surgical procedures in combination with radiation and chemotherapy are being used frequently.

Osteoclastoma

True *osteoclastoma* (giant cell tumor) is a malignant, destructive neoplasm that arises in the cancellous ends of long bones in young adults. Giant cell tumors most commonly occur between the ages of 20 and 35 years.

Common sites are the distal ends of the femur, proximal tibia, and distal radius. The giant cell tumor is a locally destructive lesion, the growth of which extends from a few months to several years.

Clinical manifestations. Manifestations include swelling, local pain, and some disturbances in joint function. X-ray evidence of giant cell tumor is variable but usually reveals local areas of bone destruction and eventual expansion of bone ends.

Treatment. Initially treatment includes a biopsy to establish a diagnosis followed by surgical curettage of the lesion with bone grafting. After treatment there is a >50% chance of recurrence. Recurrent giant cell tumors may subsequently make amputation necessary.

Ewing's Sarcoma

Ewing's sarcoma is the third most common primary malignant neoplasm of the bone, occurring most frequently in male patients under the age of 30. This neoplasm is characterized by rapid growth within the medullary cavity of long bone, especially the femur, pelvis, tibia, and ribs.

- Most frequent site of early metastasis is the lungs. Ewing's sarcoma has a poor prognosis, with a survival rate estimated at only 5%.

Clinical manifestations. These include progressive local pain, palpable soft-tissue mass, noticeable increase in the size of the affected part, fever, and leukocytosis. Initially, x-rays show periosteal bone destruction.

Treatment. Treatment usually involves radiation therapy and surgical resection or amputation. Chemotherapeutic agents commonly used are cyclophosphamide (Cytoxan), dactinomycin, vincristine (Oncovin), methotrexate, and doxorubicin (Adriamycin). Surgical resection of the tumor may help decrease the rate of recurrence.

Nursing Management

Goals

The patient with bone cancer will have satisfactory pain relief; maintain preferred activities as long as possible; accept body image changes resulting from chemotherapy, radiation, and surgery; be free from injury; and have a realistic idea of disease progression and prognosis.

Nursing Diagnoses

- Pain related to disease process, inadequate pain, or comfort measures

- Impaired physical mobility related to disease process, pain, weakness, and debility
- Body image disturbance related to possible amputation, swelling, and effects of chemotherapy
- Anticipatory grieving related to poor prognosis of disease
- Risk for injury: pathologic fracture related to disease process and improper handling or positioning of affected body part

Nursing Interventions

Nursing care of the patient with a malignant bone neoplasm does not differ significantly from care given to the patient with a malignant disease of any other body system. However, special attention is required to reduce complications associated with prolonged bed rest and to prevent pathologic fractures. The patient is often reluctant to participate in therapeutic activities because of weakness and fear of pain. Regular rest periods should be provided between activities. Careful handling of the affected extremity is important to prevent pathologic fractures.

The nurse must be able to assist the patient in accepting the guarded prognosis associated with bone cancer. The inability to accomplish age-specific developmental tasks can increase the frustrations with this condition. General nursing principles related to cancer are applicable (see Cancer, p. 88). Special attention is necessary for problems of pain and dysfunction, chemotherapy, and specific surgery, such as spinal cord decompression or amputation.

BREAST CANCER

Definition/Description

Breast cancer is the most common malignancy in North American women and is second only to lung cancer as the leading cause of death from cancer in women. This disease develops in one in eight postmenopausal women.

Although the majority of breast problems occur in women, men can have breast problems. One out of every 100 cases of breast cancer occurs in men. A thorough examination of the male breast should be a routine part of a physical examination.

Pathophysiology

Although the etiology of breast cancer is not completely understood, a number of factors are thought to be related to the development of this disease.

- Several external factors have been considered as contributory, including diet, obesity, viruses, and the use of alcohol. Environmental factors such as chemicals and radiation may also play a role.

- With increasing age, the risk of developing breast cancer also increases. The incidence of breast cancer in women less than 25 years of age is very low and increases gradually until age 60. After the age of 60 the incidence increases dramatically.
- A positive family history of breast cancer is an important risk factor, especially if the family member with breast cancer was premenopausal, had bilateral disease, and was a first-degree relative (i.e., mother, sister, daughter). As many as 5% of all breast cancer patients may have inherited a specific genetic abnormality (BRCA-1 gene), which contributed to the development of their breast cancer.

The majority of breast cancers (70% to 80%) arise from lobular or ductal epithelium. The natural history of breast cancer varies considerably from patient to patient. The cancer can range from slowly progressive to rapidly growing.

- Factors that affect growth are axillary node involvement (the more nodes involved, the worse the prognosis), tumor differentiation (morphology of malignant cells), estrogen and progesterone receptor status, tumor site, and abnormal DNA content.

Clinical Manifestations

Breast cancer is usually first detected as a single breast lump. It occurs most often in the upper outer quadrant of the breast because this is the location of most of the glandular tissue.

- On palpation, breast cancer is characteristically hard, irregularly shaped, poorly delineated, and nonmobile. Malignant lesions are characteristically painless and nontender.
- A small percentage of breast cancers have nipple discharge as a presenting symptom. The discharge is usually unilateral and may be clear or bloody. Nipple retraction may occur.
- Plugging of the dermal lymphatics can cause skin thickening and exaggeration of the usual skin markings, giving skin the appearance of an orange peel *(peau d'orange)*.
- In the late stages infiltration, induration, and dimpling (pulling in) of the overlying skin may occur.

Recurrence may be local or regional (soft tissue near mastectomy site, axillary lymph nodes) or distant (most commonly bone, lung, brain, and liver).

Diagnostic Studies

- Physical examination of breast and lymphatics
- Mammography and ultrasound
- Biopsy

- Estrogen and progesterone receptor assays
- Complete blood count (CBC), calcium and phosphate levels, liver function tests
- Chest x-ray
- Liver and bone scans

Therapeutic Management

Many prognostic factors are considered when treatment decisions are being made, including lymph node status, tumor size, and histologic classification. All these factors enter into the *staging* of breast cancer. The most widely accepted staging method is the TNM system (see Table 12, p. 71).

- Breast conservation surgery with radiotherapy and modified radical mastectomy with or without reconstruction are currently the most common options for resectable breast cancer. Ten-year overall survival with lumpectomy and radiation is approximately the same as that with modified radical mastectomy.

Axillary node dissection is usually performed regardless of the treatment option selected. Axillary lymph node involvement is one of the most important prognostic factors in breast cancer. The more nodes involved, the greater the risk of relapse. Removal of axillary nodes can prevent axillary recurrence and aid in decision making regarding adjuvant chemotherapy or hormonal therapy.

Lymphedema (accumulation of lymph in soft tissue) can occur as a result of excision or radiation of the lymph nodes. The patient may experience heaviness, pain, impaired motor function in the arm, and numbness and paresthesia of the fingers. Cellulitis and progressive fibrosis can also result.

- Frequent and sustained elevation of the arm, regular use of a custom-fitted pressure sleeve, and treatment with an inflatable sleeve (pneumomassage) are all helpful in preventing or reducing lymphedema.

Breast conservation surgery (lumpectomy) involves removal of the entire tumor along with a margin of normal tissue. An axillary node dissection is usually performed along with a lumpectomy. Radiotherapy is sometimes delivered to the entire breast, ending with a boost to the tumor bed. If there is evidence of systemic disease, chemotherapy may be given before radiation therapy.

- One of the main advantages of breast conservation surgery and radiation is that it preserves the breast, including the nipple. The goal of combined breast conservation surgery and radiation is to maximize the benefits of both cancer treatment and cosmetic outcome while minimizing the risks.

See Table 49-5 in Lewis/Collier/Heitkemper, *Medical-Surgical Nursing,* edition 4, p. 1553, for treatment options, side effects, complications, and patient issues related to common surgical procedures to treat breast cancer.

The *modified radical mastectomy* includes removal of the breast and axillary lymph nodes but preserves the pectoralis major muscle. This surgery is selected over breast conservation therapy if the tumor is too large to excise with good margins and attain a reasonable cosmetic result. Some patients may select this procedure over lumpectomy when presented with the choice of either procedure.

Follow-up care. After surgery, the woman must be followed up for the rest of her life at regular intervals. Most women have professional examinations every 3 months for the first 2 years, every 6 months for the next 3 years, and annually thereafter.

- In addition, the woman must continue to practice monthly breast self-examinations (BSE) on both breasts or the remaining breast and mastectomy site. The woman should also have yearly mammography of the remaining breast or breast tissue.
- The most common sites of recurrence are at the surgical site and in the opposite breast.

Adjuvant therapy. The decision to recommend *adjuvant (additional) therapy* after surgery depends on the number of involved nodes, the patient's menstrual status and age, cell type, size and extent of cancer, presence or absence of estrogen receptors, and other preexisting health problems that can complicate treatment.

- Adjuvant therapies include radiation therapy and systemic therapies such as chemotherapy, hormonal manipulation, and biologic response modifiers.

Radiation therapy. The three situations in which radiation therapy may be used for breast cancer are (1) as primary treatment to destroy a tumor or as a companion to surgery to prevent local recurrence, (2) to shrink a large tumor to operable size, and (3) as palliative treatment for pain caused by local recurrence and metastasis. Lumpectomy is almost always followed by radiation (see Radiation Therapy, p. 675).

Chemotherapy. Cytotoxic drugs are used to destroy cancer cells. The greatest benefits from chemotherapy have been achieved among premenopausal women with node findings that are positive for malignancy (see Chemotherapy, p. 631).

Hormonal therapy. Estrogen can promote growth of breast cancer cells if cells are estrogen-receptor positive. If the source of estrogen is removed, tumor regression may occur. The source of estrogen (especially estradiol) can be markedly reduced by surgical ablation (e.g., oophorectomy, adrenalectomy, and hypophysectomy) or with additive hormonal therapy.

- Tamoxifen (an antiestrogen) is the usual first choice of treatment in postmenopausal, estrogen-receptor–positive women with or without nodal involvement.
- Hormonal therapy is widely used to treat recurrent or metastatic cancer but may occasionally be used as an adjuvant to primary treatment.

Biologic response modifiers. The use of biologic response modifiers represents an attempt to stimulate the body's natural defenses to recognize and attack cancer cells. The use of high-dose chemotherapy and bone marrow transplant are other potential treatments. The use of these therapies is discussed in Chapter 12, Lewis/Collier/Heitkemper, *Medical-Surgical Nursing,* edition 4. For further information on adjuvant therapy for breast cancer, see *Medical-Surgical Nursing,* p. 1552.

Nursing Management
Goals
The patient with breast cancer will actively participate in the decision-making process related to treatment options, fully comply with the therapeutic plan, manage side effects of adjuvant therapy, and be satisfied with support provided by significant others and health care providers.

See the nursing care plan for the patient after a modified radical mastectomy in Lewis/Collier/Heitkemper, *Medical-Surgical Nursing,* edition 4, p. 1557.

Nursing Diagnoses/Collaborative Problems
After a diagnosis of breast cancer and before a treatment plan has been selected, the following diagnoses would apply:
- Decisional conflict related to lack of knowledge about treatment options and their effects
- Fear related to diagnosis of breast cancer
- Risk of body image disturbance related to anticipated physical and emotional effects of treatment modalities

If a *modified radical mastectomy* is planned, nursing diagnoses and collaborative problems may include:
- Pain related to surgical incision and manipulation of tissue
- Altered sexuality patterns related to loss of body part, surgical procedure, medication, and anxiety regarding diagnosis
- Fear related to diagnosis of cancer
- Impaired physical mobility related to decreased arm and shoulder mobility
- Self-esteem disturbance related to altered body image and loss of body part
- Potential complication: lymphedema related to edema on operative side and lack of knowledge of preventive measures

Nursing Interventions

The time between diagnosis of breast cancer and selection of a treatment plan is a difficult period for the woman and her family. Although the primary care provider discusses treatment options, the woman often relies on the nurse to clarify and expand on these options.

- Appropriate nursing interventions during this period include exploring the woman's usual decision-making patterns, helping the woman accurately evaluate the advantages and disadvantages of options, providing information relevant to decision making, and supporting the patient once a decision is made.
- Regardless of the surgery planned, the patient needs to be provided with sufficient information to ensure informed consent. Teaching during the preoperative phase includes instruction in turning, coughing, and deep breathing; a review of postoperative exercises; and explanation of the recovery period from the time of surgery until discharge.

The woman who has breast conservation surgery usually has an uneventful postoperative course with only a moderate amount of pain. The woman who has a modified radical mastectomy needs nursing interventions specific to this surgery.

- Restoring arm function on the affected side after mastectomy is an important nursing and patient goal.
- The woman should be placed in a semi-Fowler's position with the arm on the affected side elevated on a pillow. Flexing and extending the fingers should begin in the recovery room, with daily increases in activity.

Postoperative discomfort can be minimized by administering analgesics about 30 minutes before initiating exercises. If showering is appropriate, letting warm water run over the involved shoulder often has a soothing effect and reduces joint stiffness. Whenever possible, the same nurse should work with the woman so that progress can be commended and problems can be identified.

- Measures to prevent or reduce lymphedema must be taught. The affected arm should never be dependent, even while the person is sleeping. BP readings, venipunctures, and injections should not be done on the affected arm. The woman must be instructed to protect the arm on the operative side from even minor trauma such as a pin prick or sunburn. If trauma to the arm occurs, the area should be washed thoroughly with soap and water, and a topical antibiotic ointment and bandage should be applied. The patient must understand that she is at risk of developing lymphedema for the rest of her life.

Throughout interactions the nurse must keep in mind the extensive psychologic impact of the disease. All aspects of care must include sensitivity to the woman's efforts to cope with a life-threatening disease. The nurse can help meet the woman's psychologic needs by doing the following:

- Assisting her to develop a positive but realistic attitude
- Helping identify sources of support and strength to her such as her partner, family, and spiritual practices
- Encouraging her to verbalize anger and fears about her diagnosis
- Promoting open communication of thoughts and feelings between the patient and her family
- Providing accurate and complete answers to questions about the disease, treatment options, and reproductive/lactation issues (if appropriate)
- Offering information about community resources, such as Reach to Recovery, Encore, and local support organizations and groups

Patient Teaching

- The nurse should emphasize the importance of beginning and continuing BSE and annual mammography. Symptoms that should be reported to the clinician include new back pain, weakness, constipation, shortness of breath, and confusion.
- The nurse should stress the importance of wearing a well-fitting prosthesis.
- A preoperative sexual assessment provides baseline data that the nurse can use to plan postoperative interventions. Often, the husband, sexual partner, or family members may need assistance in dealing with their emotional reactions to the diagnosis and surgery so that they can support the patient effectively.
- Initial coping mechanisms begin to lose effectiveness at about 3 months, and a period of depression may ensue. It is important that the nurse provide anticipatory guidance.

BULIMIA

Definition/Description

Bulimia is a chronic eating disorder characterized by compulsive binge eating and purging through self-induced vomiting, laxative and exercise abuse, and diuretics. Food becomes an obsession and an addiction—an escape from the pressures of life. Unlike the person with anorexia, the patient caught up in the syndrome of bulimia usually maintains normal or near-normal body weight.

- Bulimia is increasing in incidence and may be even more prevalent than anorexia nervosa. Female students of college age are most susceptible to this disorder.

Pathophysiology

The cause of bulimia remains unclear but is thought to be similar to that of anorexia nervosa (see Anorexia Nervosa, p. 50).

Clinical Manifestations

The primary symptom of bulimia is gorging (rather than starvation as in anorexia nervosa).

- Characteristic skin lesions on the back of the hand, which are often over the metacarpophalangeal joint and are called Russell's sign, can result from repeated trauma to the skin from self-induced vomiting.
- Dental problems may develop from constant vomiting.
- Swollen glands or salivary gland hypertrophy, sore throat, facial puffiness, chronic indigestion, irregular menstrual periods, electrolyte imbalance, and dehydration can also occur.
- Sudden death from cardiac arrest or fatal dysrhythmia is not uncommon.
- Most bulimics have few, if any, noticeable signs of the illness.

Therapeutic Management

Treatment of bulimia is similar to that of anorexia nervosa. The multidisciplinary approach consists of strategies that include individual psychotherapy, nutritional counseling (with discussion of the dangers involved in binge eating and purging), cognitive behavior therapy, and drug therapy.

- Antidepressants (e.g., fluoxetine [Prozac], amitriptyline [Elavil]) are useful for the depression associated with both anorexia nervosa and bulimia.
- Vitamin, mineral, and iron supplements may be prescribed. However, iron supplementation is not generally required if amenorrhea is present.

The return to normal eating habits may take several months to years to accomplish because relapses are frequent. Recovery is difficult. The abnormal eating behavior is hard to change because binge eating and purging provide the person with a feeling of satisfaction and of control over the body.

Nursing Management

For a discussion of the nursing management of bulimia, see Malnutrition, p. 377.

BURNS

Definition/Description

Burns are a tissue injury resulting from exposure to or direct contact with hot objects, chemicals, smoke, or electric current.

Pathophysiology

Burn wounds occur when there is contact between tissue and an energy source, such as heat, chemicals, electric current, or radiation. The resulting local effects are influenced by energy intensity, duration of exposure, and type of tissue injured. Immediately after the injury occurs, there is an increase in blood flow to the area surrounding the wound. This action is followed by release of various vasoactive substances from burned tissue, which results in increased capillary permeability. Fluid then shifts from the intravascular compartment to the interstitial space, producing edema and hypovolemia.

Types of Burn Injury

Various types of burn may be seen alone or in combination with other burns.

- Thermal injury is the most common type of burn and can be caused by flame, flash, scald, or contact with hot objects.
- Chemical injury is the result of tissue injury and destruction from necrotizing substances such as acids and alkalis. Chemicals can produce respiratory, skin, eye, and systemic symptoms for up to 72 hours after injury.
- Smoke and inhalation injury can cause damage to the respiratory tract. These injuries include carbon monoxide poisoning, thermal burn above the glottis, or chemical burn below the glottis.
- Electrical injury results from coagulation necrosis caused by intense heat from an electric current.

Classification of Burn Injury

The treatment of burns is related to injury severity. A variety of methods exist for determining burn severity.

1. The *depth of burn* is described according to the depth of skin destruction (epidermis, dermis, and/or subcutaneous tissue) (Table 13).
   - Partial-thickness burn
       Superficial (first degree) with erythema, pain, mild swelling, no vesicles or blisters
       Deep (second degree) with fluid-filled vesicles, severe pain, mild to moderate edema

Table 13   Classification of Burn Injury Depth

Classification	Clinical appearance	Cause	Structure
Partial-thickness skin destruction			
• Superficial (first degree)	Erythema, blanching on pressure, pain and swelling, no vesicles or blisters (although after 24 hr skin may blister and peel)	Superficial sunburn Quick heat flash	Superficial devitalization with hyperemia. Tactile and pain sensation intact.
• Deep (second degree)	Fluid-filled vesicles that are red, shiny, wet (if vesicles have ruptured); severe pain caused by nerve injury; mild-to-moderate edema	Flame Flash Scald Contact burns	Epidermis and dermis involved to varying depth. Some skin elements, from which epithelial regeneration can occur, remain viable.
Full-thickness skin destruction			
• (third and fourth degree)	Dry, waxy white, leathery, or hard skin; visible thrombosed vessels; insensitivity to pain and pressure because of nerve destruction; possible involvement of muscles, tendons, and bones	Flame Scald Chemical Tar Electric current	All skin elements and nerve endings destroyed. Coagulation necrosis present.

- Full-thickness burn (third and fourth degree) with dry, waxy, leathery and/or hard skin, pain insensitivity, possible bone, muscle, and tendon involvement

2. The *extent of burn* is calculated as the percent of total body surface area (TBSA) that has been burned. Burn extent is determined by one of two methods:
   - Lund-Browder chart, which takes into account the patient's age and relative body area
   - Rule of Nines chart, which is easy to remember and adequate for initial assessment (Fig. 1)

3. *Burn location* has a direct relationship to the severity of the injury. For example, face and neck burns may inhibit respiratory function; burns of the hands, feet, joint, and eye may limit self-care and functioning.

4. *Age of patient* influences burn severity because infants (immature immune system) and older patients (decreased defense mechanisms) are less able to cope.

5. *Preexisting disorders* such as cardiovascular, pulmonary, or renal disease reduce the patient's ability to recover from the tremendous physiologic demands of burn injury.

A *major* adult burn is classified as >25% TBSA for a partial-thickness (second-degree) burn or as >10% TBSA for a full-thickness (third-degree) burn.

Diagnostic Studies

- Routine laboratory tests for arterial blood gases (ABGs)
- Serum electrolytes, especially sodium (Na^+) and potassium (K^+)
- X-rays, sputum, and bronchoscopy for inhalation injury

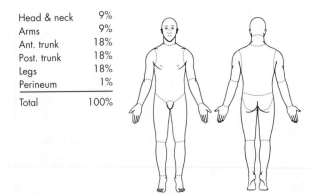

Head & neck	9%
Arms	9%
Ant. trunk	18%
Post. trunk	18%
Legs	18%
Perineum	1%
Total	100%

Fig. 1 Rule of Nines chart.

- Urine output and specific gravity to assess renal function
- White blood cell (WBC) count and wound cultures if infection is suspected

Therapeutic Management

Burn management can be classified into three phases: *emergent* (resuscitative), *acute,* and *rehabilitative.*

Emergent (resuscitative) phase is the period required to resolve the immediate problems resulting from burn injury. This phase may last from burn onset to 5 or more days, but it usually lasts 24 to 48 hours. It begins with fluid loss and edema and continues until fluid mobilization and diuresis begin.

- From the onset of the burn event until the patient is stabilized, therapy predominantly consists of airway management, fluid therapy, and wound care.
- Pharmacologic management includes administration of analgesics and narcotics for comfort and pain control and of topical antibacterial agents to prevent infection.

Acute phase begins with mobilization of extracellular fluid and subsequent diuresis. It concludes when the burned area is completely covered or when the wounds are healed. This phase may take weeks or many months.

- Predominant management in the acute phase is fluid replacement, wound care, early excision and grafting, and range-of-motion (ROM) exercises.
- Nutritional management involves minimizing energy demands and providing adequate calories (often 5000 kcal/day) to promote healing.

Rehabilitation phase begins when the burn wound is covered with skin or healed and the patient is capable of assuming some self-care activity. This phase can begin as early as 2 weeks to as long as 2 or 3 months after the injury.

- Rehabilitation goals are to assist the patient in resuming a functional role in society and to accomplish functional and cosmetic reconstruction.

Clinical Manifestations

There are three phases of burn management:

- *Emergent phase:* Characterized by possible shock from pain and hypovolemia, intense thirst, minimal urine output, shivering as a result of heat loss or anxiety, and possible disorientation. Complications may include dysrhythmias, airway obstruction, and acute tubular necrosis.
- *Acute phase:* Wounds may or may not have intact blisters and may be painful to the touch with eschar. Complications may include infection progressing to bacteremia, acute delirium at

night, contractures, Curling's ulcer, occult blood in stool, and stress diabetes.

- *Rehabilitative phase:* Contractures may occur if ROM is not adequate, and an itching sensation may be noted at the healing site, which is extremely sensitive to trauma. Complications are skin and joint contractures and hypertrophic scarring.

Nursing Management

Goals

The patient with a burn injury will have self-care activities resumed, an absence of contractures, weight loss not >10% of body weight, rapid control if wound becomes infected, no pain or a tolerable level of pain, and verbalization of realistic goals.

See the nursing care plan for the burn patient, Lewis/Collier/Heitkemper, *Medical-Surgical Nursing,* edition 4, p. 543.

Nursing Diagnoses

- Risk for fluid volume deficit related to evaporative loss, plasma loss, and fluid shift
- Pain related to burn injury and treatments
- Grieving related to change in body image
- Total self-care deficit related to pain, immobility, and perceived helplessness
- Risk for infection related to impaired skin integrity
- Impaired physical mobility related to contractures secondary to pain and immobility
- Altered nutrition: less than body requirements related to increased caloric demand

Nursing Interventions

- *Emergent phase:* It is essential to assess the adequacy of fluid replacement, provide wound care, and offer support to the patient and family.
- *Acute phase:* Wound care consumes most of the nursing care. Yet this fact should not negate the importance of supportive care, comfort and hygiene measures, and physical therapy. One of the most critical nursing functions is pain assessment and management.
- *Rehabilitative phase:* Responsibility is shared among the health care team to return the patient to optimal functioning.

Patient Teaching

- Describe to the patient and family the burn injury process and expected signs and symptoms related to phases of burn management.
- Explain therapeutic interventions, precautionary measures, gowning, and hand washing, and institution visiting policy to elicit cooperation and decrease anxiety.
- Teach the patient to watch for injuries to new skin.

- Instruct the patient and family about the signs and symptoms of infection so early treatment can be initiated.
- Teach the family how to perform dressing changes to ensure proper technique and increase their sense of control.
- Emphasize the importance of exercise and appropriate physical therapy to the patient and family. Plan a daily exercise program with the patient and offer appropriate resources to provide continuing activity program as needed.
- Assist the patient and family in setting realistic future expectations because anticipatory guidance decreases anxiety and inaccurate perceptions. The patient and family will need anticipatory guidance to know what to expect physiologically as well as psychologically during recovery.
- Provide avenues for the patient and family to maintain contact with hospital personnel after discharge to promote continuity of care and minimize anxiety.

CANCER

Definition/Description
A group of more than 200 diseases characterized by unregulated growth of cells, cancer is currently the second leading cause of death in the United States. There are differences in the incidence of certain cancers in men and women (Table 14). The death rate from cancer is leveling off or decreasing except for an increasing rate of death from lung cancer in women (Table 15).

Pathophysiology
Two major dysfunctions present in the process of cancer are *defective cellular proliferation* (growth) and *defective cellular differentiation.* The cause and development of each type of cancer is likely to be multifactorial. Tumors may have a chemical, environmental, genetic, immunologic, or viral origin.

Cancer is theorized to develop through the following stages:
- *Initiation* is the irreversible alteration in cellular genetic structure by a chemical, physical, or biologic agent.
- *Promotion* is the reversible proliferation of altered cells. Promoting factors include dietary fat, obesity, and cigarette smoking. Additional factors that promote cancer development are listed in Table 12-6, Lewis/Collier/Heitkemper, *Medical-Surgical Nursing,* edition 4, p. 266.
- *Progression* involves increased tumor growth, invasiveness, and metastasis. Metastasis refers to tumor spread to distant body parts via the vascular and lymphatic systems and by implantation (cancer cells embedded along body serosal surfaces).

Tumors can be classified according to:
- Anatomic site (e.g., leukemia originates from hematopoietic tissue)
- Histologic analysis (grading of tumor cells from well differentiated to anaplasia)
- Extent of disease (staging of cancer from 0 to IV)
- TNM classification system (see Table 12, p. 71), which is used to determine the extent of disease process according to tumor size (T), degree of regional spread to lymph nodes (N), and presence of metastasis (M)

Clinical Manifestations
Clinical manifestations are dependent on the type of cancer and may include:
- Change in respiratory status with increased frequency of infections and change in cough

- Occult bleeding, diarrhea, constipation, pain, and black tarry stools
- Dysuria and hematuria
- Abnormal uterine bleeding, pain, and change in menstrual pattern
- Sore that does not heal or change in wart or mole

Table 16 lists the seven warning signs of cancer.

Complications resulting from cancer can include infection, paraneoplastic syndrome, hypercalcemia, superior vena cava syndrome, infarction, organ failure, and spinal cord compression.

C

Table 14	Cancer Incidence by Site and Sex in 1994*		
Male		**Female**	
Type	**Percentage**	**Type**	**Percentage**
Prostate	32	Breast	32
Lung	16	Colon or rectum	13
Colon or rectum	12	Lung	13
Urinary tract	9	Uterus	8

From Cancer Statistics 1994, American Cancer Society, 1994.
*Excluding basal and squamous cell skin cancers and carcinoma in situ.

Table 15	Estimates of Cancer Deaths by Site and Sex in 1994*		
Male		**Female**	
Type	**Percentage**	**Type**	**Percentage**
Lung	33	Lung	23
Colon or rectum	10	Breast	18
Prostate	13	Colon or rectum	11

From Cancer Statistics 1994, American Cancer Society, 1994.
*Excluding basal and squamous cell skin cancers and carcinoma in situ.

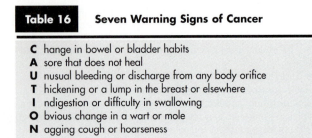

Table 16	**Seven Warning Signs of Cancer**

C hange in bowel or bladder habits
A sore that does not heal
U nusual bleeding or discharge from any body orifice
T hickening or a lump in the breast or elsewhere
I ndigestion or difficulty in swallowing
O bvious change in a wart or mole
N agging cough or hoarseness

Diagnostic Studies

Various diagnostic studies may be done, depending on the suspected primary or metastatic site(s) of the cancer, and may include:

- Cytology studies (Pap smear)
- Chest x-ray
- Oncofetal antigens or tumor cell markers such as carcinoembryonic (CEA) and alpha-fetoprotein (AFP) antigens
- Bone marrow examination for hematolymphoid malignancy
- MRI, CT scan
- Proctoscopic examination
- Radioisotope scans (liver, brain, bone, lung)
- Radiographic studies such as mammogram
- Biopsy (needle, incisional, and excisional), which can definitively diagnose cancer

Therapeutic Management

The goal of cancer treatment is cure, control, or palliation. Factors that determine treatment modality are (1) cell type of the cancer, (2) location and size of the tumor, and (3) extent of the disease. The physiologic and psychologic status and the expressed needs of the patient also have an important part in determining the treatment plan, modalities chosen, and length of treatment administration.

Cancer treatment modalities include the following:

- Surgery can be used for cure and control (e.g., mastectomy), supportive care (e.g., colostomy for rectal abcess), and palliation of symptoms (e.g., cordotomy for pain relief).
- Radiation therapy can be given externally or internally (brachytherapy), in which radioactive materials are placed in or near the tumor. Goals of therapy are cure, control, or palliation (see Radiation Therapy, p. 675).
- Chemotherapy, the systemic use of chemicals (drugs), is used to reduce the size of the primary tumor and kill metastatic cancer cells (see Chemotherapy, p. 631).

- Biologic response modifiers (BRMs) alter host biologic response to tumor cells. Two examples are α-interferon and tumor necrosis factor (TNF).

Nursing Management
Goals
The patient with cancer will maintain body weight, have adequate energy, demonstrate adequate self-care knowledge, experience adequate relief from pain, have no oral mucosal infections, and effectively communicate with family members.

See the nursing care plan for the patient with cancer, Lewis/Collier/Heitkemper, *Medical-Surgical Nursing,* edition 4, p. 300.

Nursing Diagnoses/Collaborative Problems
- Altered nutrition: less than body requirements related to anorexia, nausea, vomiting
- Altered oral mucous membranes related to chemotherapy
- Altered family processes related to cancer diagnosis of family member
- Fatigue related to effects of cancer and treatment
- Ineffective individual coping related to depression
- Body image disturbance related to hair loss, surgery, weight loss
- Risk for infection related to leukopenia
- Potential complication: bleeding related to thrombocytopenia

Nursing Interventions
- Actively listen to the patient's concerns while awaiting diagnostic study results.
- Manage the commonly experienced side effects associated with radiation therapy, chemotherapy, and biologic response modifiers.
- Assist with nutritional intake to minimize protein and calorie malnutrition.
- Monitor for signs of complications resulting from cancer.
- Facilitate development of a hopeful attitude.
- Assess and intervene for adequate relief of pain.
- Encourage relaxation techniques and humor to reduce anxiety.

Patient Teaching
A predominant role of the nurse is education of the patient in the prevention and early detection of cancer to increase survival. This teaching emphasizes the following points:
- Reduce or avoid exposure to known or suspected carcinogens.
- Eat a balanced diet that includes vegetables, fresh fruits, whole grains, and low levels of fats and preservatives.
- Participate in regular exercise and obtain adequate, consistent periods of rest (at least 6 to 8 hours/night).
- Have a health examination on a consistent basis that includes health history, physical examination, and specific diagnostic tests for common cancers.

- Learn the recommended screening guidelines for specific cancer sites (see Cancer Screening Guidelines, p. 696).
- Eliminate, reduce, or change perception of stressors.
- Learn and practice breast and testicular self-examination.
- Know the seven warning signs of cancer.
- Seek immediate medical care if cancer is suspected.

Education is an extremely important nursing role related to chemotherapy and radiation therapy. Fear and anxiety can be associated with both treatment modalities. The patient must be told what to expect during a course of treatment. The patient needs also to know the possible side effects of chemotherapy and radiation therapy. The nurse needs to provide guidance to the patient and family in setting realistic expectations.

Specific types of cancer are listed under separate headings.

CARDIOMYOPATHY

Definition/Description

Cardiomyopathy (CMP) describes a group of heart muscle diseases of unknown cause that primarily affect the structural and/or functional ability of the myocardium. The diagnosis of CMP is made based on the patient's clinical manifestations and noninvasive and invasive cardiac procedures to rule out other causes of dysfunction.

CMP can be classified as primary or secondary:

- *Primary CMP* includes those conditions in which the etiology of the heart disease is unknown. The heart muscle in this instance is the only portion of the heart involved, and other cardiac structures are unaffected.
- In *secondary CMP* the myocardial disease is known and is secondary to another disease process. Common causes of secondary CMP are ischemia, viral infections, illicit drug abuse, and pregnancy.

The World Health Organization has classified CMP conditions into three general types: *dilated (congestive), hypertrophic,* and *restrictive* (Table 17). Each of these types has its own pathogenesis, clinical presentation, and therapeutic management. All types of CMP can lead to cardiomegaly and congestive heart failure (CHF).

Dilated Cardiomyopathy

Pathophysiology. Dilated (congestive) cardiomyopathy is the most common type of CMP, accounting for >90% of all cases, and is characterized by cardiomegaly with ventricular dilatation, impairment of systolic function, atrial enlargement, and stasis of blood

C

Table 17   Characteristics of Cardiomyopathies

Dilated	Hypertrophic	Restrictive
Etiology: Idiopathic condition, alcoholism, pregnancy, myocarditis, nutritional deficiency (vitamin B_1), exposure to toxins and drugs, genetic disease	Inherited disorder (autosomal dominant), possible chronic hypertension	Amyloidosis, postradiation, post-open heart surgery, diabetes
Major manifestations: Fatigue, weakness, palpitations, dyspnea, dry cough	Exertional dyspnea, fatigue, angina, syncope, palpitations	Dyspnea, fatigue, palpitations
Cardiomegaly: Moderate to marked	Mild	Mild to moderate
Contractility: Decreased	Increased or decreased	Normal or decreased
Dysrhythmias: Sinoatrial tachycardia, atrial and ventricular dysrhythmias	Tachydysrhythmias	Atrial and ventricular dysrhythmias
Cardiac output: Decreased	Decreased	Normal or decreased
Stroke volume: Decreased	Normal or increased	Decreased
Ejection fraction: Decreased	Increased	Normal or decreased

in the left ventricle (LV). Deterioration is rapid after the development of symptoms.

- No specific cause has been identified, although dilated CMP often follows an infectious myocarditis. Thyrotoxicosis, diabetes mellitus, toxins (especially alcohol and cocaine), and drugs causing a hypersensitivity reaction have all been associated with the development of dilated CMP.

Clinical manifestations. The patient may have signs and symptoms of CHF, including fatigue, dyspnea, orthopnea, palpitations, and anorexia. Signs can include S_3, S_4, tachycardia, pulmonary crackles, edema, pallor, hepatomegaly, and jugular venous distention. The patient may also have dysrhythmias or systemic embolism.

Diagnostic studies. A diagnosis is made on the basis of patient history and ruling out conditions that cause CHF.

- Chest x-ray can demonstrate cardiomegaly.
- ECG may reveal tachycardia and dysrhythmias.
- Echocardiography is useful in distinguishing dilated CMP from other structural abnormalities, including ventricular chamber size and heart muscle thickness.
- Cardiac catheterization and coronary angiography are used to evaluate coronary arteries (normal), pulmonary capillary wedge pressure (PCWP) (elevated), and left atrial and LV end-diastolic pressures (elevated).
- Left ventriculogram may reveal abnormal wall motion caused by the dilatation within a thinned wall and dilated ventricles.

Therapeutic and nursing management. Interventions focus on controlling CHF by enhancing myocardial contractility and decreasing afterload (similar to treatment for chronic CHF).

- Digitalis is used in the presence of atrial fibrillation, diuretics are used to decrease preload, and diuretics and vasodilators such as the angiotension-converting enzyme (ACE) inhibitors are used to reduce afterload.
- Pharmacologic treatment, nutritional interventions, and cardiac rehabilitation may help to alleviate symptoms of CHF and improve cardiac output (CO.)
- A patient with secondary dilated CMP must be treated for the underlying disease process. For example, the patient with alcohol-induced dilated CMP must abstain from all alcohol intake.
- The patient with terminal end-stage cardiomyopathy may require cardiac transplantation. Approximately 50% of heart transplants are performed for the treatment of cardiomyopathic conditions.
- Patients with dilated cardiomyopathy are very ill people with a grave prognosis who need expert nursing care.

- Nursing care should focus on monitoring response to medications, monitoring for dysrhythmias, and preventing or rapidly detecting systemic emboli.
- The nurse should also educate the patient about the disease process and assist the patient in spacing daily activities to allow for periods of rest.
- This patient is in great need of emotional support. Information regarding candidacy for heart transplantation and the grave prognosis must be given honestly and empathically.
- The patient's family must learn cardiopulmonary resuscitation (CPR) and how to access emergency care in their neighborhood.
- Home health care nursing can provide the patient and family with continuous assessments and therapeutic interventions that are required to maximize and maintain functional status.

Hypertrophic Cardiomyopathy

Pathophysiology. *Hypertrophic cardiomyopathy (HCM),* also called *idiopathic hypertrophic subaortic stenosis (IHSS),* produces asymmetric myocardial hypertrophy without ventricular dilatation. HCM occurs less commonly than dilated CMP and is more common in men than in women. HCM seems to have an autosomal dominant genetic basis.

- It is usually diagnosed in young adulthood and is often seen in active athletic individuals. Degree of impairment can range from mild to severe.
- The primary defect of HCM is diastolic dysfunction. Impaired ventricular relaxation inhibits adequate filling of ventricles during diastole. Decreased ventricular filling and obstruction to outflow can result in decreased CO, especially during exertion when increased CO is needed.

Clinical manifestations. Manifestations of HCM include exertional dyspnea, fatigue, angina, and syncope. The most common symptom is dyspnea, which is caused by an elevated left ventricular diastolic pressure.

- Palpitations are common in the patient and are most often caused by dysrhythmias. Common dysrhythmias include atrial fibrillation, ventricular tachycardia, and ventricular fibrillation. Any of these dysrhythmias may lead to loss of consciousness or sudden cardiac death, which is the most common cause of death.

Diagnostic studies. Chest x-ray is usually normal except in patients with severe disease causing an increased cardiac silhouette.

- Increased voltage and duration of the QRS complex are the most common abnormalities on ECG; these findings usually indicate ventricular hypertrophy. Ventricular dysrhythmias are also frequently seen, with ventricular tachycardia the most common.

- Echocardiogram is the primary diagnostic tool revealing the classic feature of HCM, which is LV hypertrophy; the ECG may also demonstrate wall motion abnormalities and diastolic dysfunction.
- Cardiac catheterization will document a pressure gradient and depressed diastolic left ventricular compliance if HCM is present.

Therapeutic and nursing management. The primary treatment goal is to improve ventricular filling by reducing ventricular contractility and relieving left ventricular outflow obstruction. This can be accomplished with the use of β-blocking agents or calcium channel blockers.

- Antidysrhythmics are used to control dysrhythmias; however, their use has not proved to prevent sudden death in this group. An alternative treatment for ventricular dysrhythmias may be an implantable defibrillator.
- Some patients may be candidates for surgical treatment *(ventriculomyotomy* and *myectomy)* of the hypertrophied septum. Indications for surgery include severe symptoms refractory to therapy with marked obstruction to aortic outflow.
- Most patients have good symptomatic improvement after surgery and improved exercise tolerance.

Nursing interventions focus on relieving symptoms, observing for and preventing complications, and providing emotional and psychologic support.

- Education should focus on teaching the patient to adjust his/her lifestyle to avoid strenuous activity and dehydration. Any activity or procedure that causes an increase in systemic vascular resistance (SVR), thus increasing obstruction to forward blood flow, is dangerous for this patient and should be avoided. The patient should be taught to space activities and allow for rest periods.

Restrictive Cardiomyopathy

Pathophysiology. *Restrictive cardiomyopathy* is the rarest of cardiomyopathic conditions. It is a disease of the heart muscle that impairs diastolic volume and stretch.

- Although a specific etiology of restrictive CMP is unknown, a number of pathologic processes may be involved in its development. Myocardial fibrosis, hypertrophy, and infiltration produce stiffness of the ventricular wall.
- The principal characteristic of restrictive CMP is cardiac muscle stiffness characterized by the loss of ventricular compliance. The ventricles are resistant to filling and therefore demand high diastolic filling pressures to maintain CO.

Clinical manifestations

- Angina, syncope, fatigue, and dyspnea on exertion are common signs.

- Additional signs and symptoms are similar to those of CHF. The patient may have signs of both left-sided and right-sided heart failure, including peripheral edema, ascites, and hepatic dysfunction. Kussmaul's sign (bulging of internal jugular neck veins on inspiration) may also be present.

Diagnostic studies
- Chest x-ray may be normal or show cardiomegaly.
- ECG may reveal tachycardia at rest. The most common dysrhythmias are atrial fibrillation and ventricular dysrhythmias.
- Echocardiogram may reveal a thickened ventricular wall of restrictive CMP, small ventricular cavities, and a dilated atria.
- Endomyocardial biopsy and CT scan may be helpful in a definitive diagnosis.

Therapeutic and nursing management. Currently, no specific treatment for restrictive CMP exists. Interventions are directed toward improving diastolic filling and the underlying disease process. Treatment includes conventional therapy for CHF and dysrhythmias. Heart transplant may also be a consideration.

Nursing care is similar to the care of a patient with CHF. As in the treatment of patients with HCM, the patients should be taught to avoid situations that impair ventricular filling, such as strenuous activity, dehydration, and increases in SVR.

CARPAL TUNNEL SYNDROME

Definition/Description
Carpal tunnel syndrome is a condition caused by compression of the median nerve beneath the transverse carpal ligament. This compression occurs within the narrow confines of the carpal tunnel located at the wrist. This condition is frequently due to pressure from trauma or edema caused by inflammation of a tendon (tenosynovitis), neoplasm, rheumatoid synovial disease, or soft tissue masses such as ganglia.

- Carpal tunnel syndrome occurs most frequently in middle-aged or postmenopausal females and persons who are employed in occupations that require continuous wrist movement (e.g., butchers, secretaries, carpenters, computer operators).

Clinical Manifestations
Clinical manifestations include weakness, pain and numbness of the hand, impaired sensation in the distribution of the median nerve, and clumsiness in performing fine hand movements. Numbness and tingling may be present and may awaken the patient at night.

- Holding the wrist in acute flexion for 60 seconds will produce tingling and numbness over the distribution of the median nerve, palmar surface of the thumb, index finger, middle finger, and part of the ring finger. This is known as a positive *Phalen's sign.*
- In late stages there is atrophy of thenar muscles. This syndrome can result in recurrent pain and eventual dysfunction of the hand.

Therapeutic Management

Therapy is directed toward relieving the underlying cause of the nerve compression. Early symptoms can usually be relieved by placing the hand and wrist at rest by immobilizing them in a hand splint. If the cause is inflammation, injection of hydrocortisone directly into the carpal tunnel may provide relief.

- If the problem continues, the median nerve may need to be surgically decompressed by longitudinal division of the transverse carpal ligament under regional anesthesia. Endoscopic carpal tunnel release is a procedure in which decompression is done through a small puncture wound.

Nursing Management

Goals

The patient with carpal tunnel syndrome will not experience an injury as a result of impaired sensation and will have relief from associated discomfort and satisfactory mobility of the hands.

Nursing Diagnoses

- Pain related to ineffective pain or comfort measures or nerve compression
- Impaired physical mobility related to pain and weakness
- Risk for injury related to impaired sensation and clumsiness of involved hand

Nursing Interventions

Prevention of carpal tunnel syndrome involves educating employees and employers to identify risk factors.

- Adaptive devices such as wrist splints may be worn to relieve pressure on the median nerve. Special keyboard pads are available for computer operators to help prevent carpal tunnel syndrome or a worsening of symptoms if present.

Comfort should be maintained by use of medication and splints to relieve pain and protect the area. Sensation may be impaired; therefore the patient should be instructed to avoid hazards such as extreme heat because of the risk of thermal injury.

Nursing care usually occurs in the office or outpatient setting. The patient may be required to consider occupational changes because of discomfort and sensory and functional changes.

- If surgery is performed, the neurovascular status of the hand should be evaluated regularly. The patient should be instructed in assessments to perform at home since surgery is done on an outpatient basis.

CATARACTS

C

Definition/Description
Cataracts are opacities within the crystalline lens of one or both eyes.

Pathophysiology
Although most cataracts are age related (senile cataracts), they can be associated with other factors, including blunt or penetrating trauma, congenital factors (e.g., maternal rubella), radiation or ultraviolet (UV) light exposure, certain drugs such as systemic corticosteroids or long-term topical steroids, and ocular inflammation. The patient with diabetes mellitus tends to develop cataracts at a younger age than does the patient in the nondiabetic population.

Clinical Manifestations
- Complaints of a decrease in vision, abnormal color perception, and glare that worsens at night are described.
- Visual decline is gradual, but the rate of cataract development varies from patient to patient.
- Secondary glaucoma may also occur if the enlarging lens causes increased intraocular pressure.

Diagnostic Studies
- Opacity directly observable by opthalmoscopic or slit-lamp microscopic examination
- Visual acuity measurement
- Glare testing
- Keratometry and A-scan ultrasound if surgery is planned

Therapeutic Management
Presence of a cataract does not necessarily indicate the need for surgery. For many patients the diagnosis is made long before they actually may need surgery. Other therapy may postpone or even negate the need for surgery.
- Palliative measures can include changing eyeglass prescription, strong reading glasses/magnifiers, increased amount of light to read, and avoidance of nighttime driving.

- Surgery may be performed when the patient's decreasing vision interferes with normal activities such as driving, reading, and watching television. The goal of surgery is to remove the source of visual impairment and restore vision. Surgical treatment can involve lens removal (i.e., phacoemulsification) and correction (i.e., intraocular lens implantation and contact lenses).

Nursing Management
Goals
- Until surgery is necessary, the patient will wear sunglasses and avoid unnecessary radiation.
- Preoperatively the patient will make informed decisions and experience minimal anxiety.
- Postoperatively the patient will understand and comply with therapy. Comfort will be maintained and the patient will remain free of infection.

Nursing Diagnoses/Collaborative Problems
- Decisional conflict related to lack of knowledge about condition and treatment options
- Impaired self-care deficit related to visual deficit
- Anxiety related to lack of knowledge about surgical and postoperative experience
- Pain related to surgical manipulation of tissue
- Risk of infection related to presence of surgical wound
- Potential complication: increased intraocular pressure related to surgery/postoperative activities

Nursing Interventions
- For the patient who chooses not to have surgery, suggest modifying activities/lifestyle to accomodate visual deficits.
- For the patient who elects surgery, provide information, support, and reassurance about the surgical and postoperative experience to reduce or alleviate patient anxiety. Inform the patient that depth perception will not be normal until the patch is removed (usually within 24 hours).
- Postoperatively offer mild analgesics for slight scratchiness or mild pain of the eye. The physician should be notified if severe pain, increased/purulent drainage, increased redness, or decreased visual acuity is present.

Patient Teaching
- Written and verbal discharge teaching should include postoperative eye care, activity restrictions, medications, follow-up visit schedule, and signs of possible complications.
- Patient's family should be included in the teaching since some patients may have difficulty with self-care activities, especially if vision in the unoperated eye is poor. Provide an opportunity

for the patient and family to present return demonstrations of any necessary self-care activities.

- Suggest ways for the patient and family to modify activities and environment to maintain a level of safe functioning. Suggestions may include getting assistance with steps, removing area rugs and other potential obstacles, preparing meals for freezing before surgery, and obtaining audio books for diversion until visual acuity improves.

C

CEREBROVASCULAR ACCIDENT (STROKE)

Definition/Description

A cerebrovascular accident (CVA) or stroke is the abrupt or rapid onset of a neurologic deficit resulting from disease of the blood vessels that supply the brain. The term *stroke* is used to describe an event that can be caused by a number of different pathologic processes. For most persons who experience a stroke, it seems to "just happen" without warning. However, a warning sign or symptom may have occurred and gone unrecognized.

- Regardless of the cause, parts of the brain damaged by the loss of blood supply can no longer perform their specific cognitive, sensory, motor, or emotional functions. The resulting impairments can be slight or severe, temporary or permanent.
- Stroke is ranked third among all causes of death in the United States, exceeded only by heart disease and cancer.
- Approximately 60% to 75% of all strokes occur in persons more than 65 years of age.
- Approximately 30% to 50% of those who survive a stroke are left with moderate to severe disability and require assistance with activities of daily living (ADLs).

Risk Factors

Risk factors most closely associated with stroke can be divided into two categories: nonmodifiable and potentially modifiable.

- *Nonmodifiable* risk factors include gender, age, race, and heredity. Overall incidence of stroke is higher for men than for women, with risk of stroke greatly increased with advancing age. African-Americans are more likely than Caucasians to have a stroke, probably because they have a higher incidence of hypertension. There is sometimes a hereditary pattern to the occurrence of strokes, although the inherited factor(s) are not clear.

- *Potentially modifiable* risk factors are hypertension, cardiac disease, diabetes mellitus, blood lipid abnormalities, and certain lifestyle habits. The most important risk factor associated with stroke is hypertension. The treatment of hypertension is the most significant contributor to the prevention of a stroke.

Types of Stroke

Strokes may be classified as either *ischemic* or *hemorrhagic* on the basis of their underlying pathophysiology (Table 18).

- *Ischemic strokes* result from decreased blood flow to the brain secondary to partial or complete occlusion of an artery. They occur much more frequently than hemorrhagic strokes. The most common types of ischemic stroke are *thrombotic* and *embolic* (see following discussion).
- *Hemorrhagic strokes* are generally the result of spontaneous bleeding into the brain tissue itself (intracerebral or intraparenchymal hemorrhage) or into the subarachnoid space or ventricles (subarachnoid hemorrhage).

Pathophysiology

Thrombosis results from the formation of a blood clot that causes narrowing of the lumen of a blood vessel with eventual occlusion. Thrombosis is the most common cause of cerebral infarction.

- Two thirds of strokes caused by thrombosis are associated with hypertension or diabetes, both of which are conditions that accelerate the atherosclerotic process.
- Thrombosis may be preceded by prodromal warnings, such as paresthesias (abnormal sensations), paresis (decreased strength and motility of an extremity), and aphasia (disturbance of language function). These transient periods of neurologic deficit called *transient ischemic attacks* can signal a developing lesion.
- A stroke caused by thrombosis is characterized by intermittency or erratic progression of signs and symptoms.

Cerebral embolism is the occlusion of a cerebral artery by an embolus, resulting in necrosis and edema of the area supplied by the involved blood vessel. Embolism is the second most common cause of stroke.

- The majority of emboli originate from the heart, with plaques or tissue breaking off from the endocardium and entering the circulation. Emboli from the heart or extracranial arteries usually travel up through the carotid system and lodge in the middle cerebral artery or one of its branches.
- Recurrence is common unless the underlying cause is aggressively treated.

Table 18 Types of Stroke

Type	Gender/age	Warning	Time of onset	Course/prognosis
Ischemic				
Thrombotic	Men more than women, oldest median age	TIA* (30% to 50% of cases)	During or after sleep	Stepwise progression; usually some improvement; recurrence in 20% to 25% of survivors
Embolic	Men more than women	TIA (uncommon)	Lack of relationship to activity, sudden onset	Single event; usually some improvement; recurrence common without aggressive treatment of underlying disease
Hemorrhagic				
Intracerebral	Slightly higher in women	Headache (25% of cases)	Activity (often)	Progression over 24 hr; poor prognosis; fatality more likely with presence of coma
Subarachnoid	Slightly higher in women, youngest median age	Headache (common)	Activity (often), sudden onset. Most commonly related to head trauma	Single sudden event usually; fatality more likely with presence of coma

*TIA, Transient ischemic attack.

C

Classification of Stroke

Transient ischemic attack (TIA) is a brief episode of neurologic deficit that occurs without apparent residual effects. The deficits usually last less than 30 minutes but may last for up to 24 hours. There is no sign of permanent neurologic deficit between attacks.

- A widely held hypothesis is that TIAs are caused by microemboli breaking off from atherosclerotic plaques in the extracranial arteries and temporarily interrupting cerebral oxygenation.
- A TIA is considered a warning signal and is usually a sign of advanced atherosclerotic disease of the cerebral arteries.
- The signs and symptoms vary according to the part of the brain affected. If the carotid system is involved, the patient may report a temporary loss of vision in one eye, a transient hemiparesis, or a sudden inability to speak.
- Symptoms of TIA related to vertebral-basilar insufficiency are tinnitus, vertigo, darkened or blurred vision, diplopia, dysphagia, and unilateral or bilateral numbness or weakness.
- A patient with symptoms of TIA should seek medical care promptly.

Reversible ischemic neurologic deficit is a neurologic deficit that remains after 24 hours but leaves no residual signs or symptoms after days to weeks. It is considered by some to be a completed stroke with minimal to no residual deficit.

Stroke in evolution or a progressing stroke develops over a period of hours or days. A stepwise or intermittent progression of deteriorating neurologic findings is common. Progression of manifestations correlates with the degree of edema secondary to the inflammatory process.

Completed stroke (stable stroke) occurs when the neurologic deficit remains unchanged over a 2- to 3-day period. An embolic stroke may demonstrate this characteristic from the onset. With the exception of stroke secondary to a ruptured aneurysm, a completed stroke signals readiness for more aggressive rehabilitative treatment.

Clinical Manifestations

Manifestations of stroke depend on the (1) anatomic site of lesion, (2) rate of onset, (3) size of lesion, and (4) presence of collateral circulation. Table 55-2, Lewis/Collier/Heitkemper, *Medical-Surgical Nursing,* edition 4, p. 1728, lists manifestations seen when specific cerebral arteries are involved, regardless of whether the CVA is due to thrombosis, embolus, or hemorrhage.

- Physical disabilities are usually easy to identify. Language and spatial-perceptual problems are more subtle and difficult to recognize. Consequently, these problems are often ignored or misunderstood. Figure 55-3 in Lewis/Collier/Heitkemper, *Medi-*

cal-Surgical Nursing, edition 4, p. 1728, illustrates the manifestations of right-sided and left-sided stroke.

Neuromotor function. Motor deficits, the most obvious manifestations of stroke, are caused by destruction of motor neurons in the pyramidal pathway. This destruction can result in loss of skilled voluntary movements (akinesia), impairment of integration of movements, and alterations in muscle tone and reflex activity.

- Hyporeflexia that initially occurs with stroke progresses to hyperreflexia for most patients.
- The patient may have impairment of swallowing (dysphagia) because of weakness of the mouth and throat muscles; swallow reflex may also be diminished or absent. The patient may be unable to swallow secretions and consequently is susceptible to aspiration pneumonia.
- Initially, the patient may experience urinary frequency, urgency, and incontinence. Bladder training is facilitated if started immediately.
- The patient is prone to constipation, which is attributed to immobility, decreased oral intake, inability to communicate the need to defecate, and lack of response to defecation reflex.

Communication. When the stroke occurs in the dominant hemisphere, the patient may experience communication difficulties or *aphasia.*

- Language disorders involve expression and comprehension of written or spoken words.
- When the lesion involves Wernicke's area of the brain, the patient experiences *receptive* aphasia; neither sounds of speech nor its meaning can be distinguished, and comprehension of both written and spoken language is impaired.
- The lesion causing *expressive* aphasia affects Broca's area, the motor area for speech. This patient has difficulty in speaking and writing.
- Most aphasias are mixed with impairment of both expression and understanding.

Affective function. Patients with a stroke may demonstrate loss of control of their emotions; emotional responses may be exaggerated or unpredictable. Additional manifestations include impairment of memory and judgment and deficits in spatial-perceptual orientation.

Diagnostic Studies

Various tests are carried out to determine the cause of the stroke and to serve as a basis for therapeutic management.

- CT scan, the primary diagnostic test, can indicate lesion size and location and differentiate hemorrhage from infarction. MRI is the best imaging technique to differentiate types of infarcts.

- Electroencephalogram (EEG) may show low-voltage slow waves with ischemic infarction and high-voltage slow waves with hemorrhage.
- Radionuclide scan (brain scan) shows increased uptake of radioactive media in infarction.
- Angiography demonstrates cerebral and cerebrovascular occlusion, plaques, and malformations.
- Cerebrospinal fluid shows transient leukocytosis and possible blood from hemorrhage.

Therapeutic Management

Prevention.   Once a stroke has occurred, the impact of therapeutic management on modifying the extent of brain tissue damage is limited. The priority of therapy is prevention of infarction in the patient with a TIA and prevention of recurrence in the patient who has had a stroke.

- Patients with known risk factors, such as diabetes, hypertension, or cardiac dysfunction, should be followed closely. Measures designed to prevent development of a thrombus or embolus are used; the administration of aspirin (ASA) or dipyridamole (Persantine) has decreased the incidence of stroke. A newer platelet aggregation inhibitor, ticlopidine hydrochloride (Ticlid), has been shown to be more effective than aspirin. Anticoagulants are also used for patients with TIAs, although the possibility of hemorrhage must be considered.
- The most common *surgical interventions* used to reduce the frequency of TIAs and danger of impending stroke are carotid endarterectomy and extracranial-intracranial (EC-IC) bypass. Transluminal angioplasty is a third surgical procedure currently being studied. These procedures are designed to maintain cerebral blood flow and must be performed before an infarction occurs or hazards outweigh the benefits.

Acute management.   The focus of acute therapeutic management is preservation of life, prevention of additional brain damage, and lessening of disability. Treatment differs according to the type of stroke and whether the aim of treatment is prevention, management during the acute phase, or long-term rehabilitation.

- The first goal of therapeutic management is to maintain a patent airway, which may be compromised because of decreased consciousness. O_2, an artificial airway, or possibly intubation and mechanical ventilation may be indicated.
- The patient is monitored closely for signs of increasing neurologic deficit.

Three therapeutic approaches have been used with varying success to prevent additional brain damage:

- The first and most effective is the use of measures designed to reduce cerebral edema, which interferes with the metabolism of viable cells. Hyperosmotic agents, such as mannitol, may be employed. With any of these agents, the nurse must carefully monitor intake and output, body weight, electrolytes, and serum osmolality. The patient can become dehydrated.
- The second approach involves measures designed to reduce metabolic needs of the brain. Hypothermia and barbiturate therapy are among the treatments that have been attempted for this purpose, although neither has proved effective.
- The third therapeutic approach is designed to promote cerebral blood flow. Vasodilators (e.g., papaverine), hypertensive agents, and hyperventilation therapy have all been attempted but have been of little documented value.

When a cerebral hemorrhage is the result of rupture of an aneurysm, surgical intervention may be appropriate. Early surgery to decrease the danger of rebleeding and to facilitate management of vasospasm has become widely accepted.

Chronic management. After the patient's condition has stabilized for 12 to 24 hours, therapeutic management shifts from preservation of life to lessening of disability. Various members of the health care team may be involved in the effort to return the patient to optimal functioning.

- In most instances, maximal improvement is attained in 12 to 24 weeks, although some patients continue to show improvement for as long as 2 years after the stroke.

Pharmacologic Management

Anticoagulants. Heparin is used in the treatment of TIAs, thrombotic strokes, and strokes in evolution. Heparin is used as the first step in anticoagulation. Long-term anticoagulation is accomplished by oral administration of warfarin (Coumadin, Panwarfin). Duration of treatment is 3 to 6 months.

Platelet aggregation inhibitors. Drugs that interfere with platelet function are used in the management of TIAs and symptoms of progressing stroke. Aspirin, dipyridamole, and ticlopidine are three such agents.

Thrombolytic therapy. Reperfusion of acutely occluded intracranial arteries through tissue plasminogen activator (tPA) is the primary type of fibrinolytic therapy in use.

Nutritional Management

After the acute phase, the dietitian can assist in determining appropriate daily caloric intake based on the patient's overall size, weight, and activity level. Residual physical problems (e.g., paralysis of dominant arm) and psychosocial problems (e.g., depression) must also be considered.

- If the patient is unable to take in an adequate diet orally, tube feeding may be initiated, usually by the nasogastric route (see Tube Feeding, p. 685).

Nursing Management
Goals
The patient who has experienced a stroke will maintain a stable or improved level of consciousness, attain maximum physical functioning, avoid complications of immobility, have an effective pattern of bladder and bowel elimination, maximize remaining communication abilities, perform self-care activities (bathing, dressing, feeding self), remain safe without injuries, maintain desired sexual activity and relationship, and maintain effective coping (patient and family).

See the nursing care plan for the patient with a stroke in Lewis/Collier/Heitkemper, *Medical-Surgical Nursing,* edition 4, p. 1739.

Nursing Diagnoses
- Impaired physical mobility related to generalized weakness, muscle atrophy, or paralyzed extremities
- Impaired verbal communication related to residual aphasia
- Self-care deficit (partial to total) related to motor weakness, paralysis, and loss of ability to effectively perform ADLs
- Sensory/perceptual alteration: visual deficit related to visual field cut, diplopia, and ptosis secondary to decreased circulation to brain
- Impaired swallowing related to weakness or paralysis of affected muscles
- Altered pattern of urinary elimination: incontinence related to impaired impulse to void or inability to reach toilet or manage tasks of voiding
- Constipation related to immobility, inadequate fiber or bulk intake, and impaired defecation impulse
- Altered nutrition: less than body requirements related to difficulty or inability to feed self, immobility, and possible depression
- Self-esteem disturbance related to actual or perceived loss of function

Nursing Interventions
Respiratory system. During the acute phase of a stroke, the nursing priority is management of respiratory function.
- In coma the tongue tends to fall back and obstruct the airway. The patient should be positioned in a side-lying position. An oropharyngeal airway may be used during the first 24 to 48 hours.
- If the patient is unable to breathe without an airway after 48 hours, a tracheostomy is performed. A suction machine should be available in the patient's room.

Neurologic system. The patient's neurologic status needs to be monitored closely to detect stroke in evolution or increased intracranial pressure (ICP).

- Level of consciousness, mental status, pupillary responses, movement and strength of extremities, and vital signs are checked at regular intervals.
- A decreasing level of consciousness, the earliest and most sensitive sign of increasing brain ischemia, should prompt the nurse to check the patient more frequently and report this change to the physician.

Cardiovascular system. Nursing goals for the cardiovascular system are designed to maintain homeostasis.

- Fluid retention plus overhydration can result in fluid overload; it can also increase cerebral edema. The nurse, therefore, should closely monitor intake and output. IV therapy is also carefully regulated.
- After a stroke the patient is at risk for thrombophlebitis and deep-vein thrombosis in the weak or paralyzed lower extremity. The most effective prevention is to keep the patient moving. Active range-of-motion exercises should be taught if the patient has any voluntary movement in the affected extremity. For the patient with hemiplegia, passive range-of-motion exercises should be done at least several times a day.
- Additional measures often used to prevent thrombophlebitis include positioning to minimize the effects of dependent edema and use of elastic compression gradient stockings or support hose. Intermittent pneumatic compression stockings may be ordered for long-term bedridden patients.

Musculoskeletal system. Goals for the musculoskeletal system are to maintain function, which is accomplished by prevention of joint contractures and muscular atrophy.

- In the acute phase, range-of-motion exercises and positioning are important interventions. Passive range-of-motion exercise is begun on the first day of hospitalization. Muscle atrophy secondary to lack of innervation and to inactivity can develop within a month.
- The paralyzed side needs special attention when the patient is positioned. Each joint should be positioned higher than the joint proximal to it. Specific deformities on the affected side of the patient with hemiplegia are shoulder adduction; flexion contractures of the hand, wrist, and elbow; external rotation of the hip; and plantar flexion of the foot.

Integumentary system. The patient's skin is particularly susceptible to breakdown because of loss of sensation and diminished circulation.

- Pressure points should be examined and massaged with each turning. If an area of redness develops, the patient should be turned more frequently.
- The patient should not be left in any position longer than 2 hours. Time spent lying on the paralyzed side should be limited to 30 minutes.
- Special mattresses that are filled with water or air or that provide alternating pressure may help in relieving pressure areas.

Gastrointestinal system. The stress of illness contributes to a catabolic state that can interfere with recovery.

- The patient may be maintained for 5 to 7 days on IV fluids. Facial weakness on the affected side and dysphagia (difficulty swallowing) present special problems.
- If the patient is conscious, oral feeding should be considered. The first oral feeding should be approached with caution because the gag reflex may be impaired. Before initiation of feeding, the gag reflex may be assessed by gently stimulating the back of the throat with a tongue blade.
- The most common bowel problem is constipation. The patient should be checked every 2 days for impaction.
- Because diet, fluids, and exercise are limited during the acute phase of stroke, a laxative or a stool softener may be needed. Enemas are used only if suppositories and digital stimulation are ineffective because they cause vagal stimulation and increase ICP.

Urinary system. In the acute stage of stroke, the primary urinary problem is poor bladder control, resulting in incontinence.

- Efforts should be made to promote normal bladder function and avoid use of an indwelling catheter.
- Long-term use of an indwelling catheter promotes development of urinary tract infection and prolongs bladder retraining. An intermittent catheterization program may be used for patients with urinary retention.

Communication. During the acute stage, the nurse's role in meeting the psychologic needs of the patient is primarily supportive.

- An alert patient is usually very anxious because of a lack of understanding of what has happened and the inability to communicate. If the patient cannot understand words, gestures may be used to support verbal cues. It may help to speak slowly and calmly and to use relatively simple words.

Sensory-perceptual alterations. *Homonymous hemianopsia* (blindness in the same half of each visual field) is a common problem after a stroke. The patient must learn to compensate for these deficits.

- After the initial stress of the illness, the nurse may begin placing items necessary for ADLs on the affected side.

- Later the patient is instructed to attend to the neglected side consciously. The position of the affected arm or leg in space must be checked by the patient to prevent unfelt trauma.
- Visual problems may include diplopia, loss of corneal reflex, and ptosis, particularly if the stroke is in the vertebrobasilar distribution. Diplopia is often treated with the use of an eye patch. If the corneal reflex is absent, the patient is at risk of a corneal abrasion and should be observed closely and protected against eye injuries. There are no definitive interventions for ptosis.

Coping. A stroke is usually a sudden, extremely stressful event for both patient and close family members.

- Reactions vary considerably but may involve fear and apprehension, denial of severity of the stroke, depression, and anger.
- During the acute phase of caring for patient and family, nursing interventions designed to facilitate coping involve providing information and emotional support.
- Explanations to the patient about what has happened and about diagnostic and therapeutic procedures should be clear and understandable. It is particularly challenging to keep the aphasic patient adequately informed.
- Because family members usually have not had time to prepare for the illness, they may need assistance in arranging care for family members or pets and for transportation and finances.

Rehabilitative Management

The three goals of rehabilitative management are to (1) prevent deformity, (2) maintain function, and (3) restore function.

- Work toward the first two goals begins at the time the patient enters the health care system (e.g., on admission the nurse attempts to prevent deformity in the hemiplegic patient by proper positioning and range-of-motion exercises). During restoration of function the patient begins to relearn and to regain control over bodily actions and functions that are deficient or lost because of the stroke; these activities may focus on speech, walking, bowel and bladder control, and ADLs.

Rehabilitation and long-term management of the stroke patient are further described in Lewis/Collier/Heitkemper, *Medical-Surgical Nursing,* edition 4, p. 1744.

Family and Patient Teaching

- While the patient is hospitalized, the care provider needs instruction and practice in necessary areas of home care. This allows for support and encouragement as well as opportunities for feedback. Adjustments in the home environment, such as removal of a door to accommodate a wheelchair, can be made before discharge.

- Specific areas for instruction related to home care include exercise and ambulation techniques; dietary requirements; recognition of signs indicating the possibility of another stroke (e.g., headache, vertigo, numbness, visual disturbances); understanding of emotional lability and possibility of depression; medication routine; and time, place, and frequency of follow-up activities such as occupational therapy and physical therapy.
- To assist the primary care provider to stay healthy after the patient is discharged home, it is important to plan for respite or time away from caregiving activities on a regular basis.

CERVICAL CANCER

Definition/Description
Carcinoma of the cervix is the sixth most common malignancy in women. It occurs predominantly in women between the ages of 30 and 50, with the incidence higher among African-American and Hispanic women than among Caucasian women.

- An increased risk of cervical cancer is associated with low economic status, early sexual activity and marriage, several sexual partners, multiple pregnancies, venereal disease, viral infections, and smoking.

The number of deaths from cervical cancer has fallen steadily over the past 40 years. This change is attributable to better and earlier diagnosis with the widespread use of the Pap test. The high-detection efficiency of this test permits treatment at a time (stage 0) when cure is almost certain. The American Cancer Society recommends that annual Pap tests begin with onset of sexual activity.

Pathophysiology
The World Health Organization has developed an international classification for cancer of the cervix with stages from 0 to IV (see Table 51-12, in Lewis/Collier/Heitkemper, *Medical-Surgical Nursing,* edition 4, p. 1613).

- Stage 0, the preinvasive stage of carcinoma in situ, is limited to the epithelial layer. A period of 5 to 10 years may elapse between the preinvasive stage and a stage I lesion, making the prognosis good for early diagnosis and treatment.
- Stage IV involves cancer that has extended outside the reproductive tract.

Clinical Manifestations

Early cervical cancer is generally asymptomatic, but leukorrhea and intermenstrual bleeding eventually occur.

- A discharge, which is usually thin and watery, becomes dark and foul smelling as the disease advances.
- Vaginal bleeding is initially only spotting, but as the tumor enlarges, it becomes heavier and more frequent.
- Pain is a late symptom and is followed by weight loss, anemia, and cachexia.

Diagnostic Studies

- A Pap test, Schiller iodine test, colposcopy, and biopsy may be used to diagnose cancer of the cervix.
- The current trend is to use the Bethesda System for classifying the stage of cancer (see Table 51-13, in Lewis/Collier/Heitkemper, *Medical-Surgical Nursing,* edition 4, p. 1614).
- The type and extent of the biopsy may vary with the abnormality seen. A punch biopsy may be done on an outpatient basis with special punch biopsy forceps.
- Excision of a cone-shaped section of the cervix may be used for both diagnosis and treatment. Conization is accomplished using one of several techniques; choice of procedure is determined by the provider's experience and availability of equipment.
- *Cryotherapy* (freezing) and laser cone vaporization destroy the tissue. Laser cone excision and *loop electrosurgery excision procedure (LEEP)* remove identified tissue and allow for histologic examination to ensure that all microinvasive tissue has been removed.

Therapeutic Management

Treatment of cancer of the cervix is guided by the stage of tumor and by the patient's age and general state of health.

- Conization may be the only type of therapy needed for cervical intraepithelial neoplasia (CIN) if analysis of removed tissue demonstrates that a wide area of normal tissue surrounds the excised malignancy.
- Laser treatments, in which a directed infrared beam causes boiling and vaporization of intracellular water, is effective in the destruction of dysplastic tissue.
- Cautery and cryosurgery may also be used.

Invasive cancer of the cervix is treated with surgery, radiation, or a combination of the two to remove or destroy involved areas and lymphatic drainage.

- Surgical procedures commonly carried out include hysterectomy, radical hysterectomy (Wertheim), and, rarely, pelvic exenteration. Radiation may be external (e.g., cobalt) or internal (e.g., cesium or radium). Standard radiation treatment is 5 to 6 weeks of external radiation followed with one or two internal implants (see Radiation Therapy, p. 675).

- The use of chemotherapy has been disappointing in most cases of recurrent cervical cancer. Previously radiated areas are difficult to treat because the capillary blood supply is diminished, resulting in poor drug delivery to the tumor bed.

Nursing Management

For nursing management of cervical cancer, see Surgical Procedures Involving the Female Reproductive System, p. 677.

CHLAMYDIAL INFECTION

Definition/Description

Chlamydia trachomatis, a Gram-negative bacteria, is recognized as a genital pathogen responsible for a variety of illnesses.

- There are numerous strains of *C. trachomatis.* Some cause urogenital infection (e.g., nongonococcal urethritis [NGU] in men and cervicitis in women); some cause ocular trachoma, and others, lymphogranuloma venereum.
- Although it is not a reportable disease in all states, it is estimated that *C. trachomatis* infections are the most prevalent sexually transmitted diseases (STDs) in the United States.

Risk factors include age less than 25 years, multiple sex partners, history of STDs, use of nonbarrier contraception, and bleeding inducible by swabbing of the cervical mucosa.

- Because of the high prevalence of asymptomatic infections, screening of high-risk people is needed to identify those infected.

Clinical Manifestations

As with gonorrhea, chlamydial infections result in a superficial mucosal infection that can become more invasive.

- Signs and symptoms in *men* include urethritis (dysuria, urethral discharge), epididymitis (unilateral scrotal pain, swelling, fever), and proctitis (rectal discharge and pain during defecation).
- Signs and symptoms in *women* include cervicitis (mucopurulent discharge and hypertrophic ectopy [area that is edematous and bleeds easily]), urethritis (dysuria and frequent urination), bartholinitis (purulent exudate), and pelvic inflammatory dis-

ease (abdominal pain, vomiting, fever, abnormal vaginal bleeding, and menstrual abnormalities). A large number of women with chlamydial cervicitis have been found to have a male partner with NGU.

Complications often develop from poorly managed, inaccurately diagnosed, or undiagnosed chlamydial infections.

- Infection in men may result in epididymitis with possible infertility and Reiter's disease.
- Women may develop hypertrophic erosion of the cervix, salpingitis leading to pelvis inflammatory disease (PID), and infertility. Proctitis is associated with rectal intercourse.
- *Chlamydia* infection may be transmitted from mother to newborn, causing inclusion conjunctivitis or pneumonia.

Diagnostic Studies

In men a diagnosis of chlamydial infection is made by excluding gonorrhea; specifically, if no gram-negative intracellular diplococci are found on a Gram-stained smear of male urethral discharge or sediment of first-catch urine specimen, a culture is done. If results of both these tests are negative, and signs of inflammation are present (e.g., polymorphonuclear leukocytes [PMNs] on the Gram-stained smear), a diagnosis of NGU-*Chlamydia* infection can be made.

In women, screening is more effective due to the availability of nonculture tests, including direct fluorescent antibody (DFA) tests, enzyme immunoassay (EIA), and DNA hybridization tests. These tests are less specific than cultures and may produce false-positive results. Culturing for chlamydial organisms should be done if laboratory facilities are available.

Therapeutic Management

Chlamydial infections respond to treatment with tetracycline, doxycycline, or azithromycin. Erythromycin is the drug of choice for use in pregnant patients.

- *Follow-up care* should include advising the patient to return if symptoms persist or recur, treatment of sex partners, and encouraging the use of condoms during all sexual contacts.

Nursing Management

Goals

The patient with chlamydial infection will demonstrate an understanding of the mode of transmission of STDs and the risk posed by STDs, complete treatment and return for appropriate follow-up, notify or assist in notification of contacts about their need for testing and treatment, abstain from intercourse until infection is resolved, and demonstrate knowledge of safe sex practices.

Nursing Diagnoses

- Risk for infection transmission related to lack of knowledge about mode of transmission, inadequate personal and genital hygiene, and failure to practice precautionary measures
- Pain related to manifestations of infection
- Altered health maintenance related to knowledge and questions about disease process, appropriate follow-up measures and possibility of reinfection
- Anxiety related to impact of condition on relationships, disease outcome, and lack of knowledge of disease
- Risk for noncompliance because of lack of knowledge of possible complications and confusion about therapy

Nursing Interventions

The diagnosis of chlamydia or other STDs may be met with a variety of emotions such as shame, guilt, anger, and a desire for vengeance. The nurse should try to help the patient verbalize his/her feelings. A referral for professional counseling to explore the ramifications of an STD may be indicated.

All patients should return to the treatment center for repeat culture from infected sites or for serologic testing at designated times to determine the effectiveness of treatment.

- Informing the patient that cures are not always obtained on first treatment can reinforce the need for a follow-up visit.
- The patient should also be advised to inform his/her sexual partners of the need for treatment, regardless of whether they are free of symptoms or experiencing symptoms.

The patient with an STD should have certain hygiene measures emphasized.

- An important measure is frequent handwashing and bathing; this results in destruction of many of the causative organisms of STDs.
- Bathing and cleaning of involved areas can provide local comfort and prevent secondary infection. Douching may spread infection and is therefore contraindicated.
- Sexual abstinence is indicated during the communicable phase of the disease. If sexual activity occurs before treatment of the patient has been completed, the use of condoms may prevent spread of infection and reinfection.

Patient Teaching

An inspection of the sexual partner's genitals before coitus is recommended. The presence of discharge, sores, blisters, or rash should be viewed with concern.

- A patient who is aware of specific signs and symptoms of infection can intelligently make the decision to continue sexual interaction with modifications or elect not to have sexual relations.

- Men should be told that some protection is provided if they void immediately following intercourse and wash their genitals and adjacent areas with soap and water.
- Women may also benefit from postcoital voiding and washing. Spermicidal jellies and creams have a mild detergent effect that may reduce the risk of contracting STDs. These same barriers can serve as supplementary lubrication, thereby decreasing irritation and friction and the chance for development of a minor laceration, which could serve as an entry point for the organism.
- Proper use of a latex condom provides a highly effective mechanical barrier to infection. The condom should be undamaged and correctly in place throughout all phases of sexual activity. The use of a spermicide such as nonoxynol-9 (which inactivates most STD organisms) in the vagina and concurrent use of a condom can further reduce the risk of disease.
- Sexual contact with persons known or suspected to have human immunodeficiency virus (HIV) infection should be avoided. A sexually active homosexual man can reduce his risk by minimizing the number of sexual contacts. Anal intercourse should be eliminated, and condoms should be used if sexual contact continues.

CHOLELITHIASIS/CHOLECYSTITIS

Definition/Description
The most common disorder of the biliary system is *cholelithiasis* (stones in the gallbladder). *Cholecystitis* (inflammation of the gallbladder) is usually associated with cholelithiasis. The stones may be lodged in the neck of the gallbladder or in the cystic duct. Cholecystitis may be acute or chronic. Incidence of cholelithiasis is higher in women, multiparous women, and persons over 40 years of age.

Pathophysiology
The actual cause of gallstones is unknown. *Cholelithiasis* develops when the balance that keeps cholesterol, bile salts, and calcium in solution is altered so that precipitation of these substances occurs. Conditions that upset this balance include infection and disturbances in metabolism of cholesterol.

- The stones may remain in the gallbladder or migrate to the cystic duct or common bile duct. They cause pain as they pass through the ducts and may lodge in the ducts and produce an obstruction.

Cholecystitis is most commonly associated with stones. When it occurs in the absence of stones, it is thought to be caused by bacteria reaching the gallbladder via the vascular or lymphatic route or by chemical irritants in the bile.

- *Escherichia coli,* streptococci, and salmonellae are the most common causative bacteria.
- Other etiologic factors include adhesions, neoplasms, extensive fasting, frequent weight fluctuations, anesthesia, and narcotics.
- During an acute attack of cholecystitis, the gallbladder is edematous and hyperemic. It may be distended with bile or pus. The cystic duct is also involved and may become occluded.
- The wall of the gallbladder becomes scarred after an acute attack. Decreased functioning occurs if large amounts of tissue are fibrosed.

Clinical Manifestations

Cholelithiasis may produce severe symptoms or none at all. Many patients have silent cholelithiasis. The severity of symptoms depends on whether the stones are stationary or mobile and whether obstruction is present.

- When a stone is lodged in the ducts or when stones are moving through the ducts, spasms may result. This sometimes produces very severe pain, which is termed *biliary colic.* The pain can be accompanied by tachycardia, diaphoresis, and prostration. The severe pain may last up to an hour, and when it subsides, there is residual tenderness in the right upper quadrant.
- Attacks of pain frequently occur 3 to 6 hours after a heavy meal or when the patient assumes a recumbent position.
- When total obstruction occurs, symptoms related to bile blockage are manifested.

Manifestations of *cholecystitis* vary from indigestion to moderate to severe pain, leukocytosis, fever, and jaundice.

- Initial symptoms include indigestion and pain and tenderness in the right upper quadrant, which may be referred to the right shoulder and scapula.
- Pain is accompanied by restlessness, diaphoresis, and nausea and vomiting.
- Symptoms of chronic cholecystitis include a history of fat intolerance, dyspepsia, heartburn, and flatulence.

Complications of *cholecystitis* include subphrenic abscess, pancreatitis, cholangitis (inflammation of biliary ducts), fistulas, and rupture of the gallbladder, which can produce bile peritonitis. Many of the same complications can occur from *cholelithiasis,* including cholangitis, carcinoma, and peritonitis.

Diagnostic Studies

- Ultrasonography is used to diagnose gallstones.
- Oral cholecystogram detects radiopaque stones.
- IV cholangiogram outlines the gallbladder and ducts.
- Percutaneous transhepatic cholangiography (PTC) is used to diagnose jaundice and locate stones within the ducts.
- Laboratory studies may demonstrate liver function test abnormalities, elevated serum enzymes, increased white blood cell (WBC) count, elevated direct and indirect bilirubin levels, and urinary bilirubin level.

Therapeutic Management

During an acute episode of cholecystitis the focus of treatment is control of pain, control of possible infection with antibiotics, and maintenance of fluid and electrolyte balance. Treatment is mainly supportive and symptomatic.

- If nausea and vomiting are severe, gastric decompression may be used to prevent further gallbladder stimulation. Anticholinergic drugs that decrease secretions and counteract smooth muscle spasms may be administered. Analgesics are given to decrease pain.

There are currently several options for therapeutic management of cholelithiasis. These include the use of cholesterol solvents such as methyl tertiary terbutyl ether (MTBE), oral drugs that dissolve stones, endoscopic sphincterotomy, extracorporeal shock-wave lithotripsy (ESWL), and surgery. Supportive treatment, similar to that given for cholecystitis, may also be necessary.

- If stones cause an obstruction, additional treatment consists of replacement of fat-soluble vitamins, administration of bile salts to facilitate digestion and vitamin absorption, and a low-fat diet.

Surgical intervention for cholelithiasis is frequently indicated and may consist of laparoscopic cholecystectomy or open (incisional) cholecystectomy.

- Laparoscopic cholecystectomy is considered by many surgeons to be the preferred surgical procedure. This procedure is done instead of an open (incisional) surgical procedure about 80% to 85% of the time. In a laparoscopic procedure the gallbladder is removed through one of four small punctures in the abdomen. Most patients experience minimal postoperative pain and are discharged the day of surgery or the following day. In most cases they are able to resume normal activities and return to work after 2 or 3 days.
- Advantages of laparoscopic cholecystectomy include decreased postoperative pain, shorter hospital stay, and earlier return to

work and full activity. The main complication is injury to the common bile duct.

Pharmacologic management of gallbladder disease includes analgesics, anticholinergics (antispasmodics such as atropine), fat-soluble vitamins, and bile salts. Meperidine (Demerol) is used if a narcotic analgesic is required. This drug causes less spasm in the ducts than opiates such as morphine sulfate.

Nutritional management with cholelithiasis and cholecystitis is a low-fat diet, which decreases stimulation of the gallbladder. If obesity is a problem, a reduced-calorie diet is indicated.

Nursing Management
Goals
The patient with gallbladder disease will have relief of pain and discomfort, no complications postoperatively, and no recurrent attacks of cholecystitis or cholelithiasis.

For surgical management of gallbladder disease, see the nursing care plan for the patient with an incisional cholecystectomy in Lewis/Collier/Heitkemper, *Medical-Surgical Nursing,* edition 4, p. 1302.

Nursing Diagnoses/Collaborative Problems for Patient with Cholecystectomy
- Ineffective breathing pattern related to splintered or guarded respirations secondary to pain
- Pain related to surgical incision and presence of drains and bulky dressing
- Impaired management of therapeutic regimen related to lack of knowledge of postoperative management, diet, and activity restrictions
- Potential complication: paralytic ileus related to decreased peristalsis secondary to surgery and immobility

Nursing Interventions
Nursing objectives for the patient undergoing conservative therapy include relieving pain, relieving nausea and vomiting, providing comfort and emotional support, maintaining fluid and electrolyte balance and nutrition, making accurate assessments for effectiveness of treatment, and observing for complications.

The patient with cholecystitis or cholelithiasis is frequently experiencing severe pain; medications ordered to relieve pain should be given as required before the pain becomes more severe.
- The nurse should assess what medications relieve pain and how much medication is required. Observation for side effects of medications must be part of the continued assessment.
- Nursing comfort measures, such as a clean bed, comfortable positioning, and oral care, are appropriate.

Postoperative nursing care following a laparoscopic cholecystectomy include:

- Monitoring for complications such as bleeding, making the patient comfortable, and preparing the patient for discharge.
- Assessing pain, which is usually minimal and can be relieved by narcotic analgesics such as oxycodone and acetaminophen (Percocet).
- Assisting the patient with clear liquids and ambulation to the bathroom.

A common postoperative problem is referred pain to the shoulder because of carbon dioxide that was not released or absorbed by the body. Carbon dioxide can irritate the phrenic nerve and diaphragm, causing some difficulty with breathing. Placing the patient in the Sims' position (left side with right knee flexed) will help move the gas pocket away from the diaphragm.

Patient Teaching

- When the patient is undergoing conservative therapy, dietary teaching is usually necessary. The diet is ordinarily low in fat, and sometimes a weight-reduction diet is also recommended. The patient may need to take fat-soluble vitamin supplements.
- Instructions should be provided regarding observations the patient should make indicating obstruction (stool and urine changes, jaundice, and pruritus).
- The patient who undergoes a laparoscopic cholecystectomy is discharged soon after surgery, so teaching is essential. The patient should be instructed to remove bandages on the puncture sites the day after surgery and to bathe or shower.
- The patient should be instructed to report signs and symptoms of complications such as redness, swelling, or bile-colored drainage or pus from any incision; severe abdominal pain; nausea and vomiting; fever and chills.
- The patient can gradually resume normal activity and return to work within a week after surgery.

CHRONIC FATIGUE SYNDROME

Definition/Description

Chronic fatigue syndrome is a disorder characterized by debilitating fatigue and a variety of associated complaints, including fever, lymph node pain, headaches, sleep disturbance, and nonexudative pharyngitis. The case definition of chronic fatigue syndrome includes two criteria: (1) a new onset of severe and debilitating fatigue, which is present for at least 6 months, and (2) the absence of an identifiable etiology for the fatigue.

- Patients with chronic fatigue syndrome are twice as likely to be women as men and are generally ages 25 to 45 years. Prevalence of this syndrome is difficult to determine.

Pathophysiology

Despite numerous attempts to determine the etiology and pathology of chronic fatigue syndrome, the precise mechanisms remain unknown.

- A dysfunction may exist in the hypothalamus-pituitary-adrenal axis.
- Several viruses may precipitate the syndrome, including herpesviruses (e.g., Epstein-Barr virus, cytomegalovirus), and retroviruses since antibody titers to many infectious agents are elevated in patients with chronic fatigue syndrome.
- Immune alterations have been shown to occur with chronic fatigue syndrome, including decreased immunoglobulin production, altered natural killer cell activity, decreased lymphocyte proliferation, and increased CD4/CD8 ratio. These alterations do not occur in all patients and have not been shown to correlate with the severity of the disease.
- There may be a reduced production of corticotropin-releasing hormone in the hypothalamus. Serum cortisol levels are low, and adrenocorticotropic hormone (ACTH) levels are correspondingly high. These changes could cause decreased energy and altered mood states.
- Because mild to moderate depression occurs in about 70% of affected patients, it has been proposed that chronic fatigue syndrome is a psychiatric disorder. However, it is difficult to determine if depression is a cause or an effect of debilitating chronic fatigue.

Clinical Manifestations

Typical manifestations arise suddenly in a previously active, healthy individual. An unremarkable flulike illness or other acute stress is often identified as a triggering event.

- Unbearable fatigue is the problem that causes the patient to seek health care. Associated symptoms may fluctuate in intensity over time.
- The patient may become angry and frustrated with the inability of the physician to treat the problem. The disorder may have a major impact on work and family responsibilities. Some individuals may even need help with activities of daily living (ADLs).

Diagnostic Studies

Physical examination and diagnostic studies can be used to rule out other possible causes of the patient's symptoms. No laboratory test can diagnose chronic fatigue syndrome or measure its severity. In general, it remains a diagnosis of exclusion.

Therapeutic and Nursing Management

Because there is no definitive therapy for chronic fatigue syndrome, supportive management is essential. The patient should be informed about what is known about the disease, and all complaints should be taken seriously.

- Nonsteroidal antiinflammatory drugs (NSAIDs) can be used to treat headaches, muscle and joint aches, and fever. Antihistamines and decongestants can be used to treat allergic symptoms. Nonsedating antidepressants can improve mood and sleep disorders.
- Total rest is not advised because it can potentiate the self-image of being an invalid. On the other hand, strenuous exertion can exacerbate the exhaustion. Therefore it is important to plan a carefully graduated exercise program.
- Behavioral therapy may be used to promote a positive outlook as well as improve overall disability, fatigue, and other symptoms.

Chronic fatigue syndrome does not appear to progress. Although most patients recover or at least improve over time, they suffer from substantial occupational and psychosocial impairments and loss, including the social pressure and isolation from being characterized as lazy or crazy.

CHRONIC OBSTRUCTIVE PULMONARY DISEASE: EMPHYSEMA AND CHRONIC BRONCHITIS

Definition/Description

Chronic obstructive pulmonary disease (COPD) may be defined as a process characterized by the presence of chronic bronchitis and/or emphysema that may lead to the development of obstructed airways; the airway obstruction may be partially reversible and is often accompanied by airway hyperreactivity.

Etiology

Chronic lung irritation is the primary etiologic mechanism in COPD. There are three major irritants: cigarette smoking, infection, and inhaled irritants. Development of COPD is extremely variable and depends on inherent host susceptibility and the nature and severity of exposure to the irritant.

Cigarette smoking is the most common cause of COPD in the United States. Cigarette smoke has several direct effects on the respiratory tract.

- The irritating effect of smoke causes hyperplasia of cells, which subsequently results in increased production of mucus. Hyperplasia reduces airway diameter and increases the difficulty in clearing secretions. Smoking also reduces ciliary activity and produces abnormal dilatation of the distal air space with destruction of alveolar walls.
- Cigarette smoke may cause an imbalance between proteolytic enzymes that digest lung connective tissue and protease inhibitors, one of which is alpha$_1$-antitrypsin (AAT).
- Recurring respiratory tract infections are a major contributing factor to COPD. Recurring infections impair normal defense mechanisms, making the bronchioles and alveoli more susceptible to injury. The most common causative organisms are *Haemophilus influenzae, Streptococcus pneumoniae,* and *Moraxella catarrhalis.* Retained secretions provide a good medium for their proliferation.
- Incidence of COPD is higher in urban than in rural areas because of inhaled irritants. This difference may be partially explained by air pollution and occupational irritants (e.g., coal dust, potash) to which persons are exposed. Inhaled irritants cause a nonspecific inflammatory response.

A form of heredity primary emphysema is related to a deficiency of AAT that normally has an inhibitory effect on proteolytic enzymes. The level of AAT is controlled by a pair of autosomal codominant genes. Emphysema results when lysis of lung tissues by proteolytic enzymes from neutrophils and macrophages occurs because of AAT deficiency. Smoking greatly exacerbates the disease process in these patients.

Some degree of emphysema is common in the lungs of the older nonsmoker person as a result of aging, which results in changes in the lung structure, thoracic cage, and respiratory muscles. Clinically significant emphysema is usually not caused by aging alone.

Pathophysiology

It is common clinically to find a combination of emphysema and chronic bronchitis in the same person, often with one condition predominating.

Emphysema is a lung condition characterized by abnormal permanent enlargement of air spaces distal to the terminal bronchioles, accompanied by destruction of their walls and without obvious fibrosis. Structural changes include (1) hyperinflation of alveoli; (2) destruction of alveolar walls; (3) destruction of alveolar capillary walls; (4) narrowed, tortuous, small airways; and (5) loss of lung elasticity.

Chronic bronchitis is excessive production of mucus in the bronchi, accompanied by a recurrent cough that persists for at least 3 months of the year during at least 2 successive years.

- Pathologic changes in the lung consist of (1) hyperplasia of mucus-secreting glands in trachea and bronchi, (2) increase in goblet cells, (3) disappearance of cilia, (4) chronic inflammatory changes and narrowing of small airways, and (5) altered function of alveolar macrophages, leading to increased bronchial infections.
- Frequently the airways are colonized with organisms; infections can occur when organisms increase. Eventually scarring of bronchial walls may occur.
- In contrast to emphysema, with chronic bronchitis the alveolar structure and capillaries are normal.

Clinical Manifestations
Manifestations of COPD vary from those of pure emphysema to those of pure chronic bronchitis. Most patients with COPD have features of both (Table 19).

- An early symptom of *emphysema* is dyspnea, which becomes progressively more severe. The person is characteristically thin and underweight; the exact cause for this is not well understood.
- Later in the course of emphysema, secondary chronic bronchitis may develop. In advanced stages finger clubbing may be present in patients with emphysema and chronic bronchitis.
- Earliest symptom in *chronic bronchitis* is usually a frequent productive cough during most winter months. Frequent respiratory infections are another common manifestation. Somewhat later, dyspnea on exertion may develop.
- Bluish-red color of skin with chronic bronchitis results from polycythemia and cyanosis. Polycythemia develops as a result of the increased production of red blood cells (RBCs) secondary to the body's attempt to compensate for chronic hypoxemia.
- A person with chronic bronchitis is usually of normal weight or heavyset, with robust appearance. Emphysema of the centrolobular type frequently develops.

Complications
Cor pulmonale is hypertrophy of the right side of the heart, with or without heart failure, resulting from pulmonary hypertension. In COPD pulmonary hypertension is caused primarily by constriction

Table 19 Comparison of Emphysema and Chronic Bronchitis

	Emphysema	Chronic bronchitis
Clinical Features		
Age	30-40 yr (onset)	20-30 yr (onset)
	60-70 yr (disabling)	40-50 yr (disabling)
Body build	Thin	Tendency toward obesity
Health history	Generally healthy, insidious dyspnea, smoking	Recurrent respiratory tract infections, smoking
Weight loss	Often marked	Absent or slight
Dyspnea	Slowly progressive, eventually disabling	Variable, relatively late
Sputum	Scanty, mucoid	Copious, mucopurulent
Cough	Negligible	Considerable
Chest examination	Marked increase in anteroposterior diameter, quiet or diminished breath sounds, limited diaphragmatic excursion	Slight to marked increase in anteroposterior diameter, scattered crackles, rhonchi, wheezing
Cor pulmonale	Rare except terminally	Frequent with many episodes
Diagnostic Study Results		
Arterial blood gases (ABGs)	Mild $\downarrow$ PaO_2 normal or $\downarrow$ $PaCO_2$	$\downarrow$ PaO_2, $\uparrow$ $PaCO_2$
Chest x-ray	Hyperinflation, flat diaphragm, attenuated peripheral vessels, small or normal heart, widened intercostal margins	Cardiac enlargement, normal or flattened diaphragm, evidence of chronic inflammation, congested lung fields
Hematocrit and hemoglobin	Normal until late in disease	Increased

PaO_2, Partial pressure of oxygen in arterial blood; $PaCO_2$, partial pressure of carbon dioxide in arterial blood.

of pulmonary vessels in response to alveolar hypoxia, with acidosis further potentiating vasoconstriction. Overt manifestations of cor pulmonale may include jugular venous distention, hepatomegaly with right upper quadrant tenderness, ascites, epigastric distress, peripheral edema, and weight gain.

- Therapeutic management of cor pulmonale is administration of continuous low-flow O_2. Long-term O_2 therapy can reverse the progression of pulmonary hypertension in COPD. Although the use of digitalis is not indicated for cor pulmonale, it is used when congestive heart failure (CHF) is present. Dietary salt restriction is sometimes recommended, especially if overt CHF is present. Although diuretics are generally used, they are prescribed with caution because of their tendency to deplete potassium and chloride and reduce intravascular volume and cardiac output (CO).

The most common event leading to *acute respiratory failure* in COPD is acute respiratory tract infection (usually viral) or acute bronchitis.

The incidence of *peptic ulcer disease* is increased with COPD. The reason for this occurrence is not known; it may be related to the side effects of long-term use of a bronchodilator or steroid drugs or the stressful nature of the disease. It is important to test gastric aspirates and feces for occult blood (see Peptic Ulcer Disease, p. 453).

Gastroesophageal reflux, which may or may not be associated with hiatal hernia, occurs frequently with COPD and may aggravate respiratory symptoms. Reflux and accompanying heartburn may be aggravated by theophylline or β-adrenergic drugs. As a result of esophageal irritation or aspiration into the tracheobronchial tree, reflux airway constriction and obstruction may occur (see Hiatal Hernia, p. 302, and Gastroesophageal Reflux Disease, p. 244).

Pneumonia is a frequent complication of COPD, with the most common causative agents being *S. pneumoniae, H. influenzae,* and viruses. The most common manifestation is purulent sputum; systemic manifestations such as fever, chills, and leukocytosis may not be present (see Pneumonia, p. 468).

Diagnostic Studies
See diagnostic study results in Table 19, which presents a comparison of emphysema and chronic bronchitis.

Therapeutic Management
The primary goals of therapeutic management are to (1) improve ventilation, (2) promote secretion removal, (3) prevent complications and progression of symptoms, and (4) promote patient comfort and participation in care.

- Cessation of cigarette smoking in the early stages is probably the most significant factor in slowing the progression of disease. The health care provider has a responsibility to inform each smoking patient about the effects of smoking, offer suggestions and guidelines on how to quit, and refer the patient to a smoking-cessation program. The use of nicotine gum, nicotine transdermal patches, or clonidine patches may be helpful in minimizing the effects of nicotine withdrawl. These adjunctive therapies should be combined with other modalities such as support groups, educational materials, and behavior modification programs.
- Bronchodilator drug therapy is often helpful in relieving symptoms. Although patients with COPD do not respond as dramatically as those with asthma to bronchodilator therapy, a reduction in dyspnea and an increase in forced expiratory volume in 1 second (FEV_1) are usually achieved.
- Mucolytic expectorants (e.g., guaifenesin and iodinated glycerol) may be effective as adjuvant therapy in treating mucus-complicated COPD. These agents stimulate bronchial glands to secrete more fluid. Initial use may result in increased coughing, sputum production, and shortness of breath as mucus is moved from airways.
- Home O_2 therapy is the only intervention in the patient with COPD that has been shown to increase life span. O_2 may be prescribed for continuous use, only at night, or with exercise. Long-term administration of O_2 is probably the most effective therapy for prevention and treatment of cor pulmonale (see Oxygen Therapy, p. 669).
- Respiratory care is a collaborative effort involving respiratory therapists and nurses. Respiratory care includes breathing retraining, effective cough techniques, chest physiotherapy, and aerosol-nebulization therapy. See Lewis/Collier/Heitkemper, *Medical-Surgical Nursing,* edition 4, pp. 712 to 715, for further information on respiratory care and chest physiology.

Nursing Management
Goals
The patient with COPD will have a return to baseline respiratory function, the ability to perform activities of daily living (ADLs), relief from dyspnea, no complications related to COPD, and the knowledge and ability to implement a long-term treatment regimen.

See the nursing care plan for the patient with chronic obstructive pulmonary disease in Lewis/Collier/Heitkemper, *Medical-Surgical Nursing,* edition 4, p. 720.

Nursing Diagnoses
- Ineffective airway clearance related to expiratory airflow obstruction, ineffective cough, and infection in airways

- Ineffective breathing pattern related to obstruction of airflow, respiratory muscle fatigue or failure, and anxiety
- Impaired gas exchange: hypercapnia related to alveolar hypoventilation
- Impaired gas exchange: hypoxemia related to alveolar hypoventilation
- Fluid volume excess related to fluid retention secondary to cor pulmonale or steroid use
- Dyspnea related to increased airway resistance (bronchospasm and retained secretions), psychologic stress provoking and worsening dyspnea (anxiety, depression, fear), and air trapping
- Sleep pattern disturbance related to anxiety, depression, and shortness of breath
- Altered nutrition: less than body requirements related to poor appetite, lowered energy level, shortness of breath, gastric distention, and sputum production
- Risk for infection related to decreased pulmonary function, possible steroid therapy, ineffective airway clearance, and lack of knowledge regarding signs and symptoms of infection and preventive measures

Nursing Interventions

Nurses need to participate actively in developing policies establishing smoke-free working environments for themselves and others, controlling smoking in public places, requiring self-extinguishing cigarettes to prevent fire deaths and injuries, prohibiting

Table 20	Components of a Teaching Plan for the Patient with Obstructive Pulmonary Disease

- Basic understanding of lung function and pathophysiology
- Basic understanding of drug, O_2, respiratory, and other therapies
- Knowledge of the signs and symptoms of respiratory infection, heart failure, and bronchospasm; what to do if these occur
- Knowledge of good nutrition
- Knowledge of the importance of exercise
- Knowledge of energy conservation techniques
- Demonstration of abdominal breathing and pursed-lip breathing
- Demonstration of peak flow monitoring and chest physiotherapy, including vibration, percussion, and postural drainage, when indicated
- Steps for healthy psychologic coping

advertising and tobacco promotions, and mandating health warning labels on cigarette packages.

- Early diagnosis and treatment of respiratory tract infections is another way to decrease COPD incidence. Avoiding exposure to large crowds in peak periods for influenza may be necessary, especially for the older adult and the person with a history of respiratory problems. Influenza and pneumococcal pneumonia vaccines are recommended for the patient with COPD.

The patient with COPD will require acute intervention for complications such as pneumonia, cor pulmonale, and acute respiratory failure. Once the crisis in these situations has been resolved, the nurse can assess the degree and severity of the underlying respiratory problem. The information obtained will help in planning nursing care.

Patient Teaching

The most important aspect in long-term care of the patient with COPD is education. Because each COPD patient has different learning expectations, motivations, and needs, teaching must be adapted individually. Therefore it is important to assess the patient's level of knowledge and motivation before beginning to teach or develop a teaching plan.

- Help the patient understand that it is possible to plan treatment aimed at preserving lung function and slowing the progression of the disease. Patient and family participation in the treatment plan is essential. Respiratory care, as well as other related approaches, needs to be ongoing.
- A sample teaching plan on the signs of respiratory infection may include when to notify the physician, increasing fluid intake, increasing nebulizer treatments (e.g., from twice a day to four times a day) with the physician's order, beginning taking prescribed antibiotics, monitoring symptoms, and notifying the physician regarding the effects of these interventions.
- Further components of a teaching plan are discussed in Table 20.

CIRRHOSIS

Definition/Description

Cirrhosis is a chronic progressive disease of the liver characterized by extensive degeneration and destruction of liver parenchymal cells. Excessive alcohol ingestion is the most common cause of cirrhosis. The four types of cirrhosis, in order of incidence, are as follows:

1. *Alcoholic cirrhosis* (previously Laennec's), also called portal or nutritional cirrhosis, is usually associated with alcohol abuse. The first change in the liver from excessive alcohol intake is an accumulation of fat in the liver cells. Uncomplicated fatty changes in the liver are potentially reversible, if the person stops drinking alcohol.
2. *Postnecrotic cirrhosis* is a complication of viral, toxic, or idiopathic (autoimmune) hepatitis. Broad bands of scar tissue form within the liver.
3. *Biliary cirrhosis* is associated with chronic biliary obstruction and infection. There is diffuse fibrosis of the liver with jaundice.
4. *Cardiac cirrhosis* results from long-standing severe right-sided heart failure in patients with cor pulmonale, constrictive pericarditis, and tricuspid insufficiency.

Pathophysiology

In cirrhosis, cell necrosis occurs, and the destroyed liver cells are replaced by scar tissue. Eventually irregular, disorganized regeneration, poor cellular nutrition, and hypoxia caused by inadequate blood flow and scar tissue result in decreased functioning of the liver.

Clinical Manifestations

The onset of cirrhosis is usually insidious. Occasionally there is an abrupt onset of manifestations.

- *Early symptoms* include anorexia, dyspepsia, flatulence, nausea and vomiting, and a change in bowel habits (diarrhea or constipation). Other early manifestations are fever, lassitude, slight weight loss, and enlargement of the liver and spleen.
- The patient may complain of abdominal pain described as a dull, heavy feeling in the right upper quadrant or epigastrium; pain may be due to swelling and stretching of the liver capsule, spasm of biliary ducts, or intermittent vascular spasm.
- *Later symptoms* may be severe and result from liver failure and portal hypertension. Jaundice, peripheral edema, and ascites develop gradually. Other late symptoms include skin lesions, hematologic disorders, endocrine disturbances, and peripheral neuropathies. In advanced stages the liver becomes small and nodular. See Fig. 41-4 in Lewis/Collier/Heitkemper, *Medical-Surgical Nursing,* edition 4, p. 1271, for a complete description of the systemic manifestations of cirrhosis.

Complications

Major complications are portal hypertension with resultant esophageal varices, peripheral edema and ascites, hepatic encephalopathy (coma), and hepatorenal syndrome.

Portal hypertension and *esophageal varices* result from structural liver changes with cirrhosis, leading to obstruction (and destruction) of portal and hepatic veins and sinusoids. Pathophysiologic changes resulting from portal hypertension include the development of collateral circulation in an attempt to reduce high portal pressure and also to reduce increased plasma volume and lymphatic flow.

- Common areas where collateral channels form are the lower esophagus (anastomosis of left gastric vein and azygos veins), anterior abdominal wall, parietal peritoneum, and rectum.
- Varicosities may develop in areas where collateral and systemic circulations communicate, resulting in esophageal and gastric varices, caput medusae (ring of varices around the umbilicus), and hemorrhoids.

Esophageal varices are a common complication, occurring in anywhere from two thirds to three fourths of all patients with cirrhosis. These collateral vessels contain little elastic tissue and are quite fragile. They tolerate high pressure poorly, and the result is distended, tortuous veins that bleed easily.

- Bleeding esophageal varices are the most life-threatening complication of cirrhosis.
- Varices rupture and bleed in response to ulceration and irritation. Factors producing ulceration and irritation include alcohol ingestion; swallowing of poorly masticated food; ingestion of coarse food; acid regurgitation from the stomach; and increased intraabdominal pressure caused by nausea, vomiting, straining at stool, coughing, sneezing, or lifting heavy objects.
- Patient may have melena or hematemesis. There may be slow oozing or massive hemorrhage, which is a medical emergency.

Peripheral edema results from decreased colloidal osmotic pressure from impaired liver synthesis of albumin and increased portocaval pressure from portal hypertension. Peripheral edema occurs as ankle and presacral edema.

Ascites is an accumulation of serous fluid in the peritoneal or abdominal cavity. When BP is elevated in the liver, as occurs in portal cirrhosis, proteins move from the blood vessels via larger pores of the sinusoids (capillaries) into the lymph space. When the lymphatic system is unable to carry off excess proteins and water, they leak through the liver capsule into the peritoneal cavity. A second mechanism of ascites formation is hypoalbuminemia resulting from inability of the liver to synthesize albumin. A third mechanism of ascites, hyperaldosteronism, results when aldosterone is not metabolized by damaged hepatocytes, which causes increased renal reabsorption of sodium.

- Ascites is manifested by abdominal distention with weight gain. If ascites is severe, the umbilicus may be everted. Abdominal striae with distended abdominal wall veins may also be present.
- The patient will have signs of dehydration (e.g., dry tongue and skin, sunken eyeballs, muscle weakness), with a decrease in urinary output.
- Hypokalemia is common and results from an excessive loss of potassium from the effects of aldosterone and the use of diuretic therapy to treat ascites.

Hepatic encephalopathy, or coma, is a frequent terminal complication in liver disease. *Encephalopathy* is a more descriptive term than coma. Hepatic encephalopathy can occur in any condition in which liver damage causes ammonia to enter the systemic circulation without liver detoxification.

- The main pathogenic agents appear to be nitrogenous ammonia and aromatic amino acids. When blood is shunted past the liver via collateral anastomoses or the liver is unable to convert ammonia to urea, large quantities of ammonia remain in the systemic circulation. Ammonia crosses the blood-brain barrier and produces neurologic toxic manifestations.
- A number of factors may precipitate hepatic encephalopathy because they increase the amount of circulating ammonia; these include GI hemorrhage, constipation, infection, hypokalemia, hypovolemia, dehydration, and metabolic alkalosis.

Hepatorenal syndrome is a serious complication of cirrhosis. It is characterized by functional renal failure with advancing azotemia, oliguria, and intractable ascites.

- There is no structural abnormality of the kidneys, and the exact cause of decreased renal function is unknown. It is thought to be related to a redistribution of blood flow from the kidneys to the peripheral and splanchnic circulation or hypovolemia secondary to ascites.
- In the patient with cirrhosis the syndrome frequently follows diuretic therapy, GI hemorrhage, or paracentesis. Hepatic encephalopathy is also associated with deterioration in renal function.
- Treatment measures, which are usually unsuccessful, include salt-poor albumin, salt and water restrictions, and diuretic therapy.

Diagnostic Studies

- Liver function studies demonstrate an elevation in alkaline phosphatase, aspartate aminotransferase (AST) (SGOT), alanine aminotransferase (ALT) (SGPT), and gamma-glutamyltransferase (GGT)
- Liver biopsy (percutaneous needle) and scan

- Esophagogastroduodenoscopy
- Angiography (percutaneous transhepatic portography)
- Prothrombin time is prolonged.
- Serum albumin is decreased.
- Complete blood count (CBC) and stool for occult blood

Therapeutic Management

Although there is no specific therapy for cirrhosis, certain measures can be taken to promote liver cell regeneration and prevent or treat complications.

- Rest is significant in reducing the metabolic demands of the liver and allowing for recovery of liver cells. At various times during the progress of cirrhosis, rest may need to take the form of complete bed rest.

Management of *ascites* is focused on sodium restriction (250 to 500 mg/day), diuretic therapy (spironolactone is effective), and fluid removal (paracentesis). Peritoneovenous shunt insertion will provide for continuous reinfusion of ascitic fluid into the venous system.

The main therapeutic goal related to *esophageal varices* is avoidance of bleeding and hemorrhage. The patient who has esophageal varices should avoid ingesting alcohol, aspirin, and irritating foods. Upper respiratory infections should be treated promptly, and coughing should be controlled.

- Management related to bleeding esophageal varices includes the use of vasopressin (VP) and nitroglycerin (NTG), β-blockers, balloon tamponade, sclerotherapy, ligation of varices, and shunt therapy.
- Supportive measures during acute variceal bleeding include administration of fresh frozen plasma and packed red blood cells (RBCs), vitamin K (Aquamephyton), and histamine (H_2) blockers such as cimetidine (Tagamet). Neomycin administration may be started to prevent the occurrence of hepatic encephalopathy from the breakdown of blood and the release of ammonia in the intestine.

The goal of management in *hepatic encephalopathy* is the reduction of ammonia formation. This consists mainly of protein restriction and reduction of ammonia formation in the intestines. Lactulose (Cephulac) discourages bacterial growth, traps ammonia in the gut, and expels ammonia from the colon. Constipation should be prevented with cathartics and enemas to decrease bacterial action.

- Treatment of hepatic encephalopathy also involves controlling GI hemorrhage and removing blood from the GI tract to decrease protein in the intestine. Electrolyte and acid-base imbalances and infections should also be treated.

Additional management. There is no specific drug therapy for cirrhosis. A number of medications may be used to treat the symptoms and complications of advanced liver disease. Specific nutritional management varies with the degree of liver damage and the danger of encephalopathy; generally, protein and sodium are restricted.

Nursing Management
Goals
The patient with cirrhosis will have relief from discomfort, will have minimal to no complications (ascites, esophageal varices, hepatic encephalopathy), and will return to as normal a lifestyle as possible.

See the nursing care plan for the patient with cirrhosis in Lewis/Collier/Heitkemper, *Medical-Surgical Nursing,* edition 4, p. 1281.

Nursing Diagnoses/Collaborative Problems
- Ineffective breathing pattern related to pressure on diaphragm and reduced lung volume secondary to ascites
- Body-image disturbance related to changes in appearance and body function
- Risk for infection related to leukopenia and increased susceptibility to environmental pathogens
- Ineffective management of therapeutic regimen related to lack of knowledge regarding importance of follow-up care, signs and symptoms of complications, proper diet, and alcohol restrictions
- Activity intolerance related to fatigue, anemia, ascites, dyspnea, treatment schedule, and cardiac deconditioning
- Altered nutrition: less than body requirements related to anorexia, impaired utilization and storage of nutrients, nausea, and loss of nutrients from vomiting
- Total self-care deficit related to weakness, fatigue, balance and gait disturbance, and dyspnea
- Sleep pattern disturbance related to frequent assessments and treatments, discomfort, and inability to assume usual sleep position because of orthopnea
- Potential complication: hemorrhage related to bleeding tendency secondary to altered clotting factors
- Potential complication: hepatic encephalopathy related to increased formation of ammonia and aromatic amino acids

Nursing Interventions
Prevention and early treatment of cirrhosis must focus on the primary etiology.
- Alcoholism must be treated; adequate nutrition, especially for the alcoholic and other individuals at risk for cirrhosis, is essential to promote liver regeneration.
- Hepatitis must be identified and treated early so that it does not progress to chronic hepatitis.

- Biliary disease must be treated so that stones do not cause obstruction and infection.
- Underlying cause (e.g., chronic lung disease) of right-sided heart failure must be treated so that the heart failure does not lead to cirrhosis.

The focus of acute nursing interventions is conserving the patient's strength. Rest enables the liver to restore itself. Complete bed rest may not always be necessary.

- Anorexia, nausea and vomiting, pressure from ascites, and poor eating habits all create problems in the maintenance of an adequate intake of nutrients. Nursing measures relating to nutrition for patients with hepatitis also apply here, including oral hygiene and between-meal nourishment.
- A semi-Fowler's or Fowler's position allows for maximal respiratory efficiency when dyspnea is a problem. Pillows can be used to support arms and chest and may increase patient comfort and ability to breathe.
- Accurate calculation and recordings of intake and output, daily weights, and measurements of extremities and abdominal girth help in the ongoing assessment of location and extent of edema. Meticulous skin care, turning, and positioning are essential because edematous tissue is subject to breakdown.
- When a paracentesis is done, the patient must void immediately before the procedure to prevent puncture of the bladder. After the procedure, monitor for hypovolemia and electrolyte imbalances, and check the dressing for bleeding and leakage.
- If the patient has *esophageal varices* in addition to cirrhosis, it is necessary to monitor for any signs of bleeding from varices, such as hematemesis and melena. If hematemesis occurs, the patient is assessed for hemorrhage and the physician is called.
- The focus of care with *hepatic encephalopathy* is sustaining life and assisting with measures to reduce the formation of ammonia. Factors that are known to precipitate coma should be controlled as much as possible.

Patient Teaching

The patient and family need to understand the importance of continuous health care and medical supervision. They should be taught the symptoms of complications and when to seek medical attention.

- Measures to achieve and maintain remission should be encouraged, including proper diet, rest, and avoidance of potentially hepatotoxic OTC drugs such as acetaminophen.
- Abstinence from alcohol is important and results in improvement in most patients.
- Information regarding community support programs, such as Alcoholics Anonymous, should be provided.

- Other health teaching should include instruction about adequate rest periods, how to detect early signs of complications, skin care, drug therapy precautions, observation for bleeding, and protection from infection.
- Counseling information regarding sexual problems may be needed.
- Referral to a community or home health nurse may be helpful to ensure adequate patient compliance with prescribed therapy.

C

COLORECTAL CANCER

Definition/Description

Colorectal cancer is the second most common cause of cancer death in the United States. Cancer of the colon and rectum may occur at any age but is most prevalent over age 50. The 5-year survival rate for early localized cancers is 92% for colon cancer and 85% for rectal cancer, whereas a survival rate of 51% to 61% exists for cancer that has spread to adjacent organs and lymph nodes.

Pathophysiology

The causes of colorectal cancer remain unclear; however, groups at high risk of colorectal cancer have been identified.

- Age is a risk factor in both men and women. Risk for development in the general population increases slightly after age 40 and then rises rapidly in the following decades.
- The high-caloric, high-fat Western diet is the most important environmental factor that has been closely associated with the development of colon cancer.
- Adenocarcinoma is the most common type of colon cancer. Most colorectal cancers appear to arise from adenomatous polyps, which then tend to spread through the walls of the intestine and into the lymphatic system. Tumors commonly spread to the liver because venous blood flow is through the portal vein.

Clinical Manifestations

Manifestations are usually nonspecific or do not appear until the disease is advanced.

- Rectal bleeding, the most common symptom of colorectal cancer, is most often seen. Other common manifestations include alternating constipation and diarrhea, change in stool caliber (narrow, ribbonlike), and sensation of incomplete evacuation.

- Cancers of the colon may also be asymptomatic. Vague abdominal discomfort or crampy, colicky abdominal pain may be present. Iron-deficiency anemia and occult bleeding dictate further investigation. Weakness and fatigue result from anemia.

Diagnostic Studies

- Barium enema (air contrast) and sigmoidoscopy
- Colonoscopy is the procedure of choice if a questionable lesion is found on sigmoidoscopy and barium enema.
- Liver function studies to determine liver metastases
- Complete blood count (CBC) and stool testing for occult blood
- Digital rectal examination
- Carcinoembryonic antigen (CEA) level to follow progress of patient after surgery
- CT scan of abdomen
- Endorectal ultrasonography

Therapeutic Management

Prognosis and treatment correlate with the pathologic staging of disease. Several methods of staging are currently being used. The most widely known is Dukes' classification. Surgical removal of the primary lesion is the treatment for Dukes' stages A, B, and C. Prognosis for Dukes' stage A (negative nodes, lesion limited to mucosa) is 90% to 100% 5-year survival, compared with <15% with Dukes' stage D (distant, unresectable metastases). The most recent classification of colorectal cancer is the TNM system (see Table 12, p. 71).

Several noninvasive procedures may be performed through a colonoscope to treat certain types of colorectal cancer effectively.

- Endoscopic polypectomy is a highly effective and safe procedure. Adequate treatment is thought to be obtained if the resected margin of the polyp is free of cancer, the cancer is well differentiated, and there is no apparent lymphatic or blood vessel involvement.
- Laser therapy may be used to ablate nonresectable tumors. This method is usually used only as palliative therapy in patients with obstructive symptoms.

Surgical interventions. Surgery is the only curative treatment for colorectal cancer. The type of surgery performed is determined by the location and extent of cancer. The success of surgery depends on resection of tumor with an adequate margin of healthy bowel and resection of regional lymph nodes.

- *Right hemicolectomy* is performed when the cancer is located in the cecum, ascending colon, hepatic flexure, or transverse colon to the right of the middle colic artery. *Left hemicolectomy* involves resection of the left transverse colon, splenic flexure, descending colon, sigmoid colon, and upper portion of rectum.

- *Abdominal-perineal resection* is most often performed when the cancer is located within 5 cm of the anus. Complications that can occur are delayed wound healing, hemorrhage, persistent perineal sinus tracts, infections, and urinary tract and sexual dysfunction.
- Low anterior resection may be indicated for tumors of the rectosigmoid and middle to upper rectum.
- Sphincter-sparing procedures are being performed on the patient who is a poor operative risk and for the patient with early disease. In these procedures a local resection is performed and anal sphincters are left intact.

Radiation therapy and chemotherapy. Radiation may be used preoperatively or as a palliative measure for patients with advanced lesions. As a palliative measure, its primary objective is to reduce tumor size and provide symptomatic relief (see Radiation Therapy, p. 675). Chemotherapy is recommended when the patient has positive lymph nodes at the time of surgery or has metastatic disease. No drug is available that can cure malignant colon or rectal tumors. The most commonly used drugs are 5-fluorouracil (5-FU) and methotrexate. Nitrosoureas, carmustine (BCNU), levamisole, and semustine (MeCCNU) are sometimes used in combination with 5-FU (see Chemotherapy, p. 631).

Nursing Management
Goals
The patient with cancer of the colon or rectum will have no metastasis or recurrence of cancer and will have normal bowel elimination patterns, quality of life appropriate to disease progression, relief of pain, and feelings of comfort and well-being.

Nursing Diagnoses
- Diarrhea or constipation related to altered bowel elimination patterns
- Abdominal pain related to difficulty in passing stools due to partial or complete obstruction from tumor
- Fear related to diagnosis of colon cancer, surgical or therapeutic interventions, and possible terminal illness
- Ineffective individual coping related to diagnosis of cancer and side effects of treatment

Nursing Interventions
Screening recommendations from the American Cancer Society for colorectal cancer in patients who are not at high risk include annual digital rectal examination and fecal testing for occult blood beginning at age 40. Starting at age 50, flexible sigmoidoscopy should be done every 3 to 5 years, after two negative examinations done 1 year apart. Positive findings should be followed with colonoscopy or air-contrast barium enema.

- For high-risk patients screening usually begins with colonoscopy and fecal occult blood testing, and continued follow-up varies according to risk factors.

Preoperative care. Acute nursing care for patients with colon resections is similar to care of the patient having a laparotomy (see Acute Abdominal Pain, nursing management after laparotomy, p. 3). The patient should be taught side-to-side positioning and made to understand that short walks are better than sitting. The nurse should teach and assist the patient in proper positioning for taking a sitz bath.

- The patient should be told that phantom rectal sensation may be experienced because sympathetic nerves responsible for rectal control are not severed during surgery. The nurse must be astute in distinguishing phantom sensations from perineal abscess pain.

Postoperative care. After an abdominal-perineal resection there are two wounds, and a stoma has been surgically constructed in the left lower quadrant.

- Management of the perineal incision differs depending on the type of wound. Three techniques are used: (1) packing of the entire open wound, (2) partial closure with Penrose drains for open drainage, and (3) primary closure of the perineal wound with closed-suction drainage of pelvic cavity.
- A patient who has open and packed wounds requires meticulous postoperative care. During the immediate postoperative period the perineal dressing is reinforced and changed frequently because drainage can be profuse for several hours after surgery. All drainage is carefully assessed for amount, color, and consistency; drainage is usually serosanguineous.
- The nurse should examine the wound regularly and record bleeding, excessive drainage, and unusual odor. The nurse should also observe for signs of edema, erythema, drainage around the suture line, fever, and elevated white blood cell (WBC) count.
- The patient may complain of pain and itching in and around the wound. Antipruritic agents and sitz baths are usually ordered. Use of a pressure-reducing chair cushion provides comfort when sitting. Sitting on a toilet for prolonged periods is discouraged until the perineal wound is well healed.
- The perineal wound may not be completely healed before discharge. After discharge the patient is usually seen by the physician, home health nurse, and enterostomal therapist in an outpatient clinic. The wound is usually irrigated and debrided; if necessary, the infected area may be cauterized with silver nitrate. The nurse should report drainage because it may also indicate the presence of a foreign body, fistula, osteomyelitis, or

rectal tissue not removed during surgery. The patient and significant others are taught management of the wound and the procedure to take a sitz bath at home.

- Sexual dysfunction is a possible complication of an abdominal-perineal resection and should be included in the plan of care. The enterostomal therapy nurse can often provide correct and factual information concerning sexual dysfunction.
- Psychologic support for the patient and for family is important. The recovery period is long and the possibility of recurrence of cancer is always present.
- Patient and family should be aware of all community services available for assistance.

CONGESTIVE HEART FAILURE

Definition/Description
Congestive heart failure (CHF) is a cardiovascular condition in which the heart is unable to pump an adequate amount of blood to meet the metabolic needs of body tissues. CHF is not a disease; it is a syndrome caused by a variety of pathophysiologic processes including coronary artery disease (CAD), rheumatic heart disease, cor pulmonale, dysrhythmias, and anemia. CHF is characterized by left ventricular dysfunction, reduced exercise tolerance, diminished quality of life, and shortened life expectancy.

Risk factors for CHF include CAD, advancing age, hypertension, diabetes, cigarette smoking, obesity, and high cholesterol levels.
- Hypertension is a major contributing factor, increasing the risk of CHF approximately threefold. The risk of CHF increases progressively with the severity of hypertension, with systolic and diastolic values equally predicting the risk.
- Diabetes mellitus predisposes an individual to CHF regardless of the presence of concomitant CAD or hypertension. Diabetes is more likely to predispose a woman than a man to CHF.

Pathophysiology
CHF may be caused by any interference with the normal mechanisms regulating cardiac output (CO). CO depends on (1) preload, (2) afterload, (3) myocardial contractility, (4) heart rate (HR), and (5) metabolic state of the individual. Any alteration in these factors can lead to decreased ventricular function and subsequent CHF.
- Major causes of CHF may be divided into two subgroups: (1) underlying cardiac diseases such as CAD and cardiomyopathy and (2) precipitating factors such as anemia, infection, and nu-

tritional deficiencies. (See complete listing of causes in Tables 32-1 and 32-2, Lewis/Collier/Heitkemper, *Medical-Surgical Nursing,* edition 4, pp. 933 and 934.)

▪ Precipitating factors are generally more amenable to treatment than are cardiac diseases. Prompt recognition and treatment of precipitating factors can often result in successful patient outcomes.

Heart failure can be described as (1) a defect in *systolic function* that results in impaired ventricular emptying or (2) a defect in *diastolic function* that causes an impairment in ventricular filling. Patients with heart failure comprise three distinct groups: (1) those with failure of systolic ejection, (2) those with abnormal resistance to diastolic filling, and (3) those with mixed systolic and diastolic dysfunction.

Systolic failure, the most common cause of CHF, is a defect in the ability of the cardiac myofibrils to shorten, thereby decreasing the ability of the muscles to contract (pump). Systolic failure is caused by impaired contractile function (e.g., myocardial infarction [MI]), increased afterload (e.g., hypertension), or mechanical abnormalities (e.g., valvular heart disease).

Diastolic failure is characterized by high filling pressures and resultant venous engorgement in both pulmonary and systemic systems. The diagnosis of diastolic failure is based on the presence of pulmonary congestion and pulmonary hypertension in the setting of normal ejection fraction. Diastolic failure is commonly seen in older adults as a result of myocardial fibrosis and hypertension.

Mixed systolic and diastolic failure is seen in disease states such as dilated cardiomyopathy (DCM), in which poor systolic function (weakened muscle function) is further compromised by dilated left ventricular walls that are unable to relax.

The patient with ventricular failure of any type has low systemic arterial BP, low CO, and poor renal perfusion. When pulmonary congestion and edema are present, the diagnosis of CHF may be made. Whether a patient arrives at this point acutely from an MI or chronically from worsening cardiomyopathy or hypertension, the body's response to this low CO is to mobilize compensatory mechanisms to maintain CO and BP. The main compensatory mechanisms include (1) ventricular dilatation, (2) ventricular hypertrophy, (3) increased sympathetic nervous system stimulation, and (4) hormonal response.

CHF is usually manifested by biventricular failure, although one ventricle may precede the other in dysfunction.

▪ The most common form of initial heart failure is left-sided. CHF occurs in a retrograde fashion, progressing from the left ventricle (LV) to the pulmonary system to the right ventricle (RV). LV failure will usually lead to and is the main cause of right-sided failure.

- Right-sided failure can occur without preceding LV failure as a result of right ventricular MI or cor pulmonale. CHF will eventually develop in the majority of persons with moderate to severe cardiac disease.

Acute Clinical Manifestations

Regardless of the etiology, acute heart failure typically presents as *pulmonary edema,* a term used to refer to an acute, life-threatening situation in which lung alveoli become filled with serous or serosanguineous fluid. The most common factor in the onset of pulmonary edema is LV failure due to CAD.

- Manifestations of *pulmonary edema* are unmistakable: the patient may be agitated, pale, and possibly cyanotic, with clammy and cold skin.
- The patient has severe dyspnea, as evidenced by obvious use of respiratory accessory muscles, respiratory rate >30 breaths per minute, and orthopnea. Wheezing and coughing with production of frothy, blood-tinged sputum may also occur.
- Auscultation of the lungs may reveal bubbling crackles, wheezes, and rhonchi. The patient's heart rate is rapid, and BP may be elevated or decreased, depending on the severity of edema.

Chronic Clinical Manifestations

Manifestations of chronic CHF depend on the patient's age, underlying type and extent of heart disease, and which ventricle is failing to pump effectively. Table 21 lists manifestations of LV and RV failure. The patient with chronic CHF will probably have manifestations of biventricular failure.

- Fatigue is one of the earliest symptoms of chronic CHF. The patient notices fatigue after activities that normally are not tiring.
- Dyspnea is a common sign of chronic CHF. The shortness of breath makes the patient conscious of air hunger that prompts rapid, shallow respirations. Dyspnea can occur with mild exertion or at rest (orthopnea).
- *Paroxysmal nocturnal dyspnea (PND)* occurs when the patient is asleep. The patient awakens in a panic, has feelings of suffocation, and has a strong desire to seek respiratory relief by sitting up.
- Other common signs include tachycardia; edema in the legs, liver, abdominal cavity, and lungs; nocturia; cool and dusky skin; restlessness and confusion; angina-type chest pain; and weight changes.

Table 21 Clinical Manifestations of Heart Failure

Right-sided heart failure	Left-sided heart failure
Signs	**Signs**
Right ventricle heaves	Left ventricle heaves
Murmurs	Cheyne-Stokes respirations
Peripheral edema	Pulsus alternans (alternating pulses: strong, weak)
Weight gain	Increased heart rate
Edema of dependent body parts (sacrum, anterior tibias, pedal edema)	PMI displaced inferiorly and posteriorly (left ventricular hypertrophy)
Ascites	$\downarrow PaO_2$, slight $\uparrow PaCO_2$ (poor oxygen exchange)
Anasarca (massive generalized body edema)	Crackles (pulmonary edema)
Jugular venous distention	S_3 and S_4 heart sounds
Hepatomegaly (liver engorgement)	
Right-sided pleural effusion	**Symptoms**
	Fatigue
Symptoms	Dyspnea (shallow respirations up to 32-40/min)
Fatigue	Orthopnea (paroxysmal nocturnal dyspnea)
Dependent edema	Dry, hacking cough
Right upper quadrant pain	Pulmonary edema
Anorexia and GI bloating	Nocturia
Nausea	

$PaCO_2$, Partial pressure of carbon dioxide in arterial blood; PaO_2, partial pressure of oxygen in arterial blood; PMI, point of maximal impulse.

Complications

Pleural effusion results from increasing pressure in the pleural capillaries. A transudation of fluid occurs from these capillaries into the pleural space. The pleural effusion usually develops in the right lower lobe initially.

Left ventricular thrombus may occur with acute or chronic CHF in which the enlarged LV and poor CO combine to increase the chance of thrombus formation in the LV. Many physicians will initially administer anticoagulants to decrease the possibility of thrombus formation in patients with chronic CHF.

Hepatomegaly may result from CHF as liver lobules become congested with venous blood. Hepatic congestion leads to impaired liver function; eventually liver cells die, fibrosis occurs, and cirrhosis can develop.

Diagnostic Studies

- Serum chemistries, renal profile, liver profile
- Chest x-ray examination to assess and monitor heart failure
- ECG to confirm cardiac changes. Exercise-stress testing and nuclear imaging studies provide additional information to ECG findings.
- Echocardiography measures ventricular and valvular function and size of cardiac chambers.
- Hemodynamic monitoring via a pulmonary artery catheter directly assesses cardiac function.
- Cardiac catheterization and angiocardiography help detect underlying heart disease.

Therapeutic and Nursing Management of Acute CHF and Pulmonary Edema

The goal of therapy is to improve left ventricular function by decreasing intravascular volume, decreasing venous return, improving gas exchange and oxygenation, increasing CO, and reducing anxiety. Major components of management include:

- Decreasing intravascular volume with the use of diuretics by reducing venous return to the failing LV. A loop diuretic (e.g., furosemide, bumetanide) is the drug of choice for decreasing volume, because it may be administered quickly by IV push and acts within the kidney rapidly.
- The use of IV nitroglycerin (NTG), which reduces circulating volume by decreasing preload. NTG also increases the coronary artery circulation by dilating coronary arteries.
- Decreasing venous return, which reduces the amount of volume returned to the LV during diastole. This can be accomplished by placing the patient in a high Fowler's position with feet horizontal in bed or dangling at the bedside.

- The use of IV nitroprusside (Nipride), which reduces preload and afterload. Because of its potent vasodilator effects, this is the drug of choice for the patient with pulmonary edema.
- Morphine also reduces preload and afterload. It dilates both the pulmonary and systemic blood vessels, thereby decreasing pulmonary pressures and improving gas exchange.
- Administration of O_2, which helps to increase the percentage of O_2 in inspired air (see Oxygen Therapy, p. 669). In severe pulmonary edema the patient may need to be intubated and placed on a mechanical ventilator.
- Improvement of LV function by the action of digitalis, which increases contractility but also increases myocardial O_2 consumption. Newer inotropic drugs (e.g., dobutamine and amrinone) increase myocardial contractility without increasing O_2 consumption.

Hemodynamic monitoring may become necessary if rapid resolution of symptoms does not occur with diuretics, morphine, and NTG or if the patient becomes hypotensive (see Hemodynamic Monitoring, p. 654).

Nursing care focuses on continual physical assessment, hemodynamic monitoring, and monitoring the patient's response to treatment.

Therapeutic Management of Chronic CHF

One of the most important goals in the treatment of chronic CHF is to treat the underlying cause. If dysrhythmias have precipitated the failure, they should be treated accordingly. If the underlying cause is hypertension, antihypertensives should be used in treatment. Valvular defects can be treated with surgery.

- If cardiac dysfunction is a result of ischemic heart disease, specific interventions such as thrombolytic therapy, percutaneous transluminal coronary angiography (PTCA), or coronary artery bypass graft surgery (see p. 642) may be warranted.

Additional management includes:

- Administration of O_2 to improve saturation and to assist in meeting tissue O_2 needs, thereby decreasing dyspnea and fatigue.
- Physical and emotional rest so the patient may conserve energy and decrease the need for additional O_2. A patient with severe CHF needs bed rest with limited activity. A patient with mild CHF can be ambulatory with a restriction of strenuous activity.

General objectives of *pharmacologic management* for CHF are (1) identification of the type of CHF and underlying causes, (2) correction of sodium and water retention and volume overload, (3) reduction of cardiac workload, (4) improvement of myocardial contractility, and (5) control of precipitating and complicating factors. Because CHF is a complex syndrome, it is unlikely that any single pharmacologic agent would be successful alone. A combination of drugs has been the most successful in treating patients with CHF.

- Historically, LV systolic failure has been managed with positive inotropic agents (e.g., digitalis) to increase myocardial contractility and diuretic therapy to enhance sodium and water excretion, thereby controlling volume. LV volume overload (increased preload and afterload) exerts a major role in the development of LV dysfunction and has led to the addition of vasodilators (e.g., angiotensin-converting enzyme [ACE] inhibitors) in the treatment plan.

Nutritional management. Diet education and weight management are critical to the control of chronic CHF.

- The patient should be taught what foods are low and high in sodium and ways to enhance food flavors without the use of salt (e.g., substituting lemon juice and various spices). A commonly prescribed diet for a patient with mild CHF is a 2 g sodium diet. (For sample menu plans for a 2 g sodium diet, see Table 32-10 in Lewis/Collier/Heitkemper, *Medical-Surgical Nursing,* edition 4, p. 944.) For more severe CHF, sodium intake is restricted to 500 to 1000 mg.
- Fluid restrictions are not commonly prescribed for mild to moderate CHF. Diuretic therapy and digitalis preparations are effective in promoting fluid excretion. However, in moderate to severe CHF, fluid restrictions are usually implemented.
- When weight reduction is indicated to decrease the cardiac workload, the nurse and dietitian can assist the patient and family in menu planning. Patients should be instructed to weigh themselves at the same time each day, preferably before breakfast, wearing the same type of clothing. This helps to identify early signs of fluid retention.

Nursing Management of Chronic CHF
Goals
The patient with CHF will have decreased peripheral edema, decreased shortness of breath, increased exercise tolerance, compliance with medications prescribed, and no complications related to CHF. (See the nursing care plan for the patient with congestive heart failure in Lewis/Collier/Heitkemper, *Medical-Surgical Nursing,* edition 4, p. 946.)
Nursing Diagnoses
- Fluid volume excess related to pump failure
- Activity intolerance related to fatigue secondary to cardiac insufficiency, pulmonary congestion, and inadequate nutrition
- Impaired gas exchange related to increased preload, mechanical failure, or immobility

- Sleep pattern disturbance related to nocturnal dyspnea, inability to assume favored sleep position, nocturia
- Anxiety related to dyspnea or perceived threat of death
- Risk for impaired skin integrity related to edema or immobility
- Ineffective management of therapeutic regimen related to lack of knowledge regarding signs and symptoms of CHF, proper diet, medications
- Ineffective individual coping related to alterations in lifestyle, possible inability to use past coping methods, or perceived loss of control

Nursing Interventions

An important measure used to prevent heart failure is the treatment or control of underlying heart disease. For example, in rheumatic valvular disease, valve replacement should be planned before lung congestion develops.

- Prophylactic antibiotics should be given to people with a known history of rheumatic heart disease when they undergo surgery or procedures involving instrumentation (e.g., cystoscopy, tooth extraction, and tooth cleaning).
- Early and continued treatment of hypertension is important. Hyperlipidemic states in persons with CAD should be managed with diet, exercise, and medication.
- The use of antidysrhythmic agents or pacemakers is indicated for people with serious dysrhythmias or conduction disturbances.
- When a patient is diagnosed with CHF, preventive care should focus on slowing the progression of the disease. Knowledge of the importance of following the medication, diet, and exercise regimen is paramount.

Many persons with CHF do not experience an acute episode. If they do, they are usually initially managed in a critical care unit and later transferred to a general unit when their condition has stabilized. Nursing management for the patient with CHF applies to the patient with stabilized acute or chronic CHF.

CHF is a chronic illness for most persons. Important nursing responsibilities are (1) educating the patient about physiologic changes that have occurred and (2) assisting the patient to adapt to both physiologic and psychologic changes. It must be emphasized to the patient that it is possible to live productively with this health problem.

- Home health care is a vital factor in preventing future hospitalization for this patient. Home nursing care will follow up with ongoing clinical assessments and monitoring of vital signs and response to therapies.
- It must be stressed that the disease is chronic and that medication must be continued to keep the heart failure under control.

The patient must understand the importance of maintaining adequate drug levels and the danger of omitting or making up missed doses.
- The patient should also be taught to recognize signs of digitalis toxicity, how to take his/her pulse rate, to recognize symptoms of hypokalemia, and to carry out energy-saving behaviors.
- Establish small achievable goals and possible lifestyle changes with the patient and family.

CONJUNCTIVITIS

Definition/Description

Conjunctival infections may be caused by bacterial, viral, or chlamydial microorganisms with inflammation resulting from exposure to allergens or chemical irritants (including cigarette smoke). The *tarsal conjunctiva* (lining of the lid interior surface) may become inflamed as a result of a chronic foreign body in the eye, such as a contact lens or an ocular prosthesis.

Acute bacterial conjunctivitis (pinkeye) is a common infection. Although it occurs in every age group, it is often seen epidemically in children because of poor hygiene. In adults and children the most common causative microorganism is *Staphylococcus aureus.*

Clinical Manifestations

- Bacterial conjunctivitis: irritation, tearing, redness, and mucopurulent drainage. Although this typically occurs initially in one eye, it spreads rapidly to the unaffected eye.
- Viral conjunctivitis: tearing, foreign body sensation, redness, and mild photophobia. Unless other ocular structures become involved, this condition is usually mild and self-limiting.
- Allergic conjunctivitis: itching, burning, redness, and tearing with white or clear exudate. Allergic conjunctivitis is caused by exposure to an allergen and can be mild, transitory, or severe enough to cause significant swelling, sometimes ballooning the conjunctiva beyond the eyelids.

Therapeutic Management

- Bacterial conjunctivitis is usually self-limiting, but treatment with antibiotic drops will shorten the course of the disorder. Careful handwashing and using individual or disposable towels will help prevent spreading the infection.
- Viral conjunctivitis treatment is usually palliative. If the patient is severely symptomatic, topical steroids provide temporary relief

but have no benefit in the final outcome. Antiviral drops are ineffective and are therefore not indicated.

- Allergic conjunctivitis treatment includes artificial tears to dilute the allergen and wash it from the eye. Effective topical medications include antihistamines, antiinflammatory medication, and steroids.

CONSTIPATION

Description/Definition

Constipation may be defined as a decrease in the frequency of bowel movements from what is "normal" for the individual characterized by hard, difficult-to-pass stool; a decrease in stool volume; and/or retention of feces in rectum.

- Frequently constipation may be due to insufficient dietary fiber, inadequate fluid intake, medication use, and lack of exercise. Constipation may also be the result of ignoring the urge to defecate, chronic laxative abuse, and multiple organic causes. Changes in diet, mealtime, or daily routines are a few environmental factors that may cause constipation. Depression and stress can also result in constipation.

Clinical Manifestations

Clinical presentation of constipation may vary from a chronic discomfort to an acute event mimicking an "acute abdomen." Other clinical manifestations are presented in Table 22.

- *Hemorrhoids* are the most common complication of chronic constipation. They result from venous engorgement caused by repeated Valsalva maneuver (straining) and venous compression from hard impacted stool.
- *Diverticulosis* is another potential complication of chronic constipation. (See Diverticulitis/Diverticulosis, p. 196).
- In the presence of *obstipation,* or fecal impaction caused by constipation, colonic perforation may occur. Perforation, which is life threatening, causes abdominal pain, nausea, vomiting, fever, and an elevated white blood cell (WBC) count.

Therapeutic Management

- Most cases of constipation can be managed with diet therapy that includes fluids and an exercise program. Laxatives should always be used cautiously because with chronic overuse they may become a cause of constipation. Enemas are fast acting and beneficial in the immediate treatment of constipation but should be lim-

Table 22	Clinical Manifestations of Constipation

Hard, dry stool	Increased flatulence
Abdominal distention	Nausea
Abdominal pain	Anorexia
Decreased frequency	Headache
of bowel movements	Palpable mass
Straining	Stool with blood
Rectal pressure	Dizziness
Tenesmus	Urinary retention

ited for long-term treatment. Soapsuds enemas should be avoided because they may lead to inflammation of colon mucosa. Oil-retention enemas may be used to soften fecal impactions.

- The patient with severe constipation related to a motility or mechanical disorder may require more intensive treatment. In a patient with unrelenting constipation, a subtotal colectomy with ileorectal anastomosis is the procedure of choice.

- Many patients experience an improvement in their symptoms when they simply increase their intake of dietary fiber and fluids. The diet should also include a fluid intake of at least 3000 ml per day, unless contraindicated by heart or renal disease. Increasing fiber intake without increasing fluids may predispose the patient to impaction or obstruction.

Nursing Management
Goals
The patient with constipation will increase dietary intake of fiber and fluids; have passage of soft, formed stools; and have no complications, such as bleeding hemorrhoids.

See the nursing care plan for the patient with constipation in Lewis/Collier/Heitkemper, *Medical-Surgical Nursing,* edition 4, p. 1216.

Nursing Diagnoses
- Constipation related to inadequate dietary intake of fiber, inadequate fluid intake, and decreased physical activity

Nursing Interventions
Interventions should be based on assessment and the symptoms of the patient.

- Proper position is important when defecating. For a patient in bed, the head of the bed should be elevated as high as the patient can tolerate. For the person who can sit on a toilet, a footstool may be placed in front of the toilet. Placing the feet on a footstool promotes flexion of the thighs, which assists in defecation.

- The patient with poor muscle tone should be encouraged to exercise the abdominal muscles and taught to contract these muscles several times a day. Sit-ups and straight-leg raises can also be used to improve abdominal muscle tone.
- Some patients may need to be encouraged to increase their social activities as well as their physical activity; this is especially true of older adults who may become depressed and socially isolated.

Patient Teaching

- An important role of the nurse is teaching the patient the importance of dietary measures to prevent constipation. Emphasis should be placed on the maintenance of a high-fiber diet, increasing fluid intake, and a regular exercise program.
- The patient should be taught to establish a regular time to defecate and not to suppress the urge to defecate. In many persons the urge to defecate occurs after breakfast because of stimulation of the gastrocolic reflex. The patient should be discouraged from using laxatives and enemas to achieve fecal elimination.

CORNEAL DISORDERS

Definition/Description

Corneal disorders include problems that interfere with normal cornea tissue transparency resulting in diminished visual acuity.

Pathophysiology

Types of corneal disorders include keratitis and keratoconus.

Keratitis is an inflammation or infection of the cornea that can be caused by a variety of microorganisms or by other factors. This condition may involve both conjunctiva and cornea. The cornea, once infected, can develop an ulcer with a mucopurulent exudate.

- Risk factors for keratitis include soft contact lens wear (particularly with extended wear), debilitation, nutritional deficiencies, immunosuppressed states, and contaminated products (e.g., lens care solutions and cases, topical medications, and cosmetics).
- Keratitis, caused by herpes simplex virus (HSV), is the most frequently occurring infectious cause of corneal blindness in the Western hemisphere.

Keratoconus is a familial bilateral degenerative disease that can be associated with Down syndrome, atopic dermatitis, and Marfan syndrome. The anterior cornea thins and protrudes forward, a process that generally starts during adolescence. A corneal ulcer and the resulting opacity may also occur as a result of complications from ulcerative keratitis, ocular trauma, chemical injuries, or keratorefractive surgery. Opacities may also be congenital.

Clinical Manifestations

- Possible signs of keratitis include eye pain, photophobia, impaired vision, and eye exudate.
- Possible signs of keratoconus include blurred vision with variable astigmatism.

Therapeutic Management

Keratitis therapy may consist of topical antibiotics or, in severe cases, IV antibiotics. Management of HSV keratitis consists of corneal debridement followed by topical therapy. The astigmatism of keratoconus is managed with eyeglasses or rigid contact lens.

Penetrating keratoplasty (corneal transplant) may be indicated to restore vision that otherwise would be lost from scars or opacities. A rigid contact lens may correct irregular astigmatism that results from the corneal scar.

Nursing Management

Goals

The patient with a corneal disorder will maintain or improve visual acuity, maintain an acceptable level of comfort and functioning during the course of the specific ocular problem, avoid spread of infection, and comply with prescribed therapy.

Nursing Diagnoses

- Pain related to irritation or infection of external eye
- Anxiety related to uncertainty of cause of disease and outcome of treatment
- Sensory-perceptual alteration: visual related to diminished or absent vision

Nursing Interventions

- Assess hygiene techniques.
- For acute disorders (as appropriate), use warm or cool compresses, darken the room, offer analgesics, and modify activities for safety.
- If different eye drops are required, stagger their administration to promote maximum absorption.
- For compromised vision, suggest alternative ways to accomplish self-care activites.

Patient Teaching

- Emphasis is on good hygiene practices and information about ocular infection sources among the patient and family to avoid spreading infectious corneal disorders.

- Specific information about the mode of transmission should be provided for HSV keratitis if the patient has this type of infective eye disorder.
- Appropriate use and care of lenses and lens care products should be addressed.
- Giving information to the patient and family regarding medication administration and possible side effects is also recommended.

CORONARY ARTERY DISEASE

Definition/Description

Coronary artery disease (CAD) is a type of blood vessel disorder included in the general category of atherosclerosis. *Atherosclerosis* is derived from two Greek words: *athere,* meaning "fatty mush," and *skleros,* meaning "hard." Atherosclerosis is often referred to as "hardening of the arteries." Although this condition can occur in any artery in the body, the atheromas (fatty deposits) have a preference for coronary arteries.

- Arteriosclerotic heart disease (ASHD), cardiovascular heart disease (CVHD), ischemic heart disease (IHD), coronary heart disease (CHD), and CAD are used synonymously to describe this disease process.
- Cardiovascular diseases are the major cause of death in the United States. Myocardial infarctions (MIs) are the leading cause of all cardiovascular disease deaths and deaths in general.

Pathophysiology

Atherosclerosis is the major cause of CAD. It is characterized by a focal deposit of cholesterol and lipids, primarily within the intimal wall of the artery. The genesis of plaque formation is the result of complex interactions between components of the blood and elements forming the vascular wall. Table 31-1 in Lewis/Collier/Heitkemper, *Medical-Surgical Nursing,* edition 4, p. 886, summarizes the theories of atherogenesis, with endothelial injury considered to be the chief cause of atherosclerotic disease.

- The endothelial lining can be altered as a result of chemical injuries, such as hyperlipidemia (nondenuding), or high-shear stress, such as hypertension (denuding). With either type of endothelial alteration, platelets are activated and release a growth factor that stimulates smooth muscle proliferation. Smooth muscle cell proliferation entraps lipids, which are calcified throughout time and form an endothelium irritant on which platelets adhere and aggregate.

CAD takes many years to develop. When it becomes symptomatic, the disease process is usually well advanced. Stages of development in atherosclerosis are fatty streak, raised fibrous plaque resulting from smooth muscle cell proliferation, and complicated lesion.

Risk factors have been associated with atherosclerosis; the three most significant ones are elevated serum lipids, hypertension, and cigarette smoking. Risk factors in different populations may vary in prominence. For example, diabetes mellitus has been found to be a major risk factor in European populations but only a minor one in U.S. populations. Major risk factors in the United States, such as high serum cholesterol and hypertension, are less prevalent in Japanese, Puerto Rican, and Hawaiian populations.

Risk factors can be categorized as unmodifiable and modifiable (Table 23). *Unmodifiable* risk factors are age, gender, race, and genetic inheritance. *Modifiable* risk factors include elevated serum lipids, hypertension, smoking, obesity, sedentary lifestyle, and stress in daily living. Although control of diabetes is recommended, it has not been proved to decrease the incidence of CAD.

Clinical Manifestations

The three major clinical manifestations of CAD include angina pectoris (see Angina Pectoris, p. 41), acute myocardial infarction (MI) (see Myocardial Infarction, p. 397), and sudden cardiac death.

Table 23	Risk Factors in Coronary Artery Disease
Unmodifiable	**Modifiable**
Age	Major
Gender (men > women until 60 yr of age)	Elevated serum lipids
	Hypertension
Race (African-Americans < Caucasians)	Cigarette smoking
	Physical inactivity
Genetic predisposition and family history of heart disease	Minor
	Obesity (>30% overweight)
	Diabetes mellitus*
	Stressful lifestyle

*May be hereditary.

Therapeutic Management

Treatment usually begins with diet restriction, decreased dietary fat content, lower cholesterol intake, and exercise instruction. Serum cholesterol levels are redrawn after 6 months of diet therapy. If they remain elevated, drug therapy may be started.

Pharmacologic Management

Two bile acid-sequestering agents, cholestyramine (Questran) and colestipol (Colestid), are currently available. These resins primarily lower low-density lipoprotein (LDL) cholesterol and also cause an increase in high-density lipoprotein (HDL).

Nicotinic acid (niacin, a B vitamin) is highly effective in lowering cholesterol and triglyceride levels by interfering with their synthesis. Clofibrate (Atromid) is effective primarily in lowering serum triglyceride levels and has some cholesterol-lowering activity as well. It appears to act by decreasing synthesis of lipids. Gemfibrozil (Lopid) is primarily effective in lowering very low density lipoprotein (VLDL) levels and triglycerides, and it also increases high-density lipoprotein (HDL) cholesterol. Lovastatin (Mevacor) is a competitive inhibitor of the biosynthesis of cholesterol.

- Drug therapy for hyperlipidemia is likely to be prolonged, perhaps continuing for a lifetime. It is essential that diet modification be used to minimize the need for drug therapy. The patient must fully understand the rationale and goals of treatment and medication side effects.

Nursing Management

In both the acute care setting and in the community, the nurse needs to identify persons at high risk for CAD. Screening involves obtaining personal and family histories. Environmental factors, such as eating habits, type of diet, and level of exercise, are assessed to elicit lifestyle patterns. A psychosocial history is included to determine smoking habits, alcohol ingestion, life stresses, sleeping habits, and presence of anxiety or depression.

- The nurse needs to identify patient attitudes and beliefs about health and illness. This information can give some indication of how disease and lifestyle changes may affect the patient and can reveal possible misconceptions about heart disease.
- Knowledge of the patient's educational background is frequently helpful in deciding at what level to begin teaching.
- Once a high-risk person is identified, preventive measures can be taken. Risk factors such as age, gender, and genetic inheritance cannot be modified. However, the person with any of the modifiable risk factors can reduce risk by changing the additive effects of these risk factors.
- The person who has modifiable risk factors needs to be encouraged and motivated to make lifestyle changes to reduce the

risk of heart disease. For the highly motivated person, knowing how to reduce this risk may be the only information needed to prompt that person to make changes.

CROHN'S DISEASE

Definition/Description

Crohn's disease is a chronic nonspecific inflammatory bowel disorder of unknown origin that can affect any part of the GI tract. Crohn's disease may occur at any age, but it appears most often between the ages of 15 and 30 years. Similar to ulcerative colitis, it occurs more often in Jewish and upper-middle-class urban populations.

- Crohn's disease is a chronic disorder with unpredictable periods of recurrence and remission. Attacks are intermittent, usually recurring over a period of several weeks to months, with diarrhea and abdominal pain subsiding spontaneously.

Crohn's disease and ulcerative colitis are compared in Table 24.

Pathophysiology

Crohn's disease is characterized by inflammation of segments of the GI tract. It can affect any part of the GI tract but is most often seen in the terminal ileum, jejunum, and colon. Involvement of the esophagus, stomach, and duodenum is rare. The inflammation involves all layers of the bowel wall (i.e., transmural).

- Areas of involvement are usually discontinuous, with segments of normal bowel occurring between diseased portions. Typically ulcerations are deep and longitudinal and penetrate between islands of inflamed edematous mucosa, causing the classic cobblestone appearance.
- Thickening of the bowel wall occurs, as well as narrowing of the lumen with stricture development. Abscesses or fistula tracts that communicate with other loops of bowel, skin, bladder, rectum, or vagina may also develop.

Clinical Manifestations

Manifestations depend largely on the anatomic site of involvement, the extent of disease process, and the presence or absence of complications. Onset of Crohn's disease is usually insidious, with nonspecific complaints such as nonbloody diarrhea, fatigue, abdominal pain, weight loss, and fever. Pain may be severe and intermittent or constant, depending on the cause.

- Extraintestinal manifestations, such as arthritis and finger clubbing, may precede the onset of bowel disease.

Table 24   Comparison of Ulcerative Colitis and Crohn's Disease

Characteristic	Ulcerative colitis	Crohn's disease
Age	Young to middle age	Young
Location	Starts distally and spreads in continuous pattern up colon	Occurs anywhere along GI tract in characteristic skip lesions; most frequent site is terminal ileum
Distribution	Continuous	Segmental
Depth of involvement	Mucosa and submucosa	Entire thickness of bowel wall (transmural)
Small-bowel involvement	Minimal	Common
Fistulas	Rare	Common
Strictures	Rare	Common
Anal abscesses	Rare	Common
Granulomas	Absent	Common
Perforation	Common	Common
Toxic megacolon	Common	Rare

Malabsorption	Minimal incidence	Common
Diarrhea	Common	Common
Abdominal crampy pain	Possible	Common
Fever (intermittent)	During acute attacks	Common
Weight loss	Common	Severe
Rectal bleeding	Common	Infrequent
Tenesmus	Severe	Rare
Pseudopolyps	Common	Rare
Cobblestoning of mucosa	Rare	Common
Carcinoma	Increased incidence after 10 yr of disease	Slightly greater than general population
Recurrence after surgery	Cure with colectomy resections of small or large intestine	70% or more recurrence after segmental resections of small or large intestine

- As the disease progresses, there is weight loss, malnutrition, dehydration, electrolyte imbalances, anemia, increased peristalsis, and pain around the umbilicus and right lower quadrant.

Complications are common in Crohn's disease and may include the following:

- Strictures and obstruction as scar tissue from inflammation narrows the lumen of the intestine.
- Fistulas that develop between segments of the bowel occur in the perianal rectovaginal areas. Fistulas communicating with the urinary tract may cause urinary tract infections.
- Inflammation of all intestinal layers, which may result in perforation (peritonitis) and the formation of intraabdominal abscesses.
- Impaired absorption causing various nutritional abnormalities as a result of damage to the intestinal mucosa. Fat malabsorption causes a deficiency in fat-soluble vitamins and the patient may have an intolerance to gluten (a protein found in barley, rye, and wheat).
- Systemic complications are similar to those of ulcerative colitis and include arthritis, liver disease, renal disorders, cholelithiasis (especially with ileal involvement), ankylosing spondylitis, erythema nodosum, and uveitis.

Diagnostic Studies

- Complete blood count (CBC) and stool for occult blood
- Barium enema of small and large intestine to determine disease location and extent
- Flexible sigmoidoscopy and colonoscopy with biopsy to detect early inflammatory mucosal changes and presence of granulomas

Therapeutic Management

The goal of therapeutic management is to control the inflammatory process, relieve symptoms, correct metabolic and nutritional problems, and promote healing. Drug therapy and nutritional support are the mainstays of treatment.

Pharmacologic Management

- Sulfasalazine is effective when the disease involves the large intestine but is much less effective when only the small intestine is involved.
- Corticosteroid therapy is effective in reducing inflammation and suppressing the disease; dosage and route of administration depend on the severity of illness and the area involved. Once clinical symptoms subside, the dosage should be tapered.
- Immunosuppressive agents (6-mercaptopurine [6-MP], azathioprine) may be tried if repeated trials with corticosteroids fail.

- Metronidazole (Flagyl) is useful in treating Crohn's disease of the perianal area. Marked exacerbations have been reported when the drug is stopped.

Balloon dilatation of strictures may be effective in relieving symptoms; this is usually performed through a colonoscope or under fluoroscopic guidance. Strictures most often dilated are those in the colon or small bowel.

Nutritional Management

A major advance in nutrient therapy has been the elemental diet and total parenteral nutrition (TPN) (see Total Parenteral Nutrition, p. 679). The elemental diet provides a high-calorie, high-nitrogen, fat-free, no-residue substrate that is absorbed in the proximal small bowel. TPN may be given to patients with severe disease, small-bowel fistulas, or short-bowel syndrome. It is given before and after surgery to promote wound healing, reduce complications, and hasten recovery.

- Vitamin deficiencies may develop as a result of malabsorption. Vitamin B_{12} injections every month may be needed because of the inability of the terminal ileum (if affected) to absorb this vitamin.

Surgical Interventions

Surgery is used in patients with severe symptoms that are unresponsive to therapy and in those with life-threatening complications. The majority of patients eventually require surgery at least once in the course of the disease. Unlike ulcerative colitis, which can be cured by total proctocolectomy, Crohn's disease is not cured by surgery; the recurrence rate after surgery is high. The surgical procedure depends on the affected area and the condition of the patient. Conservative intestinal resection with anastomosis of healthy bowel is the procedure of choice.

Nursing Management

Acute care of the patient is very similar to that of the patient with ulcerative colitis (see Ulcerative Colitis, p. 583). As the patient's condition improves, the nurse should allow for more self-care, provide frequent rest periods, and advise the patient of the importance of rest and avoidance or control of emotional stress. Initially this may be difficult for the patient when told the nature of the disease and the limitations of treatment. Special skin care may be needed by patients who have perianal fistulas or abscesses. Postoperative care should be the same as for exploratory laparotomy (see Abdominal Pain, Acute, nursing management after laparotomy, p. 3).

Patient Teaching

- In the majority of patients the disease course is chronic and intermittent, regardless of the site of involvement. Patient and

significant others may need help in setting realistic short-term and long-term goals.
- Specific teaching strategies should include (1) importance of rest and diet management, (2) perianal care, (3) action and side effects of medications, (4) symptoms of recurrence of disease, (5) when to seek medical care, and (6) use of diversional activities to reduce stress.

CUSHING'S SYNDROME

Definition/Description

Cushing's syndrome is characterized by a spectrum of clinical abnormalities caused by excess corticosteroids. Several conditions can cause Cushing's syndrome. The most common cause is iatrogenic administration of exogenous corticosteroids. *Cushing's disease* is specifically caused by an adrenocorticotropic hormone (ACTH)-secreting pituitary tumor.
- Other causes of Cushing's syndrome include adrenal tumors and ectopic ACTH production by tumors outside the hypothalamic-pituitary-adrenal axis (usually of the lung or pancreas).

Clinical Manifestations

Manifestations can be seen in most body systems and are related to excess levels of corticosteroids (see Table 47-13 in Lewis/Collier/Heitkemper, *Medical-Surgical Nursing,* edition 4, p. 1506). Although manifestations of glucocorticoid excess usually predominate, symptoms of mineralocorticoid and androgen excess may also be seen.
- *Glucocorticoid excess* causes pronounced changes in physical appearance. Weight gain, the most common feature, results from accumulation of adipose tissue in the trunk, face, and cervical area. Transient weight gain from sodium and water retention may be present because of the mineralocorticoid effects of cortisol. Glucose intolerance occurs because of cortisol-induced resistance and increased gluconeogenesis by the liver.
- *Protein wasting* is caused by the catabolic effects of cortisol on peripheral tissue. Muscle wasting leads to muscle weakness, especially in the extremities. Loss of bone protein matrix leads to osteoporosis with pathologic fractures, vertebral compression fractures, and bone and back pain. Loss of collagen makes the skin weaker and thinner and makes it bruise more easily. The skin and mucous membranes may take on a bronze color because of the melanotropic activity of ACTH.

- *Mineralocorticoid excess* may cause hypertension, whereas adrenal androgen excess may result in pronounced acne, masculinization in women, and feminization in men. Catabolic processes predominate, and healing is delayed. Mood disturbances (irritability, anxiety, euphoria), insomnia, irrationality, and occasionally psychosis may occur.

Clinical presentation, as revealed by the health history and physical examination, is the first indication of Cushing's syndrome. Of particular importance is a combination of centripedal obesity and protein wasting, as indicated by slender extremities and thin, friable skin; "moon facies" (fullness of face); purplish-red striae on the abdomen, breast, or buttocks; premenopausal osteoporosis; and unexplained hypokalemia.

Diagnostic Studies

- Mental status examination
- Plasma cortisol levels may be elevated with loss of diurnal variations; plasma ACTH levels may be low, normal, or elevated, depending on the underlying problem.
- Complete blood count (CBC) findings reveal granulocytosis, eosinopenia, and polycythemia.
- Serum potassium and glucose levels reveal hypokalemia and hyperglycemia.
- Dexamethasone suppression test
- Twenty-four-hour urine collection for free cortisol levels
- CT scan and MRI help determine tumor localization.

Therapeutic Management

The treatment of choice for *Cushing's disease* is transsphenoidal surgical removal of the pituitary adenoma. Adrenalectomy is indicated for adrenal tumors or hyperplasia. Patients with ectopic ACTH-secreting tumors are managed with treatment of the neoplasm.

- In inoperable cases or cases in which residual disease remains, treatment with o,p'-DDD (mitotane) may be used. This drug suppresses cortisol production, alters peripheral metabolism of steroids, and decreases plasma and urine steroid levels by actually killing adrenocortical cells. The action of this drug results in a "medical adrenalectomy."
- Metyrapone and aminoglutethimide may be used to inhibit cortisol synthesis. Occasionally, bilateral adrenalectomy is necessary. Ketoconazole, which inhibits synthesis of gonadal and adrenal steroids, may also be used.

If *Cushing's syndrome* has developed during the course of prolonged administration of steroids, one or more of the following alternatives may be tried: (1) gradual discontinuance of steroid therapy to avoid potentially life-threatening adrenal insufficiency (not used when corticosteroids are given as physiologic replacements), (2) reduction of steroid dose, and (3) conversion to an alternate-day regimen.

Nursing Management

Goals

The patient with Cushing's syndrome will experience relief of symptoms with no serious complications, maintain a positive self-image, and actively participate in the therapeutic plan.

See the nursing care plan for the patient with Cushing's syndrome in Lewis/Collier/Heitkemper, *Medical-Surgical Nursing,* edition 4, p. 1509.

Nursing Diagnoses

- Risk for infection related to exposure to environmental pathogens and suppression of immune system secondary to hypercortisolism
- Altered nutrition: more than body requirements related to increased appetite and inactivity
- Self-esteem disturbance related to altered body image, emotional lability, and diminished physical capabilities secondary to hormone imbalance
- Risk for injury: fracture related to decreased muscle strength, fatigue, osteoporosis, and increased protein catabolism
- Impaired skin integrity related to excess steroids, immobility, and altered skin fragility

Nursing Interventions

Because the therapeutic interventions have many side effects, the focus of assessment is the signs and symptoms of hormone and drug toxicity and complicating conditions such as cardiovascular disease, diabetes mellitus, infection, nephrolithiasis, and pathologic fractures. Daily nursing assessment includes the following:

- Vital signs every 4 hours, particularly BP, glucose monitoring, daily weights (gain possibly indicating volume excess)
- Signs and symptoms of infection, especially pain, loss of function, and purulent drainage; other signs such as fever and redness may be minimal or absent
- Location, time, and duration of abdominal pain; bone pain or limitations of range of motion, especially in lower back
- Signs of abnormal thromboembolic phenomena, such as sudden chest pain, dyspnea, or tachypnea
- Changes in mental status, particularly the appearance of depression

The patient needs a great deal of emotional support. Changes in appearance such as centripedal obesity, multiple bruises, hirsutism in females, and gynecomastia in males can be very distressing. The nurse can help by offering respect and unconditional acceptance. The patient can be reassured that physical changes and much of the emotional lability are related to the side effects of drug therapy and will resolve when hormone levels return to normal.

If treatment involves surgical removal of a pituitary adenoma, an adrenal tumor, or one or both adrenal glands, nursing care will have an additional focus on preoperative and postoperative care. Surgery on glandular structures poses risks beyond those of other types of operations. Because glands are highly vascular, the risk of hemorrhage is increased. Manipulation of glandular tissue during surgery may release large amounts of hormone into the circulation, producing great fluctuations in metabolic processes affected by these hormones (e.g., hypertension, susceptibility to infection).

Preoperative care. Hypertension and hyperglycemia need to be controlled and hypokalemia corrected by diet and potassium supplements; a high-protein meal plan will help correct protein depletion.

- Although adrenalectomy is uncommon, patients experiencing this procedure should be aware that IV infusions and nasogastric suctioning are likely after surgery.
- Information and instruction about exercises, coughing, and deep breathing are particularly important, because patients are prone to thrombosis and infection.

Postoperative care. Because of hormone fluctuations, the patient's BP, fluid balance, and electrolyte levels tend to be unstable after surgery. High doses of cortisone are administered IV during surgery and for several days afterward to ensure adequate responses to the stress of the procedure.

- Any rapid or significant changes in BP, respiration, or heart rate should be reported. Fluid intake and output should be monitored carefully and assessed for potential imbalance.
- If cortisone dosage is tapered too rapidly after surgery, acute adrenal insufficiency may develop. Vomiting after the nasogastric tube is removed, increased weakness, dehydration, and hypotension may indicate hypocortisolism. In addition, the patient may complain of painful joints, pruritus, or peeling skin and may experience severe emotional disturbances.

The nurse must constantly be alert for signs of glucocorticoid imbalance. After surgery the patient is usually maintained on bed rest until the BP stabilizes. The nurse must also be alert for subtle signs of postoperative infections. Meticulous care must be used when changing the dressing and during any other procedures that necessitate access to body cavities, circulation, or areas under skin.

Patient Teaching

Instructions are based on the patient's lack of endogenous cortisol and resulting inability to physiologically react to stressors.

- Patients should wear a medical-alert bracelet at all times and carry medical identification and instructions in a wallet or purse. Exposure to extremes of temperature, infections, and emotional disturbances should be avoided as much as possible.
- Stress may produce or precipitate acute adrenal insufficiency because the remaining adrenal tissue cannot meet an increased hormonal demand. Many patients can be taught to adjust their corticosteroid replacement therapy in accordance with stress levels.
- If the patient cannot adjust his/her own medication or if weakness, fainting, fever, or nausea and vomiting occur, the patient should notify the physician for a possible adjustment in corticosteroid dosage. Lifetime replacement therapy is required by many patients, but it may take several months to adjust the hormonal dose satisfactorily.

CYSTIC FIBROSIS

Definition/Description
Cystic fibrosis (CF) is an autosomal recessive, multisystem disease characterized by altered function of the exocrine glands involving primarily the lungs, pancreas, and sweat glands.

Pathophysiology
The basic pathophysiologic mechanism is obstruction of the exocrine gland ducts with thick, viscous secretions that adhere to the lumen of the ducts. Thick secretions obstruct bronchioles and lead to air trapping and hyperinflation of the lungs. Stasis of mucus provides an excellent growth medium for bacteria.

- Exocrine function of the pancreas is altered and may stop completely. Pancreatic enzymes such as trypsinogen and amylase do not reach the intestine to digest nutrients. There is malabsorption of fat, protein, and fat-soluble vitamins. Fat malabsorption results in steatorrhea, and protein malabsorption results in the failure to grow and gain weight.
- Function of the reproductive system is altered; male adults are usually sterile and female adults usually have delayed menarche.
- Lung disorders can result, including pneumonia, bronchiolitis, bronchitis, bronchiectasis, atelectasis, and emphysema. There is progressive loss of lung tissue from inflammation and scarring, and chronic hypoxia leads to pulmonary hypertension and cor pulmonale. Death usually results from extensive respiratory infection.

Clinical Manifestations

Manifestations vary depending on the disease severity. Early childhood signs are failure to grow, clubbing, persistent cough with mucous production, tachypnea, and large, frequent bowel movements. A large, protuberant abdomen may develop with emaciated appearance of extremities.

The presence of small amounts of blood in the sputum is common with lung infection. Massive hemoptysis is life threatening. Respiratory failure and cor pulmonale are late complications of CF.

Diagnostic Studies

- Sweat chloride test (pilocarpine iontophoresis method)
- Chest x-ray, pulmonary function tests, fecal analysis for fat and duodenoscopy for enzyme quantification

Therapeutic Management

Major objectives of therapy are to promote clearance of secretions, control infection in the lungs, and provide adequate nutrition.

The management of pulmonary problems is focused on relieving airway obstruction and controlling infection. Drainage of thick bronchial mucus is assisted by aerosol and nebulization treatments that liquefy mucus and facilitate coughing. Aerobic exercise also seems to be effective in clearing airways. Early intervention with antibiotics for lung infection is useful with long courses of antibiotics generally prescribed.

Management of pancreatic insufficiency includes pancreatic enzyme replacement (e.g., lipase, pancrease, Cotazym-S, and Creon) administered before each meal and snack. A high-calorie, high-protein diet and multivitamins are recommended. Fat-soluble vitamins need to be supplemented. Added dietary salt is indicated whenever sweating is excessive, such as during hot weather, in the presence of fever, or from intense physical activity.

Lung transplantations have resulted in significant improvement of pulmonary function with no recurrence of lung disease.

Nursing Management

Goals

The patient with CF will have adequate airway clearance, a reduction of risk factors associated with respiratory infections, ability to perform activities of daily living (ADLs), no complications related to CF, and active participation in planning and implementing a therapeutic regimen.

Nursing Diagnoses

- Ineffective airway clearance related to thick bronchial mucus, weakness, fatigue

- Impaired gas exchange related to recurring lung infections
- Altered nutrition related to dietary intolerances, intestinal gas, and altered enzyme production
- Altered growth and development related to physical, emotional, and social effects of a serious chronic illness and shortened life span

Nursing Interventions

The nurse can assist young adults to gain independence by helping them assume responsibility for their care and for their vocational or school goals. Crises and life transitions that must be dealt with include building confidence and self-respect on the basis of achievements, persevering with employment goals, developing motivation to achieve, learning to cope with the treatment program, and adjusting to the need for dependence if health fails. For a couple considering having children, genetic counseling may be suggested.

Patient Teaching

- For the young adult a major problem that needs to be discussed is sexuality. Delayed or irregular menstruation is not uncommon. There may also be delayed development of secondary sex characteristics, such as breasts in girls, or prolonged short stature in boys.
- Home management of cystic fibrosis includes an aggressive plan of postural drainage with percussion and vibration, aerosol-nebulization therapy, and breathing retraining. The patient is taught controlled coughing techniques, deep breathing exercises, and progressive exercise conditioning such as a bicycling program or arm ergometry.
- Regardless of how well the person is coping, a normal life span is not possible. As the person continues toward adulthood, the nurse and other skilled health professionals need to be available to help the patient and family cope with complications resulting from the disease.

CYSTITIS

Definition/Description

Cystitis is a type of urinary tract infection (UTI) involving inflammation of the bladder. Although the majority of patients with cystitis are women, other groups with a high incidence are older men and young children (especially girls).

- The adult female urethra is short, and its proximity to the rectum and vagina predisposes females to the risk of bladder contamination. Bacterial bladder contamination can result from poor personal hygiene practices and sexual intercourse.

- In children and older men UTIs are often associated with other preexisting problems. In children vesicoureteral reflux is usually the preexisting abnormality. In older men infection is usually related to obstruction caused by benign prostatic hyperplasia.

Pathophysiology

Not all bacterial invasions of the bladder result in UTI or cause spread to the upper urinary tract (pyelonephritis). Once cystitis has occurred, it may remain localized in the urinary bladder for years without ascension to the kidneys or it may be completely resolved after the initial treatment. The risk of recurrent symptomatic infection is increased when urinary tract abnormalities are present.

Clinical Manifestations

- Manifestations of cystitis are frequency and urgency of urination, suprapubic pain, dysuria, and foul-smelling urine. In some persons hematuria and pyuria may be present.
- Presence of fever, nausea and vomiting, and flank tenderness usually indicates pyelonephritis.
- About one half of all persons with significant bacteriuria have no symptoms or may exhibit nonspecific signs such as increased fatigue, anorexia, or changes in cognitive ability.

Diagnostic Studies

- Urinalysis for the presence of white blood cells (WBCs) with urine culture or urine Gram stain to detect bacteriuria
- Further evaluation of urinary tract may include intravenous pyelogram (IVP), voiding cystourethrogram, cystoscopy, and pelvic examination

Therapeutic Management

Once cystitis has been diagnosed, appropriate antimicrobial therapy is initiated. Many drugs are effective against organisms that cause UTIs. These include sulfisoxazole (Gantrisin), nitrofurantoin (Furadantin, Macrodantin), ampicillin, and amoxicillin. Sulfamethoxazole combined with trimethoprim (Bactrim, Septra) has proved effective in the treatment of UTIs, especially recurrent ones, and resistance to this drug seems to develop less rapidly than to other drugs. Systemic antibiotics such as cephalosporins, aminoglycosides (gentamicin, tobramycin), and fluoroquinolones (ciprofloxacin) can also be used.

- Phenazopyridine (Pyridium) may be used in cystitis to provide an analgesic effect on urinary mucosa; this drug should relieve the burning sensation. The azo dye in the drug stains urine reddish orange. It is important to tell the patient about this color change so that he/she does not think it is related to the infection.

- Antibiotic therapy is not usually recommended for asymptomatic bacteriuria unless symptoms develop or there is evidence of obstructive uropathy. Prophylactic antibiotics may be ordered when a patient with asymptomatic bacteriuria undergoes surgery or genitourinary instrumentation.

Nursing Management

Goals

The patient with cystitis will have relief from dysuria, no upper urinary tract complications, and no recurrent episodes.

See the nursing care plan for the patient with a urinary tract infection in Lewis/Collier/Heitkemper, *Medical-Surgical Nursing,* edition 4, p. 1341.

Nursing Diagnoses

- Altered comfort: fever related to infection
- Altered patterns of urinary elimination: frequency, urgency, incontinence, or nocturia related to UTI
- Risk for reinfection related to lack of knowledge regarding prevention of recurrence and signs and symptoms of recurrence
- Pain related to dysuria, urgency, frequency, and bladder spasms secondary to inflammation and tissue trauma

Nursing Interventions

Health promotion measures include recognizing groups with a higher than normal incidence of UTIs. Especially for these individuals, health promotion activities can help decrease the frequency of infections and promote early detection of infection. These activities include teaching preventive measures, such as emptying the bladder regularly and completely, wiping the perineal area from front to back after urination and defecation, and drinking an adequate amount of liquid each day. In addition, it is important to teach the patient to seek early treatment once symptoms are identified.

- The nurse can play a major role in prevention of nosocomial infections. Debilitated persons, older adults, patients with severe underlying disease (cancer, diabetes), and patients being treated with immunosuppressive drugs or radiation are at high risk of UTIs. The patient undergoing instrumentation of the urinary tract is also at risk for nosocomial infections, and aseptic technique should always be followed for these procedures.

Acute intervention includes an adequate fluid intake (if not contraindicated). Explain to the patient that fluids will increase frequency at first but will also dilute the urine, making the bladder less irritable. Caffeine, alcohol, citrus juices, chocolate, and highly spiced foods should be avoided because they are potential bladder irritants. Treatment of cystitis does not usually require hospitalization.

If the patient has been compliant with drug therapy, relapse with bacteria suggests possible renal involvement in the infectious process. For the individual who has more than two infections every 6 months, the use of long-term antibiotic suppressive therapy may be ordered.

Patient Teaching

- The patient needs to be instructed about the prescribed drug therapy. It is important for the patient to take the full course of antibiotics. Sometimes a second medication or a reduced dose of medication is ordered to suppress bacterial growth in certain patients susceptible to recurrent UTI.
- The patient should be instructed to watch for any changes in color or consistency of urine and a decrease in or cessation of symptoms as a sign of therapy effectiveness.
- The patient must understand the need for follow-up care with a urine culture to determine if the infection has been adequately treated. Relapse with bacteria of the same species usually occurs within 1 to 2 weeks after completion of therapy.

DIABETES INSIPIDUS

Definition/Description
Diabetes insipidus (DI) is a condition that occurs when any organic lesion of the hypothalamus, infundibular stem, or posterior pituitary interferes with antidiuretic hormone (ADH) synthesis, transport, or release. Causes of DI include brain tumors, pituitary or other cranial surgery, closed head trauma, central nervous system (CNS) infections, and vascular disorders.

Clinical Manifestations
The primary characteristic is excretion of large quantities of urine (5 to 20 L/day) with a very low specific gravity. In the milder form urinary output may be lower (2 to 4 L/day).

- The patient compensates for water loss by drinking huge amounts of water so that serum osmolality is normal or only moderately elevated.
- The patient is usually fatigued from nocturia. If oral fluid intake cannot keep up with urinary losses, severe fluid volume deficit results. This deficiency is manifested by weight loss, poor tissue turgor, hypotension, tachycardia, constipation, and shock.
- The patient also shows CNS manifestations ranging from irritability and mental dullness to coma. These symptoms are related to rising serum osmolality and hypernatremia.

Therapeutic Management
Because polydipsia and polyuria may be pituitary, renal, or psychogenic in origin, identification of the cause of the DI is the initial step in management.

- A complete health history and physical examination are done. An attempt is made to rule out psychogenic DI related to emotional disturbances. *Psychogenic DI* is associated with overhydration and hypervolemia rather than with the dehydration and hypovolemia seen in other forms of DI. A water deprivation test is done to confirm the diagnosis of central DI.
- *Neurogenic DI* that results from head trauma is usually self-limiting and improves with treatment of the underlying problem. DI that follows cranial surgery may be permanent.

The goal of treatment is maintenance of fluid and electrolyte balance. This may be accomplished by IV administration of fluid (saline and glucose) and by hormone replacement with ADH administered by injection or inhalation.

- In acute DI fluids should be administered at a rate that decreases serum sodium by about 1 mEq/L every 2 hours. Chlorpropamide, clofibrate, carbamazepine, and thiazide diuretics may be prescribed.
- For long-term therapy desmopressin acetate, an analog of ADH that is administered as a nasal preparation and does not have the vasoconstrictive effect, is the preferred therapy.

Nursing Management

Nursing care of the patient with DI is based on clinical symptoms.

- Fluids must be replaced orally or intravenously, depending on the patient's condition and ability to drink copious amounts of fluids. Adequate fluids should be kept at the bedside.
- If IV glucose is used, urine should be assessed for glucose. If the glucose test result is positive, the physician should be notified because glycosuria increases fluid volume deficit.
- Accurate records of intake and output, urine specific gravity, and daily weights are mandatory in the assessment of fluid volume status. Fluid volume deficit manifested by hypotension, tachycardia, and rapid, shallow respirations can be detected early by frequent assessment.
- Polyuria and nocturia can cause disturbances in rest and sleep patterns. The patient is often listless, tired, and discouraged. Support and reassurance that the sleep disturbances are temporary can be helpful.
- Perineal care should be done at least twice daily in bedridden female patients to cleanse urine from the perineum.

When the patient affected by DI is hospitalized, often for emergency treatment of hypertonic encephalopathy, the therapeutic goal is to restore fluid balance. Desmopressin acetate is administered as a nasal or subcutaneous preparation. Adequacy of treatment is assessed by monitoring fluid intake and output and urine specific gravity. Increased urine volume with lower specific gravity is related to an inadequate pharmacologic effect, and the physician should be notified immediately.

The patient who requires long-term ADH replacement needs instruction in self-management.

- Desmopressin acetate is usually taken intranasally twice daily. Nasal irritation, headache, and nausea may indicate overdosage, whereas failure to improve may indicate underdosage.

DIABETES MELLITUS

Definition/Description

Diabetes mellitus is a group of genetically and clinically heterogeneous disorders characterized by abnormalities in glucose homeostasis resulting in hyperglycemia. The hyperglycemia associated with diabetes is caused by a decrease in the secretion or activity of insulin. These insulin alterations result in the disordered metabolism of carbohydrate, fat, and protein. In time, structural abnormalities occur in a variety of organs, especially the heart, kidneys, and eyes.

The diagnosis of diabetes mellitus is made when the fasting plasma glucose level exceeds 140 mg/dl (7.8 mmol/L) on at least two occasions or when at least two random blood glucose measurements exceed 200 mg/dl (11.1 mmol/L).

- *Type I diabetes* results from progressive destruction of β-cell function as a result of an autoimmune process in susceptible individuals. Islet cell antibodies and insulin autoantibodies cause a reduction in β cells of 80% to 90% of normal before hyperglycemia and symptoms occur.
- *Type II diabetes* is a combination of genetically determined defects in skeletal muscle, fat, and liver receptors for insulin and β-cell secretory exhaustion. Excessive hepatic glucose production eventually adds to the fasting and postprandial hyperglycemia.

A comparison of types I and II diabetes is presented in Table 25.

Pathophysiology

Type I: insulin-dependent diabetes mellitus. In type I diabetes, also called insulin-dependent diabetes mellitus or IDDM, autoimmune β-cell destruction is attributed to a genetic predisposition coupled with one or more viral agents and possibly chemical agents. It is not known conclusively that these are the only factors involved.

- Onset and progression of hyperglycemic symptoms is usually more rapid and acute in type I diabetes, and successful treatment depends on insulin replacement. If the disease process is allowed to progress without treatment, diabetic ketoacidosis with nausea and vomiting, electrolyte imbalance, weight loss, and muscle wasting may develop.
- Without treatment (i.e., insulin) ketoacidosis can progress to coma and death. Once treatment is initiated, patients with type I diabetes may go into a remission (often called *honeymoon phase*). During this time the patient needs very little insulin to control blood glucose. Eventually, blood glucose levels climb, more insulin is needed, and the honeymoon period ends.

Table 25   Characteristics of Type I and Type II Diabetes Mellitus

Factor	Type I	Type II
▪ Age at onset	Usually in young person but possible at any age	Usually >age 35 yr but possible at any age
▪ Type of onset	Signs and symptoms abrupt, but disease process may be present for several years	Insidious
▪ Genetic susceptibility	HLA-DR3, -DR4, and others	Frequent genetic background, no relation to HLA
▪ Environmental factors	Virus, toxins	Obesity, nutrition
▪ Islet cell antibody	Present at onset	Absent
▪ Endogenous insulin	Minimal or absent	Possibly excessive, adequate but delayed secretion or reduced but not absent secretion
▪ Nutritional status	Thin, catabolic state	Obese or possibly normal
▪ Symptoms	Thirst, polyuria, polyphagia, fatigue	Frequently none or mild
▪ Control of diabetes	Often difficult with wide glucose fluctuation	Variable, control with diet and exercise
▪ Insulin	Required for all	Required for 30%-40%
▪ Vascular and neurologic complications	In majority of patients after ≥5 yr diabetes	Frequent

HLA, Human leukocyte antigen.

Type II: non-insulin-dependent diabetes mellitus.　Approximately 90% of diabetes mellitus is type II non-insulin-dependent diabetes mellitus (NIDDM). There are two recognized subtypes of type II: obese and nonobese. Type II diabetes has a strong genetic influence (almost 100% concordance in monozygotic twins); no correlation with HLA (human leukocyte antigen) type has been found.

Pathophysiologic factors that have been identified in type II diabetes include decreased tissue (e.g., fat, muscle) responsiveness to insulin as a result of receptor or postreceptor defects, eventual decreased secretion of insulin resulting from β-cell exhaustion, and abnormal hepatic glucose regulation. Obesity appears to play a major role in type II diabetes by down-regulating insulin receptors in skeletal muscle and fat cells, that is, the number of insulin receptors available. These events are often referred to as *peripheral insulin resistance*.

Clinical Manifestations

Normally, insulin and its counterregulatory hormones maintain blood glucose within a range of 70 to 120 mg/dl (3.9 to 6.7 mmol/L). When an absolute insulin deficiency or decreased insulin activity occurs, glucose is not used properly. Glucose remains in the bloodstream and produces an osmotic effect on intracellular and interstitial fluid. This shift in fluid balance results in clinical symptoms of frequent urination *(polyuria)* and thirst *(polydipsia)*. Without sufficient insulin the patient may experience hunger *(polyphagia)* as the body turns to other energy sources besides glucose, first fat and then protein.

- Varying degrees of polyuria, polydipsia, and polyphagia are the hallmark symptoms of diabetes mellitus.
- In type II diabetes mellitus the onset of hyperglycemic symptoms may occur over a long period. The person may "adjust" to persistent feelings of fatigue, thirst, polyuria, and blurred vision without realizing that the diabetic disease process is producing the symptoms.

Acute Complications

The acute problems of diabetic ketoacidosis and hyperglycemia hyperosmolar nonketosis coma result from hyperglycemia and insufficient insulin. A problem that may arise from too much insulin or an excessive dose of an oral hypoglycemic agent (OHA) is *hypoglycemia* (also referred to as *insulin reaction* or *low blood glucose*), which occurs when the level of available blood glucose falls. It is important for the health care provider to be able to distinguish between hyperglycemia and hypoglycemia because hypoglycemia can constitute a serious threat and requires immediate attention.

Diabetic ketoacidosis (DKA). Also referred to as *diabetic acidosis* and *diabetic coma,* DKA may develop quickly or over several days or weeks. It can be caused by too little insulin accompanied by increased caloric intake, physical or emotional stress, or undiagnosed diabetes.

- DKA is most likely to occur in type I diabetes but may be seen in type II in conditions of severe illness or stress when the extra demand for insulin cannot be met by the pancreas.
- Manifestations include dehydration signs such as dry and loose skin, soft and sunken eyeballs, hypertension with a weak and rapid pulse, vomiting, Kussmaul's respirations, and the sweet fruity odor of acetone on the breath. Eventually renal failure and coma occur. If not treated, death is inevitable.

Hyperglycemic hyperosmolar nonketosis (HHNK). HHNK occurs in the patient with diabetes who is able to produce enough insulin to prevent DKA but not enough to prevent severe hyperglycemia, osmotic diuresis, and extracellular fluid depletion.

- This complication causes neurologic abnormalities such as somnolence, coma, seizures, hemiparesis, and aphasia.
- HHNK often occurs in the older adult patient with type II diabetes.
- There is usually a history of inadequate fluid intake, increasing mental depression, and polyuria.

Hypoglycemia. Hypoglycemia, or *low blood glucose,* occurs when proportionately too much insulin is in the blood for the available glucose. This causes the blood glucose level to drop to less than 50 mg/dl (2.8 mmol/L).

- Manifestations include cold sweats, nervousness, pallor, irritability, and increased heart rate. Other various signs may include confusion, fatigue, dizziness, and tremors.

Chronic Complications

Chronic complications are primarily those of end-organ disease from angiopathy and neuropathy. *Angiopathy* or blood vessel disease is estimated to account for the majority of deaths among patients with diabetes. Many factors are being investigated in the development of angiopathy. These chronic blood vessel dysfunctions are divided into two categories: macroangiopathy and microangiopathy.

Macroangiopathy, or disease of large and medium-sized blood vessels, is essentially atherosclerosis and arteriosclerotic vascular disease characterized by a higher frequency and earlier onset than in the nondiabetic population. The degree of vascular damage appears to be related to the duration of the diabetes, not to its severity. Tight glucose control may help delay the atherosclerotic process. Complications resulting from macroangiopathy are cerebrovascular, cardiovascular, and peripheral vascular disease.

Microangiopathy, or disease of small blood vessels, is different from macroangiopathy in that it is specific to diabetes. Although microangiopathy can be found throughout the body, areas most noticeably affected are the eyes *(retinopathy),* kidneys *(nephropathy),* and skin *(dermopathy).*

Peripheral vascular disease (PVD) is a combination of microangiopathy and macroangiopathy. The legs and feet are most often affected in diabetes mellitus. Sequelae of PVD can lead to infection, gangrene, and amputation. Signs of PVD include intermittent claudication, pain at rest, cold feet, loss of hair, delayed capillary filling, and dependent rubor.

Diabetic retinopathy refers to the microangiopathic process of the retina seen in patients with diabetes (see Diabetic Retinopathy, p. 185).

Diabetic nephropathy is now the leading cause of end-stage renal disease (ESRD) in the United States. This occurs as a result of microvascular abnormalities associated with diabetes mellitus by processes not clearly understood.

Neuropathy. Neuropathy is probably one of the most common complications of diabetes in adults; its cause is unclear.

- The two major categories of diabetic neuropathy are *neuropathic conditions* of the peripheral nervous system, including symmetric peripheral polyneuropathy, mononeuropathic disorders, and diabetic amyotrophy, and *autonomic neuropathic conditions,* including cardiovascular abnormalities, GI abnormalities, urinary bladder abnormalities, and sexual dysfunction.
- Symmetric peripheral polyneuropathy affects all the extremities but most often affects the legs. The patient has pain and paresthesias. Neuropathy in the hands causes atrophy of small muscles, limiting fine movement.

Diagnostic Tests

- Blood tests, including fasting blood glucose, postprandial blood glucose, glycosylated hemoglobin, cholesterol and triglyceride levels, blood urea nitrogen and creatinine, and electrolytes
- Urine for complete urinalysis, microalbuminuria, culture and sensitivity, glucose, and acetone
- Neurologic and funduscopic examination
- BP and monitoring of weight
- Doppler scan to determine presence and degree of PVD

Therapeutic Management

Management of diabetes mellitus is primarily aimed at pharmacologic and nutritional management together with appropriate monitoring and patient and family education.

Pharmacologic Management

Two types of glucose-lowering agents used in the treatment of diabetes are insulin and OHAs.

Insulin

Exogenous insulin is needed when a patient has inadequate insulin to meet specific metabolic needs and the combination of dietary management, exercise, and oral agents cannot maintain a satisfactory blood glucose level. Exogenous insulin is required for the management of type I diabetes. Exogenous insulin may be prescribed for patients with type II diabetes during periods of severe stress, such as illness or surgery, or when attempts at glycemic control by means of diet, exercise, or OHAs fail.

Exogenous insulin has commonly been obtained from the pancreases of pigs and cows; however, these sources have become expensive to obtain. Today, biosynthetic insulin is used almost exclusively. The advantages of these new insulins are a reduced allergic response and a more predictable insulin activity. In addition to origin and purity, insulins differ in regard to onset, peak action, and duration. The specific properties of each type of insulin are matched with the patient's diet and activity. For information on administering an insulin injection, see Table 46-6 in Lewis/Collier/Heitkemper, *Medical-Surgical Nursing,* edition 4, p. 1449.

Nursing management related to insulin therapy. Nursing responsibilities for the patient receiving insulin include proper administration, assessment of the patient's use of and response to insulin therapy, and education of the patient regarding administration, adjustment to, and side effects of insulin.

- The patient with newly diagnosed diabetes should be assessed for the ability to understand the purpose of insulin therapy; interaction of insulin, diet, and activity; and side effects.
- The patient or significant other also has to be able to prepare and inject the insulin. If the patient or family lacks the psychomotor skills to prepare insulin, the nurse may have to find additional resources to assist the patient.
- Follow-up assessment of the patient who has been using insulin therapy includes an inspection of insulin sites for allergic reactions, a review of insulin preparation and injection technique, a history pertaining to occurrence of hypoglycemic episodes, and the patient's method for handling hypoglycemic episodes.
- A review of the patient's record of urine and blood glucose tests is also important in assessing overall glycemic control.

Oral Hypoglycemic Agents

The first generation of these drugs used in the treatment of diabetes mellitus included tolbutamide (Orinase), tolazamide (Tolinase), and chlorpropamide (Diabinese). A second generation of sulfonylureas, approved for use in the United States more recently, includes glipizide (Glucotrol) and glyburide (Micronase, DiaBeta, Glynase).

- Second-generation drugs have fewer adverse effects, are about 100 times more potent by weight, and have more predictable time actions and half-lives. The main disadvantage of second-generation drugs is their increased expense.
- OHAs are not oral insulin or a substitute for insulin. The patient must have some functioning endogenous insulin for OHAs to be effective.

As with insulin, the sulfonylureas differ in dosage, absorption time, peak action, and duration. Second-generation sulfonylureas offer the advantages of lower doses, fewer side effects, and partial biliary excretion.

Nursing management related to oral hypoglycemic agents.
Nursing responsibilities for the patient taking OHAs are similar to those for the patient taking insulin. Proper administration, assessment of the patient's use of and response to the OHA, and education of patient and family about OHA are all part of the nurse's function.

- The assessment done by the nurse can be invaluable in determining the most appropriate oral agent for a patient. The assessment includes the patient's mental status, eating habits, home environment, attitude toward diabetes, and use of oral agents.
- The patient needs to understand the importance of diet and not skipping meals.
- The patient also needs to know that hypoglycemic reactions may be severe and prolonged and that physician supervision may be necessary, particularly for older patients.
- The patient should also be instructed to contact a physician if periods of illness or extreme stress occur. During such a period insulin therapy may be required to prevent or treat hyperglycemic symptoms and HHNK.

Nutritional Management

Nutritional therapy is the cornerstone of care for the person with diabetes. Today there is no one "diabetic" or "ADA" diet. The recommended diet can be defined only as a dietary prescription based on nutritional assessment and goals. Because of the complexity of nutrition issues, it is recommended that a registered dietitian with expertise in diabetes management be a member of the treatment team. Monitoring of glucose and glycohemoglobin, lipids, and renal status is essential to evaluate nutrition-related outcomes.

- *Type I Diabetes:* Meal planning should be based on the individual's usual food intake with insulin therapy integrated into the usual eating and exercise patterns. It is recommended that individuals using insulin therapy eat their meals at consistent times synchronized with the time-action of insulin preparation used.

- *Type II Diabetes:* The emphasis for nutritional therapy in type II diabetes should be placed on achieving glucose, lipid, and blood pressure goals. Weight loss and hypocaloric diets usually improve short-term glycemic levels and have potential to increase long-term metabolic control. For dietary strategies to use with type I and type II diabetes, see Lewis/Collier/Heitkemper, *Medical-Surgical Nursing,* edition 4, p. 1445.

Diet principles that both the nurse and dietitian should teach and reinforce include:

- Eat according to prescribed meal plan. A dietary prescription is individualized to reflect dietary needs related to a specific patient's body weight, occupation, age, activities, and type of diabetes. Individual responses to a dietary prescription should be monitored, and appropriate adjustments should be made when necessary.
- Never skip meals; this is particularly important for the patient taking insulin or OHAs. The body requires food at regularly spaced intervals throughout the day; omission or delay of meals can result in hypoglycemia.
- Learn to recognize appropriate food portions; practice can result in accurate portion allotments.

Nursing Management
Goals
The patient with diabetes mellitus will be an active participant in the management of the diabetes regimen; experience minimal or no episodes of DKA, HHNK, or hypoglycemia; prevent or delay the occurrence of chronic complications of diabetes; and adjust his/her lifestyle to accommodate the diabetes regimen with a minimum of stress.

See the nursing care plan for the patient with diabetes in Lewis/Collier/Heitkemper, *Medical-Surgical Nursing,* p. 1458.

Nursing Diagnoses/Collaborative Problems for Newly Diagnosed Diabetes

- Ineffective management of therapeutic regimen related to lack of knowledge of adequate exercise program, diet and weight control, administration and potential side effects and complications of glucose-lowering agents, glucose monitoring, and care during acute minor illness
- Risk for infection related to depressed immune system, inadequate circulation, and environmental pathogens
- Self-esteem disturbance related to lifestyle changes imposed by diabetes and its treatment, stigma of having a chronic illness, and frustration at progression of disease despite careful management

- Potential complication: hypoglycemia related to low blood glucose secondary to too much insulin
- Potential complication: diabetic ketoacidosis and hyperglycemic hyperosmolar nonketosis related to inadequate insulin and excess blood glucose secondary to increased caloric intake, physical or emotional stress, or undiagnosed diabetes

Nursing Interventions

The nurse may be involved in any or all aspects of management, but the focus of nursing care has two aims: to care for the patient during acute episodes and to assist the patient in learning to live with diabetes every day. Both aims require the nurse to be thoroughly familiar with diabetes and its management and to educate the patient about all aspects of the disease.

- The effect of the diagnosis of diabetes cannot be overestimated. An assessment of the patient's perception of what it means to have diabetes must be carefully assessed before patient education is designed and implemented.
- The nurse should foster a positive attitude about the prescribed regimen and assist the patient in developing an individualized management plan. Learning goals should be mutually determined by the patient and nurse on the basis of individual needs and therapeutic requirements.
- The nurse needs to assess patient feelings and facilitate acceptance of diabetes mellitus and its treatment over time.

Glucose monitoring. Glucose levels must be determined daily to monitor interactions and the effect of diet, exercise, and medication on individual diabetic regimen. Detection of extreme or episodic hyperglycemia is necessary to avoid DKA and HHNK. Urine testing for ketonuria is a valuable aid in determining the advent of DKA and is recommended for all patients with type I diabetes when they are experiencing hyperglycemia or acute illness.

- Patient self-monitoring of blood glucose with *capillary blood glucose monitoring* (CBGM) technology is the most reliable method for measuring blood glucose. CBGM patient training should be emphasized at not only the initial session but at follow-up visits with any member of the health care team. Patient technique should be reassessed after initial training.

Foot care. Proper care of the feet is crucial for the patient with diabetes. Guidelines for foot care are listed in Table 46-21 in Lewis/Collier/Heitkemper, *Medical-Surgical Nursing,* edition 4, p. 1470.

Exercise. Regular, consistent exercise is considered an essential part of diabetic management. Exercise contributes to weight loss, reduces triglycerides and cholesterol, increases muscle tone, and improves circulation.

- In *type I diabetes* exercise may increase insulin sensitivity, thereby allowing a lowering of the insulin dose. In *type II dia-*

betes exercise contributes to weight loss and improves insulin binding on cell receptors.

- Additional patient teaching information about exercise and diabetes includes (1) exercise does not have to be vigorous to be effective, (2) exercise is best done after meals, when blood glucose level is rising, (3) exercise plans should be individualized for each patient and monitored by the health care provider, (4) the patient should be encouraged to self-monitor blood glucose levels before, during, and after exercise to determine effect exercise has on blood glucose level at particular times of day, and (5) the patient should be alerted to the possibility of delayed exercise-induced hypoglycemia, which may occur several hours after completion of exercise.

D

Effects of stress. Both emotional and physical stress can increase the blood glucose level and result in hyperglycemia. Common stress-evoking situations include acute illness and the stress of surgery. The patient with diabetes who has a minor illness such as a cold or the flu should continue drug therapy and food intake.

- Blood glucose monitoring should be done every 1 to 2 hours by either the patient or a person who can assume responsibility for care during the illness. Urine output and the presence and degree of ketonuria should be monitored, particularly when fever is present. Fluid intake should be increased to prevent dehydration, with a minimum of 4 ounces per hour for an adult.
- The patient should be instructed to contact the health care provider when a blood glucose level more than 250 mg/dl (13.9 mmol/L) exists, and when fever, ketonuria, and nausea and vomiting occur. Eventually the well-informed patient will be able to make most adjustments independently on the basis of past successful experiences.
- Surgery is controlled stress, and adjustments in the diabetes regimen can be planned to ensure glycemic control. The patient is given IV fluids and insulin immediately before, during, and after surgery when there is no oral intake. The type II patient receiving OHAs usually has the OHAs discontinued 48 hours before surgery and is treated with insulin during the surgical period.
- The nurse caring for an unconscious surgical patient receiving insulin must be alert for hypoglycemic signs such as sweating, tachycardia, and tremors. The nurse should be aware that blood glucose monitoring must also be done frequently.

DKA and HHNK. When the patient is hospitalized, the nurse is responsible for monitoring blood glucose and urine for output and ketones and for using laboratory data to direct care.

- Areas that need monitoring are administration of IV fluids to correct dehydration, administration of insulin therapy to reduce

blood glucose and serum acetone, administration of electrolytes to correct electrolyte imbalance, assessment of renal status, assessment of cardiopulmonary status related to hydration and electrolyte levels, and monitoring the level of consciousness.
- The nurse must also monitor the signs of potassium imbalance resulting from hypoinsulinemia and osmotic diuresis.
- Vital signs should be assessed often to determine the presence of fever, hypovolemic shock, tachycardia, and Kussmaul's breathing.

Hypoglycemia. The preferred treatment of hypoglycemia is prevention. However, if hypoglycemia occurs, the patient should be able to reverse the situation before medical assistance is required. The patient's ability to do this depends on the state of alertness, ability to swallow, and availability of a quick-acting carbohydrate source.
- At the first sign of hypoglycemia the patient should ingest 5 to 20 g of a simple (fast-acting) carbohydrate, such as 120 to 180 ml of orange juice, 180 to 240 ml of regular soft drink, two packets of sugar, or five or six hard candies. Overtreatment with large quantities of quick-acting carbohydrates such as a whole candy bar should be avoided.
- If the symptoms are still present after 10 to 15 minutes, ingestion of 5 to 20 g of carbohydrate should be repeated. Once the symptoms have improved, the patient should eat a longer-lasting carbohydrate such as bread or milk to prevent symptoms from recurring.
- If there is little discernible improvement in the patient's condition after two to three doses of 5 to 20 g of simple carbohydrate within 30 minutes or if the patient is not alert enough to swallow, 1 mg of glucagon may be administered with the same technique used for an insulin injection. The blood glucose level must be carefully monitored during the treatment.
- With effective treatment hypoglycemia can be quickly reversed. Once acute hypoglycemia has been reversed, the nurse should explore with the patient the reasons the situation developed. This assessment may indicate need for additional education of patient and family to avoid future episodes of hypoglycemia. The danger of hypoglycemic reactions must be stressed because memory and learning impairment can result from repeated episodes of severe hypoglycemia.

Patient Teaching
- The patient should be instructed to carry diabetes identification at all times. An identification card can supply valuable information, such as the name of health care provider and type and dose of insulin or OHA. A medical-alert bracelet or necklace should be worn by all persons with diabetes.

- The major educational objective is a level of self-management appropriate to the individual patient. Ideally, the patient should be taught about the disease and encouraged to achieve self-management with guidance only from the health care provider.
- A knowledgeable patient should be able to make minor adjustments in insulin dosage and diet prescription to compensate for special circumstances such as illness or increased exercise.
- Not all patients with diabetes are capable of self-management. If the patient is not able to manage the disease, a family member may be able to assume this role. If the patient or family cannot make decisions related to diabetes management, the nurse may identify appropriate resources outside the family. These resources can assist the patient and family in outlining a feasible treatment program that meets their capabilities.

DIABETIC RETINOPATHY

Definition/Description
Diabetic retinopathy is a complication of diabetes mellitus that affects retinal blood vessels. Retinal vascular changes in persons with diabetes mellitus are probably initially caused by alterations in various biochemical processes. These alterations result in weakening of microvessel walls, microaneurysm formation, capillary dilatation, decreased capillary blood flow, and capillary atrophy. Systemic conditions that may affect the development of diabetic retinopathy include hypertension, elevated lipids and triglycerides, renal disease, elevated serum creatinine, and cardiovascular disease.

Clinical Manifestations
The earliest and most treatable stages of diabetic retinopathy often produce no visual symptoms. Because of this, the diabetic patient must have regular eye examinations for early detection and appropriate treatment.

- Retinal vascular changes are classified as *nonproliferative diabetic retinopathy (NPDR)* or *proliferative diabetic retinopathy (PDR)*. In NPDR hemorrhages and fatty deposits appear in the retina. In PDR new vessels form (neovascularization) on the retina surface and optic disc. When PDR occurs, the patient may complain of sudden and severe loss of vision.

Diagnostic Studies
- Ophthalmoscopic and slit-lamp microscopic retinal examinations can identify diabetic fundus changes.

- Fluorescein angiography demonstrates dye leakage from abnormal retinal and subretinal vessels and identifies retinal areas amenable to focal laser treatment.
- If the vitreous humor is opaque in advanced disease, ultrasonography may be useful to identify retinal detachment.

Therapeutic and Nursing Management

Current treatment includes early laser photocoagulation of the retina, focal laser treatment for vision loss from macular edema, and panretinal photocoagulation (PRP), a scatter technique of laser burns for moderate to severe neovascularization. Vitrectomy is indicated for significant vitreous or retinal hemorrhage.

- Diabetic retinopathy cannot be cured—only treated. Proper management of certain systemic diseases may help control the progression of retinopathy.

Nursing management for the patient with diabetic retinopathy has an underlying similarity to glaucoma because both disorders require long-term management and both are causes of preventable visual impairment. (See Glaucoma, nursing management, p. 251.)

DIARRHEA

Definition/Description

Diarrhea is not a disease but a symptom. The term *diarrhea* is commonly used to denote an increase in stool frequency or volume and an increase in the looseness of stool.

- Causes of diarrhea can be divided into general classifications of decreased fluid absorption, increased fluid secretion, motility disturbances, or a combination of these. Causes of acute infectious diarrhea are listed in Table 26.

Clinical Manifestations and Complications

Diarrhea may be acute or chronic. *Acute* diarrhea most commonly results from infection. Bacterial or viral infection of the intestine may result in explosive watery diarrhea, *tenesmus* (spasmodic contraction of anal sphincter with pain and persistent desire to defecate), and abdominal cramping pain. Perianal skin excoriation may also develop. Acute diarrhea is often self-limiting with symptoms continuing until the irritant or causative agent is excreted.

- Systemic manifestations may include fever, nausea, vomiting, and malaise. Leukocytes, blood, and mucus may be present in the stool, depending on the causative agent (see Table 26).

Diarrhea is considered *chronic* when it persists for at least 2 weeks or when it subsides and returns more than 2 to 4 weeks after the initial episode. Severe diarrhea may be debilitating and life-threatening.

- A patient may have severe dehydration (water and sodium loss) and electrolyte disturbances. Malabsorption and malnutrition are also sequelae of chronic diarrhea.

Diagnostic Studies

Accurate diagnosis and management require a thorough history, physical examination, and, when indicated, laboratory tests.

- A history of travel, medication use, diet, previous surgery, interpersonal contacts, and family history should be obtained.
- Blood tests may be performed to identify anemia, elevated white blood cell (WBC) count, iron and folate deficiencies, liver enzyme increases, and electrolyte disturbances.
- Stools may be examined for blood, mucus, WBCs, and parasites. Stool cultures may help in identifying infectious organisms.
- In a patient with chronic diarrhea, measurement of stool electrolytes, pH, and osmolality may help to determine whether diarrhea is related to decreased fluid absorption or increased fluid secretion (secretory diarrhea).
- Measurement of stool fat and undigested muscle fibers may be indicative of fat and protein malabsorption conditions, including pancreatic insufficiency. Elevated serum levels of GI peptides such as vasoactive intestinal polypeptide (VIP) and gastrin may be present with secretory diarrhea.
- Endoscopy may be used to examine mucosa and to obtain specimens for examination.
- Upper and lower barium studies may be helpful in detecting mucosal disease.

Therapeutic Management

The treatment of diarrhea is based on the cause and is aimed at replacement of fluid and electrolytes and decreasing the number, volume, and frequency of stools. Oral solutions containing glucose and electrolytes (e.g., Gatorade, Pedialyte) are often sufficient to replace losses due to mild diarrhea. In severe diarrhea, parenteral administration of fluids, electrolytes, and is warranted.

Once the cause has been ascertained, antidiarrheal agents may be given to coat and protect mucous membranes, inhibit GI motility, decrease intestinal secretions, and decrease central nervous system (CNS) input to the GI tract.

Table 26	Acute Infectious Diarrhea	
	Onset	**Duration**
Viral		
Rotavirus, Norwalk	18-24 hr	24-48 hr
Bacterial		
Escherichia coli	4-24 hr	3-4 days
Shigella	24 hr	7 days
Salmonellae	6-48 hr	2-5 days
Campylobacter species	24 hr	< 7 days
Clostridium perfringens	8-12 hr	24 hr
Clostridium difficile toxin	4-9 days after start of antibiotics	1-3 wk
Parasitic		
Giardia lamblia	1-3 wk	Few days to 3 months
Entamoeba	4 days	Weeks to months

- Antiperistaltic agents are not given to a patient who has infectious diarrheal syndromes because of the potential for prolonging exposure to the infectious agent. Antidiarrheal medications should not be given over a prolonged time.
- Antibiotics are usually not indicated in the treatment of diarrhea because they can cause diarrhea by altering normal bowel flora.

Nursing Management of Acute Infectious Diarrhea
Goals
The patient with diarrhea will not transmit the microorganism causing the infectious diarrhea, will cease having diarrhea and resume normal bowel patterns, will have normal fluid and electrolyte and acid-base balance, will have normal nutritional intake, and will have no perianal skin breakdown.

See the nursing care plan for the patient with acute infectious diarrhea in Lewis/Collier/Heitkemper, *Medical-Surgical Nursing*, edition 4, p. 1211.

Symptoms and Signs

Explosive, watery diarrhea; nausea; vomiting; abdominal cramps

Four or five loose stools per day, nausea, malaise, low-grade fever
Watery stools containing blood and mucus, fever, tenesmus,
    urgency
Watery diarrhea, fever, nausea
Profuse, watery diarrhea; malaise; nausea; abdominal cramps;
    low-grade fever
Watery diarrhea, abdominal cramps, vomiting

Associated with antibiotic treatment; symptoms range from mild—
    watery diarrhea—to severe—abdominal pain, fever, leukocyto-
    sis, hypoalbuminemia, leukocytes in stool

Sudden onset; foul, explosive, watery diarrhea; flatulence; epi-
    gastric pain and cramping; nausea
Frequent soft stools with blood and mucus (in severe cases, watery
    stools), flatulence, distention, cramping, fever, leukocytes in stool

Nursing Diagnoses
- Diarrhea related to acute infectious process
- Acute pain and abdominal cramping related to increased GI
  motility
- Fluid volume deficit related to excessive fluid loss and de-
  creased fluid intake secondary to vomiting or diarrhea
- Impaired skin integrity of perianal area related to contact with
  diarrheal stools and inadequate perianal hygiene
- Risk for infection transmission related to lack of knowledge in
  prevention of reinfection or transmission of infectious disease

Nursing Interventions
Adherence to infection control precautions is important because
some cases of acute diarrhea are infectious. All cases of acute diarrhea
should be considered infectious until the cause is determined.

- Handwashing is the most important measure in prevention of
  the transfer of microorganisms. Hands should be washed before and after contact with each patient and when excretions of
  any kind are handled.

- The patient should be taught the principles of hygiene, infection control precautions, and potential dangers of an illness that is infectious to themselves and others. Proper handling, cooking, and storage of food should be discussed with the patient suspected of having infectious diarrhea.

Patient Teaching

- Teach the patient to be alert for recurrence of diarrhea, fever, and other symptoms and for evidence of the same symptoms in family members.
- Assist the patient in identifying factors that precipitated diarrhea to avoid causing reinfection of self or transmission to others.
- Explain the importance of seeking medical care when diarrhea and other symptoms begin so early treatment can be initiated.

DISLOCATION AND SUBLUXATION

Definition/Description

A dislocation is a severe injury of the ligamentous structures that surround a joint. It results in the complete displacement or separation of joint articular surfaces. A *subluxation* is a partial or incomplete displacement of the joint surface. Clinical manifestations of a subluxation are similar to those of a dislocation but are less severe. Treatment of subluxation is similar to that of a dislocation, but subluxation requires less healing time.

Dislocations characteristically result from overwhelming forces transmitted to the joint that cause a disruption of the soft tissues. Joints most frequently dislocated in the upper extremity include the thumb, elbow, and shoulder. In the lower extremity the hip is vulnerable to dislocation occurring as a result of severe trauma, often associated with motor vehicle accidents.

Clinical Manifestations

The most obvious manifestation of a dislocation is asymmetry of the musculoskeletal contour. For example, if a hip is dislocated, the limb is shorter on the affected side.

- Additional manifestations include local pain, tenderness, loss of function of the injured part, and swelling of the soft tissues in the region of the joint.
- Major complications of a dislocated joint are open joint injuries, intraarticular fractures, fracture dislocation, and damage to adjacent neurovascular tissue.

Diagnostic Studies

- X-ray studies determine the extent of shifting of the involved structures.
- Joint aspiration determines the presence of fat cells. If fat cells from the exposed marrow are found in the synovial fluid, an intraarticular fracture is present.

Therapeutic Management

A dislocation requires prompt attention. The longer the joint remains unreduced, the greater the possibility of *avascular necrosis* (bone cell death as a result of inadequate blood supply). The hip joint is particularly susceptible to avascular necrosis.

The goal of therapeutic management is to realign the dislocated portion of the joint in its original anatomic position. This can be accomplished by a closed reduction, which may be performed with the patient under local or general anesthesia. In some situations open reduction may be necessary.

- After reduction the extremity is usually immobilized by taping or using a sling to allow the torn ligaments and capsular tissue time to heal.
- Observation is indicated for the patient with a posterior sternoclavicular dislocation because delayed intrathoracic complications, such as pneumothorax or subclavian vessel injury, may occur.

Nursing Management

Goals

The patient with a dislocation or subluxation will have satisfactory relief of pain and discomfort, realignment of the articular joint surfaces as quickly as possible, and a return to preinjury function.

Nursing Diagnoses

- Pain related to edema, muscle spasm, ineffective pain and/or comfort measures
- Impaired physical mobility related to pain, activity restrictions, or immobilization device

Nursing Interventions

Nursing care is directed toward symptomatic relief of pain and support and protection of the injured joint. After the joint has been immobilized, motion is usually restricted.

- A carefully regulated rehabilitation program can prevent the formation of contractures. The patient should not stretch the joint beyond its limits because the torn capsule and ligament heal in a shortened position with fibrous scar tissue that is not as strong as the original tissue.

- An exercise program slowly and methodically restores the joint to its original range of motion without causing another dislocation.
- Activity restrictions of the affected joint may be imposed to decrease the risk of dislocating the joint on a long-term basis.

DISSEMINATED INTRAVASCULAR COAGULATION

Definition/Description

Disseminated intravascular coagulation (DIC) is a serious bleeding disorder resulting from abnormally initiated and accelerated clotting. Subsequent decreases in clotting factors and platelets ensue, which may lead to uncontrollable hemorrhage. The term *coagulation* can be misleading because it suggests that blood is clotting. The paradox of this condition is that profuse bleeding results from depletion of platelets and clotting factors. DIC is always caused by an underlying disease. The underlying disease must be treated for DIC to resolve.

Pathophysiology

DIC is an abnormal response of the normal clotting cascade stimulated by a disease process or disorder. The diseases and disorders known to predispose patients to DIC include shock, septicemia, abruptio placentae, severe head injury, heat stroke, malignancy, and pulmonary emboli.

- DIC can occur as an acute catastrophic condition, or it may exist at a subacute or chronic level. Each condition may have one or multiple triggering mechanisms that start the cascade.

Initially in DIC normal coagulation mechanisms are enhanced. Intravascular thrombin is produced and it catalyzes the conversion of fibrinogen to fibrin and enhances platelet aggregation. There is widespread fibrin and platelet deposition in capillaries and arterioles, resulting in thrombosis. Excessive clotting activates the fibrinolytic system, which in turn lyses newly formed clots, creating fibrin-split (fibrin-degradation) products, which inhibit normal blood clotting. Ultimately the blood loses its ability to form a stable clot at injury sites, which predisposes the patient to hemorrhage.

- Chronic DIC is most commonly seen in patients with long-standing illnesses such as malignant disorders or autoimmune diseases.

Clinical Manifestations

There is no well-defined sequence of events in acute DIC. Bleeding in a person with no previous history or obvious cause should be questioned because it may be one of the first manifestations of acute DIC. Other nonspecific manifestations can include weakness, malaise, and fever. There are both bleeding and thrombotic manifestations in DIC.

- *Bleeding manifestations* of DIC are multifactorial and result from consumption and depletion of platelets and coagulation factors; manifestations include petechiae, oozing blood, tachypnea, hemoptysis, tachycardia, hypotension, bloody stools, hematuria, dizziness, headache, changes in mental status, and bone and joint pain.
- *Thrombotic manifestations* are a result of fibrin or platelet deposition in the microvasculature and include ischemic tissue necrosis (e.g., gangrene), acute respiratory distress syndrome, and paralytic ileus.

Diagnostic Studies for Acute DIC

- Prolonged prothrombin time (75% incidence) and partial thromboplastin time (50% to 60% incidence)
- Prolonged activated partial thromboplastin time and thrombin time
- Reduced fibrinogen, antithrombin III, and platelets
- Elevated fibrin-split products (FSP) and elevated D-dimers (cross-linked fibrin fragments)
- Decreased levels of factors V, VII, VIII, X, XIII

Therapeutic Management

It is important to diagnose DIC quickly, institute therapy that will resolve the underlying causative disease or problem, and provide supportive care for manifestations resulting from the pathologic condition of DIC itself. Treatment of DIC remains controversial and under investigation as researchers attempt to determine the most suitable means of managing this dangerous syndrome. Consequently, it is imperative that the nurse maintain an ongoing awareness of current modes of therapy. Regardless of the etiology, treating the primary disease process is essential to the resolution of DIC. Depending on its severity, a variety of different methods are used to provide supportive and symptomatic management of DIC (Fig. 2).

- If chronic DIC is diagnosed in a patient who is not bleeding, no therapy for DIC is necessary. Treatment of the underlying disease may be sufficient to reverse DIC (e.g., antineoplastic therapy when DIC is caused by malignancy). Chronic DIC does

Therapy

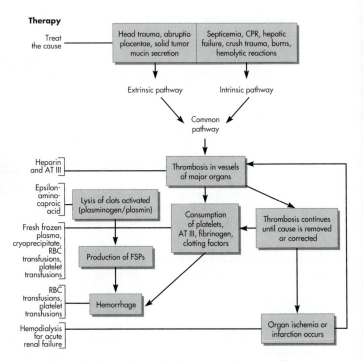

Fig. 2 Intended sites of action for therapies in disseminated intravascular coagulation. *AT III,* Antithrombin III; *CPR,* cardiopulmonary resuscitation; *FSP,* fibrin-split products; *RBC,* red blood cells. (Modified from Thelan LA and others: *Textbook of critical care nursing: diagnosis and management,* ed 2, St Louis, 1994, Mosby.)

not respond to oral anticoagulants but can be controlled with long-term, low-dose subcutaneous or IV heparin.
- When the patient with DIC is bleeding, therapy is directed toward providing support with necessary blood products while treating the primary disorder. Blood products are administered on the basis of specific component deficiencies: platelets are given to correct thrombocytopenia, cryoprecipitate replaces factor VIII and fibrinogen, and fresh frozen plasma (FFP) replaces all clotting factors except platelets and provides a source of antithrombin (see Blood Transfusion Therapy, p. 620).
- A patient with manifestations of thrombosis is often treated by anticoagulation with either unfractionated (low or high dose) or low-molecular-weight heparin. Use of heparin in the treat-

ment of DIC remains controversial. Antithrombin III (AT III), a cofactor of heparin that becomes depleted during DIC, has been used alone or in conjunction with heparin when levels of this factor are low.

- Another treatment that has been used is epsilon aminocaproic acid (EACA [Amicar]) because of its ability to inhibit fibrinolysis. The use of EACA is controversial because it can enhance thrombosis.

Therapy will stabilize a patient's condition, prevent exsanguination or massive thrombosis, and permit institution of definitive therapy to treat the underlying cause.

Nursing Diagnoses

- Altered cerebral, cardiopulmonary, renal, GI, and peripheral tissue perfusion related to bleeding and sluggish or diminished blood flow secondary to thrombosis
- Pain related to bleeding into tissues and diagnostic procedures
- Risk for decreased cardiac output related to fluid volume deficit and hypotension
- Anxiety related to fear of the unknown, disease process, diagnostic procedures, and therapy

Nursing Interventions

Nurses must be alert to the possible development of DIC and especially to the precipitating factors. This may be difficult because the nurse is focusing on the complex care often required for the primary problem that precipitated the DIC.

The nurse must remember that because DIC is the result of an underlying disease, appropriate care for managing the causative problem must be provided while providing supportive care related to manifestations of DIC. Correcting the primary disease (when possible) will help to resolve DIC.

- Nursing care plan for the patient with thrombocytopenia provides a listing of assessments and interventions appropriate for the patient with DIC (see Thrombocytopenic Purpura, p. 562).
- Early detection of bleeding, both occult and overt, must be a primary goal. The patient should be thoroughly assessed for signs of external bleeding (e.g., petechiae, oozing at IV or injection sites) and signs of internal bleeding (e.g., changes in mental status, increasing abdominal girth, pain).
- Any sites of bleeding should be carefully monitored for progression or response to supportive therapies. Tissue damage should be minimized and the patient protected from additional foci of bleeding.
- Another nursing responsibility is to administer blood products properly if they are ordered. Infusing cryoprecipitate or fresh frozen plasma (FFP) is similar to giving any other blood product (see Blood Transfusion Therapy, p. 620).

DIVERTICULITIS/DIVERTICULOSIS

Definition/Description

A diverticulum is a saccular dilatation or outpouching of the mucosa through the circular smooth muscle of the intestinal wall. Clinically, diverticular disease occurs in two forms, diverticulosis and diverticulitis. Multiple noninflamed diverticula are present with *diverticulosis*. The patient is most often free of symptoms but may have some abdominal discomfort. In *diverticulitis,* inflammation of the diverticula occurs. Diverticula may occur at any point within the GI tract but are most commonly found in the sigmoid colon.

Pathophysiology

There is no known cause of diverticular disease, but deficiency in dietary fiber has been associated with it. The disease is more prevalent in Western populations that consume diets low in fiber and high in refined carbohydrates. It is virtually unknown in areas of the world, such as rural Africa, where high-fiber diets are consumed.

- When diverticula form, the smooth muscle of the colon wall becomes thickened. Lack of dietary fiber slows transit time and more water is absorbed from the stool, making it more difficult to pass through the lumen. Decreased bulk of stool, combined with a more narrowed lumen in the sigmoid colon, causes high intraluminal pressures. These factors are believed to contribute to the formation of diverticula.

The cause of diverticulitis is related to the retention of stool and bacteria in the diverticulum, which form a hardened mass called a *fecalith*. This mass causes inflammation of the diverticulum, which spreads to the surrounding area in the intestines, causing the tissue to become edematous.

Clinical Manifestations

The majority of patients with *diverticulosis* have no symptoms. Those with symptoms typically have crampy, abdominal pain located in the left lower quadrant that is usually relieved by passage of flatus or a bowel movement. Alternating constipation and diarrhea may be present. Approximately 15% of patients with diverticulosis will progress to acute diverticulitis.

In patients with *diverticulitis* abdominal pain is localized over the involved area of the colon. A tender left lower quadrant mass may be felt on palpation of abdomen. Fever, chills, nausea, anorexia, and leukocytosis may also be present. Elderly patients with diverticulitis are frequently afebrile with little to no abdominal tenderness.

- Complications of diverticulitis include perforation with peritonitis, abscess and fistula formation, bowel obstruction, ureteral obstruction, and bleeding. Bleeding is a common complication of diverticulitis and is manifested by *hematochezia* (maroon stools). Bleeding usually stops spontaneously.

Diagnostic Studies
- Complete blood count (CBC) and stool for occult blood
- Barium enema to diagnose diverticular disease
- Sigmoidoscopy
- Colonscopy to rule out hidden polyps or lesions
- Urinalysis and blood culture

Therapeutic Management
Uncomplicated diverticular disease is treated with a high-fiber diet and bulk laxatives, such as psyllium hydrophilic mucilloid (Metamucil). Anticholinergic drugs such as dicyclomine (Bentyl) and Donnatol may be used to relieve discomfort caused by spasm of the bowel. In acute diverticulitis broad-spectrum antibiotic therapy is required. The patient is also maintained on bed rest to decrease intestinal motility and is given nothing by mouth. The white blood cell (WBC) count is monitored. A nasogastric (NG) tube may be necessary.

- Approximately 30% of patients with acute diverticulitis will require surgical intervention. Surgical intervention is necessary to drain abscesses or to resect an obstructing inflammatory mass. Usual surgical procedures involve resection of the involved colon with a temporary diverting colostomy. The colostomy is reanastomosed after the colon is healed.

Nursing Management
- Uncomplicated diverticular disease is primarily treated by a high-fiber diet. Fluids should be increased because fibers retain water, thus decreasing the amount absorbed by the body. If the patient is obese, a reduction in weight is needed.
- Increased intraabdominal pressure should be avoided because it may precipitate an attack. Factors that increase intraabdominal pressure are straining at stool, vomiting, bending, lifting, and tight, restrictive clothing.
- In acute diverticulitis the goal of treatment is to allow the colon to rest and for inflammation to subside. The patient is given nothing by mouth (NPO), kept on bed rest, and given parenteral fluids. The patient needs to be observed for signs of possible peritonitis.
- When the acute attack subsides, oral fluids progressing to a semisolid diet are allowed. Ambulation is also permitted. At this

stage the patient needs to be observed for a recurrent attack. If the patient has a bowel resection or colostomy, nursing care is the same as for these procedures.

DYSMENORRHEA

Definition/Description

Dysmenorrhea is pain or discomfort associated with menstrual flow. The degree of pain and discomfort varies with the individual. Two types of dysmenorrhea exist: *primary,* in which pelvic organs are normal, and *secondary,* in which a diagnosed pelvic disease or condition is the underlying cause of the problem.

- Approximately 50% of all women experience dysmenorrhea, making it one of the most common gynecologic problems.

Pathophysiology

Current evidence suggests that increased production of prostaglandin $F_{2\alpha}$ ($PGF_{2\alpha}$) and prostaglandin E_2 (PGE_2) released from the endometrium at the time of menstruation are associated with *primary dysmenorrhea.*

- Prostaglandins increase myometrial contractions and cause constriction of small endometrial blood vessels, with consequent tissue ischemia, endometrial disintegration, bleeding, and pain.
- Prostaglandins are also known to cause headaches, diarrhea, and vomiting, which are secondary manifestations of dysmenorrhea.
- Dysmenorrhea may be caused by excessive tissue ischemia resulting from increased intrauterine pressure, vessel constriction, and decreased uterine blood flow.
- Dysmenorrhea usually occurs in ovulatory cycles, although it has been noted in anovulatory cycles. Primary dysmenorrhea occurs in some women taking oral contraceptives, but most women experience few or no symptoms while "on the pill."

Secondary dysmenorrhea often occurs well before the onset of menses and may persist for a longer time during the flow than primary dysmenorrhea does.

- Secondary dysmenorrhea is due to pelvic diseases such as endometriosis, chronic pelvic inflammatory disease, uterine leiomyomas, and adenomyosis.

Clinical Manifestations

Primary dysmenorrhea usually occurs within 3 years of menarche.

- Characteristic manifestations include lower midabdominal pain that is colicky in nature, with radiation to the lower back and upper thighs. The abdominal pain is often accompanied by nausea, diarrhea or loose stools, fatigue, headache, and a general sense of malaise.
- The pain usually begins at the onset of menstruation and lasts for 12 to 72 hours, with the most severe pain occurring on the first day.

Secondary dysmenorrhea usually occurs after the woman has experienced problem-free periods for some time. The pain, which may be unilateral, is generally more constant in nature and may continue throughout the period.

D

Therapeutic Management

A major management goal is to distinguish primary from secondary dysmenorrhea. Taking a complete health history and performing a physical examination should be the first procedures. If the history is suggestive of dysmenorrhea and pelvic examination findings are normal, the problem is usually treated as primary dysmenorrhea.

Treatment of dysmenorrhea varies depending on the severity of symptoms and the patient's response. Many patients with dysmenorrhea respond to symptomatic therapy, including reassurance, local heat, and mild analgesics. Since dysmenorrhea is a recurring problem, the use of narcotics is discouraged because addiction is a possibility.

Pharmacologic management. Two groups of drugs considered highly effective for primary dysmenorrhea are nonsteroidal antiinflammatory drugs (NSAIDs) and oral contraceptives.

- Antiinflammatory drugs inhibit the production of prostaglandins in menstrual fluid and their subsequent action on the uterus. NSAIDs such as ibuprofen, naproxen, and mefenamic acid (Ponstel) significantly decrease the frequency and severity of symptoms.
- Oral contraceptives may be the first line of treatment if they are also the woman's contraception choice. With suppression of ovulation by oral contraceptives, production of prostaglandins is also suppressed. Because dysmenorrhea occurs most frequently in young women, there are few contraindications to the use of oral contraceptives.
- Acupuncture, exercise, and transcutaneous nerve stimulation provide varying degrees of relief. These methods may be used for women who obtain inadequate relief from medications or who prefer not to take medications.

Nursing Management

- The nurse should instruct the woman that, during acute pain, relief may be obtained by lying down for short periods, drinking hot beverages, applying heat to the abdomen, and taking an anti-inflammatory drug for mild analgesia.
- The nurse can also suggest noninvasive pain-relieving practices such as distraction and guided imagery. These practices may increase the patient's feeling of control and self-reliance.
- Other health care measures that can decrease discomfort include regular exercise, maintenance of proper nutritional habits, avoidance of constipation, maintenance of good body mechanics, and avoidance of stress and overfatigue, particularly during the time preceding menstrual periods. Staying active and interested in activities may also help.

DYSRHYTHMIAS

Definition/Description

Dysrhythmias are abnormal cardiac rhythms. Prompt assessment of an abnormal cardiac rhythm and the patient's response to the rhythm is critical. Disorders of impulse formation can initiate dysrhythmias. A pacemaker from another site may be discharged in two ways: (1) if the sinoatrial (SA) node discharges more slowly than a secondary pacemaker, electrical discharges from the secondary pacemaker may passively escape and discharge automatically at their intrinsic rates and (2) when the discharge rate is accelerated abnormally and other "pacemakers" take control of the sinus node. A premature beat or a series of premature beats can then occur from ectopic foci (abnormal cardiac impulse) in the atria, ventricles, or atrioventricular (AV) junction.

- Dysrhythmias occur as the result of various abnormalities and disease states; the cause of the dysrhythmia influences treatment of the patient. Common causes of dysrhythmias are presented in Table 27.

Types of Dysrhythmias

To assess a cardiac rhythm, the recommended approach is to note the rate, rhythm, P wave, QRS complex, relationship of P wave to QRS complex, PR interval, QRS interval, and QT interval. Examples of ECG tracings of the common dysrhythmias are presented in Figs. 33-11 through 33-20 in Lewis/Collier/Heitkemper, *Medical-Surgical Nursing,* edition 4, pp. 974-982. Descriptive characteristics of common dysrhythmias are presented in Table 33-6, p. 973.

Table 27	Common Causes of Dysrhythmias

Drug effects or toxicity
Myocardial cell degeneration
Hypertrophy of cardiac muscle
Emotional crisis
Connective tissue disorders
Coffee, tea, tobacco, alcohol
Electrolyte and acid-base imbalances
Cellular hypoxia and edema
Myocardial ischemia

Sinus bradycardia. This condition occurs because the sinus node discharges at a rate of <60 beats per minute (bpm). Sinus bradycardia is a normal sinus rhythm in aerobically trained athletes and during sleep in other individuals. It occurs in response to carotid sinus massage, Valsalva maneuver, hypothermia, increased vagal tone, and administration of parasympathomimetic drugs. Disease states associated with sinus bradycardia are hypothyroidism, increased intracranial pressure, and inferior wall myocardial infarction (MI).

- *Heart rate* (HR) is <60 bpm and *rhythm* is regular.
- Clinical significance of sinus bradycardia depends on how the patient tolerates it hemodynamically. Hypotension with decreased cardiac output (CO) may occur in some circumstances.
- Treatment consists of administration of atropine for patients with symptoms. Pacemaker therapy may be required.

Sinus tachycardia. This dysrhythmia involves an increased discharge rate from the sinus node as a result of vagal inhibition or sympathetic stimulation. The sinus rate is >100 bpm. Sinus tachycardia is associated with physiologic stressors such as exercise, fever, pain, hypovolemia, anemia, hypoxia, hypoglycemia, and congestive heart failure (CHF). It can also be an effect of drugs such as epinephrine, caffeine, theophylline, or nifedipine.

- *HR* is >100 bpm and *rhythm* is regular.
- Clinical significance depends on the patient's tolerance of increased HR. Patient may have symptoms of dizziness, and hypotension may occur.
- Treatment is determined by underlying causes. In certain settings β-blocker therapy (e.g., propranolol) is used to reduce HR and decrease myocardial O_2 consumption.

Premature atrial contraction (PAC). PAC occurs as a result of contractions originating from an ectopic focus in the atrium in a location other than sinus node. It originates in the left or right atrium and travels across the atria by an abnormal pathway, creating a distorted P wave. At the AV node it is stopped (nonconducted PAC), delayed (lengthened PR interval), or conducted normally. It moves through the AV node and in most cases is conducted normally through the ventricles. In a normal heart a PAC can result from emotional stress or the use of caffeine, tobacco, or alcohol. A PAC can also result from disease states such as infection, thyrotoxicosis, chronic obstructive pulmonary disease (COPD), and heart disease (including atherosclerotic heart disease), and valvular disease.

- *HR* varies with the underlying rate and frequency of PAC, and *rhythm* is irregular.
- Treatment depends on patient symptoms. Withdrawal of sources of stimulation such as caffeine may be warranted. Drugs such as digoxin, quinidine, procainamide, and β-blockers can be used.

Paroxysmal supraventricular tachycardia (PSVT). PSVT is a dysrhythmia originating in an ectopic focus anywhere above the bifurcation of the bundle of His. *Paroxysmal* refers to an abrupt onset and termination. Some degree of AV block may be present. In the normal heart PSVT is associated with overexertion, emotional stress, deep inspiration, and stimulants such as caffeine and tobacco. In disease states PSVT is associated with Wolff-Parkinson-White (WPW) syndrome (conduction via accessory pathways), digitalis intoxication, coronary artery disease (CAD), or cor pulmonale.

- *HR* is 100 to 300 bpm, and *rhythm* is regular.
- Clinical significance depends on the symptoms and HR. A prolonged episode and HR >180 bpm may precipitate a decreased CO with hypotension and myocardial ischemia.
- Treatment includes vagal stimulation induced by carotid massage or Valsalva maneuver. The drug of choice is adenosine, a drug with a very short half-life (10 seconds) that successfully converts PSVT to sinus rhythm in a high percentage of patients. Verapamil, digitalis, and propranolol can also be used.

Atrial flutter. This condition is an atrial tachydysrhythmia identified by recurring, regular sawtooth-shaped flutter waves. It is usually associated with a slower ventricular response. Because of the refractoriness of the AV node, there is usually some AV block in a fixed ratio of flutter waves to QRS responses (e.g., 2:1, 3:1). Atrial flutter is a relatively rare dysrhythmia and rarely occurs in a normal heart. In disease states it is associated with CAD, hypertension, mitral valve disorders, pulmonary embolus, cor pulmonale, and with the use of drugs such as digitalis, quinidine, and epinephrine.

- *Atrial rate* is 250 to 350 bpm. *Ventricular rate* varies according to the conduction ratio. In 2:1 conduction, ventricular rate is typically about 150 bpm. *Atrial* and *ventricular rhythms* are usually regular.

- High ventricular rates can decrease CO and cause serious consequences such as heart failure.
- Primary goal in treatment is to slow ventricular response by increasing AV block. Electrical cardioversion may be used to convert atrial flutter to sinus rhythm in an emergency situation. Drugs used include verapamil, digoxin, quinidine, procainamide, and β-blockers.

Atrial fibrillation. This condition involves a total disorganization of atrial electrical activity without effective atrial contraction. ECG demonstrates baseline fibrillatory waves or undulations of variable contour at a rate of 300 to 600 bpm. Ventricular response is irregular, and if the patient is untreated, the ventricular rate will be 100 to 160 bpm. The dysrhythmia may be chronic or intermittent and usually occurs in the patient with an underlying heart disease. It is also associated with alcoholism, infection, and stress.

- *Atrial rate* may be as high as 350 to 600 bpm. *Ventricular rate* can vary from 50 bpm to 180 bpm. *Atrial rhythm* is chaotic and *ventricular rhythm* is usually irregular.
- Atrial fibrillation can often result in a decrease in CO because of ineffective atrial contractions and rapid ventricular response. Thrombi may form in atria as a result of ineffective atrial contraction. Embolization to the arterial system may occur as a complication with subsequent development of a stroke.
- Goal of treatment is a decrease in ventricular response. In emergency situations cardioversion may be used to convert atrial fibrillation to normal sinus rhythm. Medications used for pharmaceutical cardioversion or a decrease in ventricular response include digoxin, verapamil, diltiazem, quinidine, and β-blockers.

First-degree AV block. In this type of AV block every impulse is conducted to the ventricles, but the duration of AV conduction is prolonged. This is manifested by a PR interval >0.2 second. After the impulse moves through the AV node, it is usually conducted normally through the ventricles. A first-degree AV block is associated with MI, chronic ischemic heart disease, rheumatic fever, hyperthyroidism, and drugs such as digitalis, β-blockers, and IV verapamil.

- *HR* is normal and *rhythm* is regular.
- First-degree AV block may be a precursor of higher degrees of AV block.
- There is no treatment for first-degree AV block.

Second-degree AV block, type I (Mobitz I, Wenckebach phenomenon). This condition includes gradual lengthening of the PR interval, which occurs because of AV conduction time that is prolonged until an atrial impulse is nonconducted and the QRS complex is dropped. Once a ventricular beat is dropped, the cycle repeats itself with progressive lengthening of PR intervals until another QRS complex is dropped. The rhythm appears on the ECG in a pattern of grouped beats. Duration of the QRS complex is normal or prolonged. Type I AV block most commonly occurs in the AV node and may result from the use of drugs such as digoxin or β-blockers. It may also be associated with ischemic cardiac disease and other diseases that can slow AV conduction.

- *Atrial rate* is normal, but *ventricular rate* may be slower as a result of dropped QRS complexes. *Ventricular rhythm* is irregular.
- Type I AV block is usually a result of inferior MI. It is almost always transient and well tolerated. However, it may be a warning signal of impending significant AV conduction disturbance.
- If the patient is symptomatic, atropine is used to increase the HR, or a temporary pacemaker may be needed, especially if patient has an acute MI.

Second-degree heart block, type II (Mobitz II).   In this type of heart block, the P wave is nonconducted without progressive antecedent PR lengthening, which occurs when a bundle branch block is present. On conducted beats, the PR interval is constant. Second-degree heart block is a more serious type in which a certain number of impulses from the sinus node are not conducted to ventricles. This occurs in ratios of 2:1, 3:1, and so on when there are two P waves to one QRS complex, three P waves to one QRS complex, and so on. It may occur with varying ratios. Type II AV block almost always occurs in the His-Purkinje system and is associated with rheumatic and atherosclerotic heart disease, acute anterior MI, and digitoxicity.

- *Atrial rate* is usually normal. *Ventricular rate* depends on the intrinsic rate and degree of AV block. *Sinus rhythm* is regular, but *ventricular rhythm* may be irregular.
- Type II AV block often progresses to third-degree AV block and is associated with a poor prognosis. Reduced HR may result in decreased CO with subsequent hypotension and myocardial ischemia. Type II AV block is an indication for therapy with a permanent pacemaker.
- Treatment before insertion of a permanent pacemaker involves the use of a temporary pacemaker (see Pacemakers, p. 671). Drugs such as atropine, epinephrine, or dopamine can be tried as temporary measures to increase HR until pacemaker therapy is available.

Third-degree AV heart block (complete heart block).   This condition constitutes one form of AV dissociation in which no impulses from the atria are conducted to the ventricles. Atria are stimulated and contract independently of ventricles. Ventricular rhythm is an escape rhythm, and the focus may be above or below the bifurcation of the bundle of His. This rhythm is associated with fibrosis or calcification of cardiac conduction system, CAD, myocarditis, cardiomyopathy, and open heart surgery.

- *Atrial rate* is usually a sinus rate of 60 to 100 bpm. *Ventricular rate* depends on the site of the block. If it is in the AV node, the rate is 40 to 60 bpm. If it is in the Purkinje system, the rate is 20 to 40 bpm. *Atrial* and *ventricular rhythms* are regular but asynchronous.
- Third-degree AV block almost always results in reduced CO with subsequent ischemia and heart failure.
- A temporary pacemaker may be inserted or an external pacemaker may be applied on an emergency basis in the patient with an acute MI. Use of drugs such as atropine, epinephrine, and dopamine are temporary treatments to increase HR and support BP before pacemaker insertion (see Pacemakers, p. 671).

Premature ventricular contractions (PVCs). These contractions originate in an ectopic focus in the ventricles. PVCs are a premature occurrence of the QRS complex, which is wide and distorted in shape. PVCs that are initiated from different foci appear different in contour from each other and are termed *multifocal PVCs.* When every other beat is a PVC, the dysrhythmia is called *ventricular bigeminy.* When every third beat is a PVC, it is called *ventricular trigeminy.* Two consecutive PVCs are called *couplets.* Three consecutive PVCs are called *triplets. Ventricular tachycardia* occurs when there are three or more consecutive PVCs. When a PVC falls on the T wave of a preceding beat, the *R on T phenomenon* occurs and is considered to be quite dangerous because it may precipitate ventricular tachycardia or ventricular fibrillation. PVCs are associated with stimulants such as caffeine, alcohol, epinephrine, and digoxin. They are also associated with hypokalemia, fever, and emotional stress. Disease states associated with PVCs include MI, mitral valve prolapse, CHF, and CAD.

- *HR* varies according to the intrinsic rate and the number of PVCs. *Rhythm* is irregular because of premature beats.
- PVCs are usually a benign finding in the patient with a normal heart. In heart disease PVCs may reduce CO and precipitate angina and heart failure. PVCs in ischemic heart disease or acute MI represent ventricular irritability.
- Indications for treatment in an appropriate clinical setting include (1) six or more PVCs occurring per minute, (2) ventricular couplets and triplets, (3) multifocal PVCs, and (4) R on T phenomenon. If treatment is not initiated, ventricular tachycardia or ventricular fibrillation may occur. For treating PVCs, lidocaine is the drug of choice. Procainamide is the second drug of choice if lidocaine is ineffective.

Ventricular tachycardia. This dysrhythmia is a run of three or more PVCs that occurs when the ectopic focus or foci fire repetitively and the ventricle takes control as the pacemaker. The ventricular rate is 110 to 250 bpm. Atria may also be depolarized by the ventricles in a retrograde fashion.

The appearance of ventricular tachycardia is an ominous sign because it usually indicates the presence of cardiac disease. It is considered a life-threatening dysrhythmia because of decreased CO and the possibility of deterioration of ventricular tachycardia to ventricular fibrillation, which is a lethal dysrhythmia. Ventricular tachycardia is associated with acute MI, CAD, significant electrolyte imbalances (e.g., potassium), cardiomyopathy, and coronary reperfusion after thrombolytic therapy. The dysrhythmia has also been observed in patients who have no evidence of cardiac disease.

- If the patient is hemodynamically stable, treatment consists of administration of a lidocaine bolus. If this treatment abolishes tachycardia, a continuous lidocaine infusion should be started. If lidocaine is ineffective, IV procainamide may be tried. If this treatment is successful, a continuous procainamide infusion should be started. A third drug of choice is IV bretylium.
- If a patient is unconscious or hemodynamically unstable, immediate cardioversion is recommended. A defibrillator is used in synchronized mode for cardioversion.

Ventricular fibrillation. This condition is a severe derangement of heart rhythm characterized on ECG by irregular undulations of varying contour and amplitude. This anomaly represents the firing of multiple ectopic foci in the ventricle. Mechanically, the ventricle is simply "quivering," and no effective contraction or CO occurs. This type of fibrillation occurs in acute MI and myocardial ischemia and in chronic diseases such as CAD and cardiomyopathy. It may occur during cardiac pacing or cardiac catheterization procedures as a result of catheter stimulation of the ventricle. Other clinical associations are accidental electrical shock, hyperkalemia, and hypoxemia.

- *HR* is not measurable. *Rhythm* is irregular and chaotic.
- Ventricular fibrillation results in unconsciousness, absence of pulse, apnea, and seizures. If left untreated, the patient will die.
- Treatment consists of immediate initiation of cardiopulmonary resuscitation (CPR) and initiation of advanced cardiac life support (ACLS) measures with the use of defibrillation and definitive drug therapy.

ENCEPHALITIS

Definition/Description

Encephalitis, an acute inflammation of the brain, is usually caused by a virus. Many different viruses have been implicated in encephalitis, some of them associated with certain seasons of the year and endemic to certain geographic areas. For example, *epidemic encephalitis* is transmitted by ticks and mosquitoes, whereas *nonepidemic encephalitis* may occur as a complication of measles, chickenpox, or mumps (see Table 28). Encephalitis is a serious, sometimes fatal disease with a mortality of 5% to 20%.

The disease is characterized by diffuse damage to nerve cells of the brain, perivascular cellular infiltration, proliferation of glia, and increasing cerebral edema. Sequelae of encephalitis includes mental deterioration, amnesia, personality changes, and hemiparesis.

Clinical manifestations resemble those of meningitis, but they have a more gradual onset, including headache, high fever, convulsions, and a change in level of consciousness. Diagnostic studies for encephalitis are described in Table 28.

Therapeutic and Nursing Management

Therapeutic and nursing management are symptomatic and supportive. Cerebral edema is a major problem with hypertonic solutions and corticosteroids used to control it. Vidarabine suspension (Vira-A) is used in the treatment of herpes simplex encephalitis. For maximal benefit, the medication must be started before the onset of coma. Acyclovir is also used for the treatment of herpes simplex encephalitis. It has fewer side effects than vidarabine and is often the preferred treatment.

Table 28   Cerebral Inflammatory Conditions

	Meningitis	Encephalitis	Brain abscess
Causative organisms	Bacteria (pneumococci, meningococci, streptococci), yeasts, fungi, viruses	Bacteria, fungi, parasites, herpes simplex virus, other viruses	Streptococci, staphylococci through bloodstream
CSF			
Pressure (normal, 60-150 mm H_2O)	Increased	Normal to slight increase, increase with increased ICP	Increased
WBC count (normal, 0-8/μL)	500/μL (mainly PMN)	<500/μL, PMN (early), lymphocytes (later)	25-300/μL (PMN)
Protein (normal, 15-45 mg/dl [0.15-0.45g/L])	High	Slight increase	Normal
Glucose (normal, 45-75 mg/dl [2.5-4.2 mmol/L])	Low or absent	Normal	Low or absent
Appearance	Turbid	Clear	Clear
Diagnostic studies	Stained smears and cultures	Viral studies	CT scan, EEG, skull x-ray
Treatment	Antibiotics with sensitivity tests	Supportive, prevention of symptoms of increased ICP, vidarabine (Vira-A)	Antibiotics, incision and drainage

CSF, Cerebrospinal fluid; EEG, electroencephalogram; ICP, intracranial pressure; PMN, polymorphonuclear cells; WBC, white blood cell.

ENDOCARDITIS, INFECTIVE

Definition/Description

Infective endocarditis, previously known as bacterial endocarditis, is an infection of the endocardial surface. Inflammation from infective endocarditis frequently affects the cardiac valves. Although the most common cause of infective endocarditis is bacterial infection, it may be caused by a variety of microorganisms. Before the era of antibiotics, infective endocarditis was almost always fatal.

Classification

Two forms of infective endocarditis, *subacute* and *acute,* have been described.

- The *subacute form* has a longer clinical course of more insidious onset with less toxicity, and the causative organism is usually of low virulence (most often *Streptococcus viridans*).
- The *acute form* has a shorter clinical course with a more rapid onset, increased toxicity, and a more virulent causative organism (usually *Staphylococcus aureus*).

Although this classification system has been used historically and may be conceptually useful, clinicians prefer to classify infective endocarditis based on the etiologic agent.

Pathophysiology

The term *bacterial endocarditis* has been replaced by *infective endocarditis* because causative organisms include fungi, chlamydiae, rickettsiae, and bacteria. Streptococci and staphylococci account for the majority of cases.

Infective endocarditis occurs when turbulence within the heart allows the causative organism to infect previously damaged valves or other endothelial surfaces. The damage may occur in individuals with underlying cardiac conditions such as rheumatic heart disease, prosthetic valves, and mitral valve prolapse with murmur. A variety of invasive procedures (e.g., surgical interventions, IV injection, and diagnostic procedures) can allow large numbers of organisms to enter the bloodstream and trigger the infectious process.

- *Vegetations,* the primary lesions of infective endocarditis, consist of fibrin, leukocytes, platelets, and microbes that adhere to the valve surface or endocardium.
- The loss of portions of these friable vegetations into the circulation results in embolization. Systemic embolization occurs from left-sided heart vegetations, progressing to organ (particularly kidney, spleen, and brain) and limb infarction. Right-sided heart lesions embolize to the lungs.

- The infection may spread locally to cause damage to valves or to their supporting structures.
- The resulting valvular incompetence and eventual invasion of the myocardium results in congestive heart failure (CHF), generalized myocardial dysfunction, and sepsis.

Clinical Manifestations

Clinical manifestations are nonspecific and can involve multiple organ systems. Fever occurs in >90% of patients with endocarditis.

- *Nonspecific manifestations* that may accompany the fever include chills, weakness, malaise, fatigue, and anorexia. Arthralgias, myalgias, back pain, weight loss, headache, and clubbing of fingers may occur in subacute forms of endocarditis.
- *Vascular manifestations* include *splinter hemorrhages* (black longitudinal streaks) that may occur in the nailbeds. Petechiae, as a result of fragmentation and microembolization of vegetative lesions, are common in the conjunctivae, lips, buccal mucosa, palate, and over the ankles, feet, antecubital, and popliteal areas. *Osler nodes* (painful, tender, red or purple, pea-size lesions) may be found on the fingertips or toes. *Janeway lesions* (flat, painless, small, red spots) may be found on the palms and soles. Funduscopic examination may reveal hemorrhagic retinal lesions called *Roth's spots.*
- Onset of a new murmur is frequently noted with infective endocarditis, with the aortic and mitral valves most commonly affected.
- Clinical manifestations secondary to embolization in various body organs may also be present: (1) embolization to the spleen may result in sharp left upper quadrant pain and splenomegaly, local tenderness, and abdominal rigidity; (2) embolization to the kidneys may cause pain in the flank, hematuria, azotemia, and glomerulonephritis; (3) emboli may lodge in small peripheral blood vessels of arms and legs and cause gangrene; (4) embolization to the brain may cause neurologic problems such as hemiplegia, ataxia, aphasia, visual changes, and change in level of consciousness; and (5) pulmonary emboli may occur in right-sided endocarditis.

Diagnostic Studies

A recent health history should be obtained with inquiry made regarding any recent dental, urologic, surgical, or gynecologic procedures, including normal or abnormal obstetric delivery. Previous history of heart disease, recent cardiac catheterization, and skin, respiratory, or urinary tract infections should also be documented.

- Blood culture and sensitivity may reveal positive cultures.

- White blood cell (WBC) count with differential may demonstrate mild leukocytosis.
- Rheumatoid factor is positive in some patients.
- Urinalysis may demonstrate hematuria.
- Chest x-ray is used to detect CHF.
- ECG may reveal changes.
- Echocardiography may identify vegetations on valves.
- Cardiac catheterization is done when surgical intervention is considered.

Prophylactic Treatment

Cardiac lesions, prosthetic valves, acquired valvular disease, mitral valve prolapse, prior endocarditis, and noncardiac diseases are the principal risk factors for infective endocarditis. Procedure-associated risks include IV injection of recreational drugs and specific dental, medical, or surgical procedures.

- Antibiotic prophylaxis is recommended for patients with specific cardiac conditions before they undergo certain dental or surgical procedures.
- Antibiotic prophylaxis should also be instituted in high-risk patients who are to undergo removal or drainage of infected tissue, have indwelling cardiac pacemakers, undergo renal dialysis, or have ventriculoatrial shunts for management of hydrocephalus.

Therapeutic Management

Accurate identification of the infecting organism is the key to successful treatment. The appropriate antibiotic (usually given intravenously) is chosen on the basis of sensitivity studies. Complete eradication of the organism generally takes weeks to achieve, and relapses are common.

- The patient's antibiotic serum levels should be monitored periodically. Subsequent blood cultures may be done to evaluate the effectiveness of antibiotic therapy. Blood cultures that remain positive indicate inadequate or inappropriate antibiotic administration, aortic root or myocardial abscess, or the wrong diagnosis (e.g., an infection elsewhere).
- Fever may persist for several days after treatment has been started and is treated with aspirin or acetaminophen, fluids, and rest.
- Complete bed rest is usually not indicated unless the patient's temperature remains elevated or there are signs of heart damage.

Results of pharmacologic management alone are generally poor in patients with fungal endocarditis and prosthetic valve endocarditis. Early valve replacement followed by prolonged pharmacologic management is recommended in these situations.

Nursing Management

Goals

The patient with infective endocarditis will have normal cardiac function with no residual cardiac damage, will perform activities of daily living (ADLs) without fatigue, and will understand the therapeutic regimen to prevent recurrence of endocarditis.

See the nursing care plan for the patient with infective endocarditis in Lewis/Collier/Heitkemper, *Medical-Surgical Nursing,* edition 4, p. 1010.

Nursing Diagnoses

- Decreased cardiac output related to valvular insufficiency and fluid overload
- Activity intolerance related to generalized weakness and alteration in oxygen transport secondary to valvular dysfunction
- Anxiety related to critical illness and prolonged hospitalization
- Altered comfort: fever related to infection of cardiac tissue
- Diversional activity deficit related to restricted mobility and activity
- Altered health maintenance related to lack of knowledge about disease and treatment process
- Altered nutrition: less than body requirements related to anorexia

Nursing Interventions

The incidence of infective endocarditis can be decreased by identifying individuals who are at risk for the development of endocarditis. Assessment of the patient's history and understanding of the disease process are crucial for planning and implementing appropriate health maintenance strategies.

Infective endocarditis generally requires treatment with antibiotics for 4 to 6 weeks. The patient usually requires in-hospital stabilization and then may be treated with outpatient parenteral antibiotic therapy (OPAT). Some patients may not be candidates for OPAT and may require a more prolonged hospitalization period.

- Fever, chronic or intermittent, is a common early sign of infective endocarditis. Frequent assessment of body temperature is important because persistent prolonged temperature elevations may mean that the drug therapy is ineffective.
- The patient needs adequate periods of physical and emotional rest. Bed rest may be necessary when fever is present or there are complications (e.g., heart damage). Otherwise the patient may ambulate and perform moderate activity.
- Laboratory data should be monitored to determine the effectiveness of long-term, high-dose antibiotic therapy.
- IV lines should be monitored for patency, and antibiotics should be given when scheduled. The patient should be monitored continuously for undesirable reactions to the drugs.

- To prevent problems because of immobility, the patient should wear elastic compression gradient stockings, perform range-of-motion (ROM) exercises, and turn, cough, and deep breathe every 2 hours.
- The patient may experience anxiety and fear associated with the illness. The nurse must recognize this problem and implement strategies to help reduce patient fears and anxieties.

Patients who receive OPAT will require vigilant home nursing care. Patients with active endocarditis are at risk for life-threatening complications such as cerebral emboli and pulmonary edema.

- Adequacy of the home environment in terms of in-home companions and hospital access must be determined for successful management.
- After therapy is completed in either the home or hospital setting, management will focus on educating the patient about the nature of the disease and on reducing the risk of reinfection.

Patient Teaching

Education is crucial for the patient's understanding of and adherence to the planned treatment regimen.

- The patient should understand the need to avoid persons with infection, especially upper respiratory, and to report cold, flu, and cough symptoms.
- The importance of avoiding excessive fatigue and the need to plan rest periods before and after activity should be carefully explained to the patient.
- Good oral hygiene, including daily care and regular dental visits, is also important.
- The patient must inform all health care providers performing dental, medical, or surgical procedures of the history of heart disease.
- The patient should understand the significance of the prophylactic antibiotic therapy given before any invasive procedure.
- Education of the patient who is at risk or has had infective endocarditis helps reduce the incidence and recurrence of the disease.
- Once therapy has been completed, the patient should be instructed about symptoms that may indicate recurrent infection such as fever, fatigue, malaise, and chills. If any of these symptoms occur, the patient should be aware of the importance of notifying the physician.

ENDOMETRIAL CANCER

Definition/Description

Cancer of the endometrium has become the most common gynecologic malignancy, accounting for about 50% of all female genital
tract neoplasms. However, it has a relatively low cause of mortality,
with approximately 75% survival.

- Highest incidence is associated with women who are between
  the ages of 50 and 70 years, nulliparous, obese, hypertensive,
  diabetic, or had a late menopause and/or prolonged unopposed
  estrogen-only replacement therapy.
- Possible external factors contributing to a current increase in
  incidence include aging of the population, better reporting of
  cases, and more widespread prescribing of estrogens for postmenopausal women.

Pathophysiology

This type of cancer arises from the lining of the endometrium. The
precursor may be a hyperplastic state that progresses to invasive
carcinoma. Direct extension develops into the cervix and through
the uterine serosa. As invasion of the myometrium occurs, regional
lymph nodes, including the paravaginal and paraaortic nodes, become involved. Hematogenous metastases develop concurrently.
The usual sites of metastases are lung, bone, liver, and brain. Most
tumors are adenocarcinomas. Endometrial cancer grows slowly,
metastasizes late, and is amenable to therapy if diagnosed early.

Clinical Manifestations

The first symptom of endometrial cancer is abnormal uterine bleeding, usually in postmenopausal women. Because perimenopausal
women have sporadic bleeding for a time, it is important that this
sign not be ignored or automatically blamed on menopause. Pain
occurs late in the disease process, and other symptoms that may
arise are related to metastasis to other organs.

Diagnostic Studies

Dilation and curettage (D & C), endometrial biopsy, and smears are
used to diagnose endometrial cancer.

- D & C and endometrial biopsy can be done as an office procedure in which endometrial tissue is "aspirated" from the uterus.
  Occurrence of breakthrough bleeding in a postmenopausal
  woman mandates obtaining a tissue sample to exclude endometrial cancer.

- The Pap test is not a reliable diagnostic tool for endometrial cancer, but it can rule out cervical cancer.

Therapeutic Management

Treatment is carried out with total hysterectomy, which includes bilateral salpingo-oophorectomy with selective node biopsies. Surgery may be followed by radiation, administered either externally with cobalt or internally with intracavitary radium (see Radiation Therapy, p. 675). Chemotherapy is reserved for recurrences or distant metastases. Progesterone therapy (e.g., Provera, Megace) is the treatment of choice when the progesterone receptor status is positive and the tumor is well differentiated. Chemotherapy is considered when progesterone therapy is unsuccessful.

Nursing Management of Malignant Tumors

See Surgical Procedures Involving the Female Reproductive System, p. 677.

E

ENDOMETRIOSIS

Definition/Description

Endometriosis is a condition characterized by the presence and proliferation of endometrial tissue in sites outside the endometrial cavity. The most frequent sites are in or near the ovaries, uterosacral ligaments, and uterovesical peritoneum. However, endometrial tissues can be in many other locations such as the stomach, lungs, and spleen.

- The tissue responds to hormones of the ovarian cycle and undergoes a mini-menstruation similar to the shedding of uterine endometrium.
- Endometriosis appears to cause infertility in 30% to 60% of cases.
- Although many theories about the cause of endometriosis have been advanced, the etiology remains unknown.

Clinical Manifestations

Symptoms may be vague and diffuse because of the multiple sites affected.

- Some patients have no symptoms, and the disease is discovered incidental to abdominal surgery.
- More commonly, the patient complains of pelvic pain that takes the form of secondary dysmenorrhea. The pain is described as dull, aching, or cramping in the lower abdominal region, oc-

curring 1 to 2 days before menses and diminishing after the onset of menstrual flow. It may be related to hemorrhagic distention of the cystlike nodules or escape of bloody discharge into the peritoneal cavity.

- Backache, abnormal uterine bleeding, dyspareunia, and painful defecation are other symptoms.
- As the ectopic endometrium sheds, blood collects in cystlike nodules that have a characteristic bluish-black look.
- When a cyst ruptures, the pain may be acute, and the resulting irritation promotes formation of adhesions, which fix the affected area to another pelvic structure. The adhesions may become severe enough to cause a bowel obstruction or painful micturition. Adhesions involving the uterus, tubes, or ovaries may result in infertility.

Diagnostic Studies

Diagnosis is frequently confirmed by the patient's health history and the palpation of firm nodular lumps in the adnexa on bimanual examination. Examination of the typical bluish nodes with culdoscopy or laparoscopy or during a laparotomy establishes a definite diagnosis.

Therapeutic Management

Treatment is influenced by the patient's age, desire to bear children, and severity of the symptoms. Pregnancy and lactation often result in relief of symptoms because menstruation ceases during this time. With menopause, ovarian atrophy begins and hormonal stimulation declines, usually leading to the disappearance of the symptoms.

- Observation and mild analgesia are used initially when symptoms are not severe or incapacitating.

Pharmacologic Management

Management with drugs is directed at imitating a state of pregnancy or menopause since both natural conditions relieve symptoms. Hormonal therapy can control, but not cure, endometriosis.

- Continuous use (for 9 months) of combined progestin and estrogen softens and causes regression of endometrial tissue. Ovulation is suppressed and *pseudopregnancy* (hyperhormonal amenorrhea) is produced. However, because of troublesome side effects, this treatment modality is used less frequently today.
- Another approach to hormonal treatment is administration of danazol (Danocrine), a synthetic androgen that inhibits the anterior pituitary. The drug produces a pseudomenopause (ovarian suppression), with consequent atrophy of ectopic endometrial tissue. Subjective relief of symptoms is noted within 6 weeks of danazol use.
- The newest and most expensive drug therapy is an injectable gonadotropin-releasing hormone agonist (leuprolide acetate

[Lupron]). It causes a hypoestrogenic state, resulting in amenorrhea.

Surgical Interventions

- *Conservative surgery* is used in the management of a young woman with infertility. It involves removal or destruction of endometrial implants and lysing or excision of adhesions by means of laparoscopic laser surgery and laparotomy. Gonadotropin-releasing hormone (GnRH) agonist therapy (e.g., Lupron) can be administered for 4 to 6 months to reduce the size of the lesions before surgery. Efforts are made to conserve all tissues necessary to maintain fertility.

- *Radical surgery* is generally performed in women approaching menopause. It involves removal of the uterus, tubes, ovaries, and as many endometrial implants as possible.

- *Hysterectomy* with removal of as many implants as possible but with preservation of all or part of the ovarian tissue is recommended for the young woman who does not want children but wishes to have cyclical ovarian function.

Nursing Management

- Nurses should encourage women to have regular physical examinations in an effort to identify early symptoms of endometriosis. Patient education about the disease process can clarify and dispel false ideas and fears.

- Dysmenorrhea after years of relatively pain-free menses and infertility after a period of trying to achieve pregnancy may serve as clues to the presence of this disease.

- When symptoms are less severe, treatment for dysmenorrhea and a "wait-and-see" approach may be used.

- Education of the patient and reassurance that a health-threatening situation does not exist may permit her to accept a conservative and progressive treatment. The nurse is often the person who counsels the patient in the use of the prescribed drugs.

- Psychologic support may be needed for the patient experiencing severe disabling pain, sexual difficulties secondary to dyspareunia, and infertility.

- If conservative surgery is the treatment selected, nursing care is similar to general preoperative and postoperative care of a patient undergoing laparotomy (see Abdominal Pain, Acute, nursing management after laparotomy, p. 3).

- If radical surgery is planned, nursing care is similar to that of the patient undergoing an abdominal hysterectomy.

See the nursing care plan for the patient with a total abdominal hysterectomy in Lewis/Collier/Heitkemper, *Medical-Surgical Nursing,* edition 4, p. 1609.

EPIDIDYMITIS

Epididymitis is an inflammatory process of the epididymis, usually secondary to an infectious process (sexually or nonsexually transmitted), trauma, or urinary reflux down the vas deferens. Swelling may progress to the point that the epididymis and testis are indistinguishable. The problem may be associated with prostatitis and is usually painful.

- Conservative treatment consists of bed rest with elevation of the scrotum, the use of ice packs, and analgesics. Ambulation places the scrotum in a dependent position and increases pain.
- The use of antibiotics is important for both partners if transmission of the infection is through sexual contact.
- Most tenderness subsides within 1 week, although swelling may last for weeks or months.

ERECTILE DYSFUNCTION

Definition/Description

Erectile dysfunction is the inability to attain or maintain an erect penis that allows satisfactory sexual performance. Erectile dysfunction is increasing in all segments of the sexually active male population. In younger men the increase is attributed to an increase in substance abuse, such as recreational drugs and alcohol. Some middle-aged men are affected by modern medical technology such as major organ transplants, bypass surgeries, and chemotherapeutic agents.

- Stress factors associated with modern lifestyles are affecting men of all ages and contribute greatly to the psychologic causes of erectile failure.
- Erectile dysfunction can occur at any age, although it is most common between the ages of 55 and 65 years. When the problem occurs during more than 25% of sexual encounters, intervention is appropriate.

Pathophysiology

Erection is a parasympathetic reflex initiated mainly by certain tactile, visual, and mental stimuli. It consists of dilatation of arteries and arterioles of the penis, which in turn fills and distends spaces in its erectile tissue and compresses its veins. Therefore more blood enters the penis through dilated arteries and then leaves it through constricted veins. Hence the penis become larger and rigid; in other words, erection occurs. Problems develop when these spaces (corporeal bodies) fail to fill when desired or when they empty before orgasm.

- There are two classifications of erectile dysfunction: *primary dysfunction* occurs when the patient has never been able to have an adequate erection with any type of sexual experience; *secondary dysfunction* occurs when the patient has lost the ability to have an erection or is able to have an erection in only a particular way.

Risk factors may be physiologic, psychologic, or both. These include anatomic anomalies (e.g., congenital deformities and cardiorespiratory disorders [emphysema]), drug-induced (e.g., caffeine and diuretics) states, endocrine imbalances (e.g., diabetes mellitus), genitourinary disorders (e.g., prostatitis), psychogenic factors (e.g., depression and fatigue), and neurologic problems (e.g., spinal cord trauma). For a summary of these risk factors, see Table 52-8 in Lewis/Collier/Heitkemper, *Medical-Surgical Nursing,* edition 4, p. 1644.

The major complication is that the man's inability to perform sexually can cause stress in his interpersonal relationships and may preclude sex role functioning. See Table 52-9 in Lewis/Collier/Heitkemper, *Medical-Surgical Nursing,* edition 4, p. 1645, for normal age-related changes in sexual performance and an explanation of these changes.

Diagnostic Studies

Rapid advances have been made in the diagnosis and treatment of erectile dysfunction. Diagnostic testing includes:

- Detailed sexual history, including practices and techniques
- Psychosocial and neurologic evaluation
- Testosterone levels; blood chemistry and profile (e.g., prolactin, follicle-stimulating hormone [FSH], luteinizing hormone [LH])
- Prostate specific antigen (PSA) levels
- Intracavernosal vasoactive drug testing
- Vascular flow studies (e.g., duplex Doppler, cavernosogram)
- Sleep tumescence studies
- Tests to exclude unrecognized systemic disease: complete blood count (CBC), urinalysis, creatinine, lipid profile, fasting blood sugar, and thyroid function studies

Therapeutic Management

Treatment of erectile dysfunction is based on the cause.

- Treatment of psychologic causes of erectile dysfunction should be carried out by a qualified therapist. The approach may be behavioral or psychologic. In some patients it may also involve therapeutic intervention to restore self-confidence. The goal of therapy is to have the man and his partner develop a satisfactory sexual relationship after treatment.

- When the problem is physical, interventions are directed at correcting or eliminating the cause or restoring function through medical means. The results of these interventions are usually satisfactory when both partners are involved in the decision-making process and have realistic expectations of the treatment.
- Suction devices applied to the flaccid penis produce a vacuum within a cylinder, thereby pulling blood up into the corporeal bodies and producing an erection. A penile ring or other device placed around the base of the penis causes vasoconstriction and prevents detumescence (subsidence of swelling).
- When these devices are used, special care must be taken to prevent tissue damage. Suction devices are sometimes used in conjunction with intracorporeal injection therapy in patients with moderate-to-severe venous leakage of penile veins.

Some patients do not require penetration for satisfactory sexual expression and may use a vibrator or dildo (rubber penis). Patients experiencing temporary loss of erection or who are awaiting surgical intervention may use a variety of methods to achieve sexual satisfaction. Sexual counselors or therapists acting as consultants can provide support and suggest alternative forms of sexual expression.

Noninvasive treatment methods should be the primary approach to care with invasive and experimental techniques limited to research centers.

- Elimination of or substitution for a medication that causes erectile dysfunction (e.g., methyldopa, propranolol) is sometimes all that is necessary to alleviate the problem. Yohimbine (Yocan) is a mild vasodilator and reported aphrodisiac. It is often used in conjunction with other forms of therapy and may serve to provide a placebo effect or boost the confidence of the man.
- When there is an established diagnosis of testicular failure (hypogonadism), androgen replacement therapy may sometimes be effective in improving erectile dysfunction. An intramuscular (IM) injection of testosterone enanthate orcypionate should be given. Effectiveness of testosterone supplementation for older men experiencing a normal, gradual decline is doubtful.
- Intracavernosal injection therapy is a diagnostic and treatment option that is gaining in popularity. Vasoactive medications (e.g., papaverine, prostaglandin E_1, phentolamine, or combinations of these) are injected directly into the corporeal body.

Surgical Interventions

Penile implants are used to treat erectile dysfunction. These paired devices can be semirigid, malleable, or inflatable. They are implanted into the corporeal bodies to provide an erection firm enough for penetration.

- All implants provide a usable erection and should be chosen carefully based on the man's mental and physical capabilities, surgical risk factors, personal lifestyle, insurance, and financial resources.
- The main problems associated with penile prostheses are mechanical failure, infection, and erosions.
- For essentially healthy men, the surgical procedure may be done on an outpatient basis, with patients being monitored by home care nurses. Complete recovery time varies from 4 to 6 weeks.
- Sexual counseling is often recommended before and after surgery to deal with unrealistic expectations and restore or promote techniques of communication.

Revascularization of the corporeal bodies may be beneficial when impotence arises from inadequate blood flow into the penis. If a venous leak occurs, ligation of the affected veins may provide a solution.

- Bypass grafts and venous ligation have limited success in older men because of rapid obstruction of the graft and the natural tendency to form collateral circulation around the ligated vessel.

Nursing Management

The patient experiencing erectile dysfunction requires a great deal of emotional support for both himself and his partner. He needs reassurance that confidentiality will be maintained.

- Men often do not feel comfortable discussing their problems with others because of society's expectations of a man's sexual abilities.
- The man may experience and demonstrate isolation from support systems, and he may also lose self-esteem, which can eventually lead to loss of role functions.
- In conjunction with therapeutic treatment, it often becomes necessary to provide counseling and therapy for the couple to establish realistic expectations and develop meaningful communication patterns.

Pain management of patients experiencing surgical intervention generally consists of administration of prescribed analgesics, elevation of the scrotum, and application of ice to the scrotum for the first 48 hours postoperatively. A normal course of healing ranges from 4 to 6 weeks.

- Resumption of sexual activities before complete healing may result in infection, extrusion, erosion, or rupture. Patients should also be instructed to use a water-soluble lubricant and approach penetration slowly and at a comfortable angle.

ESOPHAGEAL CANCER

Definition/Description
Squamous cell carcinoma is the most common form of esophageal cancer. Compared to portions of Asia in which the rate of esophageal cancer is extremely high, the incidence is low in Western societies. The incidence is higher in men and African-Americans and increases with age. Because esophageal cancer is rarely diagnosed in the early stages, the 5-year prognosis is poor.

Pathophysiology
The cause of esophageal cancer is unknown. Possible predisposing factors are cigarette smoking, excessive alcohol intake, chronic trauma, poor oral hygiene, and spicy foods. Other risk factors include exposure to asbestos and metals and a low intake of fresh fruits and vegetables.

- Certain conditions of the esophagus, such as achalasia, diverticula, and lye burns, are considered premalignant lesions.
- The malignant tumor usually appears as an ulcerated lesion. It may have advanced to this stage before the appearance of symptoms.
- The majority of tumors are located in the middle and lower portions of the esophagus, with the tumor penetrating the muscular layer and even extending outside the esophageal wall. Tumor obstruction of the esophagus occurs in the later stages.

Clinical Manifestations
The onset of symptoms is usually late in relation to the extent of the tumor.

- Progressive dysphagia is the most common symptom and may be expressed as a substernal feeling that food is not passing. Initially dysphagia occurs only with meat, then with soft foods, and eventually with liquids.
- Pain develops later and is described as occurring in the substernal, epigastric, or back areas and usually increases with swallowing. The pain may radiate to the neck, jaw, ears, and shoulders.
- If the tumor is in the upper third of the esophagus, symptoms such as sore throat, choking, and hoarseness may occur. Weight loss is fairly common.
- When esophageal stenosis is severe, regurgitation of blood-flecked esophageal contents is common.

Complications may include hemorrhage from cancer eroding the aorta and esophageal perforation and obstruction.

Diagnostic Studies

- Barium swallow with fluoroscopy may demonstrate esophageal narrowing at the site of the tumor.
- Esophagoscopy with biopsy is needed to make a definitive diagnosis.
- Endoscopic ultransonography detects tumor invasion into the muscle layer.
- Bronchoscopic examination detects malignant involvement of the trachea.
- CT scanning provides a more accurate assessment of disease extent.

Therapeutic Management

The treatment of esophageal cancer depends on the location of the tumor and whether metastasis has occurred. The best treatment results have been obtained with a combination of surgery and radiation. Chemotherapeutic agents are currently under investigation.

If the tumor is in the cervical section (upper third) of the esophagus, radiation is usually indicated (see Radiation Therapy, p. 675). A tumor in the lower third of the esophagus is usually resected surgically. Dilatation may be used to relieve dysphagia and allow for improved nutrition.

Nursing Management

Goals

The patient with esophageal cancer will have relief of symptoms (including pain and dysphagia), achieve optimal nutritional intake, understand the prognosis of the disease, and experience a quality of life appropriate to disease progression.

Nursing Diagnoses

- Altered nutrition: less than body requirements related to dysphagia, weakness, and radiation therapy
- Pain related to tumor
- Anxiety related to diagnosis of cancer, uncertain future, and poor prognosis
- Anticipatory grieving related to diagnosis of life-threatening malignancy
- Impaired home maintenance management related to lack of knowledge of disease process and therapeutic regimen, unavailability of a support system, and chronic debilitating disease

Nursing Interventions

Preoperative care should focus on general preoperative teaching and preparation, including meticulous oral care, information about chest tubes (if a thoracic approach is used), IV lines, nasogastric (NG) tube, gastrostomy feeding, turning, coughing, and deep breathing.

Postoperative care should include assessment of drainage; maintenance of NG tube; oral and nasal care; prevention of respiratory complications by turning, coughing, and deep breathing with incentive spirometry every 2 hours; and placing the patient in a semi-Fowler's position to prevent gastric reflux.

Many patients will need *chronic care,* including (1) encouragement and assistance in maintaining adequate nutrition, (2) knowledge of prognosis and appropriate counseling, and (3) referral to a community health nurse if necessary for continued care of the patient (e.g., gastrostomy teaching and follow-up wound care).

Patient Teaching

- Health counseling needs to focus on the elimination of smoking and excessive alcohol intake. Maintenance of good oral hygiene and dietary habits (intake of fresh fruits and vegetables) may also be helpful.
- Having the patient obtain treatment of esophageal problems, such as achalasia and diverticula, may be helpful because these are considered premalignant problems.
- The patient should be encouraged to have regular physical examinations and seek medical attention for any esophageal problems, especially dysphagia.

FIBROCYSTIC BREAST CHANGES

Definition/Description

Fibrocystic changes in the breast constitute the most common benign breast disorder in women. These changes include the development of excess fibrous tissue, hyperplasia of the epithelial lining of the mammary ducts, proliferation of mammary ducts, and cyst formation. Fibrocystic changes occur most frequently in women between 35 and 50 years of age but may begin in women as young as 20 years old.

Pathophysiology

- The cause of fibrocystic changes is thought to be heightened responsiveness of breast parenchyma and stroma to circulating estrogens and progesterones.
- Fibrocystic changes produce pain by nerve irritation from connective tissue edema and by fibrosis from nerve pinching.
- Masses or nodules can appear in both breasts and are often found in the upper outer quadrants and usually occur bilaterally.
- Characteristics of women affected include those with premenstrual abnormalities, nulliparous women, women with a history of spontaneous abortion, nonusers of oral contraceptives, and women with early menarche and late menopause.
- Fibrocystic changes often exacerbate in the premenstrual phase and subside after menstruation.

F

Clinical Manifestations

Manifestations of fibrocystic breast changes include one or more palpable lumps that are usually round, well delineated, and freely movable within the breast. There may be accompanying discomfort ranging from tenderness to pain.

- The lump is usually observed to increase in size and perhaps in tenderness before menstruation. Cysts may enlarge or shrink rapidly.
- Nipple discharge associated with fibrocystic breasts is often milky, watery-milky, yellow, or green.
- Pain and nodularity often increase over time but tend to subside after menopause unless high-dose estrogen replacement therapy is used.

Therapeutic and Nursing Management

With the initial discovery of a discrete mass in the breast, aspiration or surgical biopsy may be indicated. A wait of 7 to 10 days may be planned if the nodularity is recurrent to note changes through the menstrual cycle.

- An excisional biopsy should be done if no fluid is found on aspiration, fluid that is found is hemorrhagic, or a residual mass remains.
- Surgery is performed in an office or day surgery unit with local anesthesia used. About 4% of biopsy specimens contain hyperplastic changes approximating the histologic appearance of carcinoma in situ and are called atypical hyperplasia.
- The woman with cystic changes should be encouraged to return regularly for follow-up examinations. She should also be taught breast self-examination (BSE) to self-monitor the problem. Any new lumps should be evaluated, and changes in symptoms should be reported and investigated.

Many types of treatment have been suggested for a fibrocystic condition. These include dietary (low-salt diet, restriction of methylxanthines such as coffee and chocolate), therapeutic (analgesics, danocrene [Danazol], diuretics, hormone therapy, antiestrogen therapy), and surgical (subcutaneous mastectomy) approaches. The benefit of most of these treatments has not been proved.

- In the United States, danocrene has been approved as a treatment for fibrocystic changes. Danocrene decreases follicle-stimulating hormone (FSH) and luteinizing hormone (LH), which will ultimately culminate in anovulation and amenorrhea. The ensuing reduction of estrogen stimulation by this drug results in decreased pain and nodularity.

Patient Teaching

The role of the nurse in the care of the patient with fibrocystic breast changes is primarily one of teaching. A woman should be told that she may expect recurrence of the cysts in one or both breasts until menopause and that cysts may enlarge or become painful just before menstruation. Additionally, these women should be reassured that cysts do not "turn into" cancer.

- Any new lump that does not respond in a cyclic manner over 1 to 2 weeks should be examined promptly. The woman should be carefully instructed in BSE, using her own breasts. Teaching BSE with a breast model can also be helpful.

FLAIL CHEST

Definition/Description

Flail chest results from a fracture of two or more adjacent ribs in two or more places, which causes loss of stability of the chest wall. Flail chest may occur with pneumothorax, hemothorax, and tension pneumothorax (see Pneumothorax, p. 474).

Pathophysiology

The chest wall cannot provide the bony structure necessary to maintain the bellows action needed for ventilation. The affected (flail) area will move paradoxically to the intact portion of the chest during respiration. During inspiration, the affected portion is sucked inward; during expiration, it bulges outward.

- This paradoxic chest movement prevents adequate ventilation of the lung in the injured area. This defect itself does not cause hypoxia. The major difficulty is that the underlying lung has been injured.
- Associated pain and the underlying lung injury, giving rise to loss of compliance, contribute to an alteration in breathing patterns and lead to hypoxia.

Clinical Manifestations

Flail chest is usually apparent on visual examination of the unconscious patient.

- Manifestations include rapid, shallow respirations, cyanosis, and tachycardia.
- A flail chest may not be initially apparent in the conscious patient as a result of splinting of the chest wall. The patient moves air poorly, and movement of the thorax is asymmetric and uncoordinated.
- Crepitus of the rib

Diagnostic Studies

- Palpation of abnormal respiratory movements
- Chest x-ray
- Arterial blood gases (ABGs)

Therapeutic Management

Initial therapy consists of adequate ventilation, humidified O_2, and careful administration of crystalloid IV solutions. Definitive therapy is to reexpand the lung and ensure adequate oxygenation.

- Although many patients can be managed without the use of mechanical ventilation, a short period of intubation and ventilation may be necessary until the diagnosis of lung injury is complete (see Intubation, Endotracheal, p. 657, and Mechanical Ventilation, p. 662).
- Positive end-expiratory pressure (PEEP) used with mechanical ventilation to improve oxygenation will maintain positive pressure in the lungs throughout the respiratory cycle.
- Lung parenchyma and fractured ribs will heal with time.

FRACTURE

Definition/Description

A fracture is a disruption or break in the continuity of the structure of a bone. Traumatic injuries account for the majority of fractures, although some fractures are secondary to a disease process (pathologic fractures). Fractures are described and classified according to (1) type, (2) communication or noncommunication with the external environment, and (3) location.

Fractures are also described as stable or unstable. A *stable fracture* occurs when some of the periosteum is intact across the fracture and either external or internal fixation has rendered the fragments stationary. Stable fractures are usually transverse, spiral, or greenstick. An *unstable fracture* is grossly displaced during injury and is a site of poor fixation. Unstable fractures are usually comminuted or oblique.

Clinical Manifestations

The patient's history indicates an injury often associated with immediate localized pain, decreased function, and inability to use the affected part. The patient guards and protects the part against movement. The fracture may not be accompanied by obvious bone deformity.

- Manifestations include edema and swelling, pain and tenderness, muscle spasm, deformity, ecchymosis, loss of function, and crepitation.

Complications

The majority of fractures heal without complications. If death occurs after a fracture, it is usually the result of damage to underlying organs and soft tissue or of certain complications of the fracture.

- The ossification process is arrested by causes such as inadequate immobilization and reduction, excess movement, infection, and poor nutrition. For a summary of complications of fracture healing, see Table 59-4 in Lewis/Collier/Heitkemper, *Medical-Surgical Nursing,* edition 4, p. 1849.
- *Direct complications* of fractures include problems with bone union, avascular necrosis, and bone infection. *Indirect complications* are associated with blood vessel and nerve damage resulting in conditions such as compartment syndrome, venous thrombosis, fat embolism, and traumatic or hypovolemic shock (Table 29).
- Although most musculoskeletal injuries are not life-threatening, open fractures or fractures accompanied by severe blood

Table 29   Complications of Fractures

Complications	Description	Treatment
Bone infection	Devitalized and contaminated tissue is an ideal medium for many pathogens.	Open fractures should be cleaned by extensive irrigation, usually sterile saline and antibiotic solution. Antibiotics may be administered intravenously, intramuscularly, or orally.
Compartment syndrome	Compression of structures occurs within closed compartments of upper and lower extremities formed by fascial walls. Associated with fractures or extensive soft-tissue damage in an extremity.	Prevention or early recognition is critical. Affected extremity should be elevated and ice applied. May be necessary to relieve compression and restore blood supply by fasciotomy (surgically incising fascia).
Venous thrombosis	Veins of lower extremities and pelvis are highly susceptible to thrombus formation after fracture injury.	Elastic compression gradient stockings are used to prevent thrombosis. Range-of-motion exercises should be performed on unaffected extremities. Prophylactic anticoagulation may be ordered.
Fat embolism	Fat emboli from marrow of injured bones or adipose tissue embolize to lungs, brain, heart, kidneys, skin, and other places. Associated with fractures of long bones and multiple fractures associated with pelvic injuries.	Careful immobilization of long bone fracture is important in prevention. Management is symptom related and supportive.

loss and fractures that damage vital organs are medical emergencies requiring immediate attention.

Stages of Fracture Healing

The bone goes through a remarkable reparative process of self-healing (called *union*) that occurs in the following stages:

1. *Fracture hematoma:* When a fracture occurs, bleeding and edema precede development of a hematoma, which surrounds the ends of the fragments.
2. *Granulation tissue:* Active phagocytosis absorbs the products of local necrosis. The hematoma changes into granulation tissue (consisting of young blood vessels, fibroblasts, and osteoblasts), which produces a new bone substance called *osteoid.*
3. *Callus formation:* As minerals are deposited in the osteoid, an unorganized network of bone called a callus is formed. The callus is woven about the fracture parts. It usually begins to appear by the end of the first week after injury. Evidence of callus formation can be verified by x-ray.
4. *Ossification:* Ossification of the callus begins within 2 to 3 weeks postfracture and continues until the fracture has healed. Ossification of the callus is sufficient to prevent movement at the fracture site when bones are gently stressed. During this stage the patient can be converted from skeletal traction to a cast, or the cast can be removed to allow mobility.
5. *Consolidation:* As the callus continues to develop, the distance between bone fragments diminishes and eventually closes. This stage is called consolidation, and ossification continues. It can be equated with radiographic union.
6. *Remodeling:* Excess cells are absorbed, and union is completed. Gradual return of the injured bone to its preinjury structural strength and shape occurs. Remodeling of bone is enhanced as it responds to physical stress. Initially, stress is provided through exercise. Weight-bearing is gradually introduced.

Diagnostic Studies

An x-ray examination is used to determine the presence of a fracture.

Therapeutic Management of Fractures

The goals of fracture treatment are (1) anatomic realignment of bone fragments, (2) immobilization to maintain realignment, and (3) restoration of function of the part.

Fracture Reduction

Manipulation is a nonsurgical manual realignment of bones to their previous anatomic position. Traction and countertraction are manually applied to bone fragments to restore position, length, and alignment.

- *Closed reduction* is usually performed with the patient under local or general anesthesia. After reduction or manipulation the injured part is immobilized by casting or traction to maintain alignment until healing occurs.
- *Open reduction* is correction of bone alignment through a surgical incision. It may include internal fixation of the fracture with the use of wire, screws, pins, plates, intramedullary rods, or nails. If open reduction and internal fixation are used, early initiation of range of motion of the joint is indicated.

Traction devices apply a pulling force on the fractured extremity and result in realignment. The two most common types of traction are *skin traction* and *skeletal traction.*

- *Skin traction* is generally used for short-term treatment (48 to 72 hours) until skeletal traction or surgery is possible. Tape, boots, or slings are applied directly to the skin to maintain alignment, assist in reduction, and help diminish muscle spasms in the injured part.
- *Skeletal traction* is generally kept in place for longer periods of time and is used to align injured bones and joints. It provides a long-term pull that keeps injured bones and joints aligned (for comparison of types of traction, see Table 59-6 in Lewis/Collier/Heitkemper, *Medical-Surgical Nursing,* p. 1850).

Fracture alignment depends on correct positioning and alignment of the patient while traction forces remain constant. For extremity traction to be effective, forces must be pulling in the opposite direction *(countertraction)* to prevent the patient from sliding to the end of the bed.

- Countertraction may be achieved by elevating the end of the bed 8 to 12 inches, which allows the weight of the patient's own body to be used.

Fracture Immobilization

External fixation of fractures is achieved by a cast or an external fixator. Casting is a common treatment after closed reduction has been performed. It allows the patient to perform many normal activities of daily living while providing sufficient immobilization to ensure stability (see Casts, p. 628).

An *external fixator* is a metallic device used to compress fracture fragments and to immobilize reduced fragments when the use of a cast or traction is not appropriate. The external fixator is attached directly to the bones by percutaneous pins. Assessment for pin loosening and infection is critical. Infection signaled by exudate, redness, tenderness, and pain may require removal of the device.

Internal fixation devices are surgically inserted at the time of realignment. Examples of internal fixation devices include pins, plates, and screws. They are biologically inert devices that are used to realign and maintain bony fragments. Proper alignment is evaluated by x-ray studies at regular intervals.

Maintenance traction is initiation or continuation of traction and countertraction. A continuous pulling force can be applied directly to the bone with wires and pins *(skeletal traction)* or indirectly by weights attached to the skin with adhesive straps or boots *(skin traction).*

Nursing Management
Goals
The patient with a fracture will have no associated complications, obtain satisfactory pain relief, and achieve maximal rehabilitation potential.

See the nursing care plan for the patient with a fracture in Lewis/Collier/Heitkemper, *Medical-Surgical Nursing,* edition 4, p. 1856.

Nursing Diagnoses/Collaborative Problems
- Pain related to edema, movement of bone fragments, and muscle spasms
- Risk for infection related to disruption of skin integrity and presence of environmental pathogens secondary to open fracture or external fixation pins
- Activity intolerance related to prolonged immobility
- Risk for peripheral neurovascular dysfunction related to nerve compression
- Risk for impaired skin integrity related to immobility and presence of cast
- Ineffective management of therapeutic regimen related to lack of knowledge regarding muscle atrophy, exercise program, and cast care
- Potential complication: fat embolism related to fracture of a long bone

Nursing Interventions
The patient with a fracture may be treated in an emergency department or physician's office and released to home care, or the patient may require hospitalization. (Specific nursing measures depend on the type of treatment used and the setting in which the patient is placed.)

Preoperative management. If surgical intervention is required to treat the fracture, the patient will need preoperative preparation. In addition to the usual preoperative nursing measures, the nurse should inform the patient of the type of immobilization device to be used and expected activity limitations.

- Proper skin preparation is an important part of preoperative preparation. The aim of skin preparation is to clean the skin and remove debris and hair to reduce the possibility of infection.

- The patient must be assured that all needs will be met by the nursing staff until the patient can again meet his/her own needs. Assurance that pain medication will be available if needed is often beneficial.

Postoperative management. Frequent neurovascular assessments of the affected extremity are necessary to detect subtle changes. Any limitations of movement or activity related to turning, positioning, and extremity support should be monitored closely.

- Pain and discomfort can be minimized through proper alignment and positioning.
- Dressings or casts should be carefully observed for any overt signs of bleeding or drainage. Increased bleeding can be monitored by drawing a circle on the cast around an area of drainage and by noting the date and time. A significant increase in the size of the drainage area should be reported.
- If a wound-drainage system is in place, patency of the system and volume of drainage should be assessed at least once each shift. Whenever the contents of a drainage system are measured or emptied, the nurse should use sterile technique to avoid contamination.

If the patient is immobilized as a result of the fracture, the nurse must plan care to prevent constipation and renal calculi.

- Constipation can be prevented by maintenance of a high fluid intake and a diet high in bulk and roughage. If these measures are not effective in maintaining the patient's normal bowel pattern, stool softeners, laxatives, or suppositories may be necessary. Maintaining a regular time for elimination despite bed rest is effective in promoting regularity.
- Renal calculi can develop as a result of bone demineralization caused by immobilization. Unless contraindicated, a fluid intake of 2100 to 2800 ml/day is recommended. Cranberry juice is often recommended to acidify the urine and discourage development of stones.

Rapid deconditioning of the circulatory system can occur as a result of bed rest. These effects can be diminished by permitting the patient to sit on the side of the bed, allowing the lower limbs to dangle over the bedside, and performing standing transfers (unless these measures are contraindicated).

- When the patient is allowed to increase activity, careful evaluation should be made to assess for orthostatic hypotension.

Patient Teaching

Because a fracture often is cast in an outpatient setting, the patient may require only a short hospitalization or none at all. Therefore patient education is an important nursing responsibility to prevent complications. In addition to giving specific instructions for cast care and recognition of complications, the nurse should encourage the patient to contact the clinic or care provider if questions arise. The nurse should validate patient understanding of these instructions before discharge from the clinic or hospital.

For further information on rehabilitation management of fractures, see Lewis/Collier/Heitkemper, *Medical-Surgical Nursing,* edition 4, p. 1858.

See also specific types of fractures discussed in this book.

FRACTURE, HIP

Definition/Description

Hip fractures are common in older adults. A hip fracture may be expected to occur more frequently in women than in men older than 65 years because of osteoporosis. It is estimated that 30% of patients who experience a hip fracture will die within 1 year of injury because of medical complications caused by the fracture or resulting immobility. Of the survivors, 30% to 50% will never regain their prefracture functional status.

Pathophysiology

- Fractures that occur within the capsule are called *intracapsular* fractures. Intracapsular fractures are further identified by a name taken from their specific location: subcapital, transcervical, and basilar neck. These fractures are often associated with osteoporosis and minor trauma.
- *Extracapsular* fractures occur below the capsule and are termed *intertrochanteric* if they occur in a region between the greater and the lesser trochanter. They are termed *subtrochanteric* if they occur in the region below the trochanter. Extracapsular fractures are usually caused by severe direct trauma or a fall.

Clinical Manifestations

Manifestations of a hip fracture are external rotation, shortening of the affected extremity, and severe pain and tenderness in the region of the fracture site. Displaced femoral neck fractures cause serious disruption of the blood supply to the femoral head, which can result in avascular necrosis.

Complications associated with femoral neck fracture include nonunion, avascular necrosis, and degenerative arthritis. As a result of an intertrochanteric fracture, the affected leg may be shortened.

Therapeutic Management

Surgical repair is the preferred method of managing intracapsular and extracapsular hip fractures. Surgical treatment permits the patient to be out of bed sooner and decreases the major complications associated with immobility. Initially the affected extremity may be temporarily immobilized by either Buck's or Russell's traction until the patient's physical condition is stabilized and surgery can be performed. Traction also helps relieve painful muscle spasms.

- Intracapsular fractures are usually repaired with the use of a hip prosthesis. Extracapsular fractures are usually pinned. The principles of patient care for these procedures are similar.
- The intracapsular fracture is slow to heal because of interruptions in blood supply. When avascular necrosis appears imminent, the surgeon may elect to resect the femoral head and neck and insert a femoral head prosthesis. Devices such as compression screws and plates, nails, and pins are available to the surgeon for the purpose of repairing a hip fracture by pinning.

Nursing Management

Preoperative management. Because older adults are most prone to hip fractures, chronic health problems (e.g., diabetes mellitus, hypertension) must often be considered when planning treatment. Surgery may be delayed for a brief time until the patient's general health improves.

- Before surgery, severe muscle spasms that can increase pain can be managed with appropriate medications, comfortable positioning (unless contraindicated), and properly adjusted traction (if being used).
- The patient should know the method and frequency for exercising the unaffected leg and both arms. The patient should also be shown how to use the trapeze bar and opposite siderail to assist in changing positions. Practice in getting out of bed and transferring to a chair should be discussed and demonstrated.

Postoperative management. The initial management of a patient after surgical repair of hip fracture is similar to that for any older surgical patient, including monitoring vital signs and intake and output, supervising respiratory activities such as deep breathing and coughing, administering pain medication cautiously, and observing the dressing and incision for signs of bleeding and infection. Specific nursing interventions are described in the nursing care plan for the patient with fracture of the hip in Lewis/Collier/Heitkemper, *Medical-Surgical Nursing,* edition 4, p. 1865.

In the early postoperative period there is potential for impairment of circulation, movement, and sensation. The nurse should assess the patient's toes for ability to move, warmth and pink color, numbness or tingling, and edema.

- Edema may develop after the patient is out of bed and is alleviated by elevation of the leg whenever the patient is in a chair.
- Pain resulting from poor alignment of the affected extremity can be prevented by keeping pillows (or an abductor splint) between the knees when the patient is turning to either side. Sandbags and pillows are also used to prevent external rotation.

Ambulation usually begins the first or second postoperative day. The nurse needs to monitor the patient's ambulation status for proper crutch walking or use of the walker. The patient must be able to use crutches or a walker before discharge.

If the hip fracture has been treated by insertion of a femoral-head prosthesis, measures to prevent dislocation must be used.

- The patient and family must be fully aware of positions and activities that predispose the patient to dislocation (extreme flexion, adduction, or internal rotation). Many daily activities may reproduce these positions (e.g., putting on shoes and socks, crossing the legs or feet while seated, assuming the side-lying position incorrectly, standing up or sitting down while the body is flexed relative to the chair, sitting on low seats).
- Until soft tissue surrounding the hip has healed sufficiently to stabilize the prosthesis, these activities must be avoided, usually for at least 6 weeks.
- Sudden severe pain and extreme external rotation indicate prosthesis dislocation. This requires a closed reduction or open reduction to realign the femoral head in the acetabulum.

The nurse should place a large pillow between the patient's legs when turning the patient, keep leg abductor splints on the patient except when bathing, avoid extreme hip flexion in the patient, and avoid turning the patient on the affected side until approved by the surgeon.

If the hip fracture is treated by pinning, dislocation precautions are not necessary. The patient is usually encouraged to be out of bed on the first postoperative day. Weight-bearing on the involved extremity may be restricted until x-ray examination indicates adequate healing, usually within 3 to 5 months.

The nurse must assist both the patient and the family in adjusting to the restrictions and dependence imposed by the hip fracture. Depression can easily occur, but creative nursing care and awareness of the problem can do much to prevent it.

- The patient and family may need to be informed about community referral services that can assist in the postdischarge rehabilitation phase. Hospitalization averages 7 days. Regular follow-up care after discharge should be arranged.

Fracture, Humerus

Fractures involving the shaft of the humerus are a common injury among young and middle-aged adults. Prominent clinical manifestations are an obvious displacement of the humeral shaft, shortened extremity, abnormal mobility, and pain. Major complications associated with fracture of the humerus are radial nerve injury and vascular injury to the brachial artery as a result of laceration, transection, or spasm.

Treatment for a fracture of the humerus depends on location and displacement.

- Treatment may include a hanging arm cast or the sling and swathe, a type of immobilization often used for surgical repairs and shoulder dislocation.
- Skin or skeletal traction may also be used for reduction and immobilization.

When these treatment devices are used, the head of the bed should be elevated to assist gravity in reducing the fracture. The arm should be allowed to hang when the patient is sitting and standing.

Nursing management should include measures to protect the axilla and prevent skin maceration.

- During the rehabilitative phase an exercise program geared toward improving strength and motion of the injured extremity is extremely important. The program should include assisted motion of the hands and fingers. If the fracture is stable, the shoulder can also be exercised to prevent stiffness.

Fracture, Pelvis

Pelvic fractures are usually caused by vehicular accidents, although the older adult patient may sustain this injury from a fall. Pelvic fractures may cause serious intraabdominal injury such as colon laceration, paralytic ileus, hemorrhage, and rupture of the urethra or bladder.

Pelvic fractures are diagnosed and classified by x-ray study. They may range from simple undisplaced fractures to more serious fracture dislocations with the potential for serious complications. Physical examination demonstrates local swelling, tenderness, deformity, and ecchymosis. The neurovascular status of the lower extremities and manifestations of associated injuries should be assessed.

Treatment depends on the severity of the injury. Bed rest for stable pelvic fractures is maintained from a few days to 6 weeks. More complex fractures may be managed with pelvic slings, skeletal traction, hip spica casts, open reduction, or a combination of these methods. Internal fixation of a pelvic fracture may be necessary if the fracture is displaced.

- Extreme care in handling or moving the patient is important to prevent serious injury from a displaced fracture fragment. Because a pelvic fracture can damage other organs, appropriate assessments are important in the early nursing activities for this patient.
- The patient should be turned only when specifically ordered by the physician. Back care is provided while the patient is raised from the bed, either by independent use of the trapeze or with adequate assistance.
- Weight-bearing on the affected side should be avoided until healing is complete.
- If the pelvic fracture is not displaced, the patient is usually allowed to ambulate using a walker or crutches to distribute the weight-bearing between the upper and lower extremities.
- If a pelvic sling is used, elimination needs may require the use of an indwelling catheter in female patients.

FRACTURE, RIB

Rib fractures are the most common type of chest injury resulting from trauma. Ribs 4 through 9 are most commonly fractured because they are the least protected by chest muscles. If the fractured rib is splintered or displaced, it may damage the pleura and lungs.

Manifestations include pain (especially on inspiration) at the site of injury. The individual splints the affected area and takes shallow breaths to decrease the pain. Because the individual is reluctant to take deep breaths and cough, atelectasis may develop because of decreased ventilation.

The goal of treatment is to decrease pain so the patient can breathe adequately to promote good chest expansion.

- Intercostal nerve blocks with local anesthesia are most frequently used to provide pain relief. Nerves of affected ribs and the two intercostal nerves above and below the injured rib are also blocked. The effect of anesthesia lasts for a period of hours to days. It needs to be repeated as necessary to provide pain relief.

- Strapping the chest with tape or using a binder is not common practice. Most physicians believe that these measures should be avoided because they reduce lung expansion and predispose the individual to atelectasis.
- Narcotic drug therapy must be individualized and used with caution because narcotics can depress respirations.

F

GASTRITIS

Definition/Description

Gastritis is an inflammation of the gastric mucosa and one of the most common problems affecting the stomach. It may be acute or chronic and diffuse or localized. Chronic gastritis can be further classified as type A (fundal) and type B (antral).

Pathophysiology

Gastritis is the result of a breakdown in the normal gastric barrier. The mucosal barrier normally protects the stomach tissue from autodigestion by acid. When the barrier is broken, acid diffuses back into the mucosa. This action allows hydrochloric (HCl) acid to enter and increase the secretion of pepsinogen, with subsequent release of histamine from mast cells.

- The combined result of these occurrences is tissue edema, loss of plasma into gastric lumen with disruption of capillary walls, and possible hemorrhage.

Table 30 lists the causes of gastritis.

Chronic gastritis may result from repeated episodes of acute gastritis. Chronic exposure to the causes of gastritis will also result in eventual loss of viable mucosal tissue.

- Chronic gastritis, in particular *type A,* may be an autoimmune disorder. Autoimmune atrophic gastritis is associated with increased risk of gastric malignancy.
- *Type B* gastritis primarily involves the stomach antrum. The most common cause of type B gastritis is *Helicobacter pylori (H. pylori),* which promotes the breakdown process of the gastric mucosal barrier. *H. pylori* also has been correlated with other gastric disorders, including gastric and duodenal ulcers and gastric cancer.
- Progressive gastric atrophy from chronic alterations in the mucosal barrier causes chief and parietal cells to die. As the number of acid-secreting parietal cells decreases with atrophy of gastric mucosa, *hypochlorhydria* (decreased acid secretion) or *achlorhydria* (lack of acid secretion) occurs.

Clinical Manifestations

- Symptoms of *acute gastritis* include anorexia, nausea and vomiting, epigastric tenderness, and a feeling of fullness. Hemorrhage is commonly associated with alcohol abuse and at times may be the only symptom. Acute gastritis is self-limiting, lasting from a few hours to a few days, with complete healing of mucosa expected.

Table 30	Causes of Gastritis
Aspirin	Physiologic stress
Nonsteroidal anti-inflammatory drugs	Shock
	Sepsis
Corticosteroid drugs	Burns
Alcohol	Psychologic stress
Helicobacter pylori	Renal failure (uremia)
Staphylococcus organisms	Spicy, irritating food
	Trauma
Bile and pancreatic secretions	Nasogastric suction
	Large hiatal hernia
Smoking	

- Manifestations of *chronic gastritis* are similar to those for acute gastritis. Some patients have no symptoms directly associated with the gastric lesion. However, when the acid-secreting cells are lost or do not function as a result of atrophy, the source of intrinsic factor is lost and vitamin B_{12} cannot be absorbed in the ileum.

G

Diagnostic Studies

Proper diagnosis of gastritis is frequently delayed or completely missed because symptoms are nonspecific.

- Endoscopic examination with biopsy is necessary to obtain a definitive diagnosis.
- A specific analysis of gastric tissue for the presence of *H. pylori* may be performed.
- Complete blood count (CBC) may demonstrate anemia from blood loss.
- Stools are tested for occult blood.
- A gastric analysis demonstrates the amount of hydrochloric acid present, with achlorhydria being a common sign of severe atrophic gastritis.
- Serum tests for antibodies to parietal cells and intrinsic factor may be performed.
- Cytologic examination is done to rule out gastric carcinoma.

Therapeutic Management

Eliminating the cause and preventing or avoiding it in the future are generally all that is needed to treat *acute gastritis*. The plan of care is supportive and similar to that described for nausea and vomiting.

- During the acute phase, bed rest, nothing by mouth, and IV fluids may be prescribed. Fluids and electrolytes lost through vomiting and occasionally diarrhea are replaced. In severe cases a nasogastric (NG) tube may be used, either for lavage of the precipitating agent from the stomach or with suctioning to keep the stomach empty and free of noxious stimuli.
- Clear liquids are resumed when acute symptoms have subsided, with gradual reintroduction of solid bland foods.
- Antiemetics are given for nausea and vomiting. Antacids are used for relief of abdominal discomfort, and H_2 receptor antagonists such as ranitidine or cimetidine will reduce gastric hydrochloric acid secretion.

Treatment of *chronic gastritis* focuses on evaluating and eliminating the specific cause.

- Various combinations of antibiotics and bismuth salt preparations (Pepto-Bismol) are used to eradicate infection with *H. pylori.*
- For the patient with pernicious anemia, regular injections of vitamin B_{12} are needed.
- An individualized bland diet and use of antacids are recommended.
- Smoking is contraindicated with all forms of gastritis.
- The patient may need to adapt to lifestyle changes and strictly adhere to medication regimens. An interdisciplinary team approach in which the physician, nurse, dietitian, and pharmacist provide consistent information and support may increase patient success in making these alterations.

Nursing Management

Goals

The patient with gastritis will experience minimal or no symptoms of gastritis and no recurrent episodes of acute gastritis and will achieve an optimal pattern of gastric functioning relative to the disease stage.

Nursing Diagnoses

The nursing diagnoses listed for the patient with nausea and vomiting are also applicable in gastritis (see Nausea and Vomiting, p. 408).

Nursing Interventions

- Dehydration can occur rapidly in severe gastritis accompanied by vomiting. Keeping the patient on nothing by mouth (NPO) status while monitoring IV fluids is essential.
- If hemorrhage is considered likely, frequently checking vital signs and testing vomitus for blood are indicated.
- Elimination of the cause of gastritis results in rapid improvement in the patient's condition. Identification of the causative agent is important to prevent future gastric irritation.

The majority of patients with gastritis receive care in the home, and chronic management may be necessary for extended periods of time. A bland diet consisting of six small feedings a day and the use of an antacid after meals helps the patient maintain normal gastric function.

Patient Teaching

- The patient with gastritis should be encouraged to avoid causative factors and to follow a prescribed diet and medication regimen. Because the incidence of gastric cancer is higher in patients with a history of chronic gastritis, especially atrophic gastritis, close medical follow-up should be stressed.
- The patient who has gastric atrophy may need vitamin B_{12} injections included in the plan of care.

GASTROENTERITIS

Gastroenteritis is an inflammation of the mucosa of the stomach and small intestine. Causative agents are varied and include decreased fluid absorption (e.g., mucosal damage from Crohn's disease), increased fluid secretion (e.g., infectious bacterial toxins from cholera, *Escherichia coli,* or salmonella), and motility disturbances (e.g., irritable bowel syndrome, vagotomy). Most cases are self-limiting and do not require hospitalization. However, older adults and chronically ill patients may be unable to consume sufficient fluids orally to compensate for fluid loss.

Clinical manifestations include nausea and vomiting, diarrhea, abdominal cramping, and distention. Fever, leukocytosis, and blood or mucus in the stool may also be present.

Until vomiting has ceased, the patient should be on nothing by mouth (NPO) status. If dehydration has occurred, IV replacement of fluids may be necessary. As soon as tolerated, fluids containing glucose and electrolytes (e.g., Gatorade) should be given. Accurate monitoring of intake and output is important for successful replacement of lost fluid.

If the causative agent is identified, appropriate antibiotic, antimicrobial, or antiinfective medication is given. Strict medical asepsis and enteric precautions should be instituted when indicated. Symptomatic nursing care is given for nausea and vomiting and for diarrhea (see Nausea and Vomiting, p. 408, and Diarrhea, p. 186). The nurse should assess complaints of pain, vomiting, and diarrhea because gastroenteritis is often confused with appendicitis.

G

- The patient should be instructed in the importance of proper food handling and preparation of food to prevent infections such as *salmonellosis* and *trichinosis.*
- The importance of rest and increased fluid intake as symptomatic treatment measures for gastroenteritis should be stressed.
- To allay the patient's apprehension, the nurse should explain that gastroenteritis usually runs an acute course with no sequelae.

GASTROESOPHAGEAL REFLUX DISEASE

Definition/Description
Gastroesophageal reflux disease (GERD) is not a disease but a syndrome produced by conditions that result in the reflux of gastric secretions into the esophagus.

Pathophysiology
In GERD there is confirmed evidence of a reflux of gastric contents into the lower portion of the esophagus. Acidity of the gastric secretions results in esophageal irritation and inflammation (esophagitis).

One of the primary factors in GERD is an incompetent lower esophageal sphincter (LES), which is defined by a lack of high pressure in the distal portion of the esophagus. Gastric contents are then able to move from an area of higher pressure (stomach) to an area of lower pressure (esophagus) when the patient is in a supine position, or intraabdominal pressure is increased (see Hiatal Hernia, p. 302).

Clinical Manifestations
- Heartburn (pyrosis), caused by irritation of the esophagus by gastric acids, is the most common clinical manifestation. Heartburn is described as a burning, tight sensation that appears intermittently beneath the lower sternum and spreads upward to the throat or jaw.
- Regurgitation (effortless return of material from the stomach into the esophagus or mouth) is a fairly common manifestation of an incompetent LES. It is often described as hot, bitter, or sour liquid coming into the throat or mouth.
- Other manifestations include feelings of a lump in the throat or of food stopping, dysphagia, and bleeding.
- Respiratory complications, including bronchospasm or laryngospasm, may occur because of the movement of gastric contents into the upper airway.

Complications of GERD are related to the effects of gastric acid on the esophageal mucosa. As a result of repeated gastric acid exposure, there may be scar tissue formation and decreased distensibility of the esophagus, resulting in dysphagia. Esophageal metaplasia (Barrett's syndrome) may also occur.

- The potential for pulmonary complications (pneumonia) exists secondary to aspiration of gastric contents into the pulmonary system.

Diagnostic Studies

- Barium swallow for protrusion of gastric cardia
- Radionucleotide tests for esophageal clearance rate and reflux of gastric contents
- Esophagoscopy to determine LES incompetence and extent of inflammation, scarring, and/or strictures
- Biopsy and cytologic specimens for differential diagnosis
- Motility studies to measure LES pressure
- pH studies to detect acid in the normally alkaline esophagus

Therapeutic Management

Conservative management focuses on eliminating precipitating factors and using medications to relieve symptoms and reduce acid secretion.

Pharmacologic management includes:

- Antacids to relieve heartburn
- Metoclopramide (Reglan), a dopamine antagonist that increases LES pressure and gastric emptying
- Cisapride (Propulsid), a serotonin antagonist that increases LES and promotes healing
- Cholinergic drugs (e.g., Urecholine) used to increase LES pressure, improve esophageal clearance, and increase gastric emptying
- Histamine H_2 receptor blockers (ranitidine, cimetidine) that decrease gastric acid secretion.

Surgical intervention may be necessary if conservative therapy fails, a hiatal hernia is present, or complications such as stenosis, chronic esophagitis, and bleeding exist. The objective of surgery is to restore gastroesophageal integrity (see Hiatal Hernia, therapeutic and nursing management, p. 303).

Nursing Management

Goals

The patient with gastroesophageal reflux disease will avoid factors and activities that cause reflux and have restoration of gastroesophageal integrity with surgery.

Table 31	**Factors Affecting Lower Esophageal Sphincter Pressure and Reflux in Gastroesophageal Reflux Disease and Hiatal Hernia**

Substances Affecting LES Pressure and Tone

Increase pressure
  Bethanechol (Urecholine)
  Cisapride (Propulsid)
  Metoclopramide (Reglan)

Decrease pressure

Fatty foods	Diazepam (Valium)
Chocolate	Morphine sulfate
Peppermint, spearmint	β-adrenergic blocking drugs
Anticholinergics	Calcium channel blockers
Progesterone	Nitrates
Theophylline	Prostaglandins

Measures to Prevent Gastroesophageal Reflux
- *Do* eat high-protein, low-fat diet; eat small, frequent meals; sleep with head of bed elevated; lose weight if overweight
- *Do not* lie down for 2 to 3 hr after eating, wear tight clothing around waist, or bend over (especially after eating).
- *Avoid* alcohol, smoking (causes an almost immediate, marked decrease in LES pressure), and beverages that contain caffeine.

LES, Lower esophageal sphincter.

Nursing Interventions
- Observe and instruct patient about medication side effects.
- Teach and encourage the patient to follow the necessary regimen. Additionally, the nurse should elevate the head of the bed, instruct the patient not to lie down for 2 to 3 hours after eating, and help the patient understand what factors affect and prevent GERD (see Table 31).

GIGANTISM AND ACROMEGALY

Definition/Description
Gigantism or acromegaly are rare disorders characterized by soft-tissue and bony overgrowth resulting from overproduction of growth hormone (GH), which is usually caused by a benign pitu-

itary adenoma (tumor). The prognosis depends on age at onset, age when treatment is initiated, and tumor size. Usually, bone growth can be arrested and soft-tissue hypertrophy can be reversed. However, diabetic and cardiac complications may continue in spite of treatment.

Clinical Manifestations

Gigantism results when the onset of GH overproduction occurs before the closure of the epiphyses, while the long bones are still capable of longitudinal growth. This usually occurs in early childhood but may occur at puberty.

- Affected children may grow as tall as 8 feet and weigh over 300 pounds. They usually die in early adulthood.

Acromegaly is the more common abnormality caused by GH excess. Symptoms begin insidiously in the third or fourth decade of life, and both genders are affected equally. When the problem develops after epiphyseal closure, bones increase in thickness and width.

- Physical features include enlargement of hands, feet, and paranasal and frontal sinuses and deformities of the spine and mandible. Enlargement of soft tissue (e.g., tongue, skin, abdominal organs) causes speech difficulties and hoarseness, coarsening of facial features, sleep apnea, and abdominal distention.
- Persons with acromegaly may exhibit diaphoresis, oily skin, peripheral neuropathy, proximal muscle weakness, and joint pain.
- The enlarged pituitary can exert pressure on surrounding structures, leading to visual disturbances and headaches. Because GH increases free fatty acid levels in the blood, the patient is predisposed to atherosclerosis. The hormone also antagonizes the action of insulin and can cause hyperglycemia.

Diagnostic Studies

- Plasma GH and somatomedin C (insulin-like growth factor levels)
- GH response to oral glucose challenge
- Skull x-rays may show large sella turcica and increased bone density
- CT and MRI for further evaluation and tumor localization

Therapeutic Management

The therapeutic goal in gigantism and acromegaly is to return GH levels to normal. This may be accomplished by surgery, radiation, pharmacologic intervention, or a combination of these three.

- *Surgery* is the usual treatment and offers the best hope for a cure, especially for microadenomas. Surgery is most commonly accomplished with the transsphenoidal approach, in which an incision is made in the inner aspect of the upper lip and gingiva.

- *External radiation* to the tumor normalizes GH levels in most patients, although it may be months to years before GH levels return to normal. Hypopituitarism is a common sequela that often requires replacement therapy.
- *Stereotactic radiosurgery* (gamma surgery) may be applied to small surgically inaccessible pituitary tumors. This procedure consists of radiation delivered to a single site from multiple angles and can be used to occlude blood vessels feeding the tumor, thereby destroying it.
- *Pharmacologic treatment* is accomplished with bromocriptine, a dopamine agonist, or with octreotide, a somatostatin analogue, both of which reduce GH levels to within the normal range. The GH-lowering effects of these drugs are seldom complete or permanent, and they are often used as adjuncts to other therapies or to reduce tumor size before surgery.

Nursing Management

The nurse should assess for manifestations of abnormal tissue growth and physical size in each patient. Assessment of children includes evaluation of growth and development.

- Notable accelerated growth, especially if >5 to 6 inches (12 to 15 cm) per year and if inconsistent with familial patterns, constitutes cause for medical referral. Adults should be questioned about increases in hat, ring, glove, and shoe size.
- When first seen, the patient usually has experienced undesirable changes in appearance and may have substantial alterations in self-image.
- The patient needs unconditional acceptance by health care personnel and considerable emotional support during periods of diagnosis and treatment.
- The patient should be carefully monitored for hyperglycemia and cardiovascular symptoms such as angina pectoris, hypertension, and congestive heart failure.

Preoperative management. The individual treated surgically needs skilled neurosurgical nursing care. The patient should be instructed to avoid vigorous coughing, sneezing, and straining at the stool to prevent cerebrospinal fluid leakage from the point at which the sella turcica was entered.

Postoperative management. After surgery in which a *transsphenoidal approach* has been used, the head of the patient's bed should be elevated at a 30-degree angle at all times. This position avoids pressure on the sella turcica and decreases postoperative headaches.

- Mild analgesia is given for headaches. The nurse should provide mouth care every 4 hours to keep the surgical area clean and free of debris and to promote patient comfort. Tooth brushing should be avoided to prevent disrupting the suture line and creating discomfort.
- Any clear nasal drainage should be sent to the laboratory to be tested for glucose as an indicator of cerebrospinal fluid leakage. Complaints of persistent and severe generalized or supraorbital headache may indicate cerebrospinal fluid leakage into the sinuses.

If *stereotactic radiosurgery* is done, patients will usually be returned from the specialized radiation center to the neurosurgical nursing unit for overnight observation. Vital signs, neurologic status, and fluid volume status must be carefully monitored.

- Possible complications include increased headaches, nausea and vomiting, and discomfort at the pin sites. The patient with a history of seizures is at increased risk for seizures for 24 hours after the procedure.
- Anterior pin sites should be cleaned with hydrogen peroxide and covered with clean dressings; posterior pin sites should be cleaned with 3% peroxide every 6 hours for 48 hours.

If a *hypophysectomy* is performed, immediately after surgery the patient may exhibit signs of diabetes insipidus (see Diabetes Insipidus, p. 172) because of the loss of antidiuretic hormone (ADH). Vasopressin (Pitressin) is given intramuscularly as needed if the urine output is >800 to 900 ml over 2 hours or if the urine specific gravity is <1.004. This is a temporary measure. If the entire pituitary gland is removed, permanent ADH replacement will be needed.

- Because the source of adrenocorticotropic hormone (ACTH) may have been removed, cortisol replacement may be needed. Careful patient education is necessary when cortisone must be taken regularly.
- Hypopituitarism causes infertility because of deficient sex hormones secondary to loss of gonadotropin. If an individual with deficient follicle-stimulating hormone (FSH) and luteinizing hormone (LH) wishes to have children, these hormones can be replaced, with possible restoration of fertility.
- The need for continued drug therapy reduces the patient's perception of independence and requires considerable emotional adjustment.

GLAUCOMA

Definition/Description

Glaucoma is a disorder characterized by increased intraocular pressure (IOP) that ultimately damages the optic nerve, leading to visual field loss. Glaucoma may occur congenitally, as a primary disease, or secondary to other ocular or systemic conditions.

Pathophysiology

Increased IOP results from a decrease in aqueous humor outflow and in some cases may be related to an increase in production of aqueous humor. The outflow of aqueous humor can be decreased by several mechanisms.

- In *open-angle* or *chronic glaucoma,* decreased aqueous outflow is probably caused by increased resistance to outflow in the trabecular meshwork. The increased pressure affects nerve tissue of the optic disc, causing ischemia, and the patient begins to lose peripheral vision.
- In *angle-closure, closed-angle,* or *narrow-angle glaucoma,* the iridocorneal angle closes, blocking aqueous outflow. This change may occur with normal lens enlargement throughout life and can be acute, subacute, or chronic.
- In secondary glaucoma, increased IOP results from other ocular or systemic conditions that may block outflow channels in some way such as the inflammatory process.

Clinical Manifestations

- Open-angle (chronic) glaucoma develops slowly with symptoms of pain or pressure, usually noticed when peripheral vision is severely compromised (tunnel vision).
- Acute angle-closure glaucoma causes definite symptoms of sudden excruciating pain in or around the eye and can be accompanied by nausea and vomiting. Visual symptoms include seeing colored halos around lights, blurred vision, and ocular redness. The acute pressure rise may also cause corneal edema, giving the cornea a steamy appearance.
- Manifestations of subacute or chronic angle-closure glaucoma appear gradually. The patient who has had a previously unrecognized episode of subacute angle-closure glaucoma may report a history of blurred vision, colored halos around lights, ocular redness, or eye or brow pain.

Diagnostic Studies

- IOP with tonometry

- Visual acuity measurement and visual field perimetry
- Slit-lamp microscopy: in open-angle glaucoma, reveals a normal angle; in angle-closure glaucoma, reveals markedly narrow or flat anterior chamber angle, edematous cornea, and a fixed, moderately dilated pupil
- Ophthalmoscopy (direct and indirect) for optic disc cupping

Therapeutic Management

If not recognized and treated, glaucoma may cause blindness that could have been prevented in most patients. The primary focus of therapy is to keep the IOP low enough to prevent the patient from developing optic nerve damage. Specific therapies vary with the type of glaucoma.

- In open-angle (chronic) glaucoma, initial pharmacologic management can include β-adrenergic receptor blocking agents, adrenergic agents, cholinergic agents (miotics), and carbonic anhydrase inhibitors.
- Surgical management may include argon laser trabeculoplasty, trabeculectomy, cyclocryotherapy, and Molteno implant.
- Acute angle-closure glaucoma is an ocular emergency that requires immediate management, including topical cholinergic and hyperosmotic agents with laser peripheral iridotomy or surgery iridectomy.
- Secondary glaucoma is managed by treating the underlying problem and using antiglaucoma drugs.

Nursing Management

This section discusses nursing management for both glaucoma and diabetic retinopathy since both conditions are chronic and have significant long-term sight-threatening implications. Nursing management needs to focus on the chronicity of both diseases and preventing visual impairment.

Goals

The patient with glaucoma or diabetic retinopathy will have no progression of visual impairment, understand the disease process and therapeutic rationale, comply with all aspects of therapy (including medication administration and follow-up care), and have no postoperative complications.

Nursing Diagnoses

The following nursing diagnoses apply to patients with either glaucoma or diabetic retinopathy:

- Risk for noncompliance related to the inconvenience and side effects of glaucoma medications
- Risk for injury related to visual acuity deficits
- Risk for self-care deficits related to visual acuity deficits

- Pain related to pathophysiologic process and surgical correction

Nursing Interventions

The patient with acute angle-closure glaucoma requires immediate medication to lower the IOP. This patient may also be uncomfortable, and nursing comfort interventions may include darkening the environment, applying cool compresses to the patient's forehead, and providing a quiet and private space.

- Most surgical procedures for glaucoma or diabetic retinopathy are done on an outpatient basis. The patient needs postoperative instructions and nursing comfort measures to relieve discomfort.
- The patient with glaucoma and/or diabetic retinopathy needs encouragement to follow therapy recommendations, including information about the disease processes, normal course of the condition, and treatment options, including the rationale underlying each option.
- The patient with diabetic retinopathy has many nursing care needs in addition to ophthalmic considerations. See the nursing care plan for the patient with diabetes mellitus in Lewis/Collier/Heitkemper, *Medical-Surgical Nursing,* edition 4, p. 1458.

Patient Teaching

- It is important to educate the patient and family about the risk of glaucoma or diabetic retinopathy. In addition, stress the importance of early detection and treatment in preventing visual impairment.
- The patient should know that the incidence of glaucoma increases with age and that a comprehensive ophthalmic examination is invaluable in identifying persons with glaucoma or at risk for developing glaucoma.
- The patient with glaucoma needs information about prescribed antiglaucoma agents.
- The patient with diabetic retinopathy should be aware of the benefit of early laser treatment for proliferative retinopathy and the importance of early detection.

GLOMERULONEPHRITIS

Glomerulonephritis is a bilateral inflammation of renal glomeruli, resulting from immunologic processes. Two types of antibody-induced injury can initiate glomerular damage.

- In the first type, antibodies have specificity for antigens within the glomerular basement membrane (GBM). The mechanism that causes a person to develop autoantibodies against the GBM is not known.

- In the second type of immune process, antibodies react with circulating nonglomerular antigens and are randomly deposited as immune complexes along the GBM. Bacterial products appear to be important in poststreptococcal glomerulonephritis and in endocarditis. Viral agents have been recognized in certain cases of glomerulonephritis that develop after hepatitis and measles.

All forms of immune complex diseases are characterized by an accumulation of antigen, antibody, and complement in the glomeruli, which can result in tissue injury and inflammation.

There are many manifestations of glomerulonephritis, including varying degrees of hematuria (ranging from microscopic to gross) and urinary excretion of various formed elements, including red blood cells (RBCs), white blood cells (WBCs), and some granular casts. Proteinuria, elevated blood urea nitrogen (BUN), and serum creatinine levels are other manifestations.

In most cases recovery from the acute illness is complete. If progressive involvement occurs, the result is destruction of renal tissue and marked renal insufficiency.

- The patient's history provides important information related to glomerulonephritis. It is necessary to assess exposure to drugs, immunizations, microbial infections, and viral infections such as hepatitis.
- It is also important to evaluate the patient for more generalized conditions involving immune disorders, such as systemic lupus erythematosus and systemic progressive sclerosis (scleroderma).

G

GLOMERULONEPHRITIS, ACUTE POSTSTREPTOCOCCAL

Definition/Description

Acute poststreptococcal glomerulonephritis (APSGN) develops 5 to 21 days after an infection of the pharynx or skin by certain nephrotoxic strains of group A β-hemolytic streptococci (e.g., streptococcal sore throat, impetigo). Antibodies to the streptococcal antigen are produced, and the antigen-antibody complexes are deposited in the glomeruli. Complement activation causes an inflammatory reaction to the injury.

More than 95% of patients with APSGN recover completely or improve rapidly with conservative management. Prognosis for adults is less favorable than for children. Chronic glomerulonephritis develops in 5% to 15% of affected persons, with irreversible renal failure occurring in <1% of patients.

Clinical Manifestations

Manifestations appear as a variety of signs and symptoms, which may include generalized body edema, hypertension, oliguria, hematuria with a smoky or rusty appearance, and proteinuria. Fluid retention occurs as a result of decreased glomerular filtration.

- Edema appears initially in low-pressure tissues, such as the eyes (periorbital edema), but later progresses to involve the total body as ascites and/or peripheral edema in the legs.
- Smoky urine is indicative of bleeding in the upper urinary tract. The degree of proteinuria varies with the severity of the glomerulonephropathy.
- The patient with APSGN may have abdominal or flank pain. At times the patient has no symptoms, and the problem is found on routine urinalysis.

Diagnostic Studies

- Urinalysis reveals significant numbers of erythrocytes. A finding of erythrocyte casts is highly suggestive of acute glomerulonephritis. Proteinuria may be mild to severe.
- Complete blood count (CBC), blood urea nitrogen (BUN), serum creatinine, and albumin assess the extent of renal impairment.
- Decreased complement levels indicate an immune-mediated response.
- Antistreptolysin O (ASO) titer demonstrates an immune response to streptococcus.
- Renal biopsy (if indicated) may confirm the presence of disease.

Therapeutic Management

Management of ASPGN focuses on symptomatic relief.

- Bed rest is recommended until signs of glomerular inflammation (proteinuria, hematuria) and hypertension subside.
- Edema is treated by restricting sodium and fluid intake and by administrating loop diuretics such as furosemide (Lasix), ethacrynic acid (Edecrin), and bumetanide (Bumex). Severe hypertension is managed with antihypertensive drugs.
- Dietary protein intake may be restricted if there is evidence of an increase in nitrogenous wastes (e.g., elevated BUN).

Penicillin or erythromycin should be given only if streptococcal infection is still present. Steroids and cytotoxic drugs have not been shown to be of value.

Nursing Management

One of the most important ways to prevent the development of APSGN is to encourage early diagnosis and treatment of sore throats and skin lesions. If streptococci are found in the culture, treatment with appropriate antibiotic therapy (usually penicillin) is essential. The patient needs to be encouraged to take the full course of antibiotics to ensure that the bacteria have been eradicated.

- Good personal hygiene is an important factor in preventing the spread of cutaneous streptococcal infections.

Nursing management of acute glomerulonephritis is specific to the patient's symptoms. An important nursing measure is helping the patient plan adequate rest to allow the kidneys to heal. The patient may need assistance in the management of fluid and dietary restrictions.

GLOMERULONEPHRITIS, CHRONIC

Chronic glomerulonephritis is a syndrome that reflects the end stage of glomerular inflammatory disease. Most types of glomerulonephritis can eventually lead to chronic glomerulonephritis.

Chronic glomerulonephritis is characterized by proteinuria, hematuria, and the slow development of the uremic syndrome as a result of decreasing renal function. Chronic glomerulonephritis does not usually follow an acute course. It progresses insidiously toward renal failure over a few to as many as 30 years.

- Chronic glomerulonephritis is often found coincidentally when an abnormality on urinalysis or elevated BP is detected. It is quite common to find that the patient has no recollection or history of acute nephritis or any renal problems. A renal biopsy may be performed to determine the exact cause and nature of the glomerulonephritis. Ultrasonography and CT scanning may be used as diagnostic measures.

Treatment is supportive and symptomatic. Hypertension and urinary tract infections should be treated vigorously. Protein and phosphate restrictions may slow the rate of progression of renal failure (see Renal Failure, Chronic, therapeutic and nursing management, p. 502).

GONORRHEA

Definition/Description

Gonorrhea ranks first among communicable diseases in the United States. Although the overall cases of gonorrhea have been declining since 1975, the prevalence of resistant strains of gonorrhea, primarily penicillinase-producing *Neisseria gonorrhoeae* (PPNG), has been increasing steadily during the same period.

Pathophysiology

Gonorrhea is caused by *Neisseria gonorrhoeae,* a gram-negative diplococcus. Mucosa with columnar epithelium is susceptible to gonococcal infection. This tissue is present in the genitalia (urethra in men, cervix in women), rectum, and oropharynx.

- The disease is spread by direct physical contact with an infected host, usually during sexual activity. Neonates can develop a gonococcal infection after passage through an infected birth canal.
- Incubation period is 3 to 4 days. The disease confers no immunity to subsequent reinfection.
- Gonococcal infection elicits an inflammatory response, which, if left untreated, leads to the formation of fibrous tissue and adhesions. This fibrous scarring is subsequently responsible for many complications such as strictures and tubal abnormalities, which can lead to tubal pregnancy and infertility.

Clinical Manifestations

Men. The initial site of infection is usually the urethra.

- Symptoms of urethritis consist of dysuria and profuse, purulent urethral discharge developing 2 to 5 days after infection.
- Men generally seek medical assistance early in the disease because their symptoms are usually obvious and distressing. It is very unusual for men with gonorrhea to be asymptomatic.

Women. Most women who contract gonorrhea are asymptomatic or have minor symptoms that are often overlooked, making it possible for them to remain a source of infection.

- A few affected women may complain of vaginal discharge, dysuria, or frequency of urination. Changes in menstruation may be a symptom, but these changes are often disregarded by the woman.
- After the incubation period, redness and swelling occur at the site of contact, which is usually the cervix or urethra. A purulent exudate often develops with a potential for abscess formation.

- The disease may remain local or can spread by direct tissue extension to the uterus, fallopian tubes, and ovaries. Although the vulva and vagina are uncommon sites for gonorrheal infection, they may become involved when little or no estrogen is present, such as in prepubertal girls and postmenopausal women.

• • •

Anorectal gonorrhea may be present in both men and women, particularly in homosexual men, and is usually caused by anal intercourse. Gonococcal proctitis in women probably results from rectal coitus and contamination from infected vaginal secretions.

- Most patients with rectal infections have no significant symptoms. A small percentage of individuals develop gonococcal pharyngitis resulting from orogenital sexual contact. When the gonococcus can be demonstrated by culture, individuals of either gender are infectious to their sexual partners.

Because men often seek treatment early in the course of the disease, they are less likely to develop complications. Complications that do occur in men are prostatitis, urethral strictures, and sterility from orchitis or epididymitis.

Because women who are free of symptoms seldom seek treatment, complications are more common and usually constitute the reason for seeking medical attention. Pelvic inflammatory disease (PID), bartholinian abscess, ectopic pregnancy, and infertility are the main complications in women.

- A small percentage of infected persons, mainly women, may develop a disseminated gonococcal infection (DGI). In disseminated infection the appearance of skin lesions, fever, arthralgia, or arthritis usually causes the patient to seek medical help.

Diagnostic Studies

- Cultures for *N. gonorrhoeae* with gram-stained smears of urethral and endocervical exudate provide a definitive diagnosis.
- Testing for other sexually transmitted diseases (STDs) such as syphilis, HIV, and chlamydia
- No effective blood test is available for the diagnosis of gonorrhea.

Therapeutic and Nursing Management

A history of sexual contact with a partner known to have gonorrhea is considered good evidence for the presence of gonorrhea. Because of a short incubation period and high infectivity, treatment is instituted without awaiting culture results, even in the absence of signs or symptoms.

Treatment of gonorrhea in the early stage is curative. Traditionally the drug of choice has been penicillin. As a result of resistant strains of *N. gonorrhoeae,* ceftriaxone, a penicillinase-resistant cephalosporin, has become part of the treatment plan. The high frequency of coexisting chlamydial and gonococcal infections has led to the addition of doxycycline or tetracycline to the treatment regimen. Patients with coincubating syphilis are likely to be cured by the same drugs.

- All sexual contacts of patients with gonorrhea must be treated to prevent reinfection after resumption of sexual relations. The "ping-pong" effect of reexposure, treatment, and reinfection can cease only when infected partners are treated simultaneously.
- Sexual intercourse allows the infection to spread and can retard complete healing as a result of vascular congestion.
- Men should be cautioned against squeezing the penis to look for further discharge.
- Follow-up examination and reculture should be done at least once after treatment, usually in 4 to 7 days. Relapse, reinfection, and complications should be treated appropriately.

GOODPASTURE'S SYNDROME

Goodpasture's syndrome is a rare type of cytotoxic (type II) autoimmune disease characterized by the presence of circulating antibodies against alveolar and glomerular basement membranes (see Hypersensitivity Reactions, p. 314). Although the primary target organ is the kidney, the lungs are also involved.

The pathologic process of the syndrome results when binding of the antibody causes an inflammatory reaction mediated by complement fixation and activation. Type A_2 influenza viruses, hydrocarbons, and penicillamine stimulate autoantibody production. Unknown genetic factors may also be involved.

Clinical manifestations include hemoptysis, pulmonary insufficiency, rhonchi, renal involvement with hematuria and renal failure, weakness, and anemia. Pulmonary hemorrhage usually occurs and may precede glomerular abnormalities by weeks or months.

Abnormal diagnostic findings include low hematocrit and hemoglobin readings, elevated blood urea nitrogen (BUN) and serum creatinine levels, hematuria, and proteinuria.

Treatment consists mainly of corticosteroids, immunosuppressive drugs (e.g., cyclophosphamide, azathioprine), plasmapheresis, and dialysis. Renal transplantation can be attempted once the circulating anti-GBM (glomerular basement membrane) antibody titer decreases. In patients with severe pulmonary hemorrhage, bilateral nephrectomy has been helpful.

Nursing management appropriate for a critically ill patient who is experiencing symptoms of acute renal failure and respiratory distress is instituted. Death is often secondary to respiratory hemorrhage.

- Because this syndrome primarily affects previously healthy young men, support and understanding of the patient and family are of major importance.
- The patient and the family need instructions concerning current therapy, medications, and complications of the disease process.

Gout

Definition/Description

Gout is characterized by recurrent attacks of acute arthritis in association with increased levels of serum uric acid. In *primary gout* a hereditary error of purine metabolism leads to an overproduction or retention of uric acid. Primary gout occurs predominantly in middle-aged men, with almost no incidence in premenopausal women. Frequency of hyperuricemia is increased in families of patients with primary gout.

Secondary gout is usually related to another acquired disorder such as obesity, hyperlipidemia, hypertension, or intrinsic renal disease. This type of gout may also be the result of medications known to inhibit uric acid excretion.

Pathophysiology

Uric acid is the major end product of purine catabolism and is primarily excreted by the kidneys. Thus hyperuricemia may be the result of increased purine synthesis, decreased renal excretion, or both.

- About half of all patients with primary gout can be shown to produce excessive amounts of uric acid. Although high dietary intake of purine has little effect on uric acid levels, hyperuricemia may result from prolonged fasting or excessive drinking because of increased production of ketones, which then inhibit the normal renal excretion of uric acid.

Clinical Manifestations

In the acute phase, gouty arthritis may occur in one or more joints. Affected joints may appear dusky or cyanotic and are extremely inflamed and tender. The most common joint involved is the great toe. Other joints affected are the midtarsal, ankle, knee, and wrist joints and the olecranon bursa.

- Acute gouty arthritis is usually precipitated by events such as trauma, surgery, alcohol ingestion, or systemic infection. The onset of symptoms is usually rapid, with swelling and pain peaking within several hours, often accompanied by a low-grade fever.
- Individual attacks usually subside, treated or untreated, in 2 to 10 days. The affected joint returns entirely to normal, and the patient is often free of symptoms between attacks.

Chronic gout is characterized by multiple joint involvement and deposits of sodium urate crystals *(tophi)*. These are typically seen in the synovium, subchondral bone, olecranon bursa, and vertebrae; along tendons; and in skin and cartilage. Tophi are rarely present at the time of the initial attack and are generally noted only many years after the onset of disease.

The severity of gouty arthritis is variable. The clinical course may consist of infrequent mild attacks or multiple severe episodes associated with a slowly progressive disability.

Complications of chronic inflammation may result in joint deformity. Destruction of the cartilage may predispose the joint to secondary osteoarthritis (OA). Tophaceous deposits may be large and unsightly and may perforate overlying skin, producing draining sinuses that often become secondarily infected. Excessive uric acid excretion may lead to urinary tract stone formation. Pyelonephritis associated with intrarenal sodium urate deposits and obstruction may contribute to renal disease.

Diagnostic Studies
- Presence of monosodium urate monohydrate crystals in synovial fluid establishes the diagnosis.
- Serum uric acid levels are elevated.
- Twenty-four–hour urine collection for uric acid levels determines whether the patient undersecretes or overproduces uric acid.

Therapeutic Management
The management of gout has several goals. The first is to terminate an acute attack. This goal is accomplished by the use of an antiinflammatory agent such as colchicine. Future attacks are prevented by a maintenance dose of colchicine, weight reduction if necessary, avoidance of alcohol and high-purine foods, and use of drugs to reduce the serum urate concentration. Treatment is also aimed at preventing the formation of uric-acid kidney stones and other associated conditions such as hypertriglyceridemia and hypertension.

Pharmacologic Management

Acute gouty arthritis is treated with one of three types of antiin-flammatory agents: colchicine, nonsteroidal antiinflammatory drugs (NSAIDs), or corticosteroids. Corticosteroids should be reserved for cases in which colchicine or NSAIDs are contraindicated or in-effective.

- Aspirin inactivates the effect of uricosurics, resulting in urate retention, and should be avoided while patients are taking probenecid and other uricosuric drugs. Acetaminophen can be used safely if analgesia is required.
- Adequate urine volume must be maintained to prevent precip-itation of uric acid in the renal tubules. Allopurinol (Zyloprim), which blocks production of uric acid, may control the serum level and is particularly useful in patients with uric acid stones or renal impairment, in whom uricosuric drugs may be inef-fective or dangerous.

Nutritional Management

Dietary restrictions may include limiting the use of alcohol and foods high in purine. However, medication can generally control the situation without necessitating these limitations. Obese patients should be instructed in a weight-reduction program.

Nursing Management

Nursing intervention is directed at supportive care of inflamed joints.

- Bed rest may be appropriate, with affected joints properly im-mobilized. Limitation of motion and degree of pain should be assessed.
- Special care is taken to avoid causing pain to an inflamed joint by careless handling. Involvement of a lower extremity may require the use of a cradle or footboard to protect the painful area from the weight of bed clothes.

Patient Teaching

Patient and family should understand that hyperuricemia and gouty arthritis are chronic problems that can be controlled with care-ful adherence to a treatment program.

- Thorough explanations should be given concerning the impor-tance of drug therapy and the need for periodic determination of serum uric acid levels.
- The patient should be aware of precipitating factors that may cause an attack, including overindulgent intake of calories, purines, and alcohol; starvation (fasting); medication use (e.g., aspirin, diuretics); and major medical events (e.g., surgery, my-ocardial infarction).

GRAFT-VERSUS-HOST DISEASE

Graft-versus-host (GVH) disease occurs when an immunoincompetent (immunodeficient) patient undergoes transfusion or transplantation with immunocompetent cells. A GVH response may result from the infusion of any blood product containing viable lymphocytes, such as in blood transfusions, and from transplantation of a fetal thymus, fetal liver, or bone marrow. Unlike most other transplantation situations, the host's rejection of the graft is not as serious as the graft's rejection of the host.

- The GVH response may have its onset 7 to 30 days following infusion of viable lymphocytes. Once the reaction is started, little can be done to modify its course. The exact mechanism involved is not completely understood. However, it involves donor T cells attacking and destroying vulnerable host cells.

Target organs of GVH disease are the skin, gut, and liver. The skin disease may be a maculopapular rash, which can progress to a generalized erythema with bullous formation and desquamation. Liver disease may range from mild jaundice to hepatic coma. Intestinal disease may manifest as mild to severe diarrhea, severe abdominal pain, and malabsorption.

- The major complication of GVH disease is infection. Bacterial and fungal infections predominate immediately after transplantation when granulocytopenia exists. The development of interstitial pneumonitis is the predominant problem later.

There is no adequate treatment of GVH disease once it is established. Although corticosteroids are often used, they enhance susceptibility to infection. The use of methotrexate and cyclosporine has been most effective as preventive rather than treatment measures. Radiation of blood products before they are administered is another measure to prevent T-cell replication.

GUILLAIN-BARRÉ SYNDROME

Definition/Description

Guillain-Barré syndrome is an acute, rapidly progressing, and potentially fatal form of polyneuritis. It is also called *postinfectious polyneuropathy* and *ascending polyneuropathic paralysis*. This disorder affects the peripheral nervous system, resulting in edema and inflammation of affected nerves and a loss of myelin. With adequate supportive care, 85% of affected patients will recover completely.

Pathophysiology

The etiology is unknown, but it is believed to be a cell-mediated immunologic reaction directed at peripheral nerves. The syndrome is frequently preceded by stimulation of the immune system with factors such as a viral illness, trauma, surgery, viral immunizations (e.g., swine flu vaccine), or lymphoproliferative neoplasms. These stimuli are thought to cause an alteration in the immune system, resulting in sensitization of T lymphocytes to the patient's myelin and subsequent myelin damage. Demyelination occurs, and transmission of nerve impulses are stopped or slowed down. Muscle innervated by the damaged peripheral nerves undergoes denervation and atrophy.

- In the recovery phase, remyelination occurs slowly and returns in a proximal to distal pattern; lymphocytes are basically normal and return to complete functioning after the illness.
- A chronic form of Guillain-Barré syndrome has been described in which paralysis evolves more slowly. An apparent relapsing of symptoms occurs, with no involvement of respiratory function or cranial nerves. The patient with this type of polyneuritis generally does not have a full recovery.

Clinical Manifestations

Symptoms usually develop 1 to 3 weeks after the precipitating event.

- Weakness of lower extremities (evolving more or less symmetrically) occurs over hours to days to weeks, usually peaking about day 14. Distal muscles are more severely affected.
- *Paresthesia* (numbness and tingling) is frequent, and paralysis usually follows in the extremities. Hypotonia and areflexia are common persistent symptoms.
- Objective sensory loss is variable, with deep sensitivity more affected than superficial sensations.
- Autonomic disturbances are usually seen in patients with severe muscle involvement and respiratory muscle paralysis. The most dangerous autonomic dysfunctions include orthostatic hypotension, hypertension, and abnormal vagal responses (bradycardia, heart block, asystole).
- Other autonomic dysfunctions include bowel and bladder dysfunction, facial flushing, and diaphoresis. Patients may also have syndrome of inappropriate antidiuretic hormone (SIADH) secretion (see Syndrome of Inappropriate Antidiuretic Hormone, p. 542).
- Progression of Guillain-Barré syndrome to include the lower brain stem involves the facial, abducens, oculomotor, hypoglossal, trigeminal, and vagus cranial nerves. This involvement manifests itself through facial weakness, extraocular eye movement difficulties, dysphagia, and paresthesia of the face.

- Pain is a common finding. It can be categorized as paresthesias, muscular aches and cramps, and hyperesthesias. The pain appears to be worse at night. Narcotics may be indicated for those experiencing severe pain. Pain may lead to a decrease in appetite and may interfere with sleep.

The most serious complication is respiratory failure, which occurs as paralysis progresses to the nerves that innervate the thoracic area. Approximately 20% of patients will require ventilatory support. Respiratory or urinary tract infections may also occur. Fever is generally the first sign of infection, and treatment is directed at the infecting organism. Immobility from the paralysis can cause problems such as paralytic ileus, muscle atrophy, deep vein thrombosis, pulmonary emboli, and orthostatic hypotension.

Diagnostic Studies

Diagnosis is based primarily on the patient's health history and clinical signs.

- Cerebrospinal fluid is normal or has a low protein content initially, but after 7 to 10 days shows a greatly elevated protein level to 700 mg/dl (7 g/L).
- Electromyographic (EMG) and nerve conduction studies are markedly abnormal (reduced nerve conduction velocity) in affected extremities.

Therapeutic Management

Management is aimed at supportive care, particularly ventilatory support, during the acute phase.

- Plasmapheresis is used for severe Guillain-Barré syndrome that involves the respiratory muscles. It is an attempt to remove antibodies that may be present and shorten the course of the disease. Plasmapheresis appears to be more effective in younger than in older patients and when administered early (first 2 weeks) in the course of the disease.
- Corticosteroids and adrenocorticotropic hormone (ACTH) are used to suppress the immune response but appear to have little effect on the prognosis or duration of the disease.
- Monitoring BP and cardiac rate and rhythm is also important during the acute phase because transient cardiac dysrhythmias have been reported. Autonomic dysfunction is common and usually takes the form of bradycardia. Orthostatic hypotension secondary to muscle atony may occur in severe cases. Vasopressor agents and volume expanders may be needed to treat low BP.

Intake is compromised during the acute phase. The patient may experience difficulty swallowing because of cranial nerve involvement.

- Mild dysphagia can be managed by placing the patient in an upright position and flexing the head forward during feeding. For more severe dysphagia, tube feedings may be required. Later in the course of the disease, motor paralysis or weakness will affect the ability to self-feed.
- The patient's nutritional status, including body weight, serum albumin levels, and calorie counts, needs to be evaluated at regular intervals.

Nursing Management
Goals
The patient with Guillain-Barré syndrome will maintain adequate ventilation, be free from aspiration, be pain free or have pain controlled, maintain an acceptable method of communication, maintain adequate nutritional intake, and return to a normal level of physical functioning.

Nursing Diagnoses
- Risk for respiratory distress related to progression of disease process resulting in respiratory muscle paralysis
- Risk for aspiration related to dysphagia
- Pain related to paresthesias, muscle aches and cramps, and hyperesthesias
- Impaired verbal communication related to intubation or paralysis of the muscles of speech
- Fear related to uncertain outcome and seriousness of the disease
- Total self-care deficit related to inability to use muscles to accomplish activities of daily living

Nursing Interventions
The objective of nursing care is to support body systems until the patient recovers. Respiratory failure and infection are serious threats.

- Constant monitoring of the respiratory system by checking respiratory rate, depth, forced vital capacity, and negative inspiratory force provides information about the need for immediate intervention. Monitoring the vital capacity and arterial blood gases (ABGs) is essential. A tracheostomy may be done so that the patient can be mechanically ventilated (see Tracheostomy, p. 682).
- Meticulous suctioning technique is needed to prevent infection whether the patient has an endotracheal tube or tracheostomy. Thorough bronchial hygiene and chest physiotherapy help clear secretions and prevent respiratory deterioration.
- If a fever develops, sputum cultures should be obtained to identify whether the respiratory tract is the source of the pathogen. Appropriate antibiotic therapy is then initiated.

A communication system must be established using the patient's abilities. This is extremely difficult if the disease progresses to involvement of cranial nerves; at the peak of a severe episode the patient may be incapable of communicating.

- The nurse must explain all procedures before doing them and reassure the patient that muscle function will return to some part of the body so that needs and desires can be communicated.

Urinary retention is common for a few days. Intermittent catheterization is preferred to an indwelling catheter to avoid urinary tract infections. However, for the acutely ill patient receiving a large volume of fluids (>2.5 L/day), indwelling catheterization may be safer to reduce overdistension of a temporarily flaccid bladder and to prevent vesicoureteral reflux.

Physiotherapy is indicated early to help prevent problems related to immobility. Passive range-of-motion exercises and attention to body position help maintain function and prevent contractures.

Nutritional needs must be met in spite of possible problems associated with gastric dilatation, paralytic ileus development, and aspiration potential if the gag reflex is lost.

- In addition to checking for the gag reflex, the nurse should note drooling and other difficulties with secretions, which may be more indicative of an inadequate gag reflex.
- Initially, tube feedings or parenteral nutrition may be used to ensure adequate caloric intake. Fluid and electrolyte therapy must be monitored carefully to prevent electrolyte imbalances.

HEAD INJURY

Definition/Description

Head injury includes any trauma to the scalp, skull, or brain. The majority of deaths after a head injury occur immediately after the injury, either from the direct head trauma or massive hemorrhage and shock. Deaths occurring within a few hours of the trauma are caused by progressive worsening of the head injury or from internal bleeding. Observation of changes in neurologic status and surgical intervention are critical in the prevention of death at this point. Death occurring 3 weeks or more after injury results from multisystem failure.

Types of Head Injuries

Scalp lacerations. These are the most minor of the head traumas. The major complication associated with scalp laceration is infection.

Skull fractures. This type of fracture frequently occurs with head trauma. Fractures may be closed or open, depending on the presence of a scalp laceration or extension of the fracture into the air sinuses or dura.

- Type and severity of a skull fracture depends on velocity, momentum, direction of injuring agent, and site of impact. Specific manifestations of a skull fracture are generally associated with location of the injury (see Table 54-9 in Lewis/Collier/Heitkemper, *Medical-Surgical Nursing,* edition 4, p. 1701).

The major potential complications of skull fractures are intracranial infections, hematoma, and meningeal and brain tissue damage.

Minor head trauma

- *Concussion* is a sudden transient head injury associated with a disruption in neural activity and a change in level of consciousness (LOC). The patient may not lose total consciousness. Signs of concussion include a brief disruption in LOC, amnesia for the event (retrograde amnesia), and headache. The manifestations are generally of short duration.
- *Postconcussion syndrome* is seen anywhere from 2 weeks to 2 months after the concussion. Symptoms include persistent headache, lethargy, behavior changes, decreased short-term memory, and changes in intellectual ability.

Although a concussion is generally considered benign and usually resolves spontaneously, the symptoms may be the beginning of a more serious progressive problem. At discharge it is important to give the patient and family instructions for observation and accurate reporting of symptoms or changes in neurologic status.

H

Major head trauma. Contusions and lacerations are injuries that involve severe trauma to the brain. Contusions and lacerations are generally associated with closed injuries.

- A *contusion* is a bruising of brain tissue with potential for development of areas of necrosis, pulping infarction, hemorrhage, and edema. A contusion frequently occurs at the site of a fracture. Bleeding around the contusion site is generally minimal, and blood is reabsorbed slowly. Neurologic assessment demonstrates focal findings and a generalized disturbance in the LOC. Seizures are a common complication.
- *Lacerations* involve actual tearing of brain tissue and occur frequently in compound fractures and penetrating injuries. Tissue damage is severe, and surgical repair of the laceration is impossible because of the texture of the brain tissue. If bleeding is deep into the brain parenchyma, focal and generalized signs are noted.

When major head trauma occurs, many delayed responses are seen, including hemorrhage, hematoma formation, seizures, and cerebral edema (see Increased Intracranial Pressure, p. 340, and Seizure Disorders, p. 516).

- Prognosis is generally poor for a large intracerebral hemorrhage. Subarachnoid hemorrhage and intraventricular hemorrhage can also occur secondary to head trauma.

Complications

Epidural hematoma. An epidural hematoma results from bleeding between the dura and inner surface of the skull. An epidural hematoma, which is a neurologic emergency, is usually associated with a linear fracture crossing a major artery in the dura, causing a tear. It can have a venous or arterial origin.

- Venous epidural hematomas are associated with a tear of the dural venous sinus and develop slowly.
- With arterial hematomas the middle meningeal artery lying under the temporal bone is frequently torn. Because this is an arterial hemorrhage, the hematoma develops rapidly.

Clinical manifestations typically include unconsciousness, with a brief lucid interval followed by a decrease in LOC. Other symptoms may be a headache, nausea and vomiting, and focal findings. Rapid surgical intervention is needed to prevent cerebral herniation.

Subdural hematoma. A subdural hematoma occurs from bleeding between the dura mater and the arachnoid layer of the meningeal covering of the brain. A subdural hematoma usually results from injury to the brain substance and its parenchymal vessels. Because a subdural hematoma is usually venous in origin, the hematoma is much slower to develop a mass large enough to produce symptoms. Subdural hematomas may be acute, subacute, or chronic (see Table

54-10 in Lewis/Collier/Heitkemper, *Medical-Surgical Nursing,* edition 4, p. 1703).

- An *acute subdural hematoma* manifests signs within 48 hours of the injury. Manifestations are similar to those associated with brain tissue compression in increased intracranial pressure (ICP) (see Increased Intracranial Pressure, p. 340). The patient appears drowsy and confused, and the ipsilateral pupil dilates and becomes fixed.
- A *subacute subdural hematoma* usually occurs within 2 to 14 days of the injury. Failure to regain consciousness may point to this possibility.
- A *chronic subdural hematoma* develops over weeks or months after a seemingly minor head injury. Peak incidence is in the sixth and seventh decades of life, when a larger subdural space is available as a result of brain atrophy. The presenting complaints are focal symptoms rather than signs of increased ICP.

Diagnostic Studies
- Skull radiogram to rule out skull fracture
- CT scan to determine craniocerebral trauma
- MRI, positron emission tomography (PET), and evoked potential studies assist in diagnosis and differentiation of head injuries
- Transcranial Doppler study measures cerebral blood flow and velocity

Therapeutic Management

H

Emergency management of the patient with head injury includes measures to prevent secondary injury by treating cerebral edema and managing increased ICP. The principal treatment of head injuries is timely diagnosis and surgery, if necessary. For the patient with a concussion or contusion, observation and management of increased ICP are primary management strategies.

- The treatment of skull fractures is usually conservative. For depressed fractures and fractures with loose fragments, a craniotomy is necessary to elevate depressed bone and remove free fragments. If large amounts of bone are destroyed, the bone may be removed (craniectomy) and a cranioplasty will be needed at a later time (see Cranial Surgery in Lewis/Collier/Heitkemper, *Medical-Surgical Nursing,* edition 4, p. 1710).
- In cases of acute subdural and epidural hematomas the blood must be removed. A craniotomy is generally performed to visualize the bleeding vessels so that they can be properly coagulated. Burr-hole openings may be used in an emergency for more rapid decompression, followed by a craniotomy to stop all bleeding. A drain is generally placed for several days postoperatively to prevent any reaccumulation of blood.

Nursing Management
Goals
The patient with an acute head injury will maintain adequate cerebral perfusion; be free from pain, discomfort, fever, and infection; and attain maximal motor and sensory function.

Nursing Diagnoses
- Altered cerebral tissue perfusion related to interruption of cerebral blood flow associated with cerebral hemorrhage and edema
- Risk for increased ICP secondary to cerebral edema
- Hyperthermia related to increased metabolism, infection, and loss of cerebral integrative function secondary to possible hypothalamic injury
- Sensory/perceptual alterations related to cerebral injury and intensive care unit environment
- Pain related to headache
- Impaired physical mobility related to decreased LOC and treatment-imposed bed rest

Nursing Interventions
One of the best ways to prevent head injuries is to prevent car and motorcycle accidents.
- The nurse can be active in campaigns that promote driving safety and can speak to driver education classes regarding the dangers of unsafe driving and driving after drinking alcohol.
- Wearing of seat belts in cars and the use of helmets for riding on motorcycles are the most effective measures for increasing survival after accidents. Young parents should be educated in the proper use of car seats and restraints for their children.
- The nurse should also teach younger children about safety precautions for bicycle riding, skateboarding, and contact sports.

Acute nursing management may initially consist only of observation for changes in neurologic status. This action is important because the patient's condition may deteriorate rapidly, necessitating emergency surgery.
- The nurse should explain the need for frequent neurologic assessments to both the patient and family. Behavioral manifestations associated with head injury can result in a frightened, disoriented patient who is combative and resists help.
- Restraints should be avoided if possible because they often produce agitation, which further increases ICP. A family member may be available to stay with the patient and thus prevent increasing anxiety and fear.

The Glascow Coma Scale (GCS) is useful in assessing the level of arousal (see Glascow Coma Scale, p. 706). Indications of a deteriorating neurologic state, such as decreasing LOC or a lessening of motor strength, should be reported.

Much of the nursing care for the brain-injured patient relates to the unconscious state and increased ICP (see Increased Intracranial Pressure, nursing management, p. 343).

- Loss of the corneal reflex may necessitate administering lubricating eye drops, taping the eyes shut, or suturing the eyelids to prevent corneal abrasion. Periorbital ecchymosis and edema disappear spontaneously, but cold and, later, warm compresses provide comfort and hasten the process. Diplopia can be relieved by use of an eye patch.
- If cerebrospinal fluid rhinorrhea or otorrhea occurs, the nurse should inform the physician immediately. A loose collection pad may be placed under the nose or over the ear. The patient should be cautioned not to sneeze or blow the nose.
- Nausea and vomiting may be a problem and can be alleviated by antiemetic medication. Headache can usually be controlled with aspirin or small doses of codeine.

If the patient's condition deteriorates, intracranial surgery may be necessary. A burr hole or craniotomy may be indicated, depending on the underlying injury. The patient is often unconscious before surgery, making it necessary for a family member to sign the consent form for surgery. This is a difficult and frightening time for the patient's family and requires sensitive nursing management. The suddenness of the situation makes it especially difficult for the family to cope.

Once the patient's condition has stabilized, he/she is usually transferred to a general neurologic unit for rehabilitation. As with any craniocerebral problem, there may be chronic problems related to motor and sensory deficits, communication, memory, and intellectual functioning.

- Many of the principles of nursing management of the patient with a stroke are appropriate (see Cerebrovascular Accident [Stroke], p. 101). With time and patience many of the chronic problems subside or disappear. Outward appearance is not a good indicator of how well the patient will function in the home or work environment.

Progressive recovery may continue for 6 months or more before a plateau is reached and a prognosis for recovery can be made. Specific nursing management depends on residual deficits. In all cases the family must be given special consideration. They need to understand what is happening, and they must be taught appropriate interaction patterns.

- The family often has unrealistic expectations of the patient as the coma begins to recede. The nurse needs to prepare the family for the emergence of the patient from coma and must explain that the process of awakening often takes several weeks.

- Family members, particularly spouses, go through role transition as the role changes from one of spouse to that of caregiver.

Mental and emotional sequelae of brain trauma are often the most incapacitating problems. It is estimated that the majority of patients with head injuries who have been comatose for more than 6 hours undergo some personality change. They may suffer loss of concentration and memory and defective memory processing. Personal drive may decrease; apathy and apparent laziness may increase. The patient's behavior may indicate a loss of social restraint, judgment, tact, and emotional control.

HEAD AND NECK CANCER

Definition/Description

Head and neck cancer represents about 5% of all cancer cases, with more men than women diagnosed, generally after age 50. Although specific causes of head and neck cancer are not known, well-known risk factors include cigarette smoking and other forms of tobacco, heavy alcohol intake, and chronic infection with Epstein-Barr or papillomavirus.

Clinical Manifestations

Early signs and symptoms of upper airway cancers vary with the location of the tumor. Cancer of the oral cavity may cause pain that is aggravated by movement of the affected structure or with ingestion of acidic foods. Ulcers that do not heal or a change in the fit of dentures may also be early signs.

Cancers of the oropharynx, hypopharynx, and supraglottic larynx rarely produce early symptoms and are usually diagnosed in later stages.

- The patient may complain of persistent unilateral sore throat or otalgia (ear pain). Hoarseness that lasts longer than 2 weeks may be a symptom of early laryngeal cancer. Some patients experience what may feel like a lump in the throat or a change in voice quality.
- There may be thickening of the normally soft and pliable oral mucosa. *Leukoplakia* (white patch) or *erythroplakia* (red patch) may be seen and should be noted for later biopsy. Both leukoplakia and *carcinoma in situ* (localized to a defined area) may precede invasive carcinoma by many years.
- Late stages of head and neck cancers have easily detectable signs and symptoms including pain, dysphagia, decreased mobility of the tongue, airway obstruction, and cranial neuropathies.

Diagnostic Studies

- If lesions are suspected, upper airways may be examined by indirect laryngoscopy. A flexible nasopharyngoscope may also be used.
- CT scanning or MRI may be performed to detect local and regional spread.
- Multiple biopsy specimens are obtained to determine the extent of the disease.

Therapeutic Management

On the basis of information obtained, a decision will be made about the stage of the disease by means of the tumor, nodes, metastasis (TNM) system (see Table 12, p. 71). This system identifies the stage of disease (stage I to stage IV) and guides principles of treatment.

- Approximately one third of patients have highly confined stage I or II lesions. These patients can undergo surgery or radiation therapy with the goal of cure. In stage III or IV disease fewer than 30% of patients are cured.

More advanced disease is managed with combinations of surgery and radiation therapy or surgery and chemotherapy. Induction chemotherapy (i.e., chemotherapy given before surgery) may allow less extensive surgery and reduce the incidence of metastasis.

- Strategies to prevent metastasis involve chemotherapy or giving drugs such as retinoids to suppress or prevent the development of invasive cancer.
- Advanced lesions are managed by a total laryngectomy in which the entire larynx and preepiglottic region are removed and a permanent tracheostomy is performed (see Tracheostomy, p. 682). Radical neck dissection frequently accompanies total laryngectomy. Depending on the extent of involvement, extensive dissection and reconstruction may also be performed.

Nutritional Management

The patient will likely return from the operating room with a nasogastric tube in place. Initially the tube is used for gastric decompression and then later for tube feedings. It is the responsibility of the nurse to assess correct placement and function of the tube.

- Gastric distention may lead to vomiting, aspiration, stress on the suture line, or wound contamination. The patient who undergoes extensive surgical procedures may require tube feedings to maintain nutrition until healing is sufficient to permit oral intake (see Tube Feeding, p. 685).

H

Nursing Management

Goals

The patient with head or neck cancer will have a patent airway, no spread of cancer, no complications related to therapy, adequate nutritional intake, minimal to no pain, and appropriate communication methods.

See the nursing care plan for the patient having radical neck surgery or a permanent laryngectomy in Lewis/Collier/Heitkemper, *Medical-Surgical Nursing,* edition 4, p. 614.

Nursing Diagnoses

- Impaired verbal communication related to removal of vocal cords
- Anxiety related to lack of knowledge regarding surgical procedure, postoperative course, pain management, and prevention of complications
- Ineffective airway clearance related to difficulty expectorating sputum and presence of tracheostomy
- Altered nutrition: less than body requirements related to inability to ingest food secondary to pain, edema at surgical site, dysphagia, and presence of a nasogastric tube
- Pain related to surgical procedure
- Body image disturbance related to altered facial appearance

Nursing Interventions

Development of head and neck cancer is closely related to personal habits, primarily cigarette smoking and the use of chewing tobacco. The nurse should include information about these risk factors in health teaching.

- If cancer has been diagnosed, smoking cessation is still important because patients who continue to smoke during radiation therapy have lower rates of response and survival.

The nurse is in a key position to detect early signs of head and neck cancer. Early detection is critical. Symptoms are often not reported, however, because the patient does not know the significance or fears the consequences. The patient and family must be taught about the type of therapy to be performed and the care required. This teaching should include (1) changes as a result of radiation therapy or surgical intervention, (2) duration of change, (3) change in voice and ability to eat, (4) alternate methods of speech, (5) self-help groups and community resources, and (6) emotional adjustments to be anticipated. It is essential to include the patient and significant other in all aspects of teaching and care.

Preoperative care for radical neck surgery must include information about expected changes in speech after surgical intervention. The nurse or speech pathologist should demonstrate an alternative means of communicating that does not require the use of speech. This approach assists in decreasing patient anxiety about what to anticipate after surgery.

Postoperative care includes airway management as the primary concern. The patient is placed in a semi-Fowler's position to decrease edema and tension on the suture lines. Vital signs should be monitored frequently because of the risk of hemorrhage. Immediately after surgery the postlaryngectomy patient requires frequent suctioning because secretions or saliva cannot be swallowed.

- If the patient develops mucous plugs or very thick secretions, a 2 to 3 ml bolus of normal saline should be instilled into the airway to loosen the secretions enough for the patient to clear the airway either through coughing or suctioning.
- The potency of drainage tubes should be monitored every 4 hours for 24 hours to ensure that they are properly removing serous drainage. After the drainage tubes are removed, the area should be closely monitored to detect any swelling. If fluid continues to accumulate, aspiration may be necessary.

A speech therapist or speech pathologist should meet with the patient to discuss voice restoration. The International Association of Laryngectomees, an organization of laryngectomy patients, focuses on assisting patients to reestablish speech. Local groups, called "Lost Cord Clubs," identify members who can visit the patient, preferably preoperatively.

- Since the patient no longer breathes through the nose, the ability to smell smoke and food may be lost. Advise the patient to install smoke detectors in the home. It is important for food to be colorful, attractively prepared, and nutritious, because taste may also be diminished.

H

Instruct the patient on resumption of exercise, recreation, and sexual activity when able. Most patients can return to work 1 to 2 months after laryngectomy.

- Loss of speech, loss of the ability to taste and smell, inability to produce audible sounds (including laughing and weeping), and the presence of a permanent tracheal stoma that produces undesirable mucus are often overwhelming to the patient. If the patient has a significant other, the reaction of this person to the patient's altered appearance is important.
- Encouraging the patient to participate in self-care activities is an important part of rehabilitation.
- If pain is a problem, a pain control regimen should be identified to provide comfort and referral should be made to a hospice, if indicated.

Headache

Definition/Description

Headaches are one of the most common types of pain experienced by humans. Of all persons with headache, the majority have *functional* headaches, such as benign migraine or tension-type origin; the remainder have *organic* headaches caused by significant intracranial or extracranial disease.

Headaches are classified based on the characteristics of the headache and facial pain.

- Primary classifications include *tension-type, migraine,* and *cluster headaches.* The patient's health history and neurologic examination are diagnostic keys to determining the type of headache. Characteristics of these headaches are shown in Table 56-1 in Lewis/Collier/Heitkemper, *Medical-Surgical Nursing,* edition 4, p. 1752.

Tension-Type Headache

Tension-type headache has been called *muscle-contraction, tension, psychogenic,* and *rheumatic* headache. It is the most common type and is considered the most difficult to treat. This type of headache is related to abnormal neuronal sensitivity and pain facilitation at the brainstem level. The exact etiology remains obscure.

Clinical manifestations. There is no prodrome or aura (early manifestation of impending disease) in tension-type headache. Pain is usually bilateral, occurring most often in the back of the neck. It usually does not interfere with sleep. The pain is often described as a tight, squeezing, bandlike pressure. It is sustained, chronic, dull, and persistent.

- Headaches may occur intermittently for weeks, months, or even years. Many patients have a combination of migraine and tension-type headaches, with features of both types occurring simultaneously.
- Patients with migraine headaches may experience tension-type headaches between migraine attacks.

Diagnostic studies. Careful history taking is the most important diagnostic tool. Electromyography (EMG) may reveal sustained contraction of the neck, scalp, or facial muscles, but many patients do not show increased muscle tension with this test. If tension-type headache is present during physical examination, increased resistance to passive movement of the head and tenderness of the head and neck may be present.

Migraine Headache

For some individuals *migraine headaches* begin in childhood or adolescence. A family history of migraine can be found in 65% of patients with migraine. Migraine headaches often have no known precipitating events. However, the headache may be precipitated by stress, bright lights, menstruation, alcohol, or certain foods such as chocolate or cheese.

Pathophysiology. Although the exact etiology of migraine headaches is not known, recent evidence suggests that neurologic, vascular, and chemical factors are involved. Inflammation of the arterial vessels by endogenous monoamines (serotonin), peptides (substance P), estrogen, or diet (alcohol) may be responsible for migraine headaches.

- The *aura* of migraine is associated with "spreading depression," a wave of *oligemia* (diminished cerebral blood flow) beginning in the occipital lobe and spreading forward in the brain. This continues into the headache phase, during which substance P and other polypeptides are released by perivascular nerve endings. Substance P produces vasodilatation, increased capillary permeability, perivascular inflammation, and stimulation of afferent fibers.

Clinical manifestations. *Migraine without aura* is the most common type of migraine headache. The prodrome is not sharply defined and may involve psychic disturbances, GI upset, and changes in fluid balance. The prodrome may precede the headache phase by several hours or days. The headache itself may last several hours or days.

Migraine with aura occurs in only 10% of migraine headache episodes. The sharply defined aura may last 10 to 30 minutes before the start of the headache and may include sensory dysfunction (e.g., visual field defects, tingling or burning sensations, or paresthesias), motor dysfunction (e.g., weakness, paralysis), dizziness, confusion, and loss of consciousness. The classic preheadache symptom is the perception of flashing lights in one quadrant of the visual field, often referred to as *scintillating scotomata.* This type of migraine headache usually peaks in 1 hour and may last several hours.

Other clinical manifestations that occur in migraine, both with and without aura, are generalized edema, irritability, pallor, nausea and vomiting, and sweating. During the headache phase, patients with migraine tend to "hibernate"; that is, they seek shelter from noise, light, odors, people, and problems. The headache is described as a steady throbbing pain that is synchronous with the pulse. Although the headache is usually unilateral, it may switch to the opposite side in another episode.

Diagnostic studies. Diagnosis of migraine headache is usually made from the health history. Neurologic and other diagnostic examinations are often normal.

Cluster Headache

Cluster headache is one of the most severe forms of head pain. It occurs less frequently than migraine and is more common in men than in women. Onset is usually between the ages of 30 and 60 years.

Pathophysiology. Neither the cause nor pathophysiology of cluster headache is fully known. The vasodilatation that occurs in the affected part of the face is extracranial, with the trigeminal nerve implicated in the production of pain. Activation of this nerve causes release of substance P and other vasoactive substances, which cause vasodilatation, stimulation of afferent pain fibers, and neurogenic inflammation.

- Periodicity and clocklike regularity of cluster headaches indicate a dysfunction of the biologic clock mechanisms of the hypothalamus. These headaches can also be triggered by alcohol ingestion.

Clinical manifestations. The headache has an abrupt onset, usually without a prodrome. It peaks in 5 minutes and lasts 30 to 90 minutes. It is not uncommon for this type of headache to start at night, awakening the patient after a few hours of sleep. The headache may recur several times a day over a period of several days, with each cluster lasting 2 to 3 months.

- It usually affects the upper face, periorbital region, and the forehead on one side of the face and head. The headache may not recur for months or years.
- The patient may also exhibit conjunctivitis, increased lacrimation (tearing), and nasal congestion on the side of the headache. A partial *Horner's syndrome* (constriction of the pupil and *ptosis* [drooping] of the eyelid on the affected side) may be seen. The headache is described as deep, steady, and boring but not throbbing.
- Unlike the patient with migraine, who seeks isolation and quiet, the patient with a cluster headache paces the floor, cries out, does bizarre things, and resents being touched. The patient with a cluster headache does not experience systemic manifestations, such as nausea or vomiting, that accompany a migraine headache.

Diagnostic studies. Diagnosis is primarily based on the history. However, a CT scan with contrast dye and cerebral angiography may be performed to rule out an aneurysm, tumor, and infection.

Therapeutic Management of Headaches

If no underlying systemic disease is found, therapy is directed toward the functional type of headache. Table 32 summarizes current therapies for symptomatic and therapeutic relief of common headaches. These therapies can include meditation, yoga, biofeedback, and muscle relaxation training.

Pharmacologic Management

Tension-type headache. Drug treatment usually involves a nonnarcotic analgesic (e.g., aspirin, acetaminophen, ibuprofen) used alone or in combination with a sedative, a muscle relaxant, a tranquilizer, or codeine. Many of these drugs have potentially dangerous side effects.

Migraine headache. Drug treatment is aimed at treating all components of the acute attack and preventing escalation of the headache. Drugs that may relieve migraine headache include Fiorinal, Midrin, aspirin, acetaminophen, meperidine (Demerol), and codeine.

- Drugs that affect serotonin have also been found to be beneficial. Methysergide (Sansert) produces vasoconstriction, which is useful in the prevention of migraine headaches. Sumatriptan succinate (Imitrex), which is selective for vascular serotonin receptors, produces vasoconstriction, and is used for management of acute migraine headaches.
- Beta blockers (e.g., propranolol), tricyclic antidepressants, calcium channel blockers, clonidine, thiazides, and other antihypertensive drugs may be used prophylactically for very severe or frequent migraine headaches.

Cluster headache. Because these headaches occur suddenly, often at night, and are not long lasting, pharmacologic management is not as useful as it is for other types of headache. Inhalation of pure O_2 will abort the headache in approximately 50% of patients. Ergotamine and methysergide may be used prophylactically when the cluster headache recurs at a known time. However, because of its adverse side effects, methysergide is not used on a long-term basis for chronic cluster headaches. Sumatriptan (Imitrex) has been shown to shorten cluster headaches.

Nursing Management of Headaches

Goals

The patient with a headache will have reduced pain or no pain, will experience increased comfort and decreased anxiety, will understand triggering events and treatment strategies, and will use positive coping strategies to deal with chronic pain.

See the nursing care plan for the patient with headache in Lewis/Collier/Heitkemper, *Medical-Surgical Nursing,* edition 4, p. 1756.

Nursing Diagnoses

- Acute pain related to headache
- Risk for ineffective individual coping related to chronic pain behavior

Table 32	Therapeutic Management: Headache
	Tension-type headache
Diagnostic	History of neck and head tenderness, resistance to movement, EMG
Therapeutic	
■ Symptomatic	Nonnarcotic analgesics (aspirin, acetaminophen, ibuprofen) Analgesic combinations (Fiorinal) Muscle relaxants
■ Prophylactic	Tricyclic antidepressants (amitriptyline) Beta-adrenergic blockers (propranolol) Biofeedback Muscle relaxation training Psychotherapy

EMG, Electromyography.
*Only for patients suffering from one or more severe headaches per week.

- Sleep pattern disturbance related to pain
- Anxiety related to lack of knowledge of etiology and treatment of headache and uncertainty of recurrence of headache
- Hopelessness related to chronic pain, alteration of lifestyle, and ineffective treatment modalities

Nursing Interventions
- Headaches may result from an inability to cope with daily stresses. The most effective therapy may be to help the patient examine his/her lifestyle, recognize stressful situations, and learn to cope with them more appropriately. Precipitating factors can be identified, and ways of avoiding them can be developed. Daily exercise, relaxation periods, and socializing can be encouraged since each can help decrease the recurrence of headache.

Migraine headache	Cluster headache
History	History, thermography
Nonnarcotic analgesics (aspirin, acetaminophen)	Alpha-adrenergic blockers (ergotamine tartrate)
Serotonin receptor agonist (sumatriptan)	Vasoconstrictors
Alpha-adrenergic blockers (ergotamine tartrate)	O_2
Vasoconstrictors (isometheptene)	
Corticosteroids (dexamethasone)	
Beta-adrenergic blockers (propranolol)	Alpha-adrenergic blockers (ergotamine tartrate)
Serotonin antagonists* (methysergide)	Serotonin antagonists (methysergide)
Antidepressants (amitriptyline, imipramine)	Corticosteroids (prednisone)
Calcium channel blockers	Lithium
Biofeedback	Calcium channel blockers (nifedipine)
Yoga	
Meditation	
Electric counterstimulation	

H

- The nurse can suggest alternative ways of handling the pain of headache through practices such as relaxation, meditation, yoga, and self-hypnosis. Massage and moist hot packs to the neck and head can help a patient with tension-type headaches.
- The patient should learn about medications prescribed for prophylactic and symptomatic treatment of headache and should be able to describe the purpose, action, dosage, and side effects of the medication.
- For the patient whose headaches are triggered by food, dietary counseling may be provided. The patient is encouraged to eliminate foods that may provoke headaches (e.g., chocolate, alcohol, excessive caffeine, cheese, fermented foods, monosodium glutamate).

HEAT-RELATED EMERGENCIES

Definition/Description

Heat-related emergencies are a failure of the body's heat mechanism to dissipate heat relative to demands. The body is more efficient with dissipating than retaining heat. The core attempts to keep body temperature at 100° F (37.8° C). Heat illness often occurs because of strenuous activities in hot or humid environments, the wearing of clothing that interferes with perspiration, high fevers, endocrine problems, and obesity.

The basic mechanisms of heat illness are increased heat production, perspiration, and salt and water evaporation. Heat stress increases cardiac output to compensate for increased peripheral blood flow. Dehydration occurs because of increased sweating and evaporation of sweat that results in loss of salt and water. Clinical manifestations and treatment for heat-related emergencies are summarized in Table 62-8 in Lewis/Collier/Heitkemper, *Medical-Surgical Nursing,* edition 4, p. 2011.

Heat-related emergencies are common during periods of prolonged heat and high humidity. The onset may be gradual or rapid. Older adults and individuals with diabetes mellitus, chronic renal failure or cardiovascular or pulmonary disease are particularly vulnerable.

Heat stroke (hyperthermia). Heat stroke is the most serious heat-related emergency and has a high risk of mortality and morbidity. A core temperature >103° to 106° F (39.4° to 41.1° C) without sweating and with altered mentation is a true medical emergency. Prognosis is related to age, health, and length of exposure.

- Heat stroke is common during periods of prolonged heat for more than 3 days with accompanying high humidity. Fluid and electrolytes become depleted and blood vessels dilate, which results in increased cardiac output. Eventually the sweat glands stop functioning; when sweating ceases, core temperature increases rapidly.
- Patients have hot, dry skin; a greatly elevated temperature; an altered level of consciousness; ashen skin; and cardiac collapse.

Treatment requires rapid initial assessment and aggressive treatment. Airway management includes administration of 100% O_2 to compensate for the hypermetabolic state, intubation if necessary, and ventilation with a bag valve mask. IV fluids are initiated, and a central venous pressure or pulmonary artery catheter is inserted to monitor fluid status. All clothing is removed and cooling methods such as tepid water mist, fans, and ice packs to the head, groin, axillae, and neck are initiated. Shivering should be prevented because it generates muscle heat. If conventional cooling methods are not successful, more aggressive treatment can include ice water lavage, cold-water peritoneal dialysis, and cardiopulmonary bypass.

- Aggressive temperature reduction should continue until the patient's temperature reaches 101° F (38° C). If shivering occurs, diazepam (Valium) or other muscle relaxants may be administered.
- After appropriate treatment, patient teaching must be aimed at preventing recurrence. Patients who are taking phototoxic drugs (e.g., phenothiazines, tetracycline) should be warned that these drugs make them more susceptible to heat emergencies.

Heat edema. This condition involves swelling of the hands, feet, and ankles. Older people or individuals not acclimated to the environment may have pitting edema. Patients with heat edema will not have other signs and symptoms. Physical findings are due to heat-induced hyperaldosteronism. Treatment includes elevating the legs and reassurance. Diuretics should not be used to treat heat edema.

Heat cramps. These are brief, intermittent, severe muscle cramps occurring in large muscle groups fatigued by heavy work. The cramps tend to occur while the patient is resting after exercise or heavy labor. They are usually seen in athletes who are acclimated, in good health, and have good fluid intake. These patients sweat profusely and replace lost fluid with salt-poor solutions.

- Heat cramps seem to be related to salt deficiency and are rapidly relieved by administration of oral or IV crystalloid salt solutions. Additional treatment includes elevation, gentle massage, and analgesia.
- Education of the patient should emphasize including salt replacement during heavy exercise in a hot environment.

Heat exhaustion. This condition is caused by prolonged heat exposure resulting in volume and electrolyte depletion. Heat exhaustion is usually seen in people who have engaged in sports or strenuous exercise in hot, humid weather. Heat exhaustion is characterized by fatigue, lightheadedness, nausea, vomiting, diarrhea, and feelings of impending doom.

- The patient will manifest tachypnea, hypotension, tachycardia, and a moderately elevated body temperature. Additional manifestations include dilated pupils, mild confusion with impaired judgment, profuse sweating, and complaints of headache.

Treatment includes undressing the patient, IV normal saline solution, cooling, and bed rest. Fluid and electrolyte replacement depends on laboratory results of electrolyte, blood urea nitrogen, and hematocrit levels. Older or chronically ill patients should be admitted to the hospital.

H

Hemophilia

Definition/Description

Hemophilia is a hereditary bleeding disorder caused by defective or deficient coagulation factors. The two major forms of hemophilia that can occur in mild to severe forms are *hemophilia A* (classic hemophilia, factor VIII deficiency) and *hemophilia B* (Christmas disease, factor IX deficiency). *Von Willebrand disease* is a related disorder involving a congenitally acquired deficiency of the von Willebrand coagulation protein.

Hemophilia A is the most common form of hemophilia, comprising about 80% of all cases. Von Willebrand disease is considered the most common congenital bleeding disorder in humans, with estimates as high as 1 in 100.

The deficiency and inheritance patterns of these three forms of inherited coagulapathies are compared in Table 33.

Clinical Manifestations and Complications

Clinical manifestations and complications related to hemophilia include (1) slow, persistent, prolonged bleeding from minor trauma and small cuts; (2) delayed bleeding after minor injuries (the delay may be several hours or days); (3) uncontrollable hemorrhage after dental extractions or irritation of the gingiva with a hard-bristle toothbrush; (4) epistaxis, especially after a blow to the face; (5) GI bleeding from ulcers and gastritis; (6) hematuria from genitourinary trauma and splenic rupture resulting from falls or abdominal trauma; (7) ecchymoses and subcutaneous hematomas; (8) neurologic signs such as pain, anesthesia, and paralysis, which may develop from nerve compression caused by hematoma formation; and (9) *hemarthrosis* (bleeding into the joints), which may lead to joint deformity severe enough to cause unresolvable crippling (commonly in the knees, elbows, shoulders, hips, and ankles).

- All clinical manifestations relate to bleeding, and any bleeding episode in persons with hemophilia may result in death from hemorrhage.
- Many persons with hemophilia became seropositive for human immunodeficiency virus (HIV) infection transmitted by cryoprecipitates and factor concentrates. Before 1986 donated blood and blood products were not tested for HIV antibodies.
- The development of hepatitis C in hemophilia patients was also common for many years because of lack of an available test to detect it and because of the use of pooled blood products. Hepatitis C antibody screening is now routinely done on all donated blood and blood products.

Table 33 Comparison of Hemophilic States

Disorder	Deficiency	Inheritance pattern
Hemophilia A	Factor VIII	Recessive sex-linked (transmitted by female carriers, displayed almost exclusively in men)
Hemophilia B	Factor IX	Recessive sex-linked (transmitted by female carriers, displayed almost exclusively in men)
von Willebrand disease	vWF and platelet dysfunction	Autosomal dominant, seen in both sexes Recessive (in severe forms of the disease)

vWF, von Willebrand factor.

H

Diagnostic Tests

- Prolonged partial thromboplastin time from deficiency in any factor in the clotting system
- Prolonged bleeding time in von Willebrand disease because of structurally defective platelets; bleeding time is normal in hemophilia A and B because platelets are not affected
- Factor assays will reveal a reduction of factor VIII in hemophilia A, von Willebrand factor (vWF) in von Willebrand disease, and reduction of factor IX in hemophilia B.

Therapeutic Management

The goals of management are to prevent and treat bleeding. The therapeutic regimens for persons with hemophilia or von Willebrand disease focus on maintaining adequate blood levels of the deficient clotting factors. This goal is achieved by assessing clinical manifestations, determining blood levels of the involved factors, and administering the necessary factors.

- Replacement of deficient clotting factors is the primary means of supporting patients with hemophilia. In addition to treating acute crises, replacement therapy may be given before surgery and dental care as a prophylactic measure. Cryoprecipitate is commonly used and primarily contains factor VIII and fibrinogen.
- Most patients with hemophilia A use factor VIII concentrate, which is prepared from multiple donors and supplied as a lyophilized powder.
- For mild hemophilia or certain subtypes of von Willebrand disease, desmopressin acetate (DDAVP), a synthetic analog of vasopressin, may be used to stimulate an increase in factor VIII and vWF. This drug acts on endothelial cells to cause the release of vWF, which subsequently binds with factor VIII, thus increasing their concentrations. Beneficial effects (e.g., decreased bleeding time) of DDAVP, when administered intravenously, are seen within a half hour and can last more than 12 hours.

The most common difficulties with acute therapeutic management are starting factor replacement therapy too late and stopping it too soon. Generally, minor bleeding episodes should be treated for at least 72 hours. Surgery and traumatic injuries may dictate support for 10 to 14 days. Because of the short half-life of the factors, regular intermittent or continuous infusions have been used to manage bleeding episodes or expected traumatic procedures. Development of inhibitors to the factor products has occurred with long-term use and requires individualized patient management.

Nursing Management

Because of the hereditary nature of hemophilia, referral for genetic counseling is essential when preventive measures are being considered. This is especially important today because persons with hemophilia are living longer and reaching an age when reproduction is possible.

Nursing interventions for acute bleeding episodes are related primarily to controlling the bleeding and include the following:

1. Stop the topical bleeding as quickly as possible by applying direct pressure or ice, packing the area with Gelfoam or fibrin foam, and applying topical hemostatic agents such as thrombin.
2. Administer the specific coagulation factor concentrate ordered.
3. When joint bleeding occurs, it is important to rest the involved joint completely, in addition to administering antihemophilic factors to help prevent crippling deformities from hemarthrosis. The joint may be packed in ice. Analgesics are given to reduce severe pain; aspirin should *never* be used. As soon as bleeding ceases, it is important to encourage mobilization of the affected area through range-of-motion (ROM) exercises and physical therapy. Actual weight-bearing is avoided until all swelling has resolved and muscle strength has returned.
4. Manage any life-threatening complication that may develop as a result of hemorrhage. Examples include nursing interventions to prevent or treat airway obstruction from hemorrhage into the neck and pharynx and early assessment and treatment of intracranial bleeding.

Home management is a primary consideration for patients with hemophilia because the disease follows a progressive chronic course. Quality and length of life may be significantly affected by the patient's knowledge of the illness and how to live with it. The patient and family can be referred to the local chapter of the National Hemophilia Society to encourage associations with other individuals who are dealing with the problems of hemophilia. The nurse must provide ongoing assessment of the patient's adaptation to the illness. Psychosocial support and assistance should be readily available as needed.

Patient Teaching

- The patient with hemophilia must be taught to recognize disease-related problems and to learn which can be resolved at home and which require hospitalization. Immediate medical attention is required for severe pain or swelling of a muscle or joint that restricts movement or inhibits sleep and for a head injury, a swelling in the neck or mouth, abdominal pain, hematuria, melena, and skin wounds in need of suturing.

- Daily oral hygiene must be performed without causing trauma.
- The patient should understand how to prevent injuries. The patient can learn to participate in noncontact sports (e.g., golf) and wear gloves when doing household chores to prevent cuts or abrasions from knives, hammers, and other tools.
- The patient should wear a medical-alert tag to ensure that health care providers know about the hemophilia in case of an accident.
- The patient needs information about routine follow-up care and compliance with scheduled visits must be assessed.
- A reliable person can be taught to self-administer some of the factor replacement therapies at home. With the exception of intranasal DDAVP, this will require providing instructions regarding venipuncture and infusion techniques.

HEMORRHOIDS

Definition/Description
Hemorrhoids are dilated hemorrhoidal veins that may be *internal* (occurring above the internal sphincter) or *external* (occurring outside the external sphincter). They occur in all age groups and appear in affected persons periodically.

Pathophysiology
Hemorrhoids develop when the flow of blood through the veins of the hemorrhoidal plexus is impaired.

- Internal hemorrhoids may become constricted and painful. They are the most common cause of bleeding with defecation. The amount of blood lost at one time may be small but may lead to iron-deficiency anemia over time.
- External hemorrhoids are reddish blue and seldom bleed or cause pain unless a vein ruptures. If blood clots in external hemorrhoids, they become inflamed, painful, and are said to be *thrombosed*.
- Hemorrhoids may be caused by many factors, including pregnancy, prolonged constipation, straining in an effort to defecate, heavy lifting, prolonged standing and sitting, and portal hypertension.

Clinical Manifestations
Manifestations of hemorrhoids include bleeding, pruritus, prolapse, and pain.

Diagnostic Studies

Hemorrhoids are diagnosed by inspection, digital examination, proctoscopy, or examination with a flexible sigmoidoscope.

Therapeutic Management

Therapy should be directed toward the causes and relief of the patient's symptoms. A high-fiber diet and increased fluid intake will prevent constipation and reduce straining. Ointments such as Nupercainal, creams, suppositories, and impregnated pads that contain antiinflammatory agents (e.g., hydrocortisone) or astringents and anesthetics (e.g., witch hazel) may be used to shrink mucous membranes and relieve discomfort. Stool softeners may be ordered to keep stools soft, and sitz baths may be ordered to relieve pain.

Application of ice packs for a few hours, followed by warm packs, may be used for thrombosed hemorrhoids. Another treatment involves the use of a sclerosing solution, such as 5% phenol in oil, or a combined solution of quinine and urea may be injected into the submucous tissue surrounding the hemorrhoids, causing a fibrosing and shrinking of supporting tissues.

Internal hemorrhoids may be ligated with a rubber band. The constrictive effect impairs circulation, and the tissue becomes necrotic, separates, and sloughs off. There is some local discomfort with this procedure, but no anesthetic is required.

- A *hemorrhoidectomy* (surgical excision of hemorrhoids) is indicated when there is prolapse, excessive pain or bleeding, or large hemorrhoids. Surgical removal may be done by cautery, clamp, or excision.

Nursing Management

Conservative nursing management includes teaching measures for the prevention of constipation, avoidance of prolonged standing or sitting, proper use of over-the-counter medications for hemorrhoidal symptoms, and an explanation of when to seek medical care for symptoms (e.g., excessive pain and bleeding, prolapsed hemorrhoids).

- Pain is a common problem after a hemorrhoidectomy. The nurse must be aware that, although the procedure is minor, the pain is severe and narcotics are usually given initially.
- Sitz baths are started 1 to 2 days after surgery. A sponge ring in the sitz bath helps relieve pressure on the area. Initially the patient should not be left alone because of the possibility of weakness or fainting.
- Packing may be inserted into the rectum to absorb drainage. A T-binder may hold the dressing in place. If packing is inserted, it is usually removed the first or second postoperative day. The nurse should assess for rectal bleeding. The patient may be

embarrassed when the dressing is changed, and privacy should be provided.

- A stool softener such as dioctyl sodium sulfosuccinate (Colace) is usually ordered the first few postoperative days. If the patient does not have a bowel movement within 2 to 3 days, an oil retention enema is given.

- The patient usually dreads the first bowel movement and often resists the urge to defecate. Pain medication may be given before the bowel movement to reduce discomfort.

Patient Teaching

Discharge teaching includes the importance of diet, care of the anal area, symptoms of complications (especially bleeding), and avoidance of constipation and straining. Sitz baths are recommended for 1 to 2 weeks. The physician may order a stool softener to be taken for a time.

- Hemorrhoids may recur. Occasionally anal strictures develop and dilatation is necessary. Regular checkups are important in prevention of any further problems.

HEPATITIS, VIRAL

Definition/Description

Hepatitis is an inflammation of the liver. Acute viral hepatitis is the most common type of hepatitis. The types of infectious viral hepatitis are A, B, C (formerly called posttransfusion non-A, non-B), D, and E.

- Noninfectious hepatitis may be caused by drugs and other chemicals. Rarely, hepatitis is caused by bacteria, such as streptococci, salmonellae, and *Escherichia coli.*

Etiology

Viral hepatitis can be caused by one of five viruses: A, B, C, D, and E. Other viruses known to damage the liver include cytomegalovirus, Epstein-Barr virus, herpesvirus, coxsackievirus, and rubella virus.

- The only definitive way to distinguish the various forms of viral hepatitis is by the presence of the antigens and the subsequent development of antibodies to them.

- Outbreaks of hepatitis are consistently caused by hepatitis A virus; 20% to 60% of episodic or sporadic hepatitis is caused by hepatitis B virus or C virus.

- Infection with each virus provides immunity to that virus (homologous immunity). However, the patient can still develop another type of viral hepatitis.

Different characteristics of hepatitis viruses are summarized in Table 34. For a more complete description of each hepatitis virus, see Lewis/Collier/Heitkemper, *Medical-Surgical Nursing,* edition 4, p. 1259.

Pathophysiology

The pathophysiologic changes in the liver due to various types of viral hepatitis are similar. Hepatitis involves widespread inflammation of liver tissue.

- Liver cell damage consists of hepatic cell degeneration and necrosis. There is proliferation and enlargement of the Kupffer cells. Inflammation of the periportal areas may interrupt bile flow. Cholestasis may occur.
- The liver cells regenerate in an orderly manner, and if no complications occur, they should resume normal appearance and function during convalescence.
- Circulating immune complexes (antigen-antibody) activate the complement system. Manifestations of this activation are rash, angioedema, arthritis, fever, and malaise. Glomerulonephritis and vasculitis have also been found secondary to immune complex disease.

Clinical Manifestations

H

A large number of patients, especially the younger ones, have no symptoms. Manifestations of viral hepatitis may be classified into three phases: (1) preicteric or prodromal phase, (2) icteric phase, and (3) posticteric or convalescent phase (see Table 35).

- The *preicteric phase* precedes jaundice and lasts from 1 to 21 days. This is the period of maximal infectivity for hepatitis A. Patients with Hepatitis B who are hepatitis B core antigen (HBcAg)–positive can be infective for years.
- The *icteric phase* lasts 2 to 4 weeks and is characterized by jaundice. Jaundice results when bilirubin diffuses into the tissues. The urine may darken because of excess bilirubin being excreted by the kidneys.
- The convalescent stage of the *posticteric phase* begins as jaundice is disappearing and lasts weeks to months, with an average of 2 to 4 months. During this period the patient's major complaints are malaise and easy fatigability. Relapses may occur, and the disappearance of jaundice does not mean that the patient has totally recovered.

Table 34   Characteristics of Hepatitis Viruses

	Incubation period	Mode of transmission	Sources of infection and spread of disease	Infectivity
Hepatitis A (HAV)	15-50 days (average 28)	Fecal to oral route	Crowded conditions; poor personal hygiene; poor sanitation; contaminated food, milk, water, and shellfish; persons with subclinical infections; infected food handlers; sexual contact	Most infectious during 2 wk before onset of symptoms; infectious until 1-2 wk after symptoms start
Hepatitis B (HBV)	45-180 days (average 60-90)	Percutaneous (parenteral)/permucosal exposure to blood or blood products; Sexual contact; Perinatal contact	Contaminated needles, syringes, and blood products; sexual activity with infected partners; asymptomatic carriers	Before and after symptoms appear; infectious for 4-6 mo; in carriers continues for lifetime

	Incubation	Route of transmission	Source	Period of communicability
Hepatitis C (HCV)	14-180 days (average 56)	Percutaneous (parenteral)	Blood and blood products, needles and syringes	1-2 wk before symptoms; continues during clinical course; indefinitely with carriers
Hepatitis D (HDV)	Not firmly established HBV must precede HDV; chronic carriers of HBV are always at risk	Can cause infection only together with HBV, routes of transmission same as for HBV	Same as HBV	Blood is infectious at all stages of HDV infection
Hepatitis E (HEV)	15-64 days (average 26-42 days in different epidemics)	Fecal to oral route	Contaminated water; poor sanitation; found in Asia, Africa, and Mexico; not common in United States and Canada	Not known; may be similar to HAV

H

Table 35	Clinical Manifestations of the Phases of Hepatitis	

Preicteric	**Icteric**	**Posticteric**
Anorexia	Jaundice	Malaise
Nausea, vomiting	Pruritus	Easy fatigability
Right upper quad- rant discomfort	Dark urine	Hepatomegaly
Constipation or diarrhea	Bilirubinuria	
Decreased sense of taste and smell	Light stools	
	Fatigue	
Malaise	Continued hepatomegaly with tenderness	
Headache	Weight loss	
Fever		
Arthralgias		
Urticaria		
Hepatomegaly		
Splenomegaly		
Weight loss		

Additional considerations include:

- Not all patients with viral hepatitis have jaundice. This condi-
  ton is referred to as *anicteric hepatitis* and occurs more frequently in children. A high percentage of persons with hepatitis A virus are anicteric and do not have symptoms.
- There is some slight variation in manifestations between the
  types of hepatitis. In hepatitis A the onset is more acute and the
  symptoms are usually mild and flulike. In hepatitis B the onset
  is more insidious and the symptoms are usually more severe.
  There may be fewer GI symptoms.

Complications

Most patients with viral hepatitis recover completely with no complications. Complications that can occur include chronic persistent
hepatitis, chronic active hepatitis, fulminant viral hepatitis, and cirrhosis of the liver.

- The most common complication of viral hepatitis is *chronic
  persistent hepatitis* in which there is a delayed convalescent period. It is usually benign and is characterized by fatigue and
  hepatomegaly. However, no treatment is required. Liver function test results may remain abnormal for several years.

- *Chronic active hepatitis* is characterized by the persistence of signs and symptoms of hepatitis and abnormal liver function test results for more than 6 months. Chronic active hepatitis is seen only in patients with hepatitis B or C and in patients with hepatitis D who also have hepatitis B. Hepatitis B surface antigen (HBsAg) persists longer than 6 months in approximately 10% of patients with hepatitis B. It is distinguished from chronic persistent hepatitis by liver biopsy. The ongoing process of liver necrosis is likely to progress to cirrhosis. Interferon-α has been found to be effective for some patients with chronic active hepatitis B.
- *Fulminant viral hepatitis* is a clinical syndrome that results in severe impairment or necrosis of liver cells and potential liver failure. Fulminant viral hepatitis develops in a very small percentage of patients. The disorder may occur as a complication of hepatitis B or C, particularly hepatitis B accompanied by infection with hepatitis D virus. Toxic reactions to drugs and congenital metabolic disorders may also cause fulminant hepatitis. Hepatocellular failure with death usually occurs.

Diagnostic Studies

- Liver function tests show significant abnormalities
- Hepatitis serologic studies
  1. Hepatitis B surface antigen (HBsAg) and hepatitis B e antigen (HBeAg) in some cases for hepatitis B virus (HBV)
  2. Anti-HBs indicates immunity to hepatitis B; it also is a marker for response to hepatitis B vaccine
  3. Anti-HBc (IgM and IgG) for hepatitis B
  4. Anti-HAV (IgM and IgG) for hepatitis A virus (HAV)
  5. Anti-HCV for hepatitis C virus (HCV)

Therapeutic Management

There is no specific treatment for viral hepatitis. Most patients can be managed at home. Emphasis is on measures to rest the body and assist the liver in regenerating. Adequate nutrients and rest seem to be most beneficial for healing and liver cell (hepatocyte) regeneration. Dietary emphasis is on a well-balanced diet that the patient can tolerate.

- The degree of rest ordered depends on symptom severity; usually alternating periods of activity with rest is adequate.
- There are no specific drug therapies for the treatment of acute viral hepatitis. Steroid therapy is controversial. Supportive drug therapy may include antiemetics, such as dimenhydrinate (Dramamine) or trimethobenzamide (Tigan).

- An important measure in assisting hepatocytes to regenerate is adequate nutrition. No special diet is required. However, a diet high in carbohydrates and proteins with low fat content is usually recommended.

Nursing Management

Goals

The patient with viral hepatitis will have relief of discomfort, be able to resume normal activities, and return to normal liver function without complications.

See the nursing care plan for the patient with viral hepatitis in Lewis/Collier/Heitkemper, *Medical-Surgical Nursing,* edition 4, p. 1266.

Nursing Diagnoses

- Upper abdominal pain related to inflammation of the liver
- Altered nutrition: less than body requirements related to anorexia, nausea, and reduced metabolism of nutrients by liver
- Fatigue related to viral infection
- Activity intolerance related to fatigue, weakness, increased energy utilization associated with increased basal metabolic rate caused by viral infection, and inadequate nutritional status
- Ineffective management of therapeutic regimen related to lack of knowledge of follow-up care
- Anxiety related to lack of understanding of diagnosis, anticipated changes in lifestyle, and fear of prognosis and complications
- Body image disturbance related to stigma of having a communicable disease, change in appearance (jaundice), and possible alterations in roles and lifestyle (alcohol consumption, drug use, restriction of sexual activity)

Nursing Interventions

Viral hepatitis is a community health problem. The nurse must assume a significant role in the control and prevention of this disease.

Hepatitis A. Mode of transmission is fecal-oral. Preventive measures include personal and environmental hygiene and health education to promote good sanitation. Handwashing is essential and is probably the most important precaution. Health teaching should include careful handwashing after bowel movements and before eating.

- A major preventive measure for hepatitis A is administration of immune globulin. Because patients with hepatitis A are most infectious just before the onset of symptoms, those exposed through household contact or foodborne outbreaks should be given immunoglobulin within 1 to 2 weeks of exposure.
- A vaccine for HAV (Havrix) has recently become available.

Hepatitis B. HBV is transmitted percutaneously, sexually, through mucous membranes or nonintact skin, and perinatally. Control and prevention of hepatitis B focuses on identification of possible exposure through percutaneous and sexual transmission.

- The nurse must be aware of the groups at high risk of contracting hepatitis B and teach methods to reduce the risks. These include patients receiving frequent transfusions or hemodialysis, personnel in hemodialysis units and blood chemistry laboratories, IV drug users, persons with multiple sexual partners, prison inmates, and household and sexual partners of HBV carriers.
- Good hygienic practices, including handwashing and the use of gloves when expecting contact with blood, are important. A condom is advised for sexual intercourse and the partner of the person with hepatitis B should be vaccinated. Razors, toothbrushes, and other personal items should not be shared. Close contacts of the patient with hepatitis B who are HBsAg negative and antibody negative should be vaccinated.
- Immunization with hepatitis B vaccine is the most effective method of preventing HBV infection. The vaccine is 90% to 95% effective.

Hepatitis C. Risk factors for HCV infection include IV drug use, needlestick accidents, hemophilia, and hemodialysis.

- Posttransfusion HCV infection is best prevented through routine screening for anti-HCV (antibody to hepatitis C). At this time there is no test commercially available for the HCV virus (antigen) and there is no vaccine for hepatitis C.

• • •

When a patient develops hepatitis, it is important to assess for jaundice, to evaluate the patient's response to rest, and to modify care accordingly. Diversional activities may help, and the patient should be assisted to understand the temporary nature of symptoms, especially sexual abstinence, during the period of communicability.

- The patient should be assessed for any manifestations indicative of complications. Bleeding tendencies with increasing prothrombin time values, symptoms of encephalopathy, or markedly abnormal liver function tests indicate problems.

Patient Teaching

- The patient and family must learn about preventive measures and how to prevent transmission to other family members. The patient should know what symptoms need to be reported to the physician.
- The importance of regular follow-up for at least 1 year after the diagnosis of hepatitis needs to be stressed. Because relapses are fairly common with hepatitis B and C, the patient should be in-

structed about symptoms of recurrence. Alcohol should be avoided for 1 year because it is detoxified in the liver and may interfere with recovery.

- The patient with hepatitis B should be instructed to use condoms when engaging in sexual intercourse until tests for HBsAg are negative.
- The patient who is receiving interferon-α for the treatment of hepatitis B or C requires education regarding the medication. Interferon-α needs to be administered intramuscularly or subcutaneously, and thus the patient or family member needs to be taught how to administer the drug.

HERNIA

Definition/Description

A hernia is a protrusion of a viscus through an abnormal opening or a weakened area in the wall of the cavity in which it is normally contained. A hernia may occur in any part of the body, but it usually is found within the abdominal cavity.

- If the hernia can be placed back into the abdominal cavity, it is known as *reducible*. The hernia can be reduced by manipulation, or it can occur without manipulation when the person lies down.
- If the hernia cannot be placed back into the abdominal cavity, it is known as *irreducible* or *incarcerated*. In this situation intestinal flow may be obstructed. When the hernia is irreducible and intestinal flow and blood supply are obstructed, the hernia is *strangulated*. The result is an acute intestinal obstruction.

Types

The types of hernias include inguinal, femoral, umbilical, and ventral (incisional).

- *Inguinal* hernia is the most common type of hernia and occurs at the point of weakness in the abdominal wall where the spermatic cord in men and the round ligament in women emerge. An inguinal hernia is more common in men. When the protrusion escapes through the inguinal ring and follows the spermatic cord or round ligament, it is termed an *indirect* hernia. When it escapes through the posterior inguinal wall, it is a *direct* hernia.
- *Femoral* hernia occurs when there is a protrusion through the femoral ring into the femoral canal. It becomes strangulated easily and occurs more frequently in women.

- *Umbilical* hernia occurs when the rectus muscle is weak or the umbilical opening fails to close after birth. This type is found most commonly in children.
- *Ventral* or *incisional* hernias occur as a result of a weakness of the abdominal wall at the site of a previous incision. It is found most commonly in patients who are obese, who have had multiple surgical procedures in the same area, and who have had inadequate wound healing because of poor nutrition or infection.

Clinical Manifestations

A hernia commonly occurs over the involved area when the patient stands or strains. There may be some discomfort as a result of tension; severe pain occurs if the hernia becomes strangulated. In this situation the clinical manifestations of a bowel obstruction, such as vomiting, crampy abdominal pain, and distention, are found. Diagnosis is based on history and physical examination findings.

Therapeutic Management

Surgery is the treatment of choice for hernias to prevent the possible complication of strangulation. Surgical repair of a hernia is known as a *herniorrhaphy.* The reinforcement of the weakened area with wire, fascia, or mesh is known as a *hernioplasty.* When there is strangulation, necrosis and gangrene may develop if immediate care is not given. Bowel resection of the involved area or a temporary colostomy may be needed to treat a strangulated hernia. Umbilical hernia is not usually repaired surgically because it may reduce itself if left alone as the child grows older.

Nursing Management

Some patients with hernias may wear a *truss,* which is a pad placed over the hernia and held in place with a belt. The truss is worn to keep the hernia from protruding. If a patient wears a truss, the nurse should check for skin irritation caused by continual rubbing of the truss.

- After a hernia repair the patient may have difficulty voiding. Therefore the nurse should observe for a distended bladder.
- Scrotal edema is a painful complication after inguinal hernia repair. A scrotal support with application of an ice bag may help relieve pain and edema.
- Coughing is not encouraged, but deep breathing and turning should be done. If the patient needs to cough or sneeze, the incision should be splinted during coughing, and sneezing should be done with the mouth open.
- After discharge the patient may be restricted from heavy lifting or physical activities for 6 to 8 weeks.

HERPES, GENITAL

Definition/Description
There are two different strains of herpes simplex virus (HSV) that cause infection.

- *HSV type 1 (HSV-1)* generally causes infection above the waist, involving the gingivae, dermis, upper respiratory tract, and central nervous system.
- *HSV type 2 (HSV-2)* most frequently involves the genital tract and perineum (i.e., locations below the waist).

However, either strain can cause disease on the mouth or genitals. When a person is infected with HSV, the virus usually persists within the individual for life. The incubation period ranges from 1 to 45 days with an average of 6 days.

Pathophysiology
In the course of primary infection, HSV is established in the sensory nerve ganglion innervating the primary site. On activation, the virus travels down the nerve axon to the skin or mucous membranes. Additional sexual contact with an infected person is not necessary for a recurrence of HSV infection. The recurrent infection produces a syndrome similar to but less intense than the primary infection.

Because HSV is readily inactivated at room temperature and by drying, airborne and fomitic spread have not been documented as a significant means of transmission. The virus enters through the mucous membranes or breaks in the skin during contact with an infected person. There does not appear to be any period of time when viral transmission is not possible once primary HSV-2 infection has occurred. Women with recurrent symptomatic genital herpes shed the virus even when no visible lesions are present.

Clinical Manifestations
A patient with a primary HSV infection initially complains of burning or tingling at the site of inoculation. Vesicular lesions, which may occur on the penis, scrotum, vulva, perineum, perianal region, vagina, or cervix, contain large quantities of infectious viral particles. The lesions rupture and form shallow, moist ulcerations. Finally, crusting and epithelialization of the erosions occur.

- Primary infections tend to be associated with local inflammation and pain accompanied by systemic manifestations of fever, headache, malaise, myalgia, and regional lymphadenopathy.
- Urination may be painful when urine touches active lesions. Retention may occur as a result of HSV urethritis or cystitis. A purulent vaginal discharge may develop with HSV cervicitis.

- The duration of symptoms is longer and the frequency of complications are greater in women.

Many HSV-2 infections, both primary and secondary, may be asymptomatic. Therefore transmission of genital herpes can occur by means of sexual contact with an excretor of virus who is free of symptoms.

After the first infection, HSV-2 establishes latency in the sacral ganglia and may be reactivated periodically. Recurrent attacks occur in about 50% to 80% of all cases during the year after the primary episode. Stress, sexual activity, sunburn, and fever tend to trigger recurrence. Many patients can predict a recurrence by noticing early symptoms of tingling, burning, and itching at the site where lesions eventually arise. Symptoms of recurrent episodes are less severe, and the unilateral lesions heal within 8 to 12 days. With time, recurrent lesions generally occur less frequently.

Diagnostic Studies

- Diagnosis is usually based on the patient's symptoms and history.
- Viral isolation by tissue culture from active lesions confirms the diagnosis.
- Serologic methods are used for identification of specific antibody to the glycoprotein G component of HSV.

Therapeutic and Nursing Management

The skin lesions of genital herpes heal spontaneously unless secondary infection occurs. Symptomatic treatment such as good genital hygiene and the wearing of loose-fitting cotton undergarments should be encouraged. The lesions should be kept clean and dry to ensure complete drying of the perineal area; a hair dryer on a cool setting may be used.

- Frequent sitz baths may be used to soothe the area and reduce inflammation. Pain may require a local anesthetic such as lidocaine (Xylocaine) or systemic analgesics such as codeine and aspirin.
- Barrier forms of contraception, especially condoms, used during asymptomatic periods decrease transmission of the disease. When lesions are present, the patient should avoid sexual activity altogether because even barrier protection is not satisfactory in eliminating disease transmission.
- Acyclovir (Zovirax), which inhibits herpetic viral replication, is prescribed for primary infections or suppression of frequent recurrences (more than six episodes per year). Although not a cure, acyclovir shortens the duration of viral shedding and healing time of genital lesions and suppresses 75% of recurrences with daily use. Continued use of oral acyclovir for up to 5 years is safe and effective but should be interrupted after 1 year to

assess the patient's rate of recurrent episodes. (IV acyclovir is reserved for severe or life-threatening infections.)

HIATAL HERNIA

Definition/Description
Hiatal hernia is a protrusion of a portion of the stomach into the esophagus through an opening (or hiatus) in the diaphragm. It is also referred to as diaphragmatic hernia or esophageal hernia.

Hiatal hernias are classified into two types:

- A *sliding hernia* occurs at the junction of the stomach and esophagus and is located above the hiatus of the diaphragm. It "slides" into the thoracic cavity through the diaphragm's hiatal opening when the patient is supine and usually goes back into the abdominal cavity when the patient is standing upright. This is the most common type of hiatal hernia.
- A *paraesophageal* or *rolling hernia* occurs at the esophagogastric junction where the fundus and greater curvature of the stomach roll up through the diaphragm, forming a pocket alongside the esophagus.

Pathophysiology
The actual cause of hiatal hernia is unknown. Many factors may contribute to the development of hiatal hernia, including structural changes such as weakening of the muscles in the diaphragm around the esophagogastric opening. Conditions that increase intraabdominal pressure, including obesity, pregnancy, ascites, intense physical exertion, and heavy lifting on a continual basis, may also contribute to the development of a hiatal hernia. In some cases congenital weakness is a contributing factor.

Clinical Manifestations
Signs and symptoms frequently mimic gallbladder disease, peptic ulcer disease, or angina. However, some patients with hiatal hernia have no symptoms.

- The reflux and discomfort described are associated with position, occurring soon or several hours after lying down. Bending over may cause a severe burning pain, which is usually relieved by sitting or standing. Eating large meals, drinking alcohol, and smoking may precipitate pain.
- Nocturnal attacks are common, especially if the person has eaten before going to sleep.

Complications that may occur with hiatal hernia include hemorrhage from erosion, stenosis, ulcerations of the herniated portion of stomach, strangulation of the hernia, and regurgitation with tracheal aspiration.

Diagnostic Studies

- Barium swallow may show gastric mucosa protrusion through the esophageal hiatus.
- Esophagoscopy is useful to determine incompetence of the lower esophageal sphincter (LES) and whether gastric reflux is present.
- pH monitoring of gastric and esophageal secretions.
- Motility (manometry) studies may be done to determine pressure gradients.

Therapeutic and Nursing Management

Conservative management includes administration of antacids and antisecretory agents, elimination of constricting garments, avoidance of lifting and straining, and elimination of alcohol and smoking. Elevation of the bed on 4- to 6-inch blocks assists gravity in maintaining the stomach in the abdominal cavity and also helps prevent reflux and tracheal aspiration. If obese, the patient is encouraged to lose weight.

Surgical procedures are termed *valvuloplasties* or *antireflux procedures.*

- There are three slightly varied procedures: the Nissen fundoplication, the Hill gastroplexy, and the Belsey fundoplication. These three surgical procedures are all variations of fundoplication, which involves "wrapping" the fundus of the stomach around the lower portion of the esophagus in varying degrees.
- These procedures reduce the hernia, provide an acceptable LES pressure, and prevent movement of the gastroesophageal junction.
- The Nissen fundoplication procedure is being performed laparoscopically with increasing frequency.

Postoperative care focuses on prevention of respiratory complications, maintenance of fluid and electrolyte balance, and prevention of infection.

- Respiratory complications can occur in a patient treated by an abdominal approach because of the high abdominal incision. Coughing and deep breathing are essential to reexpand the lungs.
- The patient should receive only IV fluids until peristalsis returns. It is important to maintain accurate intake and output records.

H

Patient Teaching

After successful surgical intervention, minimal to no symptoms of gastric reflux should be present.

- The patient should be instructed to report symptoms such as heartburn and regurgitation. In the early postoperative period there is usually mild dysphagia caused by edema, but it should resolve.

- The patient should be told to report persistent dysphagia, epigastric fullness, and bloating. Immediately after the surgical procedure the patient cannot voluntarily vomit or belch, and this may cause the gas-bloat syndrome. If this syndrome persists, medical advice should be sought.

- It is important to emphasize that a normal diet can be resumed within 6 weeks and that the patient should avoid foods that are gas forming. Food should be thoroughly chewed.

Hodgkin's Disease

Definition/Description

Hodgkin's disease is a malignant condition characterized by proliferation of abnormal giant multinucleated cells, called *Reed-Sternberg cells,* located in the lymph nodes. The disease has a bimodal age-specific incidence, occurring most frequently in persons from 15 to 35 years of age and above age 50. In adults it is twice as prevalent in men as in women.

Pathophysiology

Although the cause of Hodgkin's disease remains unknown, several key factors are thought to play a role in its development. The main interacting factors are infection with Epstein-Barr virus (EBV), genetic predisposition, and exposure to occupational toxins.

In Hodgkin's disease the normal structure of lymph nodes is destroyed by hyperplasia of monocytes and macrophages. The disease is believed to arise in a single location (it originates in lymph nodes in 90% of patients) and to spread along adjacent lymph nodes. It eventually infiltrates other organs, especially the lungs, spleen, and liver. In about two thirds of all patients the cervical lymph nodes are the first to be affected.

Clinical Manifestations

The onset of symptoms in Hodgkin's disease is usually insidious. The initial sign is most often enlargement of cervical, axillary, or inguinal lymph nodes. The enlarged nodes are not painful unless pressure is exerted on adjacent nerves.

- The patient may notice weight loss, fatigue, weakness, fever, chills, tachycardia, or night sweats. A group of initial findings, including fever, night sweats, and weight loss (referred to as B symptoms), correlates with an unfavorable prognosis.
- Generalized pruritus without skin lesions may develop. Cough, dyspnea, stridor, and dysphagia all may reflect mediastinal node involvement.
- In more advanced disease there is hepatomegaly and splenomegaly. Anemia results from increased destruction and decreased production of erythrocytes. Intrathoracic involvement may lead to (1) superior vena cava syndrome, (2) enlarged retroperitoneal nodes, which may cause palpable abdominal masses or interfere with renal function, (3) jaundice from liver involvement, and (4) spinal cord compression leading to paraplegia (may occur with extradural involvement).
- Bone pain may occur as a result of osteoblastic bone lesions.

Diagnostic Studies

- Peripheral blood analysis often reveals microcytic hypochromic anemia, neutrophilic leukocytosis (15,000 to 28,000/μL [15 to 28 × 10^9/L]), which may be associated with lymphopenia, and an increased platelet count.
- Other blood studies may show hypoferremia caused by excessive iron uptake by the liver and spleen, elevated alkaline phosphatase from liver and bone involvement, hypercalcemia from bone involvement, and hypoalbuminemia.
- Excisional lymph node biopsy offers a definitive diagnosis. If removed, an enlarged peripheral lymph node can be examined histologically for the presence of Reed-Sternberg cells.
- Bone marrow biopsy is performed as an important aspect of staging.
- Chest x-rays, radioisotope studies, and CT scans may show mediastinal lymphadenopathy, renal displacement caused by retroperitoneal node enlargement, abdominal lymph node enlargement, and liver, spleen, bone, and brain infiltration.
- Lymphangiography, a radiographic dye study that uses blue dye injected into the lymphatic system, can be used to assess the lymph nodes and lymph vessels. This test also allows visualization of the retroperitoneal structures.

Therapeutic Management

Treatment decisions are based on the stage of the disease. Radiation therapy given to affected areas over 4 to 6 weeks can cure 95%

of patients with stage I or stage II disease. Combination chemotherapy may be used in the early stages for patients believed to have resistant disease or to be at high risk for relapse. Stage IIIA disease is treated with both radiotherapy and chemotherapy (see Radiation Therapy, p. 675, and Chemotherapy, p. 631). The role of radiation as a supplement to chemotherapy in stages III and IV varies depending on the site of disease.

Advances in treatment now enable some patients with stage IIIB and stage IV diseases to be cured with high-dose chemotherapy and bone marrow or peripheral stem cell transplantation. Intensive chemotherapy with or without the use of bone marrow transplantation and hematopoeitic growth factors is the treatment of choice for advanced Hodgkin's disease (stages IIIB and IV).

Nursing Management

Nursing care for Hodgkin's disease is largely based on managing pancytopenia and other side effects of therapy.

- Because survival of a patient with Hodgkin's disease depends on response to treatment, supporting the patient through the immunosuppressive state is extremely important.
- The patient undergoing radiotherapy will need special nursing consideration. The skin in the radiation field requires special attention. Also, the nurse must understand the concepts related to administration of radiotherapy.
- Psychosocial considerations are just as important as they are with leukemia (see Leukemia, p. 358). Although the prognosis for Hodgkin's disease is better than that for many forms of cancer or leukemia, patients must still be helped to deal with all of the physical, psychologic, social, and spiritual consquences of their disease.
- Evaluation of patients for long-term effects of therapy are important because delayed consequences of the disease and treatment may not be apparent for many years.

HUMAN IMMUNODEFICIENCY VIRUS INFECTION

Definition/Description

Human immunodeficiency virus (HIV) infection follows a highly individualized course from the time of infection to the clinical manifestations of acquired immunodeficiency syndrome (AIDS). AIDS is the final phase of a chronic, progressive immune function disorder caused by HIV.

Pathophysiology

HIV is a fragile virus that can be transmitted from human to human through infected blood, semen, vaginal secretions, and breast milk. An HIV-infected individual can transmit HIV to others starting a few days after the initial infection. The ability to transmit HIV is lifelong because HIV has no noninfectious state.

HIV is a ribonucleic acid (RNA) virus. RNA viruses are called retroviruses because they replicate in a "backward" manner, going from RNA to deoxyribonucleic acid (DNA). Like all viruses, HIV is an obligate parasite; it cannot replicate unless it is in a living cell. Although HIV can infect several types of human cells, predominately $CD4^+$ lymphocytes are infected.

Clinical Manifestations

Acute retroviral syndrome (development of HIV antibodies or seroconversion) is frequently accompanied by a flulike or mononucleosis-like syndrome of fever, pharyngitis, headache, malaise, nausea, and a diffuse rash.

- Symptoms generally occur 1 to 3 weeks after the initial infection and last for 1 to 2 weeks. $CD4^+$ lymphocyte counts fall temporarily during this syndrome but quickly return to baseline. In most individuals these symptoms are mild and may be mistaken for a cold or flu.

In *early HIV infection* the patient is generally healthy but has certain vague symptoms, including fatigue, headaches, low-grade fever, and night sweats. Demyelinating peripheral neuropathies, which resemble Guillain-Barré syndrome, may also develop during this time.

Early symptomatic disease occurs toward the end of early infection and before a diagnosis of AIDS. The $CD4^+$ lymphocyte count drops below 500 to 600 cells/μL and early symptomatic disease develops.

- Symptoms can include constitutional problems such as persistent fevers, recurrent drenching night sweats, chronic diarrhea, headaches, and fatigue. Other problems that may occur at this time include localized infections (oral candidiasis, shingles, or oral hairy leukoplakia), persistent generalized lymphadenopathy, and neurologic manifestations (headaches, myopathies, or aseptic meningitis).

A diagnosis of *AIDS* cannot be made until the HIV-infected patient meets case definition criteria established by the Centers for Disease Control and Prevention (CDC), which include the development of at least one of these additional criteria:

1. $CD4^+$ lymphocyte count below 200/μL
2. Development of an opportunistic infection (see Table 11-2 in Lewis/Collier/Heitkemper, *Medical-Surgical Nursing,* edition 4, p. 242)

H

3. Development of an opportunistic cancer (e.g., Kaposi's sarcoma)
4. Wasting syndrome (defined as a loss of 10% or more of ideal body mass)
5. Development of dementia

Diagnostic Studies

- Enzyme-linked immunosorbent assay (ELISA) test initially detects serum antibodies that bind to HIV antigen.
- Western blot or immunofluorescence assay (IFA) more specifically confirms HIV in infected cells.
- CD4+ counts are used to monitor progression of infection.
- White blood cell (WBC) count, red blood cell (RBC) count, and platelets decrease with infection.
- Chest x-ray is done.

Therapeutic Management

Management of HIV infection focuses on monitoring disease progression and immune function, preventing development of opportunistic diseases, initiating and monitoring antiretroviral therapy, detecting and treating opportunistic diseases, managing symptoms, and preventing complications of treatment.

Drugs that have been approved to treat HIV infection block reverse transcriptase, an enzyme required for HIV replication. These drugs include zidovudine (AZT, ZDV, Retrovir), didanosine (Videx), zalcitabine (ddC, HIVID), and stavudine (d4T, Zerit). None of these drugs kills HIV, and it appears that HIV can become refractory to these drugs.

Opportunistic diseases and debilitating problems associated with HIV can be delayed or prevented through prophylactic interventions, including pneumococcal and hepatitis B vaccine(s), low-dose acyclovir for herpes simplex viral infection, isoniazid (INH) for tuberculosis if reactive purified protein derivative (PPD) skin test is present, trimethoprim-sulfamethoxazole (TMP-SMX) inhalation for *Pneumocystis carinii,* rifabutin for *Mycobacterium avium* complex, and nutritional support.

Nursing Management

Goals

The patient with HIV infection will have adequate nutritional status; will have minimal to no problems with opportunistic diseases; will not transmit HIV virus to others; will maintain or develop healthy, supportive relationships; will come to terms with issues related to disease, death, and spirituality; and will maintain usual activities and productivity for as long as possible. Goals will change as HIV disease progresses and disabilities develop.

See the nursing care plan for the patient with symptomatic HIV infection and AIDS in Lewis/Collier/Heitkemper, *Medical-Surgical Nursing,* p. 251.

Nursing Diagnoses

- Chronic and acute pain related to neuropathy, arthralgia, lymphadenopathy, and opportunistic infections
- Anxiety related to multiple physical, emotional, and economic changes and losses
- Altered thought processes related to hypoxemia, fever, dehydration, and neurologic changes
- Altered nutrition: less than body requirements related to anorexia, impaired swallowing, oral lesions, fever, fatigue, and depression
- Risk for activity intolerance related to chronic HIV infection, stress, anemia, and malnutrition
- Diarrhea related to opportunistic infections and tube feeding intolerance
- Impaired gas exchange related to pulmonary infection, hypoxemia, anemia, ineffective cough, anxiety, and pain

Nursing Interventions

The initial nursing focus is to prevent infection. In the absence of a vaccination for HIV, education and behavioral change are the only effective tools for prevention.

- Promotion of early detection of HIV infection includes pretest and posttest counseling as the patient awaits the results of HIV antibody testing.
- Intervention after detection focuses on early recognition of constitutional symptoms, opportunistic diseases, and psychosocial problems.

Useful early interventions include (1) nutritional changes that maintain lean body mass, and (2) promotion of smoking and drug-use cessation, moderation or elimination of alcohol intake, regular exercise, stress reduction, avoiding exposure to new infectious agents, mental health counseling, and involvement in support groups.

- Facilitating empowerment is particularly important because the individual with HIV infection often experiences losses, including an overwhelming feeling of loss of control.
- The focus of intervention for the HIV-infected patient with symptomatic disease is quality-of-life issues and caring.
- Ongoing symptomatic care of long-term patient problems includes nutritional support for wasting syndromes and management of AIDS-dementia complex and medication side effects.

Patient Teaching

Emphasis is placed on prevention of HIV infection and risk-reducing activities related to sexual intercourse, drug use, and occupational exposure. Once the patient is infected, the focus is on education and counseling to prevent further virus transmission.

- Educate the patient and family about signs of opportunistic infections and malignancies to ensure early recognition and treatment.
- Teach about action and common side effects of medications. Provide written list of medications with times, dosages, and possible side effects to promote safe drug use.
- Teach stress reduction techniques to reduce increasing confusion.
- Explain and encourage use of alternate methods of pain relief.
- Teach energy conservation measures and use of assistive devices to increase safety and decrease fatigue.
- Discuss infection control measures with the patient, family, and visitors.
- Provide information about community resources.

HUNTINGTON'S DISEASE

Definition/Description

Huntington's disease is a genetically transmitted, autosomal dominant disorder that affects both men and women of all races. Offspring of a person with this disease have a 50% risk of inheriting it. Like that of Parkinson's disease, the pathology of Huntington's disease involves the basal ganglia and the extrapyramidal system. Huntington's disease involves a deficiency of the neurotransmitters acetylcholine (ACh) and gamma-aminobutyric acid (GABA). The net effect is an excess of dopamine, which leads to symptoms opposite those of parkinsonism.

Clinical manifestations typically appear between the ages of 35 and 45 years and are characterized by abnormal and excessive involuntary movements (chorea). These are writhing, twisting movements of the face, limbs, and body that worsen as the disease progresses.

- Facial movements involving speech, chewing, and swallowing are affected and may cause aspiration and malnutrition. The gait deteriorates, and ambulation eventually becomes impossible. Perhaps the most devastating deterioration is in mental functioning, including intellectual decline, emotional lability, and psychotic behavior.
- Death usually occurs 10 to 20 years after the onset of symptoms.

Diagnosis is based on family history, clinical symptoms, and detection of the characteristic deoxyriboncleic acid (DNA) pattern from blood samples.

Therapeutic and nursing management is palliative because there is no cure. Antipsychotic, antidepressant, and antichorea medications are prescribed and have some effect. However, they do not alter the course of the disease. This disease presents a great challenge to health care professionals.

The goal of nursing care is to provide the most comfortable environment possible for the patient and family by maintaining physical safety, treating physical symptoms, and providing emotional and psychologic support.

- Because of the choreic movements, caloric requirements are high. Patients may require as many as 4000 to 5000 calories/day to maintain body weight. As the disease progresses, meeting caloric needs becomes a greater challenge when the patient has difficulty swallowing and holding the head still. Depression and mental deterioration can also compromise nutritional intake.

HYPERPARATHYROIDISM

Definition/Description

Hyperparathyroidism is a rare condition involving increased secretion of parathyroid hormone (PTH). PTH helps regulate calcium and phosphate levels by stimulating bone resorption, renal tubular reabsorption of calcium, and activation of vitamin D.

Hyperparathyroidism is classified as primary, secondary, or tertiary.

- *Primary hyperparathyroidism* is caused by an increased secretion of PTH, leading to disorders of calcium, phosphate, and bone metabolism. Excessive concentrations of circulating hormone usually lead to hypercalcemia and hypophosphatemia. The most common cause is a benign neoplasm or a single adenoma (80% of cases). Previous head and neck radiation are predisposing factors for adenoma development.
- *Secondary hyperparathyroidism* is a compensatory response to conditions that induce or cause hypocalcemia, the main stimulus of PTH secretion. These conditions include vitamin D deficiencies, malabsorption, chronic renal failure, and hyperphosphatemia.
- *Tertiary hyperparathyroidism* occurs when there is hyperplasia of the parathyroid glands and a loss of circulating calcium

levels that cause autonomous secretion of PTH, even with normal calcium levels. It is observed in the patient who has had a kidney transplant after a long period of dialysis treatment for chronic renal failure.

Pathophysiology

Increased PTH has a multisystem effect (see Table 47-10 in Lewis/Collier/Heitkemper, *Medical-Surgical Nursing,* edition 4, p. 1500).

- In the bones decreased bone density, cyst formation, and general weakness can occur as a result of the effect of PTH on osteoclastic and osteoblastic activity.
- In the kidneys excess calcium cannot be resorbed, leading to hypercalciuria. This urinary calcium, along with a large amount of urinary phosphate, can lead to calculi formation. PTH stimulates synthesis of a form of vitamin D, which increases GI absorption of calcium. The hypercalcemia can lead to increased secretion of gastrin and pepsin, resulting in increased hydrochloric acid production and potential for ulcer development. An increase in pancreatitis is also observed because of attachment of calcium to pancreatic tissue.

Clinical Manifestations

Hyperparathyroidism has varying symptoms, including weakness, loss of appetite, constipation, increased need for sleep, and shortened attention span.

- Major signs include loss of calcium from bones (osteoporosis), broken bones, kidney stones (nephrolithiasis), and peptic ulcer. Neuromuscular abnormalities are characterized by muscle weakness, particularly in proximal muscles of the lower extremities.

Complications include renal failure, pancreatitis, collapse of vertebral bodies, cardiac changes, and long bone and rib fractures.

Diagnostic Studies

- Radioimmunoassay measurement of PTH, which is elevated.
- Serum calcium levels elevated with decreased phosphorus levels.
- Urine calcium, serum chloride, uric acid, and creatinine, all of which will be elevated.
- Amylase (if pancreatitis present) and alkaline phosphatase (if bone disease present) are both elevated.

Therapeutic Management

Treatment objectives are to relieve symptoms and prevent complications caused by excess PTH. Choice of therapy depends on the urgency of the clinical situation, degree of hypercalcemia, underlying disorder, and status of renal and hepatic function.

- Parathyroid tumors should be removed surgically. The parathyroids occasionally lie in ectopic sites such as the mediastinum. Generally, a single gland is removed if an adenoma is the cause of hyperparathyroidism. When cancer is the cause, all the parathyroids are removed.
- If symptoms are mild or if the patient is elderly or at increased surgical risk from other health problems, a conservative management approach is used. This includes an annual examination with tests for serum PTH, calcium, phosphorus, and alkaline phosphatase levels and renal function, x-ray studies to assess for metabolic bone disease, and measurement of urinary calcium excretion.

Specific management measures include maintenance of a high fluid intake, a moderate calcium intake, and phosphorus supplementation, unless contraindicated by a high risk for urinary calculi formation. Diuretics may be given to increase the urinary excretion of calcium. Continued ambulation and avoidance of immobility are critical aspects of management.

Pharmacologic Management

Mithramycin, an antihypercalcemic agent, lowers serum calcium within 48 hours. However, because of toxic side effects, its use is limited to patients with metastatic parathyroid carcinoma and severe bone disease. Estrogen therapy can reduce serum and urinary calcium levels in postmenopausal women and may retard demineralization of the skeleton. Propranolol (Inderal) may be used to inhibit the action of catecholamines at β_2 receptors, which stimulate PTH secretion.

- In severe hyperparathyroidism normal saline solution is given IV to correct fluid volume deficit and promote calcium excretion. Furosemide (Lasix) is given orally or IV to decrease renal tubular reabsorption of calcium.

Nursing Management

Goals

The patient with hyperparathyroidism will maintain a satisfactory activity level, keep a consistently high fluid intake, not experience any serious complications related to the disease or its treatment, maintain a positive self-image, and accept and comply with the long-term nature of the problem.

See the nursing care plan for the patient with hyperparathyroidism in Lewis/Collier/Heitkemper, *Medical-Surgical Nursing,* edition 4, p. 1502.

Nursing Diagnoses

- Activity intolerance related to muscle weakness and fatigue secondary to low calcium levels

- Sensory and perceptual alterations related to slowed mentation, depression, and drowsiness
- Body image disturbance related to weight loss, weakness, fatigue, and mental status changes
- Altered nutrition: less than body requirements related to loss of appetite, nausea, vomiting, and personality disturbances
- Risk for injury: fractures and joint contractures related to decreased bone density, weakness, improper body alignment, immobility
- Constipation related to dehydration and inactivity

Nursing Interventions

If surgery is performed, close monitoring of the patient's vital signs is required. Other aspects of care are similar to those of care given after thyroidectomy (see Hyperthyroidism, p. 326).

The major postoperative complications are tetany and fluid and electrolyte disturbances. Tetany is usually apparent early in the postoperative period but may develop over several days. Mild tetany, characterized by unpleasant tingling of the hands and around the mouth, may be present but should abate without problems. If tetany becomes more severe (e.g., muscular spasms or laryngospasms develop), calcium may be given intravenously.

- Strict monitoring of intake and output is necessary to evaluate fluid status. Calcium, potassium, phosphate, and magnesium levels are assessed frequently.
- Mobility is encouraged to promote bone calcification. If surgery is not performed, treatment to relieve symptoms and prevent complications is carried out.

HYPERSENSITIVITY REACTIONS

Definition/Description

The classification of hypersensitivity reactions may be done according to the source of the antigen, time sequence (immediate or delayed), or the basic immunologic mechanisms causing the injury (Gell and Coombs classification). The Gell and Coombs classification is the most comprehensive.

- Four types of hypersensitivity reactions exist. Types I, II, and III are immediate and are examples of humoral immunity, whereas type IV is a delayed hypersensitivity reaction and is related to cell-mediated immunity. Table 36 presents a summary of the four types of hypersensitivity reactions.

Type I (anaphylactoid reactions). These reactions occur only in susceptible persons who are highly sensitized to specific allergens.

Table 36 Types of Hypersensitivity Reactions

	Type I Anaphylactic	Type II Cytotoxic	Type III Immune complex-mediated	Type IV Delayed hypersensitivity
Antigen	Exogenous pollen, food, drugs, dust	Cell surface of RBC Basement membrane	Extracellular fungal, viral, bacterial	Intracellular or extracellular
Antibody involved	IgE	IgG IgM IgA	IgG IgM IgA	None
Complement involved	No	Yes	Yes	No
Mediators of injury	Histamine SRS-A	Complement lysis Neutrophils	Neutrophils Complement lysis	Lymphokines T-cytotoxic cells Monocytes/macrophages Lysosomal enzymes Contact dermatitis Tumor rejection Transplant rejection
Examples	Allergic rhinitis Asthma	Transfusion reaction Goodpasture's syndrome	Serum sickness Systemic lupus erythematosus Rheumatoid arthritis	
Skin test	Wheal and flare	None	Erythema and edema in 3-8 hr	Erythema and edema in 24-48 hr (e.g., TB test)

RBC, Red blood cell; *Ig,* immunoglobulin; *SRS-A,* slow-reacting substance of anaphylaxis; *TB,* tuberculosis.

Immunoglobulin E (IgE) antibodies, produced in response to the allergen, attach to mast cells and basophils. On first exposure to allergen, IgE antibodies are produced. On subsequent exposures the allergen links with IgE bound to mast cells or basophils and triggers degranulation of the cells. In this process mediators (e.g., histamine, serotonin) are released, which then attack target organs, causing clinical allergy symptoms.

- These reversible effects include smooth muscle contraction, increased vascular permeability, vasodilatation, hypotension, increased secretion of mucus, and itching.
- The capacity to become sensitized to an allergen appears to be inherited.
- Clinical manifestations of an anaphylactoid reaction depend on whether the mediators remain local or become systemic. When mediators remain localized, a cutaneous response called the *wheal-and-flare reaction* occurs. This reaction is characterized by a pale wheal containing edematous fluid surrounded by a red flare from hyperemia. The reaction occurs in minutes or hours and is usually not dangerous.

Anaphylactic shock (anaphylaxis) occurs when mediators are released systemically (e.g., after injection of drug or insect sting). The reaction occurs within minutes and is life threatening because of airway obstruction and vascular collapse. Initial symptoms include edema and itching at the site of exposure to allergen. Within minutes shock manifested by rapid, weak pulse; hypotension; dilated pupils; dyspnea; and cyanosis may occur. This reaction is compounded by bronchial edema and angioedema. Death will occur if emergency treatment is not initiated. (See Allergic Disorders, therapeutic and nursing management, p. 17.) Allergens leading to anaphylactic shock in hypersensitive persons may include drugs (e.g., penicillin), insect venom, animal serum (e.g., tetanus antitoxin), foods (e.g., nuts), and treatments (e.g., blood products).

Allergic rhinitis, or *hay fever,* is the most common type I hypersensitivity reaction. It may occur year round (perennial allergic rhinitis), or it may be seasonal (seasonal allergic rhinitis).

- Airborne substances are the primary cause of allergic rhinitis. Perennial allergic rhinitis may be caused by dust, molds, and animal dander. Seasonal allergic rhinitis is commonly caused by trees, weeds, or grasses.
- Target areas affected are conjunctiva of the eyes and the mucosa of the upper respiratory tract. Symptoms include nasal discharge, sneezing, lacrimation, mucosal swelling with airway obstruction, and pruritus around the eyes, nose, throat, and mouth.

Atopic dermatitis is a chronic inherited skin disorder characterized by exacerbations and remissions. It is caused by several environmental allergens that are difficult to identify. Children with infantile eczema frequently have allergic respiratory disorders. Skin lesions are generalized and involve vasodilatation of blood vessels, resulting in interstitial edema with vesicle formation.

Urticaria (hives) is a cutaneous lesion occurring in atopic persons. It is characterized by transient wheals (pink, raised edematous pruritic areas) that vary in size and shape and may occur throughout the body. Urticaria develops rapidly after exposure to an allergen and may last minutes or hours. Histamine causes localized vasodilatation (erythema), transudation of fluid (wheal), and stimulation of local axon reflexes (flaring). Internal urticaria is characterized by edema in internal organs. (Urticaria is discussed in Lewis/Collier/Heitkemper, *Medical-Surgical Nursing,* edition 4, pp. 216 and 517).

Type II (cytotoxic and cytolytic) reactions. These reactions involve direct binding of immunoglobulin G (IgG), immunoglobulin M (IgM), or immunoglobulin A (IgA) antibodies to an antigen on the cell surface. Antigen-antibody complexes activate the complement system, which mediates the reaction. Cellular tissue is destroyed in one of two ways: activation of the complement cascade resulting in cytolysis and/or enhanced phagocytosis from complement fixation.

- Target cells frequently destroyed in type II reactions are erythrocytes, platelets, and leukocytes. Pathophysiologic disorders characteristic of type II reactions include ABO- and Rh-incompatibility transfusion reaction, autoimmune and drug-related hemolytic anemias, leukopenias, thrombocytopenias, erythroblastosis fetalis (hemolytic disease of the newborn), and Goodpasture's syndrome.

Type III (immune-complex) reactions. These reactions involve antigens combining with immunoglobulins (IgG and IgM classes) to form complexes that are too small to be effectively removed by the mononuclear phagocyte system. Therefore the complexes deposit in tissue or small blood vessels. They cause fixation of complement and release of chemotactic factors that lead to inflammation and destruction of involved tissue. Type III reactions may be local or systemic and immediate or delayed.

- Clinical manifestations depend on the number of complexes and the location in the body. Common sites for deposit are the kidneys, skin, joints, and blood vessels.
- Severe type III reactions are associated with autoimmune disorders such as systemic lupus erythematosus, acute glomerulonephritis, and rheumatoid arthritis.

Type IV (delayed hypersensitivity) reactions. These reactions are called *cell-mediated immune responses.* The tissue damage in a type IV reaction is caused by sensitized T lymphocytes attacking antigens or releasing lymphokines. The macrophages and enzymes released by T lymphocytes are responsible for most of the tissue destruction. The delayed hypersensitivity response takes 24 to 48 hours. Examples of this response include contact dermatitis; hypersensitivity reactions to bacterial, fungal, and viral infections; and transplant rejections. Some drug sensitivity reactions also fit this category.

Contact dermatitis is a reaction that occurs when skin is exposed to haptens. The haptens easily penetrate the skin to combine with epidermal proteins. The hapten-carrier substance then becomes antigenic.

On subsequent exposure to the hapten, a sensitized person develops eczematous skin lesions within 48 hours. The most common haptens encountered are metal compounds (e.g., nickel, mercury); rubber compounds; catechols present in poison ivy, poison oak, and sumac; cosmetics; and some dyes.

- In the acute phase of contact dermatitis, the skin appears erythematous and edematous and is covered with papules, vesicles, and bullae. The involved area is very pruritic but may also burn or sting.
- When contact dermatitis becomes chronic, the lesions resemble atopic dermatitis because they are thickened, scaly, and lichenified.

HYPERTENSION

Definition/Description

Hypertension is a sustained elevation in BP. The diagnosis of hypertension is confirmed in the adult when the average of two or more resting BP measurements done on at least two different visits reveals a systolic BP of ≥140 mm Hg or a diastolic BP ≥90 mm Hg. In the United States 50 million people either have elevated BP or are taking antihypertensive medication. High BP is one of the major risk factors for coronary heart disease and the most important risk factor for cerebrovascular diseases.

Classification of hypertension is described in Table 37 according to stages.

The cause of hypertension can be classified as primary (essential) or secondary. Primary (essential) hypertension accounts for 90% of all cases of hypertension, with the onset usually occurring between the ages of 30 and 50 years. Although the exact cause of essential hypertension is unknown, several contributing factors, including greater than ideal body weight, sedentary lifestyle, increased sodium intake, and excessive alcohol intake, have been identified.

Table 37	Classification of Blood Pressure for Adults Age 18 Years and Older*	
Category	**Systolic (mm Hg)**	**Diastolic (mm Hg)**
Normal	<130	<85
High normal	130-139	85-89
Hypertension†		
Stage 1 (mild)	140-159	90-99
Stage 2 (moderate)	160-179	100-109
Stage 3 (severe)	180-209	110-119
Stage 4 (very severe)	≥210	≥120

From US Department of Health and Human Services: The fifth report of the Joint National Committee on Detection, Evaluation, and Treatment of High Blood Pressure (JNC-V), Washington, DC, 1993, National Institutes of Health.
*Not taking antihypertensive drugs and not acutely ill. When systolic and diastolic pressures fall into different categories, the higher category should be selected to classify the individual's blood pressure status. Isolated systolic hypertension (ISH) is defined as systolic blood pressure (SBP) ≥140 mm Hg and diastolic blood pressure (DBP) <90 mm Hg and staged appropriately (e.g., 170/85 mm Hg is defined as stage 2 ISH).
†Based on the average of two or more readings taken at each of two or more visits after initial screening.

H

Pathophysiology

The hemodynamic hallmark of hypertension is persistently increased systemic vascular resistance (SVR). This persistent elevation in SVR may come about in various ways. There is evidence that changes in the structure of blood vessel walls occur with persistent stimulation by various pressor substances. These blood vessels increase their contractility, thereby sustaining the higher BP.

There is probably no single cause of *essential hypertension*. It is multifactorial in origin, and only some factors have been identified. However, risk factors have been identified that are known to be related to the development of essential hypertension or contribute to the disease (Table 38).

Secondary hypertension is elevated BP with a specific cause that can often be corrected by surgery or medication. If an adult older than age 50 suddenly develops hypertension, especially if it is severe, a secondary cause should be suspected. Causes of secondary hypertension include (1) coarctation of congenital narrowing of the

Table 38   Risk Factors in Essential Hypertension

▪ Age	BP rises progressively with increasing age. Elevated BP is present in approximately 50% of people over 65 years of age.
▪ Sex	More prevalent in young adult/early middle aged men. After age 55, more prevalent in women.
▪ Race	The incidence of hypertension is twice as great in African-Americans as in Caucasians.
▪ Family history	BP level is strongly familial. Hypertension risk increases if a close relative has hypertension.
▪ Obesity	Weight gain is associated with increased frequency of hypertension. The risk is greatest with central abdominal obesity.
▪ Cigarette smoking	Smoking greatly increases the risk of cardiovascular disease. Hypertensive persons who smoke are at even greater risk for cardiovascular problems.
▪ Excess dietary sodium	High sodium intake can contribute to hypertension in some patients and can decrease the efficacy of certain antihypertensive medications.
▪ Elevated serum lipids	Elevated levels of cholesterol and triglycerides are primary risk factors in atherosclerosis. Hyperlipidemia is more common in hypertensive persons.
▪ Alcohol	Excessive alcohol intake is strongly associated with hypertension. Hypertensive patients should limit their daily intake to 1 oz of alcohol.
▪ Sedentary lifestyle	A regular exercise program can help control weight and may decrease BP.
▪ Diabetes	Hypertension is more common in patients with diabetes mellitus. When hypertension and diabetes coexist, complications are more severe.
▪ Socioeconomic status	Hypertension is more prevalent in lower socioeconomic groups and among the less educated.
▪ Stress	People exposed to repeated stress may develop hypertension more frequently than others. People who become hypertensive may respond differently to stress than others.

aorta; (2) renal disease such as renal artery stenosis and parenchymal disease, (3) endocrine disorders such as Cushing's syndrome and hyperaldosteronism; (4) neurologic disorders such as brain tumors, quadriplegia, and head injury; (5) medications such as sympathetic stimulants, monoamine oxidase (MAO) inhibitors taken with tyramine-containing foods, estrogen replacement therapy, oral contraceptive pills, and nonsteroidal antiinflammatory drugs (NSAIDs); and (6) pregnancy.

Clinical Manifestations

Hypertension is often called the "silent killer" because it is frequently asymptomatic, especially if the BP is mild or moderate. However, a patient with severe hypertension may experience a variety of symptoms.

- The most common symptom is headache in the occipital region that is worse in the morning on arising. In the supine position cerebrospinal fluid (CSF) pressure increases secondary to increased BP, resulting in headache. When the person stands upright, the CSF pressure gradually decreases, and the headache disappears.
- Other possible manifestations of hypertension are fatigability, dizziness, palpitations, angina, and dyspnea. Blurring of vision and epistaxis (nosebleed) may also occur.

The most common complications of hypertension are target organ damage, including hypertensive heart disease, cerebrovascular disease, peripheral vascular disease, nephrosclerosis, and retinal damage.

Coronary artery disease and congestive heart failure. Hypertension is a major risk factor for coronary artery disease and heart failure. The hypertensive patient is more susceptible to silent ischemia, unrecognized myocardial infarction, and sudden cardiac death (see Coronary Artery Disease, p. 154). Congestive heart failure (CHF) occurs when the heart can no longer pump effectively against increasing resistance. Resistance to blood flow increases cardiac workload (see Congestive Heart Failure, p. 141).

Cerebrovascular disease. Hypertension is the leading cause of stroke in the United States. As a result of hypertension, blood vessels become more rigid because of thickening of vessel walls and replacement of smooth muscle tissue with fibrous tissue. The vessel is weakened by this process and tends to rupture more easily (see Cerebrovascular Accident [Stroke], p. 101).

Peripheral vascular disease. As with other vessels, hypertension speeds up the process of atherosclerosis in peripheral blood vessels leading to the development of aortic aneurysm, aortic dissection, and peripheral vascular disease. Intermittent claudication (ischemic muscle pain precipitated by activity and relieved with rest) is a classic symptom of peripheral vascular disease.

Nephrosclerosis. Hypertension is one of the leading risk factors for end-stage renal disease, especially in African-Americans. Some degree of renal dysfunction is present in the hypertensive patient, even one with a minimally elevated BP. This disorder is the result of ischemia caused by the narrowed lumen of intrarenal blood vessels. Gradual closure of arteries and arterioles leads to destruction of glomeruli, atrophy of tubules, and eventual death of nephrons. These changes may ultimately lead to renal failure. Common laboratory abnormalities are microalbuminuria, proteinuria, elevated blood urea nitrogen (BUN) and serum creatinine levels, and microscopic hematuria. The earliest symptom of renal dysfunction is usually nocturia.

Retinal damage. The appearance of the retina provides important information about the severity and prognosis of the hypertensive process. The retina is the only place in the body where the blood vessels can be directly visualized. Therefore retinal damage provides an indication of vessel damage in heart, brain, and kidney. Manifestations of retinal damage include blurring of vision, retinal hemorrhage, and loss of vision.

Diagnostic Studies

- Routine urinalysis and BUN and serum creatinine level screens for renal involvement
- Uric acid levels and serum electrolytes (especially K^+ to detect aldosteronism)
- Blood glucose (fasting, if possible) levels to identify endocrine causes of hypertension (e.g., diabetes mellitus, Cushing's syndrome)
- Serum lipid profile, cholesterol, and triglycerides levels to assess for atherogenesis risk factors
- Chest x-ray to determine heart size and if coarctation of aorta exists
- ECG to provide cardiac status baseline

Therapeutic Management

The goal in treating a hypertensive patient is to prevent morbidity and mortality associated with high BP and to control BP by the least intrusive means possible. Lifestyle modifications are indicated for the individual with either borderline or sustained hypertension. These modification measures include dietary management, smoking cessation, regular exercise, and limitation of alcohol intake.

- If BP remains ≥104/90 mm Hg after 3 to 6 months of lifestyle changes, drug therapy is indicated.
- Follow-up monitoring of BP is very important. After the BP has stabilized, it should be monitored every 4 to 6 months to ensure control and to assess for target organ damage.

- Dietary management of hypertension consists of sodium restriction, caloric restriction if the patient is overweight, and restriction of cholesterol and fat. Alcohol consumption is strongly associated with hypertension, and studies suggest that consumption of three or more alcoholic drinks daily is a definite risk factor. The patient should be advised to limit alcohol intake to 1 oz per day (amount of alcohol in 2 oz of 100-proof whiskey, 8 oz of wine, or 24 oz of beer).
- Aerobic exercise such as walking, jogging, or swimming can help control BP, promote relaxation, and decrease or control body weight. For a sedentary patient moderate activity, such as 30 to 45 minutes of brisk walking three to five times per week, is recommended. The patient should be advised to increase exercise levels gradually. The patient with heart disease or other serious health problems needs a thorough physical examination, possibly including a stress test, before beginning an exercise program.
- Although cigarette smoking does not contribute to the development of hypertension, it is a major risk factor for cardiovascular disease, and avoidance of tobacco is essential. Everyone, especially a hypertensive patient, should be strongly advised not to smoke.

Pharmacologic Management

The general goals of pharmacologic management of hypertension are to reduce and maintain diastolic BP at <90 mm Hg and to keep the disabling side effects of medications to a minimum. The drugs currently available for treating hypertension have two main actions: reduction of SVR and decreased volume of circulating blood.

- Drugs used in the treatment of hypertension include diuretics, adrenergic (sympathetic)-inhibiting agents, vasodilators, angiotensin-converting enzyme (ACE) inhibiting agents, and calcium channel blockers (antagonists). See Lewis/Collier/Heitkemper, *Medical-Surgical Nursing,* edition 4, Table 30-7, p. 872, for a description of antihypertensive drug therapy and p. 871 for drug recommendations for the stages of hypertension.

Nursing Management
Goals
The patient with hypertension will have a decrease in BP, no target organ damage, and minimal or no unpleasant side effects of therapy.

Nursing Diagnoses/Collaborative Problems
- Altered health maintenance related to lack of knowledge of pathology, complications, and management of hypertension

- Anxiety related to complexity of management regimen, possible complications, and lifestyle changes associated with hypertension
- Ineffective management of therapeutic regimen (specify) related to unpleasant side effects of medication, subsiding of symptoms, lack of motivation, and inconvenient schedule for taking medications
- Body image disturbance related to diagnosis of hypertension
- Potential complication: hypertensive crisis
- Potential complication: cerebral vascular accident

Nursing Interventions

The nurse in routine screening settings is in an ideal position to assess for the presence of hypertension, identify risk factors for hypertension and coronary artery disease, and educate the patient regarding hypertension.

- Effort and resources should be focused on controlling BP in the person already identified as having hypertension; identifying and controlling BP in high-risk groups such as African-Americans, obese persons, and blood relatives of people with hypertension; and screening those with limited access to the health care system.

The majority of patients with hypertension are managed on an outpatient basis. The patient with a severely elevated BP, especially with significant target organ damage, may be hospitalized. The purpose of hospitalization is to lower BP, determine the underlying cause of hypertension, prevent or limit target organ damage, and treat the cause if it is secondary hypertension. The primary goal of the nurse at this stage of intervention is to assist in reducing BP and to begin patient education.

For the patient with severe hypertension, BP should be monitored every 1 to 2 hours and then with decreasing frequency as the BP stabilizes. Antihypertensive drug therapy at this time may be given parenterally; this requires frequent (every 2 to 5 minutes) BP checks. Careful monitoring of vital signs provides information regarding effectiveness of drugs and patient response to therapy.

- Frequent neurologic checks, including level of consciousness, pupillary size and reaction, movement of extremities, and reaction to stimuli, help to detect changes in the patient's condition. Cardiac, pulmonary, and renal systems should be monitored for decompensation caused by the severe elevation in BP (e.g., pulmonary edema, CHF, angina, and renal failure).
- If the patient has headaches, it is important to assess when the headaches occur and what precipitating factors are present. In addition to lowering BP, nursing interventions for headache include modification of any environmental or emotional factors that may be contributing to the headache. Appropriate inter-

ventions include encouraging the patient to verbalize fears, answering questions concerning hypertension, and eliminating excess noise in the patient's environment.

Patient Teaching

Beginning and continuing patient education includes diet therapy, drug therapy, exercise, and if appropriate, BP home monitoring and smoking cessation.

Diet therapy. The patient and family, especially the member who prepares the meals, should be educated about sodium-restricted diets. They need to be instructed on reading the labels of over-the-counter drugs and packaged foods to identify hidden sources of sodium. It is helpful to review the patient's normal diet and to identify foods high in sodium.

Drug therapy. Side effects of antihypertensive drug therapy are common. The number or severity of side effects may be related to dosage, and in certain cases it is necessary to change the drug or decrease the dosage. Side effects may be caused by an initial response to drug and may decrease with its long-term use. With some drugs side effects can be alleviated by arranging a convenient schedule.

Exercise. The patient needs assistance in developing a graduated exercise program. An aerobic exercise program based on the patient's current exercise activities can be planned. The patient needs to be monitored for long-term adherence to the program.

Home monitoring. Patients should be assessed individually about the feasibility of being taught, or having a family member taught, to take BP readings at home. Often home BP measurement gives a more valid indication of BP than does that done in a clinical setting because the patient is more relaxed.

- The development of an individual plan is essential and needs to be compatible with the patient's personality, habits, and lifestyle. Active patient participation increases the likelihood of adherence to the treatment plan. Measures such as involving the patient in scheduling the medications for convenience in a daily routine, helping the patient link pill taking with another daily activity, and involving family members (if necessary) help increase patient compliance.

- It is important to help the patient and family understand that hypertension is a chronic condition that cannot be cured but can be controlled with drug therapy, diet therapy, an exercise program, periodic evaluation, and other relevant lifestyle changes.

Hyperthyroidism

Definition/Description

Hyperthyroidism is hyperfunction of the thyroid that results from excess circulating levels of thyroxine (T_4), triiodothyronine (T_3), or both. The incidence of hyperthyroidism is six times greater in women than in men. Iodine deficiency is believed to predispose the patient to hyperthyroidism and other thyroid diseases with a greater incidence in iodine-poor geographic locations.

- The most common form of hyperthyroidism is Graves' disease, followed by multinodular goiter. A *goiter* is an enlargement of the thyroid gland.

Types

Graves' disease is an autoimmune disease of unknown etiology marked by an increased production of thyroid hormone. Patients who are genetically susceptible become sensitized to and develop antibodies against various antigens within the thyroid gland.

Most patients with Graves' disease have hyperthyroidism and diffuse thyroid hyperplasia caused by antibodies that attack thyroid tissue and thus stimulate hyperplasia. These antibodies, known collectively as *thyroid-stimulating antibodies* (TSAbs), stimulate the thyroid-stimulating hormone (TSH) receptor and activate production of thyroid hormones.

- The disease is characterized by remissions and exacerbations, with or without treatment. It may progress to destruction of thyroid tissue, causing hypothyroidism.
- Precipitating factors such as insufficient iodine supply, infections, and emotions may interact with genetic factors to cause Graves' disease.

Multinodular goiter is characterized by small, discrete autonomously functioning nodules that secrete thyroid hormone. These nodules may be benign or malignant. If associated with signs of hyperthyroidism, a nodule is termed *toxic adenoma.*

- The frequency of toxic multinodular goiter is highest in women in the sixth and seventh decades of life. There is usually a history of preexisting simple goiter for years before the onset of demonstrable hyperthyroidism.
- Manifestations are slower to develop and usually less severe than in Graves' disease.

Clinical Manifestations

Manifestations of hyperthyroidism are related to the effects of excess thyroid hormones. Manifestations are numerous and include dysrhythmias, angina, tachypnea, fatigue, insomnia, weight loss, increased appetite, diarrhea, diaphoresis, goiter, intolerance to heat, and menstrual irregularities.

- Exophthalmos (proptosis), in which the eyeballs protrude from the orbits, is due to impaired venous drainage from the orbit leading to increased deposits of fat and fluid (edema) in the retroorbital tissues. This sign is seen in 20% to 40% of patients with Graves' disease. When the eyelids do not close completely, exposed corneal surfaces become dry and irritated. Serious consequences, such as corneal ulcers and eventual loss of vision, can occur.

- A patient with advanced disease may exhibit many symptoms, whereas a patient in the early stages of hyperthyroidism may exhibit only weight loss and increased nervousness. For a comparison of the features of hyperthyroidism in young and geriatric patients, see Table 47-5 in Lewis/Collier/Heitkemper, *Medical-Surgical Nursing,* edition 4, p. 1489.

Complications

Hyperthyroid crisis (thyrotoxic crisis) is an acute but rare condition in which all hyperthyroid manifestations are heightened. The cause is presumed to be stressors such as infection, trauma, or surgery in a patient with preexisting hyperthyroidism. This condition is potentially fatal, but death is rare when treatment is vigorous and initiated early.

- Manifestations include severe tachycardia, heart failure, shock, hyperthermia (up to 105.3° F [40.7° C]), restlessness, agitation, abdominal pain, nausea, vomiting, diarrhea, delirium, and coma.

- Measures must be taken to prevent death. Treatment is aimed at reducing circulating thyroid hormone levels by appropriate drug therapy and extracorporeal removal of thyroid hormone. Therapy is directed at fever reduction, fluid replacement, and elimination or management of the initiating stressor(s).

Diagnostic Studies

- Ophthalmologic examination.
- ECG may show tachycardia, atrial fibrillation, and alterations in P and T waves.
- Serum T_3RU, T_4, free T_3, and TSH levels will be elevated.
- Thyroid-releasing hormone (TRH) stimulation test and thyroid scan.

Therapeutic Management

The goals of management are to block the adverse effects of thyroid hormones and to stop their oversecretion. Therapy involves pharmacotherapy with antithyroid drugs and β-adrenergic receptor blockers, thyroid ablation with radioactive iodine, and subtotal thyroidectomy after adequate preparation.

Pharmacologic Management

Antithyroid drugs. The most commonly used antithyroid drugs are classified as thioamides; propylthiouracil (PTU) and methimazole (Tapazole) are the most commonly used drugs. These drugs inhibit the synthesis of thyroid hormones. PTU also blocks the peripheral conversion of T_4 to T_3.

- Indications for the use of antithyroid drugs include Graves' disease in the young patient, thyrotoxicosis during pregnancy, and the need to make a patient euthyroid before surgery or irradiation.

Iodine. In large doses iodine (e.g. Lugol's solution, potassium iodide) inhibits the synthesis of T_3 and T_4 and blocks release of these hormones into the circulation. Iodine decreases thyroid size and vascularity, making resection safer and easier. Administration of PTU, with iodine therapy added 10 days before surgery, is a common method for surgical preparation of a patient with hyperthyroidism.

β-Adrenergic blockers. Propranolol (Inderal) is the most frequently used ß-adrenergic blocker. It relieves symptoms of hyperthyroidism that result from increased ß-adrenergic receptors caused by excess thyroid hormones.

Radioactive iodine. Radioiodine limits thyroid hormone secretion by damaging or destroying thyroid tissue. It is administered orally, with the dose determined by estimated thyroid weight. This treatment is effective but often results in hypothyroidism.

Nutritional Management

The potential for nutritional deficits is high when an increased metabolic rate is present. A high-calorie diet (4000 to 5000 kcal/day) may be ordered to satisfy hunger and prevent tissue breakdown. This is accomplished with six full meals a day and snacks high in protein, carbohydrates, minerals, and vitamins (particularly vitamin A, thiamine, vitamin B_6, and ascorbic acid). The nurse should weigh the patient daily to monitor the adequacy of diet since weight increases are usually desirable. Offering fluids frequently prevents volume deficit related to diaphoresis and insensible loss. Highly seasoned and high-fiber foods should be avoided because they stimulate the already hypermotile GI tract.

Nursing Management

Goals

The patient with hyperthyroidism will experience relief of symptoms, have no serious complications related to the disease or treatment, and cooperate with the therapeutic plan.

See the nursing care plan for the patient with hyperthyroidism in Lewis/Collier/Heitkemper, *Medical-Surgical Nursing,* edition 4, p. 1492.

Nursing Diagnoses

- Activity intolerance related to fatigue, exhaustion, and heat intolerance secondary to hypermetabolism
- Altered nutrition: less than body requirements related to hypermetabolism and inadequate diet
- Anxiety related to lack of knowledge about management and course of disease, hypermetabolism, and presence of hypertension
- Risk for trauma related to fine muscle tremors, fatigue, inattentiveness, incoordination
- Sleep pattern disturbance related to anxiety, environmental stimulation, disruption of normal sleep pattern, and caffeine intake
- Risk for injury: corneal ulceration related to decreased blinking or inability to close eyelids secondary to exophthalmos

Nursing Interventions

A restful, calm, quiet room should be provided because increased metabolism causes sleep disturbances. Provision of adequate rest may be a challenge because of the patient's irritability and restlessness.

- Interventions may include placing the patient in a cool room, away from very ill patients and noisy, high-traffic areas; using light bed coverings and changing the linen frequently if the patient is diaphoretic; encouraging and assisting with exercise involving the large muscle groups (tremors can interfere with small-muscle coordination) to allow release of nervous tension and restlessness; and establishing a supportive, trusting relationship to help the patient cope with aggravating events and lessen anxiety.

If exophthalmos is present, there is potential for corneal injury related to irritation and dryness. The patient may also have orbital pain. Interventions to relieve eye discomfort and prevent corneal ulceration include applying artificial tears to soothe and moisten the conjunctival membranes, salt restriction and elevation of the patient's head to reduce periorbital edema, dark glasses to reduce glare and prevent irritation from smoke, air currents, dust, and dirt. If the eyelids cannot be closed, they should be lightly taped shut for sleep.

- To maintain flexibility, the patient should be taught to exercise the intraocular muscles several times a day by turning the eyes in a complete range of motion.

Nursing Management of Patient Receiving Radioactive Iodine Therapy

Radioactive iodine therapy (ablation) is usually done on an outpatient basis and is the therapy of choice for adults beyond the childbearing years. Because the usual therapeutic dose of iodine is only 7 to 10 millicurie (mCi), no radiation safety precautions are necessary.

- The patient should be instructed that radiation thyroiditis and parotiditis are possible and may cause dryness and irritation of the mouth and throat. Relief may be obtained with frequent sips of water, ice chips, or the use of a salt and soda gargle three to four times per day. Discomfort should subside in 3 to 4 days.
- Because of the high frequency of hypothyroidism after radioactive iodine therapy, the patient and significant others should be taught the symptoms of hypothyroidism and should be instructed to seek medical help if these symptoms occur.

Nursing Management of Patient Having Thyroid Surgery

Preoperative care. When subtotal thyroidectomy is the treatment of choice, the patient must be adequately prepared to avoid postoperative complications. Preoperative teaching should include comfort and safety measures in which the patient can participate and the practice and importance of coughing, deep breathing, and leg exercises. The patient should also be taught how to support the head manually while turning in bed to minimize stress on the suture line. Range-of-motion exercises of the neck should be practiced, and the patient should be told that talking is likely to be difficult for a short time after surgery.

Postoperative care. The hospital room must be prepared before the patient's return from surgery. O_2, suction equipment, and a tracheostomy tray should be readily available.

- Recurrent laryngeal nerve damage leads to vocal cord paralysis. If there is paralysis of both cords, spastic airway obstruction will occur, requiring an immediate tracheostomy.
- Respiration may become difficult because of excess swelling of the neck tissues, hemorrhage, and hematoma formation.
- Laryngeal stridor (harsh, vibratory sound) may occur during respiration as a result of tetany, which occurs if the parathyroid glands are removed or damaged during surgery. To treat tetany, calcium salts should be readily available for IV administration.

After a thyroidectomy the nurse should do the following:

- Assess the patient every 2 hours for 24 hours for signs of hemorrhage or tracheal compression, such as irregular breathing, neck swelling, frequent swallowing, sensations of fullness at the incision site, choking, and blood on the anterior or posterior dressings.
- Place the patient in a semi-Fowler's position and support the head with pillows, avoiding flexion of the neck and any tension on suture lines.
- Monitor vital signs. Check for signs of tetany secondary to hypoparathyroidism (e.g., tingling in toes, fingers, or around the mouth; muscular twitching; apprehension) and by evaluating

difficulty in speaking and hoarseness. Some hoarseness is expected after surgery because of edema.

- Control postoperative pain by giving medication.

The neck incision should be lubricated and range-of-motion exercises should be carried out three or four times daily to promote comfort and return of full range of motion.

- The appearance of the incision may be distressing, but the patient can be reassured that the scar will fade in color and eventually look like a normal neck wrinkle. A scarf, jewelry, or other covering can effectively camouflage a fresh scar.

Patient Teaching

Follow-up care is important for the patient who has undergone thyroid surgery. Hyperthyroidism may recur after a period of time, requiring further treatment.

- Hormone balance should be monitored periodically to ensure that normal function has returned.
- Caloric intake must be reduced substantially below the amount required before surgery to prevent weight gain.
- Adequate iodine is necessary to promote thyroid function, but an excessive amount inhibits the thyroid. Seafood once or twice a week or normal use of iodized salt should provide sufficient intake.
- Regular exercise helps stimulate the thyroid and should be encouraged.
- High environmental temperature should be avoided because it inhibits thyroid regeneration.
- If a complete thyroidectomy has been performed, the patient needs instruction in lifelong pharmacologic thyroid replacement.
- The patient should be taught the signs and symptoms of progressive thyroid failure and instructed to seek medical care if these develop.

H

HYPOPARATHYROIDISM

Definition/Description

Hypoparathyroidism is an uncommon condition characterized by inadequate circulating parathyroid hormone (PTH), resulting in hypocalcemia. PTH resistance at the cellular level may also occur. This is caused by a genetic defect resulting in hypocalcemia in spite of normal or high PTH levels and is often associated with hypothyroidism and hypogonadism.

Pathophysiology

The most common cause of hypoparathyroidism is accidental removal of the parathyroids or damage to the vascular supply of the glands during neck surgery (e.g., thyroidectomy, radical neck surgery).

- Idiopathic hypoparathyroidism resulting from the absence, fatty replacement, or atrophy of the glands is a rare disease that usually occurs early in life and may be associated with other endocrine disorders. Affected patients may have antiparathyroid antibodies.
- Hypomagnesemia is increasingly being recognized as a cause of hypoparathyroidism. Hypomagnesemia, as seen in alcoholism or malabsorption, impairs PTH secretion and its action on bone and kidneys.

Clinical Manifestations

The clinical features of acute hypoparathyroidism are due to a low serum calcium level (see Table 47-10 in Lewis/Collier/Heitkemper, *Medical-Surgical Nursing*, edition 4, p. 1500).

- Sudden decreases in calcium concentration give rise to a syndrome called *tetany*. This state is characterized by tingling of the lips, finger tips, and occasionally feet and increased muscle tension leading to paresthesias and stiffness. Dysphagia, painful tonic spasms of smooth and skeletal muscles (particularly of extremities and face), and laryngospasms are also present. Chvostek's sign (facial muscle spasm when the face is tapped below the temple) and Trousseau's phenomenon (carpopedal spasm when arterial circulation is interrupted by applying a BP cuff for 3 minutes) are usually positive.
- Respiratory function may be severely compromised by accessory muscle spasm– and laryngeal spasm–induced airway obstruction. Patients are usually anxious and apprehensive.

Abnormal diagnostic laboratory findings include decreased serum calcium and PTH levels and increased serum phosphate levels.

Therapeutic Management

The main objectives of treatment are to treat tetany when present and to prevent long-term complications by maintaining eucalcemia. Tetany is treated with IV infusion or slow push of calcium salts. Long-term therapy consists of administration of vitamin D and possibly supplemental calcium and oral phosphate binders.

- Emergency treatment of tetany requires administration of IV calcium. Calcium salts can cause hypotension and cardiac arrest; thus a slow IV push is required. For long-term management oral calcium supplements may be prescribed.
- Specific hormone replacement of PTH is not used to treat hypoparathyroidism because of the possibility of antibody for-

mation to PTH, the expense, and the need for parenteral administration.

- Vitamin D is used in chronic and resistant hypocalcemia to enhance intestinal calcium absorption and bone resorption. Preferred preparations are dihydrotachysterol (Hytakerol) and calcitriol (Rocaltrol). These drugs are potent, raise calcium levels rapidly, and are quickly metabolized. Rapid metabolism is desired because vitamin D is a fat-soluble vitamin and toxicity can cause irreversible renal impairment.

Nursing Management
Goals
The patient with hypoparathyroidism will develop no complications such as tetany or dysrhythmias, recognize signs and symptoms of hypoparathyroidism and hyperparathyroidism, and comply with periodic assessment of calcium level.

Nursing Diagnoses/Collaborative Problems
- Impaired skin integrity related to dry, scaly skin
- Activity intolerance related to fatigue, weakness, and painful muscle cramps
- Altered thought processes related to personality and psychiatric changes and memory impairment
- Ineffective management of therapeutic regimen related to lack of knowledge regarding signs and symptoms of calcium deficiency, calcium-rich foods and supplements, and chronic nature of the problem
- Potential complication: dysrhythmia
- Potential complication: tetany

Nursing Interventions
If tetany or generalized muscle cramps develop, rebreathing may partially alleviate the symptoms. The patient who can cooperate should be instructed to breathe in and out of a paper bag or breathing mask. This reduces carbon dioxide excretion from the lungs and lowers body pH. Because an acidic environment enhances both solubility and degree of ionization of calcium, ionized calcium is increased, temporarily relieving the hypocalcemia.

- IV calcium salts should be available at the bedside for treatment of acute tetany. Calcium salts must be infused slowly because high blood levels can cause serious cardiac dysrhythmias or cardiac arrest. The patient who has been digitalized is particularly vulnerable. ECG monitoring is indicated.
- Siderails should be padded as a seizure precaution. Patients should be kept in a nonstimulating environment, assisted with hygienic needs, and given support and encouragement until they are free of symptoms.

H

Patient Teaching

The patient with hypoparathyroidism needs instruction in the management of long-term nutrition and drug therapy.

- A high-calcium meal plan includes foods such as dark-green vegetables, soy beans, and tofu. The patient should be told that foods containing oxalic acid (e.g., spinach and rhubarb), phytic acid (e.g., bran and whole grains), and phosphorus reduce calcium absorption.
- Calcium supplements of at least 1 g/day for patients less than 40 years of age and 2 g/day for the patient more than 40 years of age are usually prescribed. These supplements are best administered 2 to 3 hours after meals. Calcium carbonate often leads to constipation and flatulence. Nursing interventions include providing stool softeners, adequate fluids, and fresh fruits.

The patient should be instructed about the signs and symptoms of hypocalcemia and hypercalcemia through written handouts and told to report these to a clinician as soon as possible if they occur.

- If manifestations of hypocalcemia occur, calcium supplementation should be increased. The need for lifelong treatment and health supervision should be stressed.
- Patient calcium levels should be monitored three to four times a year. Treatment modification is often necessary because hypercalcemia can develop.
- Thorough patient instruction and frequent serum calcium assessment should allow a normal life expectancy. The patient needs support and encouragement to continue with the regimen.

HYPOPITUITARISM

Definition/Description

Hypopituitarism is a rare disorder that involves a decrease in one or more of the anterior pituitary hormones. Primary hypofunction may be due to infections, autoimmune disorders, tumors, or destruction of the gland through irradiation or surgical procedures. Failure to secrete growth hormone is the most common abnormality, followed by deficiencies of the gonadotropins, thyroid-stimulating hormone (TSH), corticotropin, and prolactin.

Manifestations of hypopituitarism depend on the specific pituitary hormones that are lacking. Thus infertility may be caused by primary gonadal failure or may be the first indication of pituitary hypofunction (gonads lack tropic hormone stimulation).

Clinical Manifestations

Clinical findings associated with pituitary hypofunction vary with the degree and speed of onset of pituitary dysfunction and are related to hyposecretion of the target glands. Symptoms are often nonspecific and commonly include weakness, fatigue, headache, sexual dysfunction, fasting hypoglycemia, dry and sallow skin, diminished tolerance for stress, and poor resistance to infection.

- In the adult, premature fine wrinkling around the eyes and mouth is common. Psychiatric symptoms include apathy, mental slowness, and delusions. Orthostatic hypotension may also occur.
- If a pituitary tumor exerts pressure on the optic chiasma, there may be asymmetric visual field changes. If the tumor is large, blindness in one or both eyes may occur.
- When pituitary hypofunction affects follicle-stimulating hormone (FSH) and luteinizing hormone (LH), sexual development is impaired and features remain childlike. FSH and LH deficiencies in the adult woman are first manifested as menstrual irregularities, diminished libido, and changes in secondary sex characteristics. Men with FSH and LH deficiencies experience testicular atrophy, loss of libido along with impotence, and decreased facial hair and muscle mass.

If hypopituitarism is not detected and treated, the patient eventually develops deficiencies of thyroid hormone and the adrenal corticosteroids. The latter deficiency causes a tendency toward shock and may result in an episode of acute adrenal insufficiency (refractory and life-threatening shock resulting from sodium and water depletion).

Therapeutic and Nursing Management

Treatment of hypopituitarism consists of surgery or irradiation for tumor removal, permanent target gland hormone replacement, and dietary management. Replacement therapy is carried out with corticosteroids, thyroid hormone, and sex hormones. Gonadotropins can sometimes restore fertility.

A primary nursing role in anterior pituitary insufficiency is assessment and recognition of subtle signs and symptoms.

- The patient with hypopituitarism may first exhibit symptoms in stressful situations such as trauma or surgery. In addition, hypopituitarism may be detected in patients with complaints of failure to grow, infertility, or amenorrhea.

HYPOTHYROIDISM

Definition/Description

Hypothyroidism usually results from insufficient circulating thyroid hormone caused by a variety of abnormalities. Hypothyroidism may occur in infancy *(cretinism),* childhood, or adulthood. Although the typical patient with hypothyroidism is a woman more than 50 years old, the disease can occur at any age and in either sex.

Pathophysiology

- Cretinism is caused by thyroid hormone deficiencies during fetal or early neonatal life. It can be caused by maternal iodine deprivation or congenital thyroid abnormalities.
- In the adult the most common cause of primary hypothyroidism is atrophy of the thyroid gland. This condition is considered to be the end result of both Hashimoto's thyroiditis and Graves' disease. These autoimmune diseases destroy the thyroid gland. Thyroid deficiency also occurs when pituitary thyroid-stimulating hormone (TSH) production is inadequate. Iatrogenic causes of hypothyroidism include surgical removal of the thyroid, destruction of thyroid gland by radiation, and surgical removal of the pituitary gland.

Clinical Manifestations

The major manifestations of *cretinism* are defective physical development and mental retardation. Although affected infants usually appear normal at birth, cretinism should be suspected when there is a long gestational period and a large infant who fails to thrive.

- Cretinism causes irreversible mental retardation and dwarfism. When treatment with hormone replacement is begun soon after birth, normal physical and intellectual development will ensue.

In the adult, hypothyroidism is characterized by an insidious and nonspecific slowing of body processes, personality changes, fatigue, and lethargy. Mental changes include impaired memory, slowed speech, and somnolence. In addition, cold intolerance, hair loss, dry and coarse skin, brittle nails, muscle weakness and swelling, constipation, weight gain, and menorrhagia are common. Hypothyroid heart disease includes cardiomyopathy, pericardial effusion, and coronary atherosclerosis.

- Symptoms are so insidious that medical attention is seldom sought. The patient and family are often unaware of the changes. Severity of symptoms depends on the degree of thyroid hormone deficiency.

- The term *myxedema* is often used synonymously with hypothyroidism but actually connotes severe long-standing hypothyroidism. With myxedema there is accumulation of hydrophilic mucopolysaccharides in the ground substance of the dermis and other tissues. This mucinous edema causes the characteristic facies of hypothyroidism, including facial puffiness, periorbital edema, and masklike affect.

The mental sluggishness, drowsiness, and lethargy of hypothyroidism may progress gradually or suddenly to a notable impairment of consciousness or coma. This situation, termed *myxedema coma,* constitutes a medical emergency. Myxedema coma can be precipitated by infection, drugs (especially narcotics, tranquilizers, and barbiturates), exposure to cold, and trauma. It is characterized by subnormal temperature, hypotension, and hypoventilation. For the patient to live, vital functions must be supported, and IV thyroid hormone must be administered.

Diagnostic Studies

- Serum triiodothyronine (T_4), thyroxine (T_3), and T_3RU levels are low.
- Serum TSH levels help determine the cause of hypothyroidism. If levels are high, the thyroid is diseased; if low, the pituitary is diseased.
- ECG shows bradycardia and low voltage.
- Serum cholesterol is increased.
- Thyroid-releasing hormone (TRH) stimulation test will show an increase in TSH if the hypothalamus is diseased and no change in TSH if the pituitary is diseased.

H

Therapeutic Management

The therapeutic objective in hypothyroidism is restoration of a euthyroid state as safely and rapidly as possible with hormone replacement therapy. Synthetic oral thyroxine (Synthroid, Levothroid) is the drug of choice to treat hypothyroidism. In the young, otherwise healthy patient, the maintenance replacement dose can be started at once. In the older adult patient and the person with compromised cardiac status, a small initial dose is recommended because the usual dose may overstimulate the cardiovascular system. Any chest pain experienced by a patient starting thyroid replacement should be reported immediately, and ECG and serum cardiac enzyme tests must be performed. The dose is increased at 1- to 4-week intervals. It is important that the patient take replacement medication regularly.

- With treatment striking transformations occur in both appearance and mental function. Most adults return to a normal state.

Cardiovascular conditions and (occasionally) psychosis may persist despite corrections of the hormonal imbalance. Relapses occur if treatment is interrupted.

Nursing Management
Goals

The patient with hypothyroidism will experience relief of symptoms, maintain a euthyroid state, maintain a positive self-image, and comply with lifelong thyroid replacement therapy.

See the nursing care plan for the patient with hypothyroidism in Lewis/Collier/Heitkemper, *Medical-Surgical Nursing,* edition 4, p. 1499.

Nursing Diagnoses

- Altered comfort related to cold intolerance
- Altered thought processes related to diminished cerebral blood flow secondary to decreased cardiac output
- Activity intolerance related to decreased metabolic rate and mucin deposits in joints and interstitial spaces
- Constipation related to gastrointestinal hypomotility
- Altered nutrition: more than body requirements related to weight gain

Nursing Interventions

- Provide a comfortable, warm environment because of the patient's intolerance to cold.
- Take measures to prevent skin breakdown. Use soap sparingly and apply an emollient or lotion. An alternating-pressure mattress may be helpful.
- Avoid using sedatives. If they must be given, give the lowest possible dose and closely monitor mental status, level of consciousness, and respirations.
- Prevent constipation by gradually increasing exercise, increasing fiber in meal plan, administering stool softeners, and promoting regular bowel habits. Avoid enemas because they produce vagal stimulation, which can be hazardous to the patient with cardiac disease.
- Note the patient's energy level and mental alertness. These should increase within 2 to 14 days and continue to rise steadily to normal levels.

For assessment of the patient's progress, vital signs, body weight, fluid intake and output, and visible edema should be monitored. Cardiac assessment is especially important because the cardiovascular response to the hormone determines the medication regimen.

Patient Teaching

Repeated patient education is imperative. Initially the hypothyroid patient needs more time than usual to comprehend all the necessary information.

- The need for lifelong drug therapy must be stressed. The signs and symptoms of hypothyroidism or hyperthyroidism that indicate hormone imbalance should be included in the teaching plan. It is sometimes difficult for the patient to recognize signs of overdosage or underdosage; therefore a family member or friend should be included in the instruction process.
- The patient must be taught to contact a clinician immediately if signs of overdose such as orthopnea, dyspnea, rapid pulse, palpitations, nervousness, or insomnia appear.
- The patient with diabetes mellitus should test his/her capillary blood glucose at least daily because return to the euthyroid state frequently increases insulin requirements.
- In addition, thyroid preparations potentiate the effects of other common drugs such as anticoagulants, antidepressants, and digitalis.

H

Increased Intracranial Pressure

Definition/Description

Increased intracranial pressure (ICP) is a life-threatening situation that results from an increase in any or all of the three components of the skull: brain tissue, blood, and cerebrospinal fluid (CSF). Cerebral edema is an important factor related to increased ICP. Regardless of the cause, cerebral edema results in an increase in tissue volume that has the potential for increased ICP. The extent and severity of the original insult are factors that determine the degree of cerebral edema.

Three types of cerebral edema—vasogenic, cytotoxic, and interstitial—have been identified. More than one type may be present from one insult in the same patient.

- *Vasogenic cerebral edema* is the most common type of edema. It occurs mainly in the white matter and is attributed to changes in the endothelial linings of cerebral capillaries.
- *Cytotoxic cerebral edema* results from local disruption of the functional or morphologic integrity of cell membranes and occurs most often in the gray matter. This type of edema develops from destructive lesions or trauma to brain tissue.
- *Interstitial cerebral edema* is the result of periventricular diffusion of ventricular CSF in a patient with uncontrolled hydrocephalus. It can also be caused by enlargement of the extracellular space as a response to systemic water excess (hyponatremia).

Pathophysiology

Increased ICP can be caused by several clinical problems, including a mass lesion (e.g., hematoma), cerebral edema associated with brain tumors, hydrocephalus, head injury, or brain inflammation, or by metabolic coma. These cerebral insults may result in hypercapnia, cerebral acidosis, impaired autoregulation, and systemic hypertension, which promote the formation and spread of cerebral edema. This edema distorts brain tissue, further increasing ICP, which leads to even more tissue hypoxia and acidosis. (For an illustration of the progression of increased ICP, see Fig. 54-4 in Lewis/Collier/Heitkemper, *Medical-Surgical Nursing,* edition 4, p. 1689.)

Unless there is a reduction in ICP, brain stem compression occurs. As the intracranial mass continues to increase, herniation of the brain from one compartment to another can occur.

With brain displacement and herniation, ischemia and edema are further increased. Compression of the brain stem and cranial nerves may be fatal. (For an illustration of the symptoms of supratentorial increased ICP from the early phase through herniation of the brain, see Lewis/Collier/Heitkemper, *Medical-Surgical Nursing,* edition 4, p. 1690.) Supratentorial lesions occur below the tentorium (a fold of dura) and include epidural and subdural hematomas, cerebral infarction, brain tumors, and abscesses.

- Herniation forces the cerebellum and brain stem downward through the foramen magnum. If compression of the brain stem is unrelieved, respiratory arrest may occur.

Clinical Manifestations

Manifestations of increased ICP can take many forms, depending on the cause, location, and rate at which the pressure increase occurs. The earlier the condition is recognized and treated, the better the prognosis. Manifestations of increased ICP associated with supratentorial lesions include the following:

- *Change in level of consciousness (LOC):* LOC is a sensitive and important indicator of the patient's neurologic status. The change in consciousness may be dramatic, as in coma, or subtle, such as a change in orientation or a decrease in level of attention.
- *Change in vital signs:* Although the complex of increasing systolic pressure (widening pulse pressure), bradycardia with a full and bounding pulse, and irregular respiratory pattern (Cushing's triad) may be present, these symptoms often do not appear until ICP has been increased for some time. A change in body temperature may also be noted.
- *Ocular signs:* Compression of the oculomotor nerve (CN III) results in dilatation of the ipsilateral pupil, sluggish or no response to light, inability to move the eye upward, and ptosis of the eyelid. A fixed, unilaterally dilated pupil is a neurologic emergency that indicates transtentorial brain herniation. Other cranial nerves may also be affected, with signs of blurred vision, diplopia, and changes in extraocular eye movements. Papilledema is also seen and is a nonspecific sign associated with long-standing increased ICP.
- *Decrease in motor function:* As ICP continues to rise, the patient manifests changes in motor ability. A contralateral hemiparesis or hemiplegia may be seen. If painful stimuli to elicit a motor response is used, the patient may exhibit a localization to the stimuli or a withdrawal from it. *Decorticate* (flexor) and *decerebrate* (extensor) posturing may also be elicited by noxious stimuli (see Fig. 54-7 in Lewis/Collier/Heitkemper, *Medical-Surgical Nursing,* edition 4, p. 1691).
- *Headache:* Although the brain itself is insensitive to pain, compression of other intracranial structures such as the walls of ar-

teries and veins and the cranial nerves can produce a headache. The headache is often continuous but worse in the morning; straining or movement may accentuate the pain.

- *Vomiting:* Vomiting that is usually not preceded by nausea is often a nonspecific sign of increased ICP.

Diagnostic Studies

- Vital signs, neurologic checks, ICP measurements (via intraventricular catheter, subdural bolt, or epidural transducer) every hour
- Skull, chest, and spinal x-ray studies
- CT, electroencephalogram, electrocardiogram, angiography
- Cerebral blood flow and velocity studies, MRI, positron emission tomography (PET)
- Laboratory studies, including complete blood cell count (CBC), coagulation profile, electrolytes, creatinine, arterial blood gases (ABGs), ammonia level, general drug and toxicology screen, CSF protein

Therapeutic Management

The goals of management are to identify and treat the underlying cause of increased ICP and to support brain function. A careful history is an important diagnostic aid that can direct the search for the underlying cause.

While the cause of increased ICP is being sought, the condition itself must be treated aggressively to interrupt the cycle. Ensuring adequate oxygenation to support brain function is the first step in management. An endotracheal tube or tracheostomy may be necessary to maintain adequate ventilation. It may be necessary to maintain the patient on ventilatory support to ensure adequate oxygenation.

- If the condition is caused by a mass lesion, such as a tumor or hematoma, surgical removal of the mass is the best management.
- Nonsurgical intervention for the reduction of tissue volume related to cerebral tissue swelling and edema includes the use of diuretics, corticosteroids, and fluid restriction.

Pharmacologic Management

Drug therapy plays an important part in the management of increased ICP. Osmotic and loop diuretics are used to reduce the volume of brain water, and corticosteroids are thought to control the cerebral edema. Osmotically active agents such as mannitol (Osmitrol), glycerol, and urea are used. Fluid and electrolyte status must be monitored when these drugs are used. Loop diuretics such as furosemide (Lasix) and ethacrynic acid (Edecrin) cause a decrease in CSF production, thus lowering ICP. Corticosteroids have been used extensively in the treatment of cerebral edema. Dexamethasone (Decadron) is the most commonly used steroid to reduce vasogenic cerebral edema. High-dose barbiturates (e.g., pentobarbital and thiopental) are used to produce a decrease in cerebral metabolism and a subsequent decrease in increased ICP.

Nursing Management

Goals

The patient with increased ICP and unconsciousness will have decreased ICP to within normal limits, maintain a patent airway, and demonstrate normal fluid and electrolyte balance. (See the nursing care plan for the unconscious patient in Lewis/Collier/Heitkemper, *Medical-Surgical Nursing,* edition 4, p. 1696.)

Nursing Diagnoses

- Altered cerebral tissue perfusion related to cerebral tissue swelling
- Ineffective breathing patterns related to loss of central nervous system integrative function and immobility
- Ineffective airway clearance related to unconsciousness, immobility, and inability to mobilize secretions
- Altered nutrition: less than body requirements related to hypermetabolism and inability to ingest food and fluids
- Impaired skin integrity related to nutritional deficit, self-care deficit, and immobility
- Self-care deficit (total) related to altered mental state
- Risk of infection related to immobility, invasive monitoring devices and lines, and compromised immune system
- Risk for injury related to seizure activity and environmental hazards
- Anxiety of family members related to lack of knowledge concerning nature and prognosis of coma

Nursing Interventions

Airway patency. With increased ICP, maintenance of a patent airway is critical and is a primary nursing responsibility. As LOC decreases, the patient is at increased risk of airway obstruction. Altered breathing patterns may become evident.

- Airway patency can be aided by keeping the patient lying on one side, with frequent position changes. Snoring sounds, which may indicate obstruction, should be noted. Accumulated secretions should be removed by suctioning. An oral airway facilitates breathing and provides an easier suctioning route in the comatose patient.

The nurse must use measures to prevent hypoxia and hypercapnia. Proper positioning of the head is important.

- Elevation of the head of the bed by 30 degrees enhances respiratory exchange and aids in decreasing cerebral edema.

- Suctioning and coughing can cause transient increases in ICP and decreases in the partial pressure of oxygen in arterial blood (PaO_2). Suctioning should be kept to a minimum.
- Abdominal distention can interfere with respiratory function and should be prevented. Insertion of a nasogastric tube to aspirate the stomach contents can prevent distention, vomiting, and possible aspiration.
- Arterial blood gases (ABGs) should be measured and evaluated regularly.
- Unless the patient is on ventilatory support, the use of narcotic sedatives and opiates should be evaluated on an individual basis. Besides depressing respiration, these agents can also cloud the patient's LOC. A narcotic that does not increase ICP, depress respiration, or cloud LOC should be selected to control pain.

Fluid and electrolyte balance. Fluid and electrolyte disturbances can have an adverse effect on ICP. IV fluids should be closely monitored. Intake and output, with insensible losses and daily weights taken into account, are important parameters in the assessment of fluid balance.

- Electrolyte determinations should be made daily. It is especially important to monitor glucose, sodium, potassium, and serum osmolality. Urinary output is monitored for problems related to diabetes insipidus and the syndrome of inappropriate antidiuretic hormone (see Diabetes Insipidus, p. 172, and Syndrome of Inappropriate Antidiuretic Hormone, p. 542).

Monitoring of ICP. Measurement of ICP is valuable in detecting the early rise of ICP and patient response to treatment.

Body position. The patient should be maintained in the head-up position. The nurse must take care to prevent extreme neck flexion, which can cause venous obstruction and increased ICP. The bed should be positioned so that it lowers the ICP while maintaining cerebral perfusion pressure (CPP).

- Care should be taken to turn the patient with slow, gentle movements because rapid changes in position may increase ICP. Caution should be used to prevent discomfort in turning and positioning of the patient because pain or agitation also increases pressure. Increased intrathoracic pressure contributes to increased ICP; thus coughing, straining, and the Valsalva maneuver should be avoided.

Protection from injury. The patient with increased ICP and a decreased LOC needs protection from self-injury. Confusion, agitation, and the possibility of seizures can put the patient at risk of injury. Restraints should be used judiciously in the agitated patient. A quiet, nonstimulating environment is beneficial. Touching and talking to the patient, even one who is in coma, is always an appropriate approach. The nurse needs to create a balance between sensory deprivation and sensory overload.

Psychologic considerations. Anxiety over the diagnosis and prognosis for the patient with neurologic problems can be distressing to the patient, family, and nursing staff. Short, simple explanations are appropriate and allow the patient and family to acquire the amount of information they desire. Support, information, and education of both patients and families are needed beginning with the traumatic event and continuing for years after the event.

- The nurse should assess the family members' desire and need to assist in providing care for the patient and allow for their participation as appropriate.

INFERTILITY

Definition/Description
Infertility is the failure to conceive after a year or more of unprotected, adequately timed sexual intercourse. Approximately 15% of couples in the United States are involuntarily infertile. Professional intervention can help about 40% of these couples achieve a pregnant state. In determining the cause of infertility and in treating this condition, both the man and woman need to be evaluated.

Etiology
- Causes of female infertility include anovulation, tubal or uterine disease, and abnormalities of the cervical mucus.
- Male infertility can be caused by disorders of the hypothalamic-pituitary system, disorders of the testes, and abnormalities of the ejaculatory system.
- Other possible causes include systemic illnesses, marital and sexual difficulties, and lack of knowledge about reproductive functioning.
- The fertility problem can be attributed to the couple rather than to one of the partners. Immune factors (antisperm agglutinating and immobilizing antibodies found in either partner), infrequent intercourse, and nonoptimal sexual techniques may be implicated.

Diagnostic Studies
After a detailed history is obtained and a general physical examination of the woman and man is performed to rule out any related medical or gynecologic disease, several basic tests can be performed. These include the following:

- *Women:* Ovulatory studies, tubal patency studies, and postcoital studies
- *Men:* Semen analysis, plasma testosterone, serum luteinizing hormone (LH) and follicle-stimulating hormone (FSH) levels, testicular biopsy

Therapeutic and Nursing Management

The management of infertility problems depends on the cause. If infertility is secondary to an alteration in ovarian function, supplemental hormone therapy to restore and maintain ovulation may be attempted. Drugs used to induce ovulation include clomiphene citrate (Clomid), human menopausal gonadotropin (Pergonal), and bromocriptine (Parlodel).

When an actual mechanical tubal blockage exists, a reparative microsurgical procedure can be done. Poor cervical mucus may be a result of chronic cervicitis or inadequate estrogen stimulation. Cauterization of the cervix may eradicate chronic cervicitis, and the administration of estrogens can improve the quantity and quality of cervical mucus.

- Improving the patient's general health may help, especially when a debilitating or chronic illness is present. Removing or reducing psychologic stress can improve the emotional climate, making it more conducive to achieving a pregnancy.
- Education of the couple regarding the probable time of ovulation and appropriate coital technique may also be indicated.

When a couple has not succeeded in conceiving during infertility management, another option is intrauterine insemination with the husband's or a donor's sperm. If this technique does not succeed, *in vitro fertilization (IVF)* may be used. IVF is the removal of mature oocytes from the woman's ovarian follicle by laparoscopy, followed by fertilization of the ova with the partner's sperm in a petri dish. When fertilization and cleavage have occurred, the resulting embryos are transferred into the woman's uterus. The procedure requires 2 to 3 days to complete and is used in cases of fallopian tube obstruction, oligospermia, and unexplained infertility.

Assisted reproductive technologies (ART) consist of IVF, *gamete intrafallopian transfer (GIFT), zygote intrafallopian transfer (ZIFT), cryopreserved embryo transfer (CPE),* and *donor oocyte programs (DOP).*

The nurse has a major responsibility for teaching and providing emotional support throughout the infertility testing and treatment period.

- Feelings of anger, frustration, sadness, and helplessness between partners and between the couple and health care providers may heighten as more and more tests are performed. The problem of infertility can generate great tension in a marriage as the couple exhaust their financial and emotional resources. Few insurance carriers cover the cost of infertility testing or the therapeutic measures associated with infertility.

- Shame and guilt may be precipitated when other persons become involved in this intimate area of a relationship. Recognizing and taking steps to deal with the psychologic and emotional factors that surface can assist the couple to cope with the situation better.

- Couples should be encouraged to participate in a support group for infertile couples in addition to undergoing individual therapy. Provisions for giving information and emotional support by the nurse continue as therapeutic measures are attempted.

INFLAMMATORY BOWEL DISEASE

Crohn's disease and *ulcerative colitis* are immunologically related disorders referred to as *inflammatory bowel disease (IBD)*. These disorders are characterized by chronic, recurrent inflammation of the intestinal tract. For both conditions clinical manifestations are varied, with long periods of remission interspersed with episodes of acute inflammation. Both diseases can be debilitating.

Although extensive research has been done on the etiology of IBD, the cause of both ulcerative colitis and Crohn's disease remains unknown. Possible causes include (1) an infectious agent (e.g., virus, bacteria) because IBD produces mucosal changes in the colon similar to those of infectious diarrhea, although no consistent pathogen has been identified; (2) an autoimmune reaction resulting from the presence of other immune-related disorders, such as systemic lupus erythematosus, ankylosing spondylitis, and erythema nodosum in patients with IBD; (3) food allergies (although this has not been substantiated); and (4) heredity (familial recurrences have been documented). Both Crohn's disease and ulcerative colitis run in related families.

See Ulcerative Colitis, p. 583, and Crohn's Disease, p. 157, for a more detailed discussion.

INTESTINAL OBSTRUCTION

Definition/Description

Intestinal obstruction occurs when the intestinal contents cannot pass through the GI tract. The obstruction may be partial or complete. The causes of intestinal obstruction can be classified as *mechanical* or *nonmechanical.*

Mechanical obstruction may be caused by an occlusion of the lumen of the intestinal tract. Most intestinal obstructions occur in the small intestine. Mechanical obstruction accounts for 90% of all intestinal obstructions. Adhesions normally develop after abdominal surgery. Obstruction can occur within days of surgery or years later. Carcinoma is the most common cause of large bowel obstruction, followed by volvulus and diverticular disease.

Nonmechanical obstruction may result from a neuromuscular or vascular disorder. Paralytic (adynamic) ileus is the most common form of nonmechanical obstruction. It occurs to some degree after any abdominal surgery. Other causes of paralytic ileus include inflammatory reactions (e.g., acute pancreatitis, acute appendicitis), electrolyte abnormalities, and thoracic or lumbar spinal fractures.

Pathophysiology

When fluid, gas, and intestinal contents accumulate proximal to the intestinal obstruction, distention occurs, and the distal bowel may collapse. As the fluid increases, so does the pressure in the lumen of the bowel. The increased pressure leads to an increase in capillary permeability and extravasation of fluids and electrolytes into the peritoneal cavity. Edema, congestion, and necrosis from impaired blood supply and possible rupture of the bowel may occur. Retention of fluid in the intestine and peritoneal cavity can lead to a severe reduction in circulating blood volume and result in hypotension and hypovolemic shock.

- Strangulation and gangrene are likely to develop if treatment is not immediate. A strangulated obstruction occurs when the circulation to the obstructed intestine is impaired. This is the most dangerous form of obstruction because it may lead to necrosis of the intestine (incarcerated). It is most commonly caused by volvulus, hernias, or adhesions.

Clinical Manifestations

Manifestations vary, depending on the location of intestinal obstruction, and include nausea, vomiting, abdominal pain, distention, inability to pass flatus, and obstipation.

- Obstruction located high in the small intestine produces rapid-onset, (sometimes projectile) vomiting with bile-containing vomitus. Vomiting from more distal obstructions of the small intestine is more gradual in onset. Vomitus may be orange-brown and foul smelling because of bacterial overgrowth. In some cases it may be feculent. Vomiting may be entirely absent in large bowel obstruction if the ileocecal valve is competent; otherwise, the patient may eventually vomit feculent material.

- Abdominal pain in high intestinal obstructions is usually relieved by vomiting. Persistent, colicky abdominal pain is seen with lower intestinal obstruction. A characteristic sign of mechanical obstruction is pain that comes and goes in waves. This is caused by intestinal peristalsis in the attempt to move bowel contents past the obstructed area. In contrast, paralytic ileus produces a more constant generalized discomfort. Strangulation causes severe, constant pain that is rapid in onset.

- Abdominal distention is a common manifestation of all intestinal obstructions. It is usually absent or minimally noticeable in high obstructions of the small intestine and greatly increased in lower intestinal obstructions. Abdominal tenderness and rigidity are usually absent unless strangulation or peritonitis has occurred.

- Auscultation of bowel sounds reveals high-pitched sounds above the area of obstruction. Audible borborygmi are often noted by the patient. The patient's temperature rarely rises above 100° F (37.8° C) unless strangulation or peritonitis has occurred.

Diagnostic Studies

- Abdominal x-rays are the most useful diagnostic aids. Upright and lateral abdominal x-rays show the presence of gas and fluid in the intestines. The presence of intraperitoneal air indicates perforation.

- Barium enemas are helpful in locating large intestinal obstructions.

- Sigmoidoscopy or colonoscopy may provide direct visualization of obstruction in the colon.

- Elevated white blood cell (WBC) count may indicate strangulation or perforation; elevated hematocrit values may reflect hemoconcentration; decreased hemoglobin and hematocrit values may indicate bleeding from a neoplasm or strangulation with necrosis.

- Serum sodium, potassium, and chloride concentrations are decreased in a small bowel obstruction. Blood urea nitrogen (BUN) values may be increased because of dehydration. Stools should be checked for occult blood.

Therapeutic Management

Treatment is directed toward decompression of the intestine by removal of gas and fluid, correction and maintenance of fluid and electrolyte balance, and relief or removal of the obstruction.

- Nasogastric (NG) or intestinal tubes may be used to decompress the bowel. NG tubes should be inserted before surgery to empty the stomach and relieve distention. They are also used instead of nasointestinal tubes to treat partial or complete small bowel obstruction.
- Sigmoidoscopy may successfully reduce a sigmoid volvulus. Colon-decompression catheters may be passed through partially obstructed areas via a colonoscope to decompress the bowel before surgery.

IV infusions that contain normal saline solution and potassium should be given to maintain fluid and electrolyte balance. Total parenteral hyperalimentation may be necessary in some cases to correct nutritional deficiencies, improve the patient's nutritional status before surgery, and promote postoperative healing.

Most mechanical obstructions are treated surgically. The procedure may involve simply resecting the obstructed segment of bowel and anastomosing the remaining healthy bowel. Partial or total colectomy, colostomy, or ileostomy may be required when extensive obstruction or necrosis is present. Occasionally obstructions can be removed nonsurgically. A colonoscope can be used to remove polyps, dilate strictures, and remove and necrose tumors with a laser.

Nursing Management

The patient should be monitored closely for signs of dehydration and electrolyte imbalance.

- A strict intake and output record should be maintained. All vomitus and tube drainage should be included. IV fluids should be administered as ordered.
- Serum electrolyte levels should be monitored closely. A patient with a high obstruction is more likely to have metabolic alkalosis. A patient with a low obstruction is at greater risk of metabolic acidosis.
- A patient is often restless and constantly changing position to relieve the pain. Analgesics may often be withheld until the obstruction is diagnosed because they may mask other signs and symptoms and decrease intestinal motility.
- The nurse should provide comfort measures, promote a restful environment, and keep distractions and visitors to a minimum.
- Nursing care of the patient after surgery for an intestinal obstruction is similar to care of the patient after a laparotomy (see Abdominal Pain, Acute, nursing management after laparotomy, p. 3).

Care of NG and Intestinal Tubes

Although the physician usually inserts intestinal tubes, the nurse assists with the procedure. Insertion is easier if the patient relaxes, takes deep breaths, and swallows when instructed.

- Once the tube is in place, mouth care is extremely important. Vomiting leaves a terrible taste in the patient's mouth, and fecal odor may be present. When an NG tube is in place, the patient breathes through the mouth, drying the mouth and lips. The nurse should encourage and assist the patient to brush the teeth frequently. Mouthwash and water for rinsing the mouth and petroleum jelly or water-soluble lubricant for moistening the lips should be provided at the bedside.
- The patient's nose should be checked for signs of irritation from the NG tube. This area should be cleaned and dried daily, with application of a water-soluble lubricant and retaping of the tube.
- NG and intestinal tubes should be checked every 4 hours for patency.

Intracranial Tumors

Definition/Description

Tumors of the brain may be primary, arising from tissues within the brain, or secondary, resulting from a metastasis of a malignant neoplasm located elsewhere in the body. Brain tumors are generally classified according to the tissue from which they arise: those arising inside the brain substance (e.g., gliomas, vascular tumors) or those arising outside the brain substance (e.g., meningiomas, cranial nerve tumors).

- Unless treated, all intracranial tumors eventually cause death from increasing tumor volume, which leads to increased intracranial pressure (ICP). (For a comparison of the major intracranial tumors, see Table 54-12 in Lewis/Collier/Heitkemper, *Medical-Surgical Nursing,* edition 4, p. 1707.)

Clinical Manifestations

Manifestations are generally caused by local destructive effects of the tumor, displacement of structures, obstruction of cerebrospinal fluid flow, and effects of edema and increased ICP on the cerebral function. The appearance of manifestations depends on location, size, and rate of tumor growth.

A wide range of clinical manifestations are associated with brain tumors. In some circumstances a slight decrease in mental acuity may be the only symptom. In other cases there may be a dramatic event such as a seizure, whereas in others increased ICP signs may be apparent.

- Manifestations may clearly indicate the location of the tumor by an alteration in the function controlled by the affected area (see Table 54-13 in Lewis/Collier/Heitkemper, *Medical-Surgical Nursing,* edition 4, p. 1709).

If the tumor mass obstructs the ventricles or occludes the outlet, ventricular enlargement *(hydrocephalus)* can occur. Surgical treatment, which is needed to relieve pressure, involves placement of a ventriculoatrial, ventriculopleural, or ventriculoperitoneal shunt. The physician should be notified if signs of increased ICP, such as headache, blurred vision, vomiting without nausea, decreasing level of consciousness, or restlessness, occur. Signs of an infected shunt, such as high fever, persistent headache, and stiff neck, warrant investigation.

Diagnostic Studies

- MRI allows for detection of very small tumors.
- Cerebral angiography determines blood flow and localization of tumor.
- CT and brain scanning assist in tumor location.
- Other useful diagnostic studies include skull x-ray, electroencephalogram (EEG), and positron emission tomography (PET).

Therapeutic Management

Treatment goals are aimed at identifying the tumor type and location, removing or decreasing tumor mass, and preventing or managing increased ICP.

Surgical intervention is the preferred treatment for brain tumors (see Cranial Surgery in Lewis/Collier/Heitkemper, *Medical-Surgical Nursing,* edition 4, p. 1710). Surgical outcome depends on type and location of tumor. Meningiomas and oligodendrogliomas can usually be completely removed, whereas more invasive gliomas and medulloblastomas can be only partially removed. Tumors located in deep central areas of the dominant hemisphere, posterior corpus callosum, or upper brain stem cause extensive neurologic damage and are considered inoperable. Surgery can reduce the tumor mass, which decreases ICP and provides relief of symptoms with an extension of survival time.

Radiation therapy lengthens survival in patients with malignant gliomas, especially when it is combined with partial surgical removal. Patients with less malignant tumors respond to radiation with longer survival time and decreased recurrence of tumor. Cerebral edema and rapidly increasing ICP may be complications of radiation therapy, but they can be managed with high doses of corticosteroids.

Normally the blood-brain barrier prohibits entry of most drugs into the brain parenchyma. The most malignant tumors cause a breakdown of the blood-brain barrier in the tumor area, allowing chemotherapeutic agents to be used to treat the malignancy. Carmustine (BCNU) and lomustine (CCNU) are particularly effective in treating brain tumors. Other drugs being used include methotrexate and procarbazine (Matulane). (See also Radiation Therapy, p. 675, and Chemotherapy, p. 631.)

Brain tumors that cannot be totally removed may be treated with a combination of steroids, surgery, radiation, and chemotherapy. Many techniques to control and treat brain tumors are under investigation, including radium implants into the tumor bed, local hyperthermia, and biologic response modifiers.

- Although progress in treatment has increased the length and quality of survival of patients with gliomas, death is almost always inevitable.

Nursing Management
Goals
The patient with a brain tumor will maintain normal ICP, maximize neurologic functioning, be free from pain and discomfort, and be aware of the long-term implications with respect to prognosis and cognitive and physical functioning.
Nursing Diagnoses/Collaborative Problems
- Altered cerebral tissue perfusion related to cerebral edema
- Pain (headache) related to cerebral edema and increased ICP
- Self-care deficit related to altered neuromuscular function secondary to tumor growth and cerebral edema
- Anxiety related to diagnosis and treatment
- Potential complication: seizures related to abnormal electrical activity of the brain
- Potential complication: increased intracranial pressure from presence of tumor and failure of normal compensatory mechanisms

Nursing Interventions
Behavioral changes such as loss of emotional control, confusion, memory loss, and depression are often not perceived by the patient but can be very disturbing and frightening to the family. Assisting and supporting the family in understanding what is happening through this phase are very important roles for the nurse.

- The confused patient with behavioral instability can be a challenge. Close supervision of activity, use of siderails, judicious use of restraints, padding of rails, and a calm, reassuring approach to care are all essential care techniques.

- Minimization of environmental stimuli, creation of a routine schedule, and the use of reality orientation can be incorporated into the care plan for the confused patient.

- Motor and sensory dysfunctions are problems that interfere with activities of daily living. Alterations in mobility must be managed, and the patient needs to be encouraged to provide as much self-care as physically possible. Self-image often depends on the patient's ability to participate in care within the limitations of the physical deficits.

- Motor (expressive) and/or sensory (receptive) dysphasias may occur. Disturbances in communication can be frustrating for the patient and may interfere with the nurse's ability to meet patient needs. Attempts should be made to establish a communication system that can be used by both patient and staff.

- Nutritional intake may be decreased because of the patient's feeding inability, loss of appetite, or loss of desire to eat. Assessing the nutritional status of the patient and ensuring adequate nutritional intake are important aspects of care. The patient may need encouragement to eat or, in some cases, may need to be fed orally, parenterally, by gastrostomy or nasogastric tube, or by total parenteral nutrition (see Tube Feeding, p. 685, and Total Parenteral Nutrition, p. 679).

The patient with a brain tumor who undergoes cranial surgery requires complex nursing care. (See Cranial Surgery in Lewis/Collier/Heitkemper, *Medical-Surgical Nursing,* edition 4, p. 1710.)

IRRITABLE BOWEL SYNDROME

Definition/Description

Irritable bowel syndrome (IBS) is a symptom complex characterized by intermittent and recurrent abdominal pain associated with an alteration in bowel function (diarrhea or constipation). Other symptoms commonly found include abdominal distention, excessive flatulence, the urge to defecate, and a sensation of incomplete evacuation.

IBS is a common problem affecting approximately 10% to 17% of the population in the United States. In Western societies approximately two times as many women as men seek health care services for IBS. Stress, psychologic factors, and specific food intolerances have been identified as major factors that precipitate IBS symptoms.

Diagnostic studies include a thorough health history and physical examination. Emphasis should be on presenting symptoms, past health history (including psychosocial aspects), family history, and drug and dietary history. Tests should be selectively used to rule out life-threatening disorders with symptoms similar to those of IBS, such as colon cancer, peptic ulcer disease, and malabsorption disorders.

- The patient needs reassurance that the symptoms are functional and should be encouraged to verbalize concerns and anxiety.
- A diet containing at least 20 g per day of dietary fiber should be initiated. The diet may also include the addition of psyllium-containing products (e.g., Metamucil). The patient whose primary symptoms are abdominal distention and increased flatulence should be advised to eliminate common gas-producing foods such as broccoli and cabbage from the diet and to substitute yogurt for milk products if lactose intolerance is present.
- If taken before meals, anticholinergic agents such as dicyclomine (Bentyl) may be helpful in alleviating the pain associated with ingestion of food.
- Additional therapies include relaxation and stress management techniques, although no single therapy has been found to be effective for all patients with IBS. For the patient with a high level of anxiety, a mild sedative or tranquilizer may be ordered but should be prescribed for only a short time.

I

KAPOSI'S SARCOMA

Kaposi's sarcoma is characterized by multiple vascular neoplasms that appear on the skin, mucous membranes, and viscera. These neoplasms occur frequently in HIV-infected individuals.

Clinical manifestations initially include small reddish-purple nodules on the skin ranging in size from a few millimeters to several centimeters. These lesions can cause lymphedema and disfigurement, particularly when confluent. Systemic manifestations are associated with the organ involved (e.g., lung involvement results in shortness of breath). The diagnosis is based on biopsy results of the suspicious lesion(s).

Treatment depends on the severity of the lesions and the patient's immune status. Initially an attempt is made to avoid treatments that further suppress the immune system in HIV-infected individuals. Localized radiation, intralesional vinblastine, combination chemotherapy, α-interferon, and cryotherapy may be used to suppress the growth of the neoplasm.

See nursing management of the patient with cancer, p. 91, and/or human immunodeficiency virus (HIV) infection, p. 308.

LACTASE DEFICIENCY

Definition/Description
Lactase deficiency is a condition in which lactase, the enzyme that breaks down lactose into two simple sugars (glucose and galactose), is deficient or absent.

Although primary lactase deficiency seems to be hereditary, milk intolerance may not become clinically evident until late adolescence or early adulthood. About 5% of the adult population has primary lactase deficiency, with the highest incidence found in African-Americans, Native Americans, Mexican-Americans, and Jewish Americans.

Acquired lactase deficiency is often seen in GI diseases in which the mucosa has been damaged, including ulcerative colitis, Crohn's disease, gastroenteritis, and sprue syndrome.

Clinical Manifestations
Symptoms of lactose intolerance include bloating, flatulence, crampy abdominal pain, and diarrhea. They may occur within one-half hour to several hours after drinking a glass of milk or ingesting a milk product.

Diagnostic Studies
A lactose intolerance test can be performed to rule out milk allergies. The patient is given 50 to 100 mg of lactose orally. Blood samples are drawn before the consumption of lactose and at 15-, 30-, 60-, and 90-minute intervals. Failure of the blood glucose level to increase more than 20 mg/dl is suggestive of lactase deficiency. Results of a hydrogen breath test after ingestion of lactose are abnormal.

Therapeutic and Nursing Management
- Treatment consists of eliminating lactose from the diet by avoiding milk and milk products. A lactose-free diet is given initially and is gradually advanced to a low-lactose diet as tolerated by the patient. The objective of care is to teach the importance of adherence to the diet. Many lactose-intolerant persons may not exhibit symptoms if lactose is taken in small amounts. In some persons lactose may be tolerated better if taken with meals.
- The patient needs to be aware that milk, ice cream, cottage cheese, and cheese have a high lactose content. If the milk has been fermented (e.g., cultured buttermilk, yogurt, sour cream), the patient with low lactase levels may tolerate it better.
- Lactase enzyme (Lactaid) is available commercially as an over-the-counter product. It is mixed with milk and breaks down the lactose before the milk is ingested.

L

LEIOMYOMAS (FIBROIDS)

Leiomyomas (fibroids, myomas, fibromyomas, fibromas) are the most common benign tumors of the female genital tract. By 30 years of age, 10% of Caucasian women and 30% of African-American women will have uterine leiomyomas.

- The cause of leiomyomas is unknown, but they are thought to depend on ovarian hormones, growing slowly during the reproductive years and undergoing atrophy with the advent of menopause. These tumors are composed mainly of smooth muscle and fibrous connective tissue.

From 20% to 50% of women with leiomyomas develop symptoms, the most common being menorrhagia. Although rarely experienced with leiomyomas, pain is associated with infection or twisting of the pedicle from which the tumor is growing. Dysmenorrhea and dyspareunia may occasionally occur. Pressure on surrounding organs may result in rectal, bladder, and lower abdominal discomfort. Large tumors may cause a general enlargement of the lower abdomen. These tumors are sometimes associated with abortion and infertility.

Diagnosis is usually based on the characteristic pelvic findings of an enlarged uterus distorted by nodular masses. The presence of a malignant tumor is ruled out before treatment is begun.

Treatment depends on the patient's symptoms, age, and desire to bear children and the location and size of the tumor(s). If the symptoms are minor, the health care provider may elect to follow up the patient closely for a time. In the young woman who wishes to have children, a myomectomy is performed. In cases of large leiomyomas the treatment is hysterectomy. Gonadotropin-releasing hormone agonist (Lupron) may be used preoperatively to shrink the size of the leiomyomas.

LEUKEMIA

Definition/Description

Leukemia is a general term used to describe a group of malignant disorders affecting the blood and blood-forming tissues of the bone marrow, lymph system, and spleen. It results in an accumulation of dysfunctional cells because of a loss of regulation in cell division. Leukemia follows a progressive course that is eventually fatal if untreated. Although often thought of as a disease of children, the number of adults affected with leukemia is 10 times that of children.

Table 39 summarizes the relative incidences of the different subtypes and their characteristic features.

Regardless of the specific type of leukemia, there is generally no
single causative agent in the development of leukemia. Most
leukemias result from a combination of factors, including genetic
and environmental influences.

Classification

Acute leukemia is characterized by clonal proliferation of immature
undifferentiated hematopoietic cells (blasts). The most prominent
characteristic of the neoplastic cell in acute leukemia is a defect in
maturation beyond the myeloblast or promyelocyte level in *acute
myelogenous leukemia (AML)* and the lymphoblast level in *acute
lymphocytic leukemia (ALL)*. Acute leukemia has an abrupt and dramatic onset and requires immediate and aggressive intervention.

Chronic lymphocytic leukemia (CLL) is a neoplasm of activated
lymphocytes. CLL cells, which morphologically resemble mature
small lymphocytes of the peripheral blood, accumulate in the bone
marrow, blood, lymph nodes, and spleen in large numbers. Many individuals in the early stages of CLL require no treatment. As the disease progresses, various treatments can be used to control symptoms.

Chronic myelogenous leukemia (CML) is a clonal stem cell disorder characterized by greatly increased myelopoiesis and the presence of the Philadelphia chromosome in 90% of patients. The
chronic phase of CML can persist for 2 to 4 years and can usually be
well controlled with treatment.

Hairy cell leukemia is a chronic disease of lymphoproliferation
predominantly involving B lymphocytes that infiltrate the bone marrow and spleen. Complete remissions are rare, but retreatment of
recurrent disease is often successful.

Clinical Manifestations

Manifestations of leukemia are varied (see Table 39). Essentially
they relate to problems caused by bone marrow failure and the formation of masses composed of leukemic infiltrates. Bone marrow
failure results from inadequate production of normal marrow elements and bone marrow crowding by abnormal cells, leading to
marrow suppression. The patient is predisposed to anemia, thrombocytopenia, and decreased numbers and function of white blood
cells (WBCs).

- Increased numbers of WBCs can lead to infiltration and damage to the bone marrow, lymph nodes, spleen, and other organs, including the central nervous system (CNS). Leukemic
  infiltration leads to problems such as splenomegaly, hepatomegaly, lymphadenopathy, bone pain, meningeal irritation,
  and oral lesions.

Table 39 Types of Leukemia

Type/incidence*	Age of onset	Clinical manifestations	Diagnostic findings
Acute myelogenous leukemia—23%	Increase in incidence with advancing age	Fatigue and weakness, headache, mouth sores, anemia, bleeding, fever, infection, sternal tenderness	Low RBCs, Hb, Hct; low platelet count; low to high WBCs with myeloblasts; greatly hypercellular bone marrow with myeloblasts
Acute lymphocytic leukemia—14%	Before 14 yr of age, peak incidence between 2-9 yr of age	Fever; pallor; bleeding; anorexia; fatigue and weakness; bone, joint, and abdominal pain; generalized lymphadenopathy; infections; weight loss; hepatosplenomegaly; headache; mouth sores; neurologic manifestations, including increased intracranial pressure secondary to meningeal infiltration	Low RBC count, Hb, Hct; low platelet count; low, normal, or high WBCs; hypercellular bone marrow with lymphoblasts; lymphoblasts also possible in cerebrospinal fluid

Chronic myelogenous leukemia—17%	25-60 yr of age, peak incidence around 45 yr of age	No symptoms early in disease, fatigue and weakness, fever, sternal tenderness, weight loss, joint pain, bone pain, massive splenomegaly	Low RBCs, Hb, Hct; high platelet count early, lower count later; increase in polymorphonuclear neutrophils, normal number of lymphocytes, low leukocyte alkaline phosphatase; presence of Philadelphia chromosome in 90% of patients
Chronic lymphocytic leukemia—29%	50-70 yr of age, predominance in men	No symptoms usually; detection of disease often during examination for unrelated condition; chronic fatigue, anorexia, splenomegaly and lymphadenopathy, hepatomegaly	Mild anemia and thrombocytopenia with disease progression; increase in peripheral lymphocytes; increase in presence of lymphocytes in bone marrow

CNS, Central nervous system; *Hb,* hemoglobin; *Hct,* hematocrit; *RBC,* red blood cell; *WBC,* white blood cell.
*This is the incidence of all leukemias; the number does not add up to 100% because approximately 17% are unclassifiable.

L

Diagnostic Studies

The goal is to define the subclass or specific type of leukemia so that the appropriate treatment and prognosis can be determined (see Table 39).

- Peripheral blood evaluation and bone marrow examination are the primary methods of diagnosing and classifying the acute and chronic subtypes of leukemia. (See Tables 28-25 and 28-26 for these classifications in Lewis/Collier/Heitkemper, *Medical-Surgical Nursing,* edition 4, p. 812.)
- Morphologic, histochemical, immunologic, and cytogenetic methods are all used to identify cell subtypes and the stage of development of leukemic cell populations.
- Further studies such as lumbar puncture and CT scan can determine the presence of leukemic cells outside of the blood and bone marrow.

Therapeutic Management

Management includes remission induction with chemotherapeutic drugs and, sometimes, radiation therapy (see Chemotherapy, p. 631, and Radiation Therapy, p. 675). Other considerations include regular examination of patients on an ongoing basis to evaluate their progress and supportive interventions to prevent complications of the disease and the therapy (e.g., hemorrhage, infection).

- The nurse needs to understand the principles of cancer chemotherapy, including cellular kinetics, the use of multiple drugs rather than single agents, and the cell cycle (see Chemotherapy, p. 631).
- Corticosteroids and radiation therapy can also have a role in therapeutic plans for the patient with leukemia. Total body radiation may be used to prepare a patient for bone marrow transplantation, or it may be restricted to certain areas (fields) such as the liver and spleen or other organs affected by infiltrates.
- In acute lymphocytic leukemia, prophylactic intrathecal methotrexate is given to decrease the chance of CNS involvement, which is common in this particular type of leukemia. When CNS leukemia does occur, cranial radiation is given. The use of biologic response modifiers in the treatment of leukemia is being investigated (see Lewis/Collier/Heitkemper, *Medical-Surgical Nursing,* edition 4, p. 303).

Chemotherapeutic agents used to treat leukemia vary. The choice of drugs and the sequence of therapy depend on the preference of the oncologist and on current research findings.

Bone marrow transplantation (BMT) is another form of therapy used for patients with different forms of leukemia, including ALL,

AML, CML. This treatment modality is also used for other hematologic malignancies such as Hodgkin's disease, non-Hodgkin's lymphoma, solid tumors (e.g., breast cancer), and some nonmalignant disorders, including aplastic anemia and congenital immunodeficiencies. The goal of BMT is to totally eliminate leukemic cells from the body with combinations of chemotherapy and total body irradiation. This treatment also eradicates the patient's bone marrow stem cells, which are then replaced with those of a human leukocyte antigen (HLA)–matched sibling or volunteer donor (allogeneic) or an identical twin (syngeneic) or with the patient's own marrow (autologous) removed (harvested) before the intensive therapy.

Bone marrow stem cells are aspirated from the pelvis of the donor, usually from the iliac crest, but they can also be obtained from the sternum or ribs. A newer method of obtaining bone marrow stem cells is through an apheresis procedure that separates them from circulating blood. Regardless of the harvesting method, the specially prepared marrow is infused intravenously into the recipient following intensive chemotherapy and radiation therapy. Usually 2 to 4 weeks are required for the transplanted marrow to start producing hematopoeitic blood cells, with a lesser period of time when peripheral blood stem cells have been used.

During this pancytopenic period it is critical for the patient to be in a protective isolation environment receiving supportive care. Red blood cell (RBC) and platelet transfusions may be necessary to maintain circulating blood cells during this time. Primary complications of patients with allogeneic BMT are graft-versus-host disease (GVHD), relapse of leukemia (especially ALL), and infection (especially interstitial pneumonia). GVHD is mediated by competent T cells infused with the donor marrow that mount an attack against the recipient's immune system (see Graft-versus-Host Disease, p. 262). The intent of BMT is cure. Because it is a highly toxic therapy, the patient must weigh the significant risks of treatment-related death or treatment failure (relapse) with the hope of cure.

Nursing Management
Goals
The patient with leukemia will understand and cooperate with the treatment plan, experience minimal side effects and complications associated with both the disease and its treatment, and feel hopeful and supported during the periods of remission and relapse.
Nursing Diagnoses
Nursing diagnoses related to leukemia include those appropriate for anemia and thrombocytopenia (see Anemia, p. 22, and Throm-

bocytopenic Purpura, p. 562), and neutropenia (see Lewis/Collier/Heitkemper, *Medical-Surgical Nursing,* edition 4, p. 809).

Nursing Interventions

The nursing role during the acute phases of leukemia is extremely challenging because the patient has many physical and psychosocial needs. As with other forms of cancer, the diagnosis of leukemia can evoke great fear and be equated with death. The nurse has a special responsibility in helping patients and families deal with these feelings.

- The nurse must help the patient realize that although the future may be uncertain, one can have a meaningful quality of life while the disease is in remission or under control.
- Families also need help in adjusting to the stress of this abrupt onset of serious illness (e.g., dependence, withdrawal, changes in role responsibilities, alterations in body image) and the losses imposed by the sick role. The diagnosis of leukemia often brings with it the need to make difficult decisions at a time of profound stress for the patient and family.

The nurse is an important advocate in helping the patient and family understand the complexities of treatment decisions as well as the expected side effects and toxicities. A patient may require isolation or may need to temporarily relocate to an appropriate treatment center. These situations can lead patients to feel deserted and isolated at the time when they need the most support. The nurse has contact with patients 24 hours a day and can help reverse feelings of abandonment and loneliness by balancing the demanding technical needs with a humanistic, caring approach.

- From a physical care perspective, the nurse is challenged to make astute assessments and plan care to help the patient survive the severe side effects of chemotherapy. The life-threatening results of bone marrow suppression (anemia, thrombocytopenia, neutropenia) require aggressive nursing interventions.
- The nurse must be knowledgeable about all drugs being administered. In addition, the nurse must know how to assess laboratory data reflecting the effects of the drugs. Patient survival and comfort during aggressive chemotherapy are significantly affected by the quality of nursing care.
- Long-term management following treatment for leukemia affects the quality of the patient's life.

Patient Teaching

The patient and significant other must be educated to understand the importance of their continued diligence in disease management and the need for follow-up care. At a minimum the patient must be taught about the drugs and when to seek medical attention.

- Assistance may be needed to reestablish the various relationships that are a part of the patient's life. Friends and family may not know how to interact with the patient.
- Involving the patient in survivor networks, support groups, or services such as CanSurmount and Make Today Count may help the patient adapt to living after a life-threatening illness. Exploring resources in the community (e.g., American Cancer Society, Leukemia Society, Meals-on-Wheels, wheelchair taxis) may reduce the financial burden and feelings of dependence.
- Spiritual support may give the patient inner strength and peace.
- Vigilant follow-up care by providers who are aware of the unique needs of a cancer survivor is of the utmost importance for early recognition and treatment of long-term or delayed physical, psychologic, and social effects. Often these needs require the initiation of a referral or consultation. They can also include issues such as growth and development concerns for childhood survivors, vocational retraining, and reproductive concerns for patients of childbearing age.

LIVER CANCER

Definition/Description

Primary hepatocellular carcinoma is the most common malignant tumor of the liver, although it is quite rare. Some cases of hepatocellular carcinoma are associated with chronic hepatitis B or C. A high percentage of patients with primary liver cancer have cirrhosis of the liver, with men having a higher incidence than women.

Metastatic carcinoma of the liver is more common than primary carcinoma. The liver is a common site of metastatic growth because of its high rate of blood flow and extensive capillary network. Cancer cells in other parts of the body are commonly carried to the liver via the portal circulation.

- The prognosis for liver cancer is very poor. The cancer grows rapidly, and death may occur within 4 to 7 months as a result of hepatic encephalopathy or massive blood loss from GI bleeding. Primary liver tumors commonly metastasize to the lung.

L

Clinical Manifestations

It is difficult to diagnose carcinoma of the liver. It is particularly difficult to differentiate it from cirrhosis in its early stages because many of the clinical manifestations (e.g., hepatomegaly, weight loss, peripheral edema, ascites, portal hypertension) are similar.

- Other common manifestations include dull abdominal pain in the epigastric or right upper quadrant region, jaundice, anorexia, nausea and vomiting, and extreme weakness. Patients frequently have pulmonary emboli.

Diagnostic Studies

Tests used to assist in the diagnosis are liver scan, hepatic arteriography, endoscopic retrograde cholangiopancreatography (ERCP), and liver biopsy. The test for α-fetoprotein (AFP) may be positive in hepatocellular carcinoma. AFP helps to distinguish primary cancer from metastatic cancer.

Therapeutic and Nursing Management

Treatment of liver cancer is largely palliative. Surgical excision (lobectomy) is sometimes performed if the tumor is localized to one portion of the liver. Only 30% to 40% of patients have surgically resectable disease. Usually surgery is not feasible because the cancer is too far advanced when it is detected. Surgical excision offers the only chance for cure of liver cancer. Management is very similar to that for cirrhosis (see Cirrhosis, p. 130). Chemotherapy may be used, but there is usually a poor response. Portal vein or hepatic artery perfusion with 5-fluorouracil may be attempted.

Nursing intervention focuses on keeping the patient as comfortable as possible. Because this patient manifests the same problems as any patient with advanced liver disease, the nursing interventions discussed for cirrhosis of the liver apply (see Cirrhosis, p. 130, and Cancer, p. 88).

LOW BACK PAIN, ACUTE

Definition/Description

Low back pain is common and has probably affected every adult at least once during a lifetime. Risk factors associated with low back pain include smoking, low educational level, tension, and anxiety. Jobs that require repetitive heavy lifting, vibration (e.g., jackhammer operator), and extended periods of driving are also associated with low back pain.

Pathophysiology

Pain in the lumbar region is a common problem because this area (1) bears most of the weight of the body; (2) is the most flexible region of the spinal column; (3) contains nerve roots, which are vulnerable to injury or disease; and (4) has an inherently poor biomechanical structure.

Low back pain is most often due to a musculoskeletal problem. Other causes such as metabolic, circulatory, gynecologic, urologic, or psychologic problems, which may refer pain to the lower back, must not be overlooked.

- The causes of low back pain of musculoskeletal origin include (1) acute lumbosacral strain, (2) instability of lumbosacral bony mechanism, (3) osteoarthritis of the lumbosacral vertebrae, (4) intervertebral disk degeneration, and (5) herniation of the intervertebral disk.

Clinical Manifestations

Acute low back pain is usually associated with some type of activity that causes undue stress on the tissues of the lower back. Often symptoms do not appear at the time of injury but develop later because of a gradual buildup of paravertebral muscle spasms. Few definitive diagnostic abnormalities are present with paravertebral muscle strain. The straight-leg raise test may produce pain in the lumbar area without radiation along the sciatic nerve.

Therapeutic Management

If the muscle spasms are not severe, the patient may be treated on an outpatient basis with a combination of the following: analgesics, nonsteroidal antiinflammatory drugs (NSAIDs), muscle relaxants, and use of a corset. A corset prevents rotation, flexion, and extension of the lower back.

- If the spasms and pain are severe, a period of hospitalization may be necessary. Since paravertebral muscle spasms are worse when the patient is upright, bed rest is maintained for 5 to 10 days or until the patient can move and turn from side to side with minimal discomfort. At this time, gradually increasing activity is initiated. The patient is discharged to continue bed rest and activity restrictions at home when comfortable on oral pain medication.

If conservative treatment is ineffective and the cause of the pain is nerve root irritation, an epidural steroid injection may be performed. Epidural steroids have been shown to decrease pain, speed return of function, and improve objective neurologic signs. Epidural injections typically consist of a series of one to three injections over a span of several days to several weeks.

L

Nursing Management
Goals

The patient with low back pain will have satisfactory pain relief, avoid constipation secondary to medication and immobility, learn back-sparing practices, and return to previous level of activity within prescribed restrictions. See the nursing care plan for the patient with low back pain in Lewis/Collier/Heitkemper, *Medical-Surgical Nursing,* edition 4, p. 1884.

Nursing Diagnoses

- Acute pain related to specific physical problem, muscle spasms, and ineffective comfort measures
- Impaired physical mobility related to pain
- Constipation related to immobility, inadequate fluids and fiber, and pain medications
- Ineffective individual coping related to effects of pain on lifestyle
- Ineffective management of therapeutic regimen related to lack of knowledge regarding posture, body mechanics, and weight reduction
- Body image disturbance related to impaired mobility and chronic pain

Nursing Interventions

Primary nursing responsibilities are to assist the patient to maintain bed rest, promote comfort, and educate the patient about the disease process. Whether the patient is at home or hospitalized, measures to ensure bed rest should be enforced.

- Although actual muscle-strengthening exercises are often taught by the physical therapist, it is the nurse's responsibility to ensure that the patient understands the type and frequency of exercise prescribed, and the rationale for the program.
- The frustration, pain, and disability imposed on the patient with low back pain problems require emotional support and understanding care by the nurse.

One goal of management is to make an episode of acute low back pain an isolated incident. If the lumbosacral mechanism is unstable, repeated episodes can be anticipated. Intervention is aimed at strengthening the supporting muscles by exercise and the use of a corset to limit extremes of movement. In addition, weight reduction decreases the mechanical demands on the lower back.

Patient Teaching

The nurse is a significant role model and teacher for patients with low back problems. The nurse should use proper body mechanics at all times. This should be a primary consideration when teaching patients and care providers transfer and turning techniques. The nurse should assess the patient's use of body mechanics and offer advice when activities that could produce back strain are used (see Table 59-17 in Lewis/Collier/Heitkemper, *Medical-Surgical Nursing,* edition 4, p. 1883).

- Patients are advised to maintain appropriate weight. Excess body weight places extra stress on the lower back and weakens the abdominal muscles that support the lower back.
- Position assumed while sleeping is also important in preventing low back pain. Sleeping in a prone position should be avoided because it produces excessive lumbar lordosis, placing excessive stress on the lower back. A firm mattress is recommended. The patient should sleep in either a supine or side-lying position with the knees and hips flexed to prevent unnecessary pressure on support muscles, ligamentous structures, and lumbosacral joints.

LOW BACK PAIN, CHRONIC

Definition/Description
Chronic low back pain is caused by degenerative disk disease, lack of physical exercise, obesity, structural and postural abnormalities, and systemic disease. Structural degeneration of the intervertebral disk results in degenerative disease manifested by low back pain. Degeneration can also occur in the cervical spine area. The degeneration results in intervertebral narrowing and a lessening of the efficiency of the intervertebral disks in acting as shock absorbers. As stresses on the degenerated disk continue and eventually exceed the strength of the disk, herniation of the intervertebral disk may result, causing compression or tension on a lumbar or sacral spinal nerve root.

Clinical Manifestations
The most characteristic feature of a lumbar herniated intervertebral disk is back pain with associated buttock and leg pain along the distribution of the sciatic nerve. (Manifestations based on level of lumbar disk herniation are summarized in Table 59-19 in Lewis/Collier/Heitkemper, *Medical-Surgical Nursing,* edition 4, p. 1887.)

- Back and/or leg pain may be reproduced by raising the leg and flexing the foot at 90 degrees. Low back pain from other causes may not be accompanied by leg pain.
- Reflexes may be depressed or absent, depending on the spinal nerve root involved, and numbness or tingling in the toes and feet may be felt by the patient.
- If the disk ruptures in the cervical area, stiff neck, shoulder pain radiating to the hand, and paresthesias and sensory disturbances of the hand are evident.

L

Diagnostic Studies

- X-rays to note any structural defects
- Myelogram, MRI, and CT scan to help localize the site of herniation; diskogram, if other methods of diagnosis are unsuccessful
- Electromyogram (EMG) of the lower extremities to determine the severity of nerve irritation caused by herniation

Therapeutic Management

Degenerative disk disease is managed conservatively with pelvic traction, rest, limitation of extremes of spinal movement (corset), local heat, ultrasound, transcutaneous electrical nerve stimulation, and NSAIDs. If herniation of the disk occurs, more aggressive treatment is indicated.

Conservative treatment sometimes results in a healing over of the herniated area with a decrease in pain of nerve-root irritation. Complete bed rest is often encouraged during this phase. Traction may be used to decrease muscle spasms. Once symptoms subside, back-strengthening exercises are begun. Extremes of flexion and torsion are strongly discouraged.

- Most patients with herniated disks recover with a conservative treatment plan. However, if conservative treatment is unsuccessful, surgery may be indicated.

Surgical Treatment

- A *percutaneous diskectomy* is a surgical procedure in which a tube is passed through the retroperitoneal soft tissues to the lateral border of the disk with the aid of fluoroscopy. The herniated portion of the disk is shaved and removed in small portions. Although there is no incision, small stab wounds are made.
- A *diskectomy* may be performed to decompress the nerve root. It involves partial removal of the lamina. *Microsurgical diskectomy* is a version of the standard diskectomy in which a surgeon uses a microscope to allow better visualization of the disk and disk space during surgery.
- A *laminectomy* is the traditional and most common procedure performed. It involves surgical excision of part of the posterior arch of the vertebra (referred to as the lamina) to gain access to part or all of the protruding disk to remove it. A laminectomy may be performed in combination with a diskectomy.
- A *spinal fusion* may be performed if an unstable bony mechanism is present. The spine is stabilized by creating an ankylosis (fusion) of contiguous vertebrae with a bone graft from the patient's fibula or iliac crest or from donated bone. If vertebral instability exists, metal fixation with rods, plates, or screws may be done at the time of spinal surgery to provide more stability and decrease vertebral motion.

Nursing Management

For nursing management of chronic low back pain, see Low Back Pain, Acute, nursing management, p. 367).

LUNG CANCER

Definition/Description

Primary lung cancer is the leading cause of death in men and women who have malignant disease in the United States. The overall 5-year survival rate is 13%, which is the poorest prognosis for any cancer other than cancers of the pancreas, liver, and esophagus. The disease is found most frequently in persons 40 to 75 years of age.

Risk factors for lung cancer include cigarette smoking, inhaled carcinogens, and preexisting pulmonary diseases.

- Cigarette smoking as a chronic respiratory irritant is by far the greatest risk factor. Smoking is responsible for approximately 80% to 90% of all lung cancers. Cigarette smoking causes a change in bronchial epithelium, which usually returns to normal when smoking is discontinued.
- Inhaled carcinogens include asbestos, nickel, iron and iron oxides, uranium, polycyclic aromatic hydrocarbons, arsenic, and air pollution. The incidence of lung cancer correlates with the degree of urbanization and population density. One reason for this may be increased exposure to irritants and pollutants.
- Preexisting pulmonary diseases such as tuberculosis, pulmonary fibrosis, bronchiectasis, and chronic obstructive pulmonary disease (COPD) are also possible risk factors. Chronic inflammatory conditions often precede cancer.

Pathophysiology

Pathogenesis of primary lung cancer is not well understood. More than 90% of cancers originate from the epithelium of the bronchus (bronchogenic). They grow slowly, and it takes 8 to 10 years for a tumor to reach 1 cm in size, which is the smallest detectable lesion on x-ray. Lung cancers occur primarily in the segmental bronchi or beyond and have a preference for the upper lobes of the lungs.

Pathologic changes in the bronchial system show nonspecific inflammatory changes with hypersecretion of mucus, desquamation of cells, reactive hyperplasia of basal cells, and metaplasia of normal respiratory epithelium to stratified squamous cells. Lung cancers metastasize primarily by direct extension and via the blood circulation and lymph system. Common sites for metastatic growth are the liver, brain, bones, lymph nodes, and adrenal glands.

L

Clinical Manifestations

Manifestations are usually nonspecific, dependent on the type of primary lung cancer, and usually appear late in the disease process. Often extensive metastasis occurs with the appearance of symptoms.

- Persistent pneumonitis as a result of obstructed bronchi may be one of the earliest manifestations, causing fever, chills, and cough.
- One of the most significant symptoms, and often the one reported first, is a persistent cough that may be productive of sputum. Blood-tinged sputum may be produced because of bleeding, but hemoptysis is not a common early symptom.
- Chest pain may be localized or unilateral and may range from mild to severe. Dyspnea and an auscultatory wheeze may be present if there is bronchial obstruction.

Later manifestations may include nonspecific systemic symptoms such as anorexia, fatigue, weight loss, and nausea and vomiting. Hoarseness may be present as a result of involvement of the recurrent laryngeal nerve. Unilateral paralysis of the diaphragm, dysphagia, and superior vena cava obstruction may occur because of intrathoracic spread of malignancy. Palpable lymph nodes may be present in the neck or axilla. Mediastinal involvement may lead to pericardial effusion, cardiac tamponade, and dysrhythmias.

Paraneoplastic syndrome is caused by certain lung cancers. It is characterized by various manifestations resulting from certain substances (e.g., hormones, enzymes) produced by tumor cells. Small cell carcinomas are most commonly associated with paraneoplastic syndrome. Systemic manifestations may include hormonal syndromes (Cushing's syndrome of inappropriate secretion of antidiuretic hormone [SIADH]), neuromuscular signs (peripheral neuropathy), vascular and hematologic signs (anemia, thrombophlebitis), and connective tissue disease (arthralgias, digital clubbing).

Diagnostic Studies

- Chest x-ray for diagnosis, evidence of metastasis, and presence of pleural effusion
- Lung tomograms to locate tumor
- CT and MRI scans for detection of lymph node enlargement and mediastinal involvement
- Positron emission tomography (PET) scan for early detection and staging
- Additional diagnostic studies: sputum specimens, biopsy, fiberoptic bronchoscope, radionuclide scans to determine metastasis

Therapeutic Management

Surgical resection is usually the only hope for cure in lung cancer. Unfortunately, detection is often so late that the tumor is no longer localized and is not amenable to resection. Oat cell (small cell) carcinomas usually have widespread metastasis at the time of diagnosis. Therefore surgery is usually contraindicated. Squamous cell carcinomas are more likely to be treated with surgery because they remain localized; or, if they metastasize, they primarily do so by local spread. The type of surgery is lobectomy (one or more lung lobes removed) or pneumonectomy (the entire lung removed).

Radiation therapy is used as a curative approach in the individual who has a resectable tumor but is considered a poor surgical risk. Adenocarcinomas are the most radioresistant type of lung cancer cell.

- Radiation is also done as a palliative procedure to reduce distressing symptoms such as cough, hemoptysis, bronchial obstruction, and superior vena cava syndrome (see Radiation Therapy, p. 675).

Chemotherapy may be used for nonresectable tumors or as adjuvant therapy to surgery in non–small cell lung cancer with distant metastases. Multidrug regimens have increased the survival rate in oat cell carcinoma. Chemotherapy has not shown any significant results when used for treatment of squamous cell carcinoma and adenocarcinoma (see Chemotherapy, p. 631).

Nursing Management
Goals
The patient with lung cancer will have effective breathing patterns, adequate airway clearance, adequate oxygenation of tissues, and minimal to no pain.
Nursing Diagnoses
- Ineffective airway clearance secondary to increased tracheobronchial secretions
- Anxiety related to lack of knowledge of diagnosis or unknown prognosis and treatments
- Pain from pressure of tumor on surrounding structures and erosion of tissues
- Altered nutrition: less than body requirements related to increased metabolic demands, weakness, and anorexia
- Altered health maintenance related to lack of knowledge about disease process and therapeutic regimen
- Ineffective breathing pattern related to decreased lung capacity
Nursing Interventions
When obtaining a health history, it is important to obtain information related to respiratory carcinogens. The patient should be asked about occupational exposure to carcinogens and excessive exposure to air pollution.
- A detailed history of cigarette smoking should also be obtained. This information should be used to evaluate the patient's risk of

lung cancer and to teach about early recognition of symptoms. Anyone with a history of exposure to respiratory carcinogens who has pneumonitis that persists for longer than 2 weeks in spite of antibiotic therapy should be evaluated for the possibility of lung cancer.

- Screening chest x-rays every 6 to 12 months may be of value for individuals who are considered at high risk for lung cancer.
- During diagnostic evaluation, the patient and family may require support and reassurance.

Another major responsibility of the nurse is to help patients and their families deal with the diagnosis of lung cancer. Patients may feel guilty about their cigarette smoking having caused the cancer and may need to discuss this feeling with someone who has a nonjudgmental attitude. Questions regarding each patient's condition should be answered honestly. Additional counseling from a social worker, psychologist, or member of the clergy may be needed.

Specific care of the patient will depend on the treatment plan.

- Postoperative care for the patient having surgery is discussed in Lewis/Collier/Heitkemper, *Medical-Surgical Nursing,* edition 4, see Chapter 16. For care of the patient undergoing radiation therapy, see p. 675; for chemotherapy, see p. 631. The nurse has a major role in providing patient comfort, in teaching methods to reduce pain, and in assessing indications for hospitalization (see Cancer, p. 88).

Patient Teaching

Discharge instructions for the patient who has had a surgical resection with the intent to cure should focus on the manifestations of metastasis. The patient and family should be told to contact the physician if symptoms such as hemoptysis, dysphagia, chest pain, and hoarseness develop.

For many individuals who have lung cancer, very little can be done to significantly prolong their lives. Radiation therapy and chemotherapy can be used to provide palliative relief from distressing symptoms. Constant pain becomes a major problem.

LYME DISEASE

Definition/Description

Lyme disease is a spirochetal infection transmitted by the bite of an infected tick. It is the most common vector-borne disease in the United States. The peak season for human infection is the summer months. Most cases occur in three U.S. endemic areas: along the northeastern coast from Maryland to Massachusetts; in the midwestern states of Wisconsin and Minnesota; and along the north-western coast of California and Oregon.

Clinical Manifestations

The most characteristic sign of Lyme disease is a skin lesion, *ery-thema migrans (EM),* which occurs at the site of the tick bite in 80% of patients. This lesion begins as a red macule or papule that slowly expands to form a large round lesion with a bright-red border and central clearing. The EM lesion is often accompanied by other acute symptoms, such as intermittent fever, headache, fatigue, stiff neck, and migratory joint and muscle pain.

- If not treated, Lyme disease can progress in several weeks or months to debilitating arthritis; atrioventricular conduction defects such as palpitations, bradycardia or myocarditis; and neurologic abnormalities, including meningitis, facial palsy, and radiculoneuropathy.

Diagnosis is based on the clinical manifestations, history of exposure in an endemic area, and a positive serologic test for *Borrelia burgdorferi.* Other illnesses are frequently misdiagnosed as Lyme disease, particularly chronic fatigue syndrome and fibromyalgia. Serologic testing is not standardized, and false-positive results are common.

Therapeutic and Nursing Management

Active infection and lesions can be treated with antibiotic therapy. Oral doxycycline or amoxicillin is often effective in early-stage infection and in prevention of later stages of the disease. More diffuse infection may require 20 to 30 days of therapy. Intravenous ceftriaxone (Rocephen) is used for cardiac or neurologic abnormalities. Lyme disease arthritis usually responds to oral antibiotic therapy.

- Public education for the prevention of Lyme disease is outlined in Table 60-9 in Lewis/Collier/Heitkemper, *Medical-Surgical Nursing,* edition 4, p. 1916.

L

Malabsorption Syndrome

Malabsorption results from the impaired absorption of fats, carbohydrates, proteins, minerals, and vitamins. Lactose intolerance is the most common malabsorption disorder, followed by inflammatory bowel disease, nontropical (celiac) and tropical sprue, and cystic fibrosis.

The stomach, small intestine, liver, and pancreas regulate normal digestion and absorption. Nutrients are broken down so that absorption can take place through the intestinal mucosa and nutrients can enter the bloodstream. If there is an interruption in this process at any point, malabsorption may occur.

- Malabsorption can be caused by (1) biochemical or enzyme deficiencies, (2) bacterial proliferation, (3) disruption of the mucosa of the small intestine, (4) disturbed lymphatic and vascular circulation, and (5) surface area loss.

The most common clinical manifestation of malabsorption is *steatorrhea* (fatty stools). Bulky, foul-smelling stools that float in water and are difficult to flush are characteristic of steatorrhea.

Diagnostic studies include qualitative examination of stool for fat (Sudan stain), a 72-hour stool collection for quantitative measurement of fecal fat, and the D-xylose absorption-excretion test. Additional studies may include (1) the bile acid breath test to evaluate bile-salt malabsorption or malabsorption from bacterial overgrowth; (2) the triolein breath test, which measures carbon dioxide excretion after ingestion of a radioactive triglyceride; and (3) the excretion of breath hydrogen after ingestion of lactose, which is a sensitive, specific, and noninvasive test for detection of lactase deficiency.

- A pancreatic secretin test may be performed to rule out pancreatic insufficiency. Endoscopy may be used to obtain a small-bowel biopsy specimen for diagnosis. Radiographic studies of the esophagus, stomach, and small intestine may be indicated. A small-bowel barium enema is frequently performed to identify abnormal mucosal patterns.

See the specific disorders of Crohn's Disease, p. 157, Cystic Fibrosis, p. 166, Lactase Deficiency, p. 357, Sprue, p. 538, and Ulcerative Colitis, p. 583.

Malnutrition

Definition/Description

Malnutrition is an excess, deficit, or imbalance in the essential components of a balanced diet. Malnutrition is also described as undernutrition or overnutrition.

Pathophysiology

Protein-calorie malnutrition (PCM) is the most common form of undernutrition and can result from primary factors (poor eating habits) or secondary factors (alteration/defect in ingestion, digestion, absorption, or metabolism).

In states of increased stress, such as severe trauma, sepsis, anxiety, or uncontrolled pain, more calories and protein are required for healing. Additionally, nitrogen loss is accelerated when fever is present; and despite the return of body temperature to normal, the rate of protein breakdown and resynthesis may be accelerated for several weeks.

- In the early phase of starvation, the only use of protein is in its obligatory participation in cellular metabolism. Once carbohydrate stores are depleted, protein begins to be converted to glucose for energy. As protein depletion continues, liver function is impaired, with albumin leaking into the interstitial compartment, with edema then resulting.

Clinical Manifestations

Signs of malnutrition are evident in many body systems and include conjunctival and corneal dryness; dental caries, loose teeth, and discolored enamel; constant hunger, diarrhea, and flatulence; hepatomegaly; decreased BP; increased number of infections; and depression, confusion, and motor weakness.

Diagnostic Studies

- Serum albumin, prealbumin, and transferrin levels are decreased.
- Serum electrolytes are often elevated, especially potassium.
- Red blood cell (RBC) count and hemoglobin level may indicate anemia.
- White blood cell (WBC) count and total lymphocyte count are decreased.
- Liver enzyme studies reflect hepatic dysfunction.
- Serum levels of fat and water-soluble vitamins are often decreased.

M

Therapeutic Management

Early management of uncomplicated PCM is usually achieved with hospitalization and a diet high in calories and protein. In severe PCM the hospitalized patient may also be treated for correction of fluid and electrolyte imbalances and for infections secondary to a compromised immune system. Enteral feeding, both oral and tube feedings, can be used to supplement the diet. In cases of severe PCM total parenteral nutrition (TPN) may be initiated (see Tube Feeding, p. 685, and Total Parenteral Nutrition, p. 679).

Nursing Management

Goals

The patient with malnutrition will achieve weight gain to within normal range for height and age, consume a specified number of calories a day (with a diet individualized for the patient), and have no adverse consequences related to malnutrition.

Nursing Diagnoses

- Altered nutrition: less than body requirements related to decreased ingestion, digestion, or absorption of food or to anorexia
- Deficit in self-feeding related to decreased strength and endurance, fatigue, and apathy
- Altered bowel elimination: constipation, diarrhea, or impaction related to poor eating patterns, immobility, or medication effects
- Risk for fluid volume deficit related to deviations affecting access to or absorption of fluids
- Risk for impaired skin integrity related to poor nutritional state
- Risk for noncompliance with treatment regimen related to alteration in perception, lack of motivation, or incompatibility of regimen with lifestyle or resources
- Activity intolerance related to weakness, fatigue, and inadequate caloric intake

Nursing Interventions

The nurse must not ignore a patient's nutritional state by focusing attention on other physical problems of the patient. The incidence of nutritional deficiency, especially PCM, is high in hospitalized patients. It is important to know who is at risk, and why and how to intervene appropriately.

- The nurse must have a thorough understanding of nutritional support and rationale; a dietitian should assist with the plan of care.
- The nurse should assess for any psychosocial problems that may have led to the undernourished state.

Patient Teaching

- Discuss with the patient and family the importance of high-caloric, high-protein foods.

- Provide education for both the patient and family, including (1) the cause of the undernourished state and ways to avoid the problem in the future, (2) the need for continuous follow-up care if successful rehabilitation is to be accomplished, and (3) the importance of dietary change. The patient's understanding needs to be assessed, and information provided by the dietitian should be reinforced whenever possible.

MENIÈRE'S DISEASE

Definition/Description

Menière's disease is an inner ear disease characterized by a triad of symptoms: episodic vertigo, tinnitus, and fluctuating sensorineural hearing loss. Symptoms are incapacitating because of sudden, severe vertigo.

Pathophysiology

The cause of the disease is unknown, but it results in an excessive accumulation of endolymph in the membranous labyrinth. The volume of endolymph increases until the membranous labyrinth ruptures, mixing high-potassium endolymph with low-potassium perilymph. These changes lead to degeneration of delicate vestibular and cochlear hair cells. Menière's disease generally occurs in only one ear.

Clinical Manifestations

- Attacks of vertigo are sudden and often occur without warning. Attacks may be preceded by an aura consisting of a sense of fullness in the ear, increasing tinnitus, and decrease in hearing. Before vertigo attacks the patient may report inner ear "fullness."
- The patient complains that the environment is whirling wildly and experiences the feeling of being pulled to the ground (often called "drop attacks").
- Autonomic symptoms include pallor, sweating, nausea, and vomiting.
- The duration of the attacks may be hours or days, and attacks may occur several times a year. The clinical course is highly variable. Low-pitched tinnitus may be present continuously in the affected ear or intensified during an attack. Hearing loss fluctuates but decreases with each vertigo attack.

Diagnostic Studies

- Audiogram for low-tone hearing loss

M

- Vestibular test indicating decreased functioning
- Glycerol test supports the diagnosis if hearing improvement is obtained.
- Neurologic testing to rule out central nervous system (CNS) disease

Therapeutic and Nursing Management

During the acute attack, diazepam (Valium) or atropine may be given to decrease autonomic nervous system function. Acute vertigo is treated symptomatically with bed rest, sedation, and antiemetics or drugs for motion sickness. Diazepam (Valium) and Antivert (Bonamine plus nicotinic acid) are commonly used to reduce the dizziness. Most patients respond to the prescribed medications but must learn to live with the unpredictability of the attacks.

Management between attacks may include vasodilators, diuretics, antihistamines, and a low-sodium diet. Surgical management is used for frequent incapacitating attacks and reduced quality of life. Surgical options include endolymphatic shunt, vestibular nerve section, and labyrinth ablation. Careful therapeutic management can decrease the possibility of progressive sensorineural loss in many patients.

During an acute attack a patient needs reassurance that the condition is not life-threatening. The nurse should focus on providing only essential care since motion aggravates vertigo. If the patient is in bed, the siderails should be up and the bed in low position. Avoid the use of lights and television, which exacerbates symptoms. Have an emesis basin available because vomiting is common. Assist with ambulation because unsteadiness remains after an attack. Inform the patient after the attack that severe tinnitus and vertigo may exist for days to weeks.

MENINGITIS

Definition/Description

Meningitis is an acute inflammation of the pia mater and arachnoid membrane surrounding the brain and spinal cord. Meningitis usually occurs in the fall, winter, or early spring and is often secondary to viral respiratory disease. *Staphylococcus pneumoniae* causes about 30% of the cases. Children under 6 years of age, older adults, and persons who are debilitated are more often affected than the general population. Table 28, p. 208, compares meningitis and encephalitis.

Pathophysiology

Organisms usually gain entry to the central nervous system (CNS) through the upper respiratory tract or bloodstream, but they may enter by direct extension from penetrating wounds of the skull or through fractured sinuses in basal skull fractures.

The inflammatory response to the infection increases cerebrospinal fluid (CSF) production with a moderate increase in pressure. The purulent secretion produced quickly spreads to other areas of brain through the CSF.

- All patients must be observed closely for manifestations of increased intracranial pressure (ICP), which is a result of swelling around the dura, increased CSF volume, and endotoxins produced by the bacteria (see Increased Intracranial Pressure, p. 340).

Clinical Manifestations

Fever, severe headache, nausea and vomiting, and nuchal rigidity (resistance to flexion of the neck) are key signs of meningitis.

- A positive Kernig's sign, a positive Brudzinski's sign, photophobia, decreased level of consciousness (LOC), and signs of increased ICP may also be present.
- If the infecting organism is a meningococcus, a skin rash is common and petechiae may be seen.
- Coma is associated with a poor prognosis and occurs in 5% to 10% of patients with bacterial meningitis. Seizures occur in 20% of all cases.

Complications

In bacterial meningitis cranial nerve dysfunction, which usually disappears within a few weeks, often occurs with cranial nerves III, IV, VI, VII, or VIII.

- Cranial nerve irritation can have serious sequelae; the optic nerve is compressed by increased ICP. Papilledema is often present, and blindness may occur.
- When oculomotor, trochlear, and abducens nerves are irritated, ocular movements are affected. Ptosis, unequal pupils, and diplopia are common.
- Irritation of the trigeminal nerve is evidenced by sensory losses and loss of the corneal reflex, with irritation of the facial nerve resulting in facial paresis. Irritation of the vestibulocochlear nerve causes tinnitus, vertigo, and deafness.
- Hemiparesis, dysphasia, and hemianopsia may also occur, with these signs resolving over time. Acute cerebral edema may occur with bacterial meningitis, causing seizures, optic nerve palsy, bradycardia, hypertensive coma, and death.

M

- Hearing loss may be permanent after bacterial meningitis, but it is not a complication of viral meningitis.
- A complication of meningococcal meningitis is the *Waterhouse-Friderichsen syndrome*. The syndrome is manifested by petechiae, disseminated intravascular coagulation, and adrenal hemorrhage.

Diagnostic Studies

- Analysis of CSF includes (1) cultures, (2) protein levels (high in bacterial meningitis), (3) glucose concentration (decreased in bacterial meningitis), and (4) gross examination (purulent and turbid in bacterial meningitis).
- Skull x-rays may detect infected sinuses.
- CT scan may reveal increased ICP or hydrocephalus.

Therapeutic Management

A rapid diagnosis based on health history and physical examination is crucial because the patient is usually in a critical state when health care is sought. When meningitis is suspected, antibiotic therapy is instituted after collection of specimens for cultures, even before the diagnosis is confirmed. Penicillin and ampicillin are the drugs of choice. Chloramphenicol is used for persons who are allergic to penicillin. Nafcillin can be used for gram-negative organisms.

Nursing Management

Prevention of respiratory infections through vaccination programs for pneumococcal pneumonia and influenza should be supported by nurses. In addition, early and vigorous treatment of respiratory and ear infections is important. Persons who have close contact with anyone who has meningitis should be given prophylactic antibiotics.

The patient with meningitis is acutely ill. The fever is high and resistant to aspirin, and head pain is severe. Irritation of the cerebral cortex may result in seizures, with changes in mental status and LOC dependent on the level of ICP.

- The initial assessment should include vital signs, neurologic evaluation, fluid intake and output, and evaluation of lung fields and skin. These should be reassessed at frequent intervals based on the patient's condition.
- Head and neck pain secondary to movement require appropriate interventions. Codeine provides some pain relief without undue sedation for most patients. A darkened room and cool cloth over the eyes relieves the discomfort of photophobia. For the delirious patient, additional low lighting may be necessary to decrease hallucinations.
- All patients suffer some degree of mental distortion and hypersensitivity. They may be frightened and misinterpret the en-

vironment. Every attempt should be made to minimize environmental stimuli and the resulting exaggerated perception.

If seizures occur, protective measures should be taken. Anticonvulsant medications are administered as ordered. Problems associated with increased ICP need to be managed (see Increased Intracranial Pressure, p. 340). Restraints should be avoided. Padded siderails with sheets tied to the four corners to keep the patient from getting out of bed may be used to prevent injury. The presence of a familiar person at the bedside has a calming effect.

Fever must be vigorously managed because it increases cerebral edema and the frequency of seizures. Aspirin is useful in reducing fever. However, if the fever is resistant to aspirin, more vigorous means are necessary. An automatic cooling blanket is most efficient. If a cooling blanket is not available, tepid sponge baths with water may be effective. Because high fever greatly increases the metabolic rate, the patient should be assessed for dehydration and adequacy of intake. Supplemental feedings to maintain adequate nutritional intake via tube or oral feedings may be necessary.

- In most cases the patient with meningitis no longer requires isolation, with the exception of meningococcal meningitis.

In the recovery period good nutrition should be stressed, with an emphasis on a high-protein, high-caloric diet in small frequent feedings.

- Muscle rigidity may persist in the neck and the back of the legs. Progressive range-of-motion exercises and warm baths are useful. Activity should be gradually increased as tolerated, but adequate bed rest and sleep should be encouraged. Quiet activities based on an assessment of the patient's individual interests should be encouraged to prevent boredom.

- Residual effects are uncommon in meningococcal meningitis, but pneumococcal meningitis can result in sequelae such as dementia, epilepsy, deafness, hemiplegia, and hydrocephalus. Vision, hearing, cognitive skills, and motor and sensory abilities should be assessed after recovery, with appropriate referrals as indicated.

- Throughout the acute and recovery periods, the nurse should be aware of the anxiety and stress experienced by individuals close to the patient. The family needs to be supported and involved in care as much as possible.

M

MENSTRUAL IRREGULARITIES

Definition/Description

The ovarian cycle is more unstable and vulnerable to disruptive influences in its early (adolescent) and late phases (premenopausal). Therefore abnormal bleeding is more common at the beginning and end of an active menstrual life. When irregular bleeding becomes a problem for the patient, whether amenorrhea, menorrhagia, or metrorrhagia, a systematic investigation should be done to determine the cause of dysfunctional uterine bleeding.

Types of Dysfunctional Uterine Bleeding

Amenorrhea. The absence of menses refers to failure to menstruate before 17 years of age *(primary amenorrhea)* and cessation of menses for 6 months or more after they have become established *(secondary amenorrhea).* Amenorrhea probably occurs in less than 5% of females. Common causes of amenorrhea include autoimmune disease, polycystic ovary disease, tumors, congenital conditions, infection, and irradiation. Changes in lifestyle, such as marriage, death in the family, financial stress, and other emotional crises, can cause amenorrhea or unusual bleeding.

Menorrhagia. This condition is an increased duration or amount of menstrual bleeding at the time of a normal period. In the early reproductive years it may be associated with anovulatory cycles or uterine growths. A single episode of excessive bleeding may indicate a spontaneous abortion or ectopic pregnancy. Uterine tumors, including carcinoma, are common causes of menorrhagia. Pelvic inflammatory disease, endometriosis, the use of an intrauterine device (IUD), and drugs such as anticoagulants and thiazides (secondary to the thrombocytopenia) can also produce heavy menses.

Metrorrhagia. Bleeding or spotting between menstrual periods is called metrorrhagia. The most common cause of intramenstrual bleeding (breakthrough bleeding) is the use of hormonal contraceptives. Intramenstrual blood loss may also be caused by uterine lesions such as fibroids, polyps, hyperplasia, and carcinoma; cervical inflammation or lesions; and pelvic inflammatory disease.

Therapeutic Management

Because the causes of menstrual irregularities are multiple and varied, diagnostic and therapeutic measures also vary. A detailed health history and physical examination, including a pelvic examination, will limit possible diagnoses. The treatment of menstrual irregularities depends on a woman's need for contraception, her desire to conceive, or her wish to regulate irregular bleeding. The goal is to stop the current episode of bleeding, to prevent recurrence, and to preserve ovulation if pregnancy is desired.

Conservative treatment consists of hormonal therapy. For a woman wishing to conceive, progesterone is given to return normal ovarian function and control excessive bleeding. For recurrent irregular bleeding, low-dose oral contraceptives are the treatment of choice. For chronic recurrent bleeding, microsurgical techniques with a laser or electrocautery are safe and effective alternatives to hysterectomy when conservative therapy has failed. However, this therapy may result in no return of menses.

In the treatment of amenorrhea, pregnancy should be ruled out before any further endocrine workup is undertaken. Depending on the cause, treatment may involve hormone replacement therapy (e.g., estrogens, thyroid hormone, corticosteroids, gonadotropins) or a corrective procedure, such as surgical removal of the pituitary tumor(s).

Surgical interventions for the treatment of menstrual irregularities include a variety of procedures such as dilatation and curettage (D & C), polypectomy, cauterization (destruction of tissue by a chemical or by heat), myomectomy (removal of a uterine tumor without removal of the uterus), and hysterectomy. These procedures may be performed using standard surgical techniques, but more often microsurgical techniques, using a hysteroscope or a laparoscope and laser or electrocautery, are done. Microsurgery reduces bleeding and postoperative infection. Patients have fewer recovery days from these less invasive techniques.

- D & C is the most frequently performed gynecologic procedure. *Dilatation* is the widening of the cervical canal with a dilator. *Curettage* is the scraping of the lining of the uterus with a curette. A diagnostic D & C is performed to identify a lesion in the endocervix or endometrium, whereas a therapeutic D & C is done for an incomplete abortion or to correct excessive or prolonged bleeding. Dilatation of the cervix may be done to treat dysmenorrhea or sterility caused by cervical stenosis.

Nursing Management

The amount of vaginal bleeding the patient experiences should be accurately assessed. The number and size of pads or tampons used and the degree of saturation should be reported and recorded. The patient's fatigue level, along with variations in BP and blood count, should be noted because anemia and hypovolemia may be present.

When a patient is scheduled for a D & C, food intake is restricted after midnight the evening before the procedure. The procedure may be done in the operating room, in a free-standing surgery center, or in the physician's office. Either local or general anesthesia may be used. Postoperatively, the patient's vital signs should be checked ev-

M

ery 15 minutes until stable. The amount of vaginal bleeding should be noted, and a pad count should be kept. Some abdominal cramping, pelvic discomfort, or back pain is usual. These problems should be relieved with mild antiinflammatory analgesics (e.g., aspirin, ibuprofen). Persistent pain should be reported to the physician because the uterus is occasionally perforated during the procedure.

Treatment of menstrual problems is not always adequate. For example, a D & C for metrorrhagia may be helpful for a time, but the problem may recur. Continued use of contraceptives may become undesirable because of the patient's age or state of health. If abnormal bleeding persists, the patient generally becomes frustrated and worried and wants something done to correct the condition.

- It is critical that the nurse take time to provide an extensive explanation of common variations of menstruation. Irregular menstruation during adolescence should not be construed as something abnormal. Young women in particular need reassurance that this irregularity does not indicate future reproductive problems.
- If fibroids are noted and abdominal bleeding persists, hysterectomy may be the treatment of choice. The nurse can play an important role in addressing concerns some women express about physical, sexual, and emotional changes after a hysterectomy. The woman who does not wish to become pregnant may be relieved to have an end to persistent bleeding. Assessment of the individual woman provides the direction for counseling.

Patient Teaching
- Because the patient is discharged within 1 to 6 hours after a D & C operation, teaching is especially important. Specific instructions for self-care must be provided, including the following:
  1. Avoid the use of tampons or douching and refrain from sexual intercourse until the examination the second week after operation.
  2. Expect vaginal discharge during the healing process. It should be lighter in amount than the usual menses. Color varies from dark red to dark brown. Discharge should last no longer than 1 week.
  3. Avoid strenuous activity for 1 week, but a return to usual activities 2 days after recovery from anesthesia is usually appropriate.
  4. Report any signs of infection, such as fever, chills, foul-smelling discharge, heavy bleeding, and pelvic pain. Explain that the subsequent menstrual period is not usually affected.

MULTIPLE MYELOMA

Definition/Description

Multiple myeloma, or plasma cell myeloma, is a condition in which neoplastic plasma cells infiltrate the bone marrow and destroy bone. If the disorder is untreated, the patient usually lives for about 2 years after diagnosis. The incidence of multiple myeloma is about 2 to 3 per 100,000 people, which is similar to that of Hodgkin's disease or chronic lymphocytic leukemia. The disease is twice as common in men as in women. It usually develops after 40 years of age, with a peak incidence around 55 years of age.

Pathophysiology

There are many hypotheses regarding the etiology of multiple myeloma (e.g., chronic inflammation, chronic hypersensitivity reactions, viral influences), but no actual cause has been identified.

- The disease process involves excessive production of plasma cells that infiltrate the bone marrow and produce abnormal and excessive amounts of immunoglobulin (usually IgG, IgA, IgD, or IgE). This abnormal immunoglobulin is known as a *myeloma protein.*
- Plasma cell production of excessive and abnormal amounts of cytokines (IL-4, IL-5, IL-6) also contributes to the pathologic process of bone destruction.
- Ultimately, plasma cells destroy bone and invade the lymph nodes, liver, spleen, and kidneys.

Clinical Manifestations

Multiple myeloma develops slowly and insidiously.

- The patient often does not manifest symptoms until the disease is advanced, at which time skeletal pain is the major manifestation. Pain in the pelvis, spine, and ribs is particularly common.
- Diffuse osteoporosis develops as the myeloma protein destroys more bone. Osteolytic lesions are seen in the skull, vertebrae, and ribs. Vertebral destruction can lead to collapse of vertebrae with ensuing compression of the spinal cord, requiring emergency measures (e.g., radiation, surgery, chemotherapy) to prevent paraplegia.
- Loss of bone integrity can lead to the development of pathologic fractures.
- Bony degeneration causes calcium to be lost from bones, resulting in hypercalcemia. Hypercalcemia may cause renal, GI, or neurologic changes such as polyuria, anorexia, and confusion.

M

- Cell destruction contributes to the development of hyperuricemia, which, along with the high protein levels caused by the myeloma protein, can result in renal failure from renal tubular obstruction and interstitial nephritis from uric acid precipitates.
- The patient may display symptoms of anemia, thrombocytopenia, and granulocytopenia, all of which are related to the replacement of normal bone marrow elements with plasma cells.

Diagnostic Studies

- High serum protein may be present as evidenced by an "M" spike on serum electrophoresis.
- Pancytopenia, hyperuricemia, hypercalcemia, and elevated creatinine may be found.
- An abnormal globulin known as *Bence Jones protein* is found in the urine of patients with multiple myeloma.
- Radiologic studies, including bone scans, are done to establish the degree of bone involvement. The studies identify diffuse bony lesions, demineralization, and osteoporosis in affected skeletal areas.
- Bone marrow analysis shows significantly increased numbers of plasma cells. Other marrow components, particularly megakaryocytes, may be normal.

Therapeutic Management

The therapeutic approach involves managing both the disease and its symptoms because with treatment the chronic phase of multiple myeloma may last for more than 10 years.

- Symptoms of multiple myeloma remit and exacerbate. Consequently, acute care is needed at various times during the course of the illness. The final acute phase is unresponsive to treatment and usually short in duration.

Ambulation and adequate hydration are used to treat hypercalcemia, hyperuricemia, and dehydration. Weight bearing helps the bones reabsorb some calcium, and fluids dilute calcium and prevent protein precipitates from causing renal tubular obstruction.

Control of pain is another goal of therapeutic management. Analgesics, orthopedic supports, and localized radiation help to reduce the skeletal pain (e.g., melphalan [Alkeran], cyclophosphamide [Cytoxan], chlorambucil [Leukeran], carmustine [BCNU]). Chemotherapy is used to reduce the number of plasma cells (see Chemotherapy, p. 631). Corticosteroids may be added because they exert an antitumor effect in some patients. Radiotherapy is another important component of treatment, primarily because of its palliative effect on localized lesions (see Radiation Therapy, p. 675).

- Drugs may be used to treat the complications of multiple myeloma. For example, allopurinol (Zyloprim) may be given to reduce hyperuricemia, and IV furosemide promotes renal excretion of calcium. Calcitonin and pamidronate (Aredia) may be used to treat moderate to severe hypercalcemia.

Nursing Management

Maintaining adequate hydration is a primary nursing consideration to minimize problems from hypercalcemia. Fluids are administered to attain a urinary output of 1.5 to 2 L/day. This may require an intake of 3 to 4 L. In addition, weight bearing helps bones to reabsorb some of the calcium, and steroids may augment the excretion of calcium.

Once chemotherapy is initiated, uric acid levels increase because of increased cell destruction. Hyperuricemia must be resolved by ensuring adequate hydration and using allopurinol.

- Because of the potential for pathologic fractures, the nurse must be careful when moving and ambulating the patient. A slight twist or strain in the wrong area (e.g., a weak area in the patient's bones) may be sufficient to cause a fracture.

Pain management requires innovative and knowledgeable nursing interventions. If radiotherapy is used to diminish pain from localized myeloma lesions, appropriate skin care techniques must be used. Mild analgesics, such as nonsteroidal antiinflammatory drugs, acetaminophen, or acetaminophen with codeine, may be more effective than potent analgesics in diminishing bone pain. Braces, especially for the spine, may also help control pain. As in any pain management situation, the nurse is responsible for assessing the patient and for implementing necessary nursing measures to reduce pain.

- The patient's psychosocial needs require sensitive, skilled management. As with leukemia (see Leukemia, p. 358), it is important to help the patient and significant others adapt to changes fostered by chronic sickness and to adjust to the losses related to the disease process.
- The way in which patients and families deal with confronting death may be affected by the manner in which they learned to accept and live with the chronic nature of the disease.

MULTIPLE SCLEROSIS

Definition/Description

Multiple sclerosis is a chronic, progressive, degenerative disorder of the central nervous system (CNS). It is considered an autoimmune disease of young adults, with the onset usually between 15 and 50 years of age. Women are affected more often than men.

M

Multiple sclerosis (MS) primarily affects Caucasian persons of northern European descent. The incidence is highest in the temperate zones of the globe (between 45 and 65 degrees of latitude), especially northern Europe, Canada, and the northern United States. It is also associated with place of birth: an individual born and reared in one of the regions listed above who moves to a warmer climate (nearer the equator) after 15 years of age carries the same risk of MS as others in the country of origin.

Pathophysiology

The cause of MS is unknown, although research findings suggest that MS is related to infectious (viral), immunologic, and genetic factors and perpetuated as a result of intrinsic factors (e.g., faulty immunoregulation). Susceptibility to MS appears to be inherited; first-, second-, and third-degree relatives of patients with MS are at slightly increased risk. Possible precipitating factors include infection, physical injury, emotional stress, and pregnancy.

MS is characterized by CNS demyelination. The primary neuropathologic condition is an immune-mediated inflammatory demyelinating process, which some believe may be triggered by a virus in genetically susceptible individuals.

- Activated T cells responding to environmental triggers (e.g., infection) enter the CNS in increased numbers. Oligodendrocytes are damaged, resulting in demyelination. Macrophages are recruited and cause further cell damage.
- The process consists of loss of myelin, disappearance of oligodendrocytes (cells that make myelin), and proliferation of astrocytes. These changes result in characteristic plaque formation, or *sclerosis,* with plaques scattered throughout *multiple* regions of the CNS.
- As the disease progresses, myelin is totally disrupted and is replaced by glial scar tissue, which forms hard sclerotic plaques in multiple regions of the CNS. Without myelin, nerve impulses slow down. With destruction of nerve axons, impulses are totally blocked, resulting in permanent loss of function.

Clinical Manifestations

Because the onset is often insidious and gradual, with vague symptoms that occur intermittently over months or years, the disease may not be diagnosed until long after the onset of the first symptoms.

- Because the disease process has a spotty distribution in the CNS, signs and symptoms vary over time. The disease is characterized by chronic progressive deterioration in some persons and by remissions and exacerbations in others.
- Some patients have severe, long-lasting symptoms early in the course of the disease, whereas others may experience only oc-

casional and mild symptoms for several years after onset of the disease. The average life expectancy after the onset of symptoms is more than 25 years.

Common signs and symptoms include motor, sensory, cerebellar, and emotional phenomena.

- Motor symptoms include weakness or paralysis of limbs, trunk, or head; diplopia; and spasticity of muscles.
- Sensory symptoms include numbness and tingling, patchy blindness *(scotomas),* blurred vision, vertigo, tinnitus, and decreased hearing.
- Cerebellar signs include nystagmus, ataxia, dysarthria, and dysphagia.
- Bowel and bladder function can be affected if the sclerotic plaque is located in areas of the CNS that control elimination. Problems usually involve constipation and a *spastic* (uninhibited) bladder.
- Sexual dysfunction occurs in many persons. Physiologic impotence may result from spinal cord involvement in men. Women may experience decreased libido, difficulty with orgasmic response, painful intercourse, and decreased vaginal lubrication.
- Although intellectual functioning generally remains intact, emotional stability may be affected. Persons may be easily angered, depressed, or euphoric. Signs and symptoms are aggravated or triggered by physical and emotional trauma, fatigue, and infection.

Death usually occurs because of the infectious complications (e.g., pneumonia) of immobility or because of unrelated disease. Occasionally, suicide is a cause.

Diagnostic Studies

Because there is no definitive diagnostic test for MS, diagnosis is based primarily on history and clinical manifestations. Laboratory tests are adjuncts to the clinical examination.

- Cerebrospinal fluid (CSF) analysis may show an increase in immunoglobulin (IgG) or a high number of lymphocytes and monocytes.
- Evoked response testing is often delayed due to decreased nerve conduction.
- CT and MRI may detect sclerotic plaques.

Therapeutic Management

Because there is no cure for MS, therapeutic management is aimed at treating the disease process and providing symptomatic relief. The disease process is treated with drugs, and the symptoms are controlled with a variety of medications and other therapy.

- Spasticity is primarily treated with antispasmodic drugs. However, surgery (e.g., neurectomy, rhizotomy, cordotomy) or dorsal-column electrical stimulation may be required.
- Intention tremor that becomes unmanageable with medication is sometimes treated through stereotactic surgery on the thalamus.
- Neurologic dysfunction sometimes improves with physical therapy, speech therapy, and hypothermia, which normalizes body temperature if it is above normal.

Pharmacologic Management

Adenocorticotropic hormone (ACTH), methylprednisolone, and prednisone are helpful in treating acute exacerbations. Immunosuppressive drugs, such as azathioprine (Imuran), cyclosporine, and cyclophosphamide (Cytoxan), have produced some beneficial effects in patients with severe and relapsing MS. For ambulatory patients with exacerbating and remitting MS, interferon-ß (Betaseron) has decreased the number of exacerbations and the number of new lesions seen on an MRI scan.

Nutritional Management

A nutritious, well-balanced diet is essential. Although there is no standard prescribed diet, a high-protein diet with supplementary vitamins is often advocated. A diet high in roughage may help relieve constipation.

Nursing Management

Goals

The patient with MS will maximize neuromuscular function, maintain independence in activities of daily living for as long as possible, and optimize psychosocial well-being.

See the nursing care plan for the patient with multiple sclerosis in Lewis/Collier/Heitkemper, *Medical-Surgical Nursing,* edition 4, p. 1772.

Nursing Diagnoses

- Altered patterns of urinary elimination (incontinence) related to sensorimotor deficits or possible urinary tract infection
- Risk for impaired skin integrity related to immobility, sensorimotor deficits, and inadequate nutrition
- Sensory or perceptual alteration related to visual disturbances
- Self-concept disturbance related to prolonged debilitating condition
- Sexual dysfunction related to uncompensated neuromuscular deficits
- Constipation related to immobility, inadequate fluid intake, improper diet, and neuromuscular impairment
- Self-care deficit related to muscle spasticity and uncompensated neuromuscular deficits

- Risk for ineffective management of therapeutic regimen related to compromised functioning
- Impaired physical mobility related to muscle weakness or paralysis and muscle spasticity
- Altered family processes related to changing family roles, potential financial problems, and fluctuating physical condition

Nursing Interventions

The patient with MS should be aware of triggers that may cause exacerbations or worsening of the disease. Exacerbations of MS are triggered by infection (especially upper respiratory infections), trauma, delivery after pregnancy, stress, fatigue, and climactic changes. The nurse should help the patient identify particular triggers and develop ways to avoid them or minimize their effects.

The most common reasons for hospitalization are for a diagnostic workup and treatment of an acute exacerbation of complications such as bladder dysfunction.

- During the diagnostic phase, the patient needs reassurance that even though there is a tentative diagnosis of MS, certain diagnostic studies must be made to rule out other neurologic disorders. The patient with recently diagnosed MS may need assistance with the grieving process.
- During an acute exacerbation, the patient is often immobile and confined to bed for 2 to 3 weeks. The focus of nursing intervention at this phase is to prevent hazards of immobility, such as respiratory and urinary tract infections and decubitus ulcers.

Home management focuses on helping the patient adjust to the illness, teaching the patient how to avoid factors that precipitate exacerbations, maximizing self-care in light of current neurologic deficits, and meeting the needs for activities of daily living. The main goal is to keep the patient active and maximally functional.

- Physical therapy is important in keeping the patient as functionally active as possible. The purpose of therapy is to relieve spasticity, increase coordination, and train the patient to substitute unaffected muscles for impaired ones. An especially beneficial type of physical therapy is water exercise.

Patient Teaching

Patient education should focus on building general resistance to illness. This includes avoiding fatigue, extremes of heat and cold, and exposure to infection.

- It is important to teach the patient to achieve a good balance of exercise and rest, to eat nutritious and well-balanced meals, and to avoid the hazards of immobility (contractures and pressure sores).
- Patients should know their treatment regimens, the side effects of medications and how to watch for them, and the expected drug interactions with over-the-counter medications.

M

- Increasing dietary fiber may help some patients achieve regularity in bowel habits.
- The patient should be informed about the National Multiple Sclerosis Society in the United States and its local chapters, which offer a variety of services to meet the needs of patients with MS.

Muscular Dystrophy

Muscular dystrophy (MD) is an inherited progressive degeneration of skeletal muscle. Types of MD include Duchenne, Becker, and myotonic. These disorders result from abnormalities in the dystrophin gene, which leads to defects in the plasma membrane of muscle fiber; subsequent muscle fiber degeneration then occurs.

Duchenne dystrophy is an X-linked recessive disorder seen only in males. Manifestations, which occur by age 5 years, include symmetric and progressive weakness of pelvic and shoulder girdle muscles, leading to difficulties in running and climbing, contractural deformities of tendons and muscles, cardiomyopathy, and intellectual impairment. By 12 years of age, most patients are nonambulatory, with survival rare beyond age 25.

Becker dystrophy, an X-linked recessive disorder seen in males, is less common and less severe than Duchenne. Onset is between ages 5 and 15 with a slower course of pelvic and shoulder muscle wasting. Inability to walk may occur 25 years after onset.

Myotonic dystrophy is an autosomal dominant disorder seen in either gender in which slowly progressive weakness in the eyelids, neck, face, and distal limb muscles is seen. Myotonia is also noted. Multiple organ involvement with muscle atrophy can affect the heart, lungs, and endocrine system.

Diagnostic studies for MD include elevation of muscle enzymes (creatine kinase, aldolase), electromyogram (EMG) testing, muscle fiber biopsy, and electrocardiogram (ECG) abnormalities reflective of cardiomyopathy.

Definitive therapy is not available. Corticosteroid therapy may significantly halt the disease progression for up to 3 years. Myotonia may be treated with phenytoin and procainamide for patients without underlying heart problems. Leg and spinal braces may control foot drop and stabilize the ankle and spinal column, thereby preserving ambulation for several years.

Nursing care is supportive and should be directed toward maintenance of daily living activities as much as possible, including the avoidance of contractures, skeletal deformities, and obesity.

MYASTHENIA GRAVIS

Definition/Description

Myasthenia gravis (MG) is a disease of the neuromuscular junction characterized by fluctuating weakness of certain skeletal muscle groups. Women are affected slightly more often than men, although among patients with both thymoma and myasthenia (15% to 20% of all persons with myasthenia gravis), the majority are men over the age of 50. Peak age at onset in women is 20 to 30 years.

Pathophysiology

MG is caused by an autoimmune process that results in the production of antibodies directed against the acetylcholine (ACh) receptors. A reduction in the number of ACh receptor sites at the neuromuscular junction prevents ACh molecules from attaching and stimulating muscle contraction. Anti-ACh receptor antibodies are detectable in the serum of most patients with MG. Thymic tumors are found in about 10% of all patients with MG.

- Although a viral infection is suspected as precipitating an attack, a single specific cause for all MG cases has not been found.

Clinical Manifestations

The primary feature of MG is easy fatigability of skeletal muscle during activity. Strength is usually restored after a period of rest. The muscles most often involved are those used for moving the eyes and eyelids, chewing, swallowing, speaking, and breathing. The muscles are generally the strongest in the morning and become exhausted with continued activity. By the end of the day, muscle fatigue is prominent.

- In more than 90% of cases, the levator palpebrae (eyelid muscles) or extraocular muscles are involved. Facial mobility and expression can be impaired. There may be difficulty in chewing and swallowing food. Speech is affected, and the voice often fades after a long conversation.
- No other signs of neural disorder accompany MG; there is no sensory loss, reflexes are normal, and muscle atrophy is rare.

The course of the disease is highly variable. Some patients may have short-term remissions, others may stabilize, and others may have severe progressive involvement. Restricted ocular myasthenia, usually seen only in men, has a good prognosis.

- Exacerbations and initial onset of MG can be precipitated by emotional stress, pregnancy, temperature extremes, hypokalemia, and ingestion of drugs with neuromuscular blocking properties.

M

Complications result from muscle weakness in areas that affect swallowing and breathing. Aspiration, respiratory insufficiency, and respiratory infection are the major complications. An acute exacerbation of this type is sometimes called *myasthenic crisis.*

Diagnostic Studies

- Physical examination demonstrates fatigability with prolonged upward gaze (2 to 3 min) and muscle weakness
- EMG may show muscle fatigability with repeated stimulation of hand muscles
- Tensilon test reveals improved muscle contractility after an IV injection of anticholinesterase inhibitor

Therapeutic Management

Major therapies are anticholinesterase drugs, alternate-day corticosteroids, immunosuppressants, and plasmapheresis. Because the thymus gland appears to enhance the production of ACh receptor antibodies, removal of the thymus gland results in improvement in 85% of patients. Plasmapheresis removes anti-ACh receptor antibodies. Plasmapheresis can yield short-term improvement in symptoms and is indicated for patients in crisis or in preparation for surgery when corticosteroids need to be avoided.

- Acetylcholinesterase is the enzyme responsible for the breakdown of ACh in the synaptic cleft. Acetylcholinesterase inhibitors prolong the action of ACh and facilitate transmission of impulses at the neuromuscular junction. Neostigmine (Prostigmin) and pyridostigmine (Mestinon) are the most successful drugs of this group.
- Because of the autoimmune nature of MG, corticosteroids (specifically prednisone) are used to suppress immunity. Cytotoxic drugs such as azathioprine (Imuran) and cyclophosphamide (Cytoxan) may also be used for immunosuppression.

Nursing Management

Goals

The patient with myasthenia gravis will have a return of normal muscle endurance, avoid complications, and maintain a quality of life appropriate to disease progression.

Nursing Diagnoses

- Ineffective breathing patterns and airway clearance related to intercostal muscle weakness and impaired cough and gag reflexes
- Impaired verbal communication related to weakness of the larynx, lips, mouth, pharynx, and jaw

- Altered nutrition: less than body requirements related to impaired swallowing, weakness, and inability to prepare food or feed self
- Sensory/perceptual visual alterations related to ptosis, decreased eye movements, and dysconjugate gaze
- Activity intolerance related to muscle weakness and fatigability
- Body image disturbance related to inability to maintain usual lifestyle and role responsibilities

Nursing Interventions

The patient who is admitted to the hospital usually has a respiratory tract infection or is in an acute myasthenic crisis. Nursing care is aimed at maintaining adequate ventilation, continuing drug therapy, and watching for side effects of therapy. The nurse must be able to distinguish cholinergic from myasthenic crisis because the causes and treatment of the two differ greatly (see Table 56-18 in Lewis/Collier/Heitkemper, *Medical-Surgical Nursing,* edition 4, p. 1781).

As with other chronic illnesses, care focuses on the neurologic deficits and their impact on daily living.

- A balanced diet of food that can be chewed and swallowed easily should be prescribed. Semisolid foods may be easier to eat than solids or liquids. Scheduling doses of medication so that peak action is reached at mealtime may make eating less difficult.
- Diversional activities that require little physical effort and match the interests of the patient should be arranged.

Patient Teaching

Education should focus on the importance of following the medical regimen, potential adverse reactions to specific drugs, planning activities of daily living to avoid fatigue, the availability of community resources, and complications of the disease and therapy (crisis conditions) and what to do about them.

- Contact with the Myasthenia Gravis Society or an MG support group may be helpful and should be explored.

MYOCARDIAL INFARCTION

Definition/Description

A myocardial infarction (MI) occurs when ischemic intracellular changes become irreversible and necrosis results. Angina as a result of ischemia causes reversible cellular injury, and infarction results from sustained ischemia, causing irreversible cellular death.

M

Prehospital mortality in patients with acute MI is approximately 30% to 50%. Mortality among patients who reach the hospital is about 5%. Most of these deaths occur within the first 3 to 4 days after the event.

Pathophysiology

Cardiac cells can withstand ischemic conditions for approximately 20 minutes before cellular death (necrosis) begins. Contractile function of the heart stops in the areas of myocardial necrosis. The degree of altered function depends on the area of the heart involved and the size of the infarct. Most infarcts involve the left ventricle. A transmural MI occurs when the entire thickness of the myocardium in a region is involved. A subendocardial MI (nontransmural) exists when the damage has not penetrated the entire thickness of the myocardial wall.

- Infarctions are described by the area of occurrence as anterior, inferior, lateral, or posterior wall infarctions. Common combinations of areas are the anterolateral or anteroseptal MI. An inferior MI is also called a diaphragmatic MI.
- The degree of preestablished collateral circulation also determines the severity of infarction. In an individual with a history of heart disease, adequate collateral channels may have been established that provide the area surrounding the infarction site with blood supply and O_2.

The body's response to cell death is the inflammatory process. Within 24 hours leukocytes infiltrate the area. Enzymes are released from the dead cardiac cells. The proteolytic enzymes of the neutrophils and macrophages remove all necrotic tissue by the second or third day. Collagen matrix that will eventually form scar tissue is laid down.

- The necrotic zone is identifiable by ECG changes within 4 to 10 days and by technetium scanning 24 to 72 hours after the onset of symptoms.
- At 10 to 14 days after MI, beginning scar tissue is still weak. The myocardium is considered to be especially vulnerable to increased stress because of the unstable state of the healing heart wall.
- By 6 weeks after MI, scar tissue has replaced necrotic tissue. At this time the injured area is said to be healed. The scarred area is often less compliant than the surrounding fibers. This condition may be manifested by uncoordinated wall motion, ventricular dysfunction, or pump failure.

Clinical Manifestations

Severe, immobilizing, and persistent chest pain not relieved by rest or nitrate administration is the hallmark of an MI. The pain is caused by inadequate O_2 supply to the myocardium. Persistent and unlike any other pain, it is usually described as a heaviness, tightness, or constriction.

- Common locations are substernal or retrosternal, radiating to the neck, jaw, and arms or to the back. Pain may occur while the patient is active or at rest, asleep or awake and commonly occurs in the early morning hours.
- The pain usually lasts for 20 minutes or more and is described as more severe than anginal pain. It may be located atypically in the epigastric area. The patient may have taken antacids without relief.
- Some patients may not experience pain but may have "discomfort," weakness, or shortness of breath.

Additional manifestations may include nausea and vomiting, diaphoresis and vasoconstriction of peripheral blood vessels "cold sweat," fever within the first 24 hours up to 100.4° F (38° C), which may continue for 1 week, and BP and pulse rate initially elevated. BP then drops, with decreased urine output, lung crackles, hepatic engorgement, and peripheral edema.

Complications

Dysrhythmias are the most common complication after an MI. They are caused by any condition that affects the myocardial cell's sensitivity to nerve impulses, such as ischemia, electrolyte imbalances, and sympathetic nervous system stimulation. The intrinsic rhythm of the heartbeat is disrupted, causing the heart rate to be either very fast (tachycardia) or very slow (bradycardia) or to have an irregular beat. Life-threatening dysrhythmias occur most often with anterior wall infarction, pump failure, and shock. Complete heart block is seen in massive infarction (see Dysrhythmias, p. 200).

- Ventricular fibrillation, a common cause of sudden death, is a lethal dysrhythmia that most often occurs within the first 4 hours after the onset of pain. Premature ventricular contractions (PVCs) may precede ventricular tachycardia and fibrillation. Ventricular dysrhythmias need immediate treatment.

Congestive heart failure (CHF) occurs when the pumping power of the heart has diminished. It is common to see some degree of left ventricular dysfunction in the first 24 hours.

- Depending on the severity and extent of the injury, CHF occurs initially with subtle signs such as slight dyspnea, restlessness, agitation, or slight tachycardia. Jugular vein distention from right-sided heart failure, crackles in the lungs, and the presence of an S_3 or S_4 heart sound may indicate the onset of heart failure.

Cardiogenic shock occurs when inadequate O_2 and nutrients are supplied to the tissues because of left ventricular failure. It occurs

M

when there is dysfunction of much of the left ventricle as a result of infarction. Cardiogenic shock occurs in 10% to 15% of patients hospitalized with acute MI and has a high mortality.

Papillary muscle dysfunction may occur if the infarcted area includes or is adjacent to these structures.

- Papillary muscle dysfunction causes mitral regurgitation, which increases the volume of blood in the left atrium. Papillary muscle rupture is a severe complication causing massive mitral regurgitation, which results in dyspnea, pulmonary edema, and decreased cardiac output (CO).
- Treatment consists of rapid afterload reduction with nitroprusside or intraaortic balloon pumping and immediate open heart surgery with mitral valve replacement.

Ventricular aneurysm results when the infarcted myocardial wall becomes thinned and bulges out during contraction. Ventricular aneurysms are identified by bulges seen on x-ray, echocardiogram, or fluoroscopy or by persistent long-term ST segment changes on an ECG. The patient with a ventricular aneurysm may experience intractable congestive heart failure (CHF), dysrhythmias, and angina. Ventricular aneurysms also harbor thrombi, cause dysrhythmias, and promote left ventricular dysfunction.

- Surgical excision is the treatment for ventricular aneurysms severe enough to cause dysfunction.

Acute pericarditis is an inflammation of the visceral or parietal pericardium, or both, and may result in cardiac compression, lowered ventricular filling and emptying, and cardiac failure. It may occur 2 to 3 days after an acute MI as a common complication of the infarction. Chest pain, which may vary from mild to severe, is aggravated by inspiration, coughing, and movement of the upper body. The pain may radiate to the back and down to the left arm and may be relieved by sitting in a forward position. Assessment of the patient may reveal a friction rub over the pericardium, with fever also present.

- Diagnosis of pericarditis can be made with serial 12-lead ECGs. Treatment may include pain relief by aspirin, corticosteroids, or indomethacin.

Additional complications include pulmonary embolism and Dressler syndrome (antigen-antibody reaction to necrotic myocardium and right ventricular infarction).

Diagnostic Studies

Three noninvasive diagnostic parameters are used to determine whether a person has sustained an acute MI.

- Patient's history of pain, risk factors, and health history
- Twelve-lead ECG consistent with acute MI (ST-T wave elevations of greater than 1 mm or more in two contiguous leads)

- Measurement of serial myocardial serum enzymes, creatine kinase (CK), lactic dehydrogenase (LDH), and aspartate aminotransferase (AST)

Other diagnostic measures include initial chest x-ray to assess cardiac size and pulmonary congestion, leukocytosis, radionucleotide imaging to assess coronary blood flow, and technetium pyrophosphate scanning, which can localize areas of acute necrosis.

Therapeutic Management

Initial management of the patient with MI is best accomplished in a cardiac care unit (CCU), where constant monitoring is available. Dysrhythmias may be detected by nurses trained in continuous ECG monitoring techniques, and appropriate treatment can be instituted. An IV route is established to provide an accessible means for emergency drug therapy. Morphine sulfate or meperidine may be given intravenously for relief of pain. O_2 is usually administered by nasal cannula at a rate of 2 to 4 L/min. A continuous IV infusion of lidocaine may be given prophylactically to prevent ventricular fibrillation, which is the greatest threat to life after MI.

- Vital signs are taken frequently during the first few hours after admission and monitored closely thereafter. Bed rest and limitation of activity are usual initially, with a gradual increase in activity.
- A pulmonary artery catheter and intraarterial line may be used to accurately monitor intracardiac, pulmonary artery, and systolic arterial pressures in complicated MI so that the most effective mode of treatment in the acute phase can be determined.
- Thrombolytic therapy is the standard of practice in the treatment of acute MI. The goal is to salvage as much myocardial muscle as possible. Most commonly used thrombolytics are streptokinase, urokinase, and tissue plasminogen activator (tPA). To be of most benefit, thrombolytics must be given as soon as possible, preferably within the first 6 hours after the onset of pain. Contraindications and complications with thrombolytic therapy are described in Lewis/Collier/Heitkemper, *Medical-Surgical Nursing,* edition 4, p. 912.

Surgical intervention can include a percutaneous transluminal coronary angioplasty (PTCA), which may be performed in the patient exhibiting signs of cardiogenic shock or in the patient in whom thrombolytic therapy was unsuccessful. Coronary artery bypass graft (CABG) surgery may be a treatment choice in a select group of patients with acute MI (see Coronary Artery Bypass Graft Surgery, p. 642).

Pharmacologic management may include IV nitroglycerin, antidysrhythmic drugs, positive inotropic drugs, ß-blockers, calcium-channel blockers, angiotensin-converting enzyme (ACE) inhibitors, and stool softeners.

M

Nursing Management

Goals

The patient with an MI will experience relief of pain, have no progression of MI, receive immediate and appropriate treatment, cope effectively with associated anxiety, cooperate with the rehabilitation plan, and alter high-risk behaviors.

See the nursing care plan for the patient with myocardial infarction, Lewis/Collier/Heitkemper, *Medical-Surgical Nursing,* edition 4, p. 919.

Nursing Diagnoses

- Acute pain related to lactic acid production from myocardial ischemia and altered myocardial O_2 supply
- Altered cardiac tissue perfusion related to myocardial damage, ineffective CO, and potential pulmonary congestion
- Impaired gas exchange related to ineffective breathing pattern and decreased systemic tissue perfusion secondary to decreased CO
- Anxiety related to present status and unknown future, possible lifestyle changes, pain, and perceived threat of death
- Activity intolerance related to fatigue secondary to decreased CO and poor lung and tissue perfusion
- Self-esteem disturbance related to lack of control, illness event, and perceived or actual role changes
- Constipation related to immobility, change in diet, possible fluid restriction, and medications
- Ineffective management of therapeutic regimen related to lack of knowledge of disease process, rehabilitation, home activities, diet, and medications
- Grieving related to actual or perceived losses secondary to cardiac condition

Nursing Interventions

Acute interventions include the initial CCU stay (2 to 3 days) and the rest of hospitalization (5 to 7 days). Priorities for nursing interventions in the initial phase of recovery after MI include pain assessment and relief, physiologic monitoring, promotion of rest and comfort, alleviation of stress and anxiety, and understanding of the patient's emotional and behavioral reactions. Proper management of these priorities decreases the O_2 needs of a compromised myocardium. In addition, the nurse needs to institute measures to avoid the hazards of immobility while encouraging rest.

- Morphine should be given as needed to eliminate or reduce chest pain. The nurse should instruct the patient to rate the pain on a scale of 1 to 10 to assist in the assessment and treatment of pain.
- The nurse should be trained in ECG interpretation so that dysrhythmias causing further deterioration of the cardiovascular status can be identified and eliminated.

- In addition to frequent vital signs, intake and output should be evaluated at least once a shift, and physical assessment should be carried out to detect deviations from the patient's baseline parameters. Included is the assessment of lung sounds and heart sounds and inspection for evidence of fluid retention (e.g., distended neck veins, hepatic engorgement). Because a patient is on strict bed rest initially, dorsiflexion of the feet (Homans' sign) to elicit deep calf pain should also be done to evaluate the presence of deep-vein thrombosis.

- Assessment of the patient's oxygenation status is helpful, especially if the patient is receiving O_2. Also, the nares should be checked for irritation or dryness (see Oxygen Therapy, p. 669).

- It is important to plan nursing and therapeutic actions to ensure adequate rest periods free from interruption. Comfort measures that can promote rest are smooth bedclothes, frequent oral care, adequate warmth, dim lighting, a quiet atmosphere, and assurance that personnel are nearby and responsive to the patient's needs.

- Anxiety is present in all patients in various degrees. The nurse's role is to identify the source of anxiety and assist the patient in reducing it. If the patient is afraid of being alone, a family member should be allowed to sit quietly by the bedside or to check the patient frequently. If a source of anxiety is fear of the unknown, the nurse should explore these concerns with the patient and help with appropriate reality testing.

The phases of cardiac rehabilitation are outlined in Table 40. The patient must realize that recovery takes time. Resumption of physical activity after MI is slow and gradual. However, with appropriate and adequate supportive care, recovery is more likely to occur. For a sample rehabilitation program, see Table 31-21 in Lewis/Collier/Heitkemper, *Medical Surgical Nursing,* edition 4, p. 923.

Patient Teaching

Teaching begins with the CCU nurse and progresses through the staff nurse to the community health nurse. Careful assessment of the patient's learning needs helps the nurse to set realistic goals and objectives.

- In addition to teaching the patient and family what they want to know, there are several types of information that are considered necessary in achieving health. A teaching plan for the patient with MI should include the following:

  1. Anatomy and physiology of the heart and vessels
  2. Cause and effect of atherosclerosis
  3. Definition of terms (e.g., coronary artery disease, angina, MI, sudden death, congestive heart failure)
  4. Signs and symptoms of angina and MI and reasons they occur

M

Table 40	Phases of Cardiac Rehabilitation

Phase I—Time when patient is in CCU: Activity level depends on severity of MI; patient may rest in bed or chair; attention focuses on management of pain, anxiety, dysrhythmias, and cardiogenic shock.

Phase II—Time from transfer from CCU to discharge from hospital: Resumption of activities begins to point of self-care at time of discharge; information giving and teaching are appropriate at this time.

Phase III—Time of convalescence at home: Patient and family examine and possibly restructure lifestyles and roles; exercise program begins, commonly a walking program, which progresses daily during first week and then weekly; patient undergoes exercise treadmill test at about 8 wk to determine workload of recovering myocardium.

Phase IV—Time of recovery and maintenance: Involvement with community rehabilitation program for physical training and fitness continues.

CCU, Cardiac care unit; MI, myocardial infarction.

5. Healing after infarction
6. Identification of risk factors
7. Rationale for tests and treatment, including ECG, blood tests, and angiography, rest, diet, and medications
8. Appropriate expectations about recovery and rehabilitation (anticipatory guidance)
9. Measures to take to promote recovery and health
10. Importance of the gradual, progressive resumption of activity

- Anticipatory guidance involves preparing the patient and family for what to expect in the course of recovery and rehabilitation. By learning what to expect during treatment and recovery, the patient gains a sense of control over his/her life.
- Because of the short hospitalization, it is critical to give the patient specific guidelines for activity and exercise so that overexertion will not occur. It is helpful to stress that when the patient "listens to what the body is saying" uncomplicated recovery should proceed.
- It is important to include sexual counseling for cardiac patients and their partners. Reading material on resumption of sexual activity may be presented to the patient to facilitate discussion. The nurse should return to clarify and explain as necessary.

MYOCARDITIS

Definition/Description

Myocarditis is a focal or diffuse inflammation of the myocardium that has been associated with a variety of etiologic agents. Viruses are the most common etiologic agent in the United States and Canada, with a predominance of RNA viruses (coxsackievirus A and B), echovirus, influenza A and B, and mumps. Certain medical conditions such as metabolic disorders and collagen-vascular diseases (e.g., systemic lupus erythematosus) may also precipitate myocarditis.

- Myocarditis is frequently associated with acute pericarditis, particularly when it is caused by coxsackievirus B strains or echoviruses.

Pathophysiology

Pathophysiologic mechanisms of myocarditis are poorly understood because there is usually a period of several weeks after the initial infection before the development of manifestations of myocarditis. Immunologic mechanisms may play a role in the development of myocarditis. The majority of infections are benign, self-limiting, and subclinical.

Clinical Manifestations

The clinical features for patients with myocarditis are variable, ranging from a benign course without any overt manifestations to severe heart involvement or sudden death. Fever, fatigue, malaise, myalgias, pharyngitis, dyspnea, lymphadenopathy, and GI complaints are early systemic manifestations of the viral illness.

- Early cardiac manifestations appear 7 to 10 days after viral infection and include pericardial chest pain with an associated friction rub because pericarditis often accompanies myocarditis. Cardiac symptoms may progress to congestive heart failure (CHF) with the presence of a third heart sound (S_3), crackles, jugular venous distention, peripheral edema, pericardial effusion, syncope, and possibly ischemic pain.
- The majority of individuals with myocarditis recover spontaneously. Occasionally, acute myocarditis progresses to chronic dilated cardiomyopathy.

Diagnostic Studies

Electrocardiogram (ECG) changes are often nonspecific and reflect associated pericardial involvement, including diffuse ST-segment

M

abnormalities. Dysrhythmias and conduction disturbances may be present.

Laboratory findings are often inconclusive, with the presence of mild to moderate leukocytosis and atypical lymphocytes, elevated viral titers (virus is generally only present in tissue and fluid samples during the initial 8 to 10 days of illness), increased enrythrocyte sedimentation rate, and elevated levels of enzymes such as the transaminases, creatine kinase, and lactic dehydrogenase.

- Histologic confirmation is possible through endomyocardial biopsy (EMB). A biopsy done during the initial 6 weeks of acute illness is most useful for diagnosis because this is the period in which lymphocytic infiltration and myocyte damage indicative of myocarditis are present.
- Special myocardial imaging techniques may also be used in the diagnostic evaluation of myocarditis.

Therapeutic Management

The specific treatment for myocarditis has yet to be established but usually consists of managing associated cardiac decompensation.

- Digoxin is often used to treat ventricular failure because it improves myocardial contractility and reduces ventricular rate. Digoxin should be used cautiously in patients with myocarditis because of the increased sensitivity of the heart to the adverse effects of this drug and potential toxicity even with minimal doses.
- O_2 therapy, bed rest, restricted activity, and maintenance of standby emergency equipment are general supportive measures used for management of myocarditis.

Immunosuppression therapy, with agents such as prednisone, azathioprine, and cyclosporine, has been used to reduce myocardial inflammation and to prevent irreversible myocardial damage. Administration of immunosuppressive agents is recommended only during the postinfectious stage of the disease, approximately 10 days after the onset of initial symptoms. If used early in the course of viral myocarditis, these drugs can actually increase tissue necrosis.

- The use of corticosteroids for the treatment of myocarditis remains controversial because of the associated serious side effects and lack of clear documentation for their efficacy.

Nursing Management

Interventions focus on assessment for the signs and symptoms of CHF and instituting measures to decrease cardiac workload (e.g., use of semi-Fowler's position, spaced activity and rest periods, and provisions for a quiet environment). Prescribed medications that increase the heart's contractility and decrease the preload, afterload, or both are administered. Careful monitoring and evaluation of the patient taking these medications is necessary.

The patient may be anxious about the diagnosis of myocarditis, recovery from myocarditis, and therapy. Nursing measures include assessing the level of anxiety, instituting measures to decrease anxiety, and keeping the patient and family informed about therapeutic measures.

The patient who receives immunosuppressive therapy may have additional problems of alteration in immune response, with the potential for infection and complications related to the therapy. Guidelines for care include monitoring for complications and providing the patient with a clean, safe environment according to proper infection control standards.

M

Nausea and Vomiting

Definition/Description

Nausea and vomiting are the most common manifestations of GI diseases. Although each symptom can occur independently, they are closely related and usually treated as one problem. They are also found in a wide variety of conditions unrelated to GI disease, including pregnancy, infectious diseases, central nervous system (CNS) disorders (e.g., meningitis), cardiovascular problems (e.g., myocardial infarction, congestive heart failure), side effects of drugs (e.g., digitalis, antibiotics), metabolic disorders (e.g., uremia), and psychologic factors (e.g., stress, fear).

Nausea is a feeling of discomfort in the epigastrium, with a conscious desire to vomit. Anorexia usually accompanies nausea and is brought on by unpleasant stimulation involving any of the five senses. Generally, nausea occurs before vomiting and is characterized by contraction of the duodenum and a slowing of gastric motility and emptying.

Vomiting is the forceful ejection of partially digested food and secretions from the upper GI tract. It occurs when the gut becomes overly irritated, excited, or distended. Vomiting can be a protective mechanism to rid the body of spoiled or irritating foods and liquids.

Pathophysiology

The vomiting center in the brainstem coordinates the multiple components involved in vomiting. Neural impulses reach the vomiting center via afferent pathways through branches of the autonomic nervous system. Visceral receptors for these afferent fibers are located in the GI tract, kidneys, heart, and uterus. When stimulated, these receptors relay information to the vomiting center, which initiates the vomiting reflex.

In addition, the chemoreceptor trigger zone (CTZ) located in the brain responds to chemical stimuli of drugs and toxins. Once stimulated (e.g., motion sickness) CTZ transmits impulses to the vomiting center.

Emotions, stress, unpleasant sights and odors, and pain can also trigger vomiting. Severe nausea and vomiting may also be caused by a metabolic crisis. For example, nausea and vomiting are frequently associated with uremia, hyperthyroidism, hyperparathyroidism and hypoparathyroidism, diabetic acidosis, Addison's disease, and hypertensive crisis.

Clinical Manifestations

Signs of severe or prolonged nausea and vomiting include rapid dehydration with essential electrolytes (e.g., potassium) lost. As vomiting persists, there may be severe electrolyte imbalances, loss of extracellular fluid (ECF) volume, decreased plasma volume, and eventually circulatory failure. Weight loss may occur in a short time.

Diagnostic Studies

- Abdominal x-rays
- Serum electrolytes, which may be altered (especially hypokalemia)
- Decreased urine output and concentrated urine
- Amount, frequency, character (projectile), content (feces, bile, blood), and color of vomitus (red, "coffee ground") to determine the etiology

Therapeutic Management

Goals of management are to determine and treat the underlying cause of nausea and vomiting and to provide symptomatic relief. Determining the cause is often difficult because nausea and vomiting are manifestations of many conditions of the GI tract and of disorders of other body systems.

Antiemetic medications are used with caution until the cause of vomiting is determined. These may include scopolamine, chlorpromazine, diphenhydramine, metoclopramide, and promethazine.

The patient with severe vomiting requires IV fluid therapy with electrolyte replacement until able to tolerate oral intake. In some cases a nasogastric (NG) tube and suction are used to decompress the stomach. Once symptoms have subsided, oral nourishment beginning with clear liquids is started. As the patient's condition improves, a diet high in carbohydrates and low in fat is preferred.

Nursing Management

Goals

The patient with nausea and vomiting will experience minimal or no further nausea and vomiting, have normal electrolyte levels, and return to a normal pattern of fluid balance and nutrient intake.

See the nursing care plan for the patient with nausea and vomiting in Lewis/Collier/Heitkemper, *Medical-Surgical Nursing,* edition 4, p. 1173.

Nursing Diagnoses

- Nausea and vomiting related to multiple etiologies
- Fluid volume deficit related to prolonged vomiting
- Anxiety related to lack of knowledge of etiology of the problem, treatment plan, and follow-up care

- Risk for altered nutrition: less than body requirements related to nausea and vomiting

Nursing Interventions

Until a diagnosis is confirmed, the patient is kept on nothing by mouth (NPO) and IV status. An NG tube may be necessary if persistent vomiting occurs.

- The patient who cannot adequately manage self-care should be put in a semi-Fowler's or side-lying position to prevent aspiration.
- The environment should be quiet, free of noxious odors, and well ventilated.

With prolonged vomiting, interventions include accurate intake and output with vital signs, assessment for dehydration, proper positioning to prevent aspiration, and observation for changes in comfort and mentation.

Patient Teaching

- Instruct the patient to take several deep breaths, prevent sudden changes in position, and keep the head of the bed elevated to decrease stimulation of the vomiting center.
- Provide explanations for diagnostic tests and procedures.
- For chronic nausea and vomiting, instruct the patient and family on how to deal successfully with unpleasant sensations of nausea, methods for preventing nausea and vomiting, and strategies to maintain fluid and nutritional intake during periods of nausea.
- When food is identified as the precipitating cause of nausea and vomiting, help the patient with problem solving. What food was it? When was it eaten? Has this food caused problems in the past? Is anyone else in the family sick?

NEPHROTIC SYNDROME

Definition/Description

Nephrotic syndrome is characterized by a clinical course of increased glomerular membrane permeability, which is responsible for a massive urinary excretion of protein. Causes of nephrotic syndrome include primary glomerular disease, infections (e.g., hepatitis, streptococcus), neoplasms (e.g., Hodgkin's disease), allergens (e.g., bee sting, drugs), and multisystem disease (e.g., diabetes mellitus).

Pathophysiology and Manifestations

Diminished plasma oncotic pressure from the decreased serum proteins being excreted in urine stimulates hepatic lipoprotein synthesis, which results in hyperlipidemia. Fat bodies (fatty casts) commonly appear in the urine.

Immune responses, both humoral and cellular, are altered in nephrotic syndrome. As a result, infection is a major cause of morbidity and mortality.

Hypercoagulability with thromboembolism is potentially the most serious complication of nephrotic syndrome. The renal vein is the most commonly involved site for thrombus formation. Pulmonary emboli occur in about 40% of nephrotic patients with thrombosis.

- Skeletal abnormalities may occur, including hypocalcemia, blunted calcemic response to parathyroid hormone, hyperparathyroidism, and osteomalacia.

Therapeutic Management

Treatment of nephrotic syndrome is symptomatic. The goals are to relieve edema and cure or control the primary disease. Management of edema includes the cautious use of loop diuretics and a low-sodium (2 to 3 g/day), high-protein diet (1.5 to 2.0 g/kg/day).

- IV albumin may be of value in the patient with symptomatic hypovolemia and hypotension or with edema resistant to therapy with diuretic drugs. Long-term therapy with albumin is not a practical approach because it is lost in the urine. However, an increase in dietary protein or IV albumin may ameliorate the hypoalbuminemia if either angiotensin-converting enzyme inhibitors or nonsteroidal antiinflammatory agents are administered concomitantly.
- Treatment of hyperlipidemia is frequently unsuccessful. However, treatment with lipid-lowering agents, such as colestipol, probucol, and lovastatin may result in moderate decreases in serum cholesterol levels.
- Corticosteroids and cyclophosphamide (Cytoxan) may be used for the treatment of severe cases. Prednisone has been effective in some persons with membranous glomerulonephritis, proliferative glomerulonephritis, and lupus nephritis.
- Management of diabetes and treatment of edema are the only measures used for diabetic nephrosis.

Nursing Management

The major focus of care is related to edema. It is important to assess edema by weighing the patient daily, accurately recording intake and output, and measuring abdominal girth or extremity size. Comparing this information daily provides the nurse with a tool for assessing the effectiveness of treatment. Edematous skin needs careful cleaning. Trauma should be avoided, and the effectiveness of diuretic therapy must be monitored. The person is often ashamed of his/her edematous appearance and may need support in dealing with an altered body image.

The patient has the potential to become malnourished from the excessive loss of protein in the urine. Maintaining a high-protein diet that is also low in sodium is not always easy. Protein intake should be 1.0 to 1.5 g/kg of body weight. The patient is usually anorexic. Serving small, frequent meals in a pleasant setting may encourage better dietary intake.

- Because the patient is susceptible to infection, measures should be taken to avoid exposure to persons with known infections.

NEUROGENIC BLADDER

Neurogenic bladder refers to any bladder dysfunction resulting from a central nervous system (CNS) neurologic disorder. There are numerous causes of this condition, including CNS tumors, cerebrovascular accidents, multiple sclerosis, diabetic neuropathy, and spinal cord injury.

A person with a neurogenic bladder may have problems with urgency, frequency, incontinence, inability to urinate, and obstruction-like symptoms. Long-term problems include formation of calculi, urinary tract infection, and progressive deterioration in renal function.

A simple way to classify neurogenic dysfunction is to identify whether there is a failure to store, failure to empty, or both problems and whether the dysfunction is of the bladder or urethra. Either or both problems lead to urinary tract damage if not treated.

The type of dysfunction usually depends on where the problem affects the brain or spinal cord (e.g., cerebral centers, suprasacral spinal cord, or sacral cord area).

- Lesions in the brain or upper spinal cord usually cause hyperreflexic symptoms, whereas lesions in the sacral cord cause arreflexia. Detrusor sphincter dyssynergia (the bladder and sphincter contract at the same time) is often associated with lesions in the suprasacral spinal cord. (For further information, see Chapter 57 in Lewis/Collier/Heitkemper, *Medical-Surgical Nursing,* edition 4, p. 1814.)

NON-HODGKIN'S LYMPHOMA

Definition/Description

Non-Hodgkin's lymphomas (NHL) are a heterogenous group of malignant neoplasms of the immune system that affect all ages. They are classified according to different cellular and lymph node characteristics (see Table 28-33 in Lewis/Collier/Heitkemper, *Medical-Surgical Nursing,* edition 4, p. 821). NHLs can originate outside the lymph nodes, the method of spread can be unpredictable, and the majority of patients have widely disseminated disease at the time of diagnosis.

As more information about the cell types is discovered, evolving schemas have been used to describe different subtypes. A variety of clinical presentations and courses are recognized from indolent to rapidly progressive disease. Common names for different types of NHL include *Burkitt's lymphoma, reticulum cell sarcoma,* and *lymphosarcoma.*

Clinical Manifestations

There is no hallmark feature in NHLs that parallels the Reed-Sternberg cell of Hodgkin's disease. However, all NHLs involve lymphocytes arrested in various stages of development. The primary clinical manifestation is painless lymph node enlargement. Because the disease is usually disseminated when it is diagnosed, other symptoms will be present, depending on where the disease has spread (e.g., hepatomegaly with liver involvement).

- Patients with high-grade lymphomas may have lymphadenopathy and constitutional ("B") symptoms such as fever, night sweats, and weight loss. The peripheral blood is usually normal, but some lymphomas may occur in a "leukemic" phase.

Diagnostic Studies

Diagnostic studies used for NHL resemble those used for Hodgkin's disease. Lymph node biopsy establishes the cell type and pattern. Staging, as described for Hodgkin's disease, is used to guide therapy.

Therapeutic Management

Treatment for NHL involves radiotherapy and chemotherapy. (See Radiation Therapy, p. 675, and Chemotherapy, p. 631.) Ironically, more aggressive lymphomas are more responsive to treatment and more likely to be cured. In contrast, indolent lymphomas have a naturally long course but are difficult to treat effectively.

- Radiotherapy alone may be effective for treatment of stage I disease, but combination radiation therapy and chemotherapy are used for other stages. Initial chemotherapy uses alkylating agents such as cyclophosphamide and chlorambucil.
- High-dose chemotherapy with peripheral blood stem cell or bone marrow transplantation is commonly employed. Biologic response modifiers (BRMs), such as α-interferon, interleukin-2, and tumor necrosis factor, are also being investigated for treatment of NHL. (BRMs are discussed in Chapter 12 in Lewis/Collier/Heitkemper, *Medical-Surgical Nursing,* edition 4, p. 303.)

OBESITY

Definition/Description
Obesity is the most common nutritional problem in North America. Twenty-four percent of all men and 27% of all women are considered overweight. The calculated body mass index (BMI), a clinical index of obesity, classifies women with a BMI value of 23 to 29 and men with a BMI value of 25 to 30 as obese. Obese persons have a higher rate of hypertension, gout, degenerative joint disease, diabetes mellitus, stroke, and breast cancer.

Pathophysiology
Many factors have been identified as critical elements in the development and maintenance of obesity. Environmental and genetic factors are considered important. Children of obese parents tend to be obese, and obesity tends to affect several persons within a family. Evidence of a genetic component is suggested in twin and adoptive children.

- Obesity may be modulated by a variety of factors, including energy intake, level of habitual physical activity, and the tendency to store ingested energy in the form of lean or fat tissue.

It is hypothesized that the hypothalamus has a set point for energy balance, above which energy conservation becomes increasingly less efficient and below which energy conservation becomes increasingly more efficient.

- This homeostatic mechanism accounts for the fact that most adults keep their weight remarkably constant, despite large swings in energy input and expenditure.
- This mechanism could also account for why the obese person tends to remain overweight.
- An emotional tendency to overeat beyond satiety is also powerful for some persons.

Complications
The medical problems associated with obesity are numerous and frequently include cardiovascular and respiratory signs such as dyspnea on exertion, paroxysmal nocturnal dyspnea, orthopnea, drowsiness, and somnolence. There is a high risk for polycythemia, which results in occluded vessels, sluggish vessel flow, varicose veins, hypertension, and increased heart size. Pickwickian syndrome or obesity hypoventilation leads to chronic hypercapnia with cyanosis, dyspnea, edema, and somnolence.

Impaired glucose intolerance leads to non–insulin dependent diabetes mellitus (NIDDM). Gallstones may occur with increased serum cholesterol and triglyceride levels. Excessive weight on multiple joints contributes to degenerative joint disease.

- Long-standing emotional and social problems may lead to poor self-esteem and body image.

Diagnostic Studies

- The presence of obesity is commonly calculated by BMI, standardized height-weight charts, anthropometric measurements, or hip-to-waist ratio.

  Assessment of etiologic factors includes testing for hypothyroidism, hypothalamic tumors, Cushing's syndrome, hypogonadism (men), and polycystic ovarian disease (women).

Therapeutic Management

When no organic cause can be found for obesity, it should be considered a chronic complex illness. Any supervised plan of care should be directed at:

- Successful weight loss
- Successful weight control, requiring long-term behavior changes
- A multipronged approach, with attention to dietary intake, physical activity, behavioral-cognitive modification, and perhaps drug therapy; restricting dietary intake so that intake is below energy requirements; and following a sensible, well-balanced, low-caloric diet

Surgical management for treating morbid obesity may include:

- Lipectomy (adipectomy) to remove unsightly adipose folds
- Liposuction for cosmetic purposes and not weight reduction
- Jaw wiring with a change in eating patterns once the wires are removed
- Intragastric balloon to control oral intake by reducing stomach size
- GI surgery such as vertical banded gastroplasty and Roux-en-Y gastric bypass to reduce gastric capacity

Nursing Management

Goals

The patient with obesity should achieve and maintain weight loss to a specified level, modify eating habits, and participate in a regular physical activity program.

Nursing Diagnoses

- Altered nutrition: more than body requirements related to excessive intake in relation to metabolic need and activity level
- Impaired physical mobility related to excessive body weight

- Social isolation related to alterations in physical appearance and perceived unattractiveness
- Risk for impaired skin integrity related to alterations in nutritional state (obesity), immobility, excess moisture, and multiple skin folds
- Ineffective breathing pattern related to decreased lung expansion from obesity
- Risk for noncompliance with treatment regimen related to alteration in perception or lack of motivation
- Body image disturbance related to deviation from usual or expected body size and inability to lose or sustain weight loss

Nursing Interventions

When assessing the obese patient, the nurse needs to consider several different types of questions, such as the following:

- What is the psychologic importance of food to the patient?
- Is the patient's food intake influenced by hunger?
- Does the taste and appearance of food or other physical factors in the environment stimulate the patient to eat?
- Is there an emotional problem that stimulates the patient to eat?
- Are there any stressors influencing the patient's eating patterns?

Preoperative care for gastric surgery includes planning for special needs such as large-size BP cuff, oversized bed and chair, reinforced trapeze bar, meat or freight scales for weighing, and special gowns.

Postoperative care includes administration of pain medications, facilitating patient respiratory efforts (elevate head of bed, and turn, cough, and deep breathing), monitoring the abdominal wound for healing, and monitoring NG tube patency.

- Several potential psychologic problems after surgery need to be anticipated and recognized. Some patients express guilt feelings because the only way they could lose weight was by surgical means rather than by the "sheer willpower" of reduced dietary intake. The nurse should be ready to provide support so that such a patient does not dwell on negative feelings.
- Discharge postoperative gastric surgery teaching includes the importance of a diet high in protein and low in carbohydrates, fat, and roughage, with six small feedings daily, and prompt recognition of complications such as anemia, diarrhea, vitamin deficiencies, and psychiatric problems, especially episodes of depression.

The nurse needs to reinforce participation in physical activity programs and cognitive training such as self-help support groups or professional counseling.

ORAL CANCER

Definition/Description

Carcinoma of the oral cavity may occur on the lips or anywhere within the mouth (e.g., tongue, floor of mouth, buccal mucosa, hard palate, soft palate, pharyngeal walls, tonsils). Carcinoma of the lips has the most favorable prognosis of any of the oral tumors because lip lesions are more apparent to the patient than other oral lesions and are usually diagnosed earlier.

Pathophysiology

Although the cause of oral cancers is not definitive, there are a number of predisposing factors, including constant overexposure to ultraviolet radiation from sun, tobacco use (cigar, cigarette, pipe, snuff), excessive alcohol intake, and chronic irritation such as from a jagged tooth or poor dental care. A positive history of use of tobacco (cigar, cigarette, pipe, snuff) and alcohol, in the past or currently, is the most significant etiologic factor.

Clinical Manifestations

- *Leukoplakia,* called "white patch" or "smoker's patch," is a whitish precancerous lesion on the mucosa of the mouth or tongue that results from chronic irritations such as smoking. The patch becomes keratinized (hard and leathery) and is sometimes described as hyperkeratosis.
- *Erythroplasia (erythroplakia),* seen as a red velvety patch on the mouth or tongue, is also considered a precancerous lesion.
- Cancer of the lip appears as an indurated painless lip ulcer.
- The first sign of carcinoma of the tongue is an ulcer or area of thickening. Soreness or pain of the tongue may occur, especially when hot or highly seasoned foods are eaten. Some patients experience limitation of movement of the tongue. Later symptoms of cancer of the tongue include increased salivation, slurred speech, dysphagia, toothache, and earache.
- Approximately 30% of patients with oral cancer are first seen with an asymptomatic neck mass.

Diagnostic Studies

- Biopsy of suspected lesion with cytologic examination for definitive diagnosis
- Oral exfoliative cytology and toluidine blue test to screen for oral cancer
- CT and MRI scans to detect metastases

Therapeutic Management

Management usually consists of surgery, radiation, chemotherapy, or a combination of these. Surgery remains the most effective treatment, especially for removing the tumor central core. Many of the operations are radical procedures involving extensive resections. Various surgical procedures may be performed, including hemiglossectomy (half the tongue), glossectomy (entire tongue), and radical neck dissection. A tracheostomy (see Tracheostomy, p. 682) is commonly done with radical neck dissection to prevent airway obstruction.

Radiation (internal or external) therapy is sometimes used before surgery to decrease the tumor size. Radiation may also be used postoperatively or palliatively (see Radiation Therapy, p. 675). Chemotherapy and radiation are used together when the lesions are more advanced or involve several structures of the oral cavity. Chemotherapy may also be used when surgery and radiation fail or as the initial therapy for smaller tumors (see Chemotherapy, p. 631).

Palliative treatment may be indicated when the prognosis is poor, cancer is inoperable, or the patient decides against mutilating surgery. These treatments may include gastrostomy and adequate amounts of analgesic medication.

Nursing Management

Goals

The patient with oral cancer will have a patent airway, be able to communicate, have adequate nutritional intake to promote wound healing, and achieve relief from pain and discomfort.

Nursing Diagnoses

- Altered nutrition: less than body requirements related to oral pain, difficulty swallowing, surgical resection, and radiation treatment
- Pain related to the tumor
- Anxiety related to the diagnosis of cancer, uncertain future, and the potential for disfiguring surgery
- Impaired home maintenance management related to lack of knowledge of the disease process and therapeutic regimen, and unavailability of a support system

Nursing Interventions

The nurse has a significant role in early detection and treatment of carcinoma of the oral cavity. Inspection of a patient's oral cavity to detect suspicious lesions should be included in a routine physical examination.

Preoperative care for the patient who is having radical neck dissection involves consideration of the patient's physical and psychosocial needs (see the nursing care plan for the patient after a radical neck dissection in Lewis/Collier/Heitkemper, *Medical-Surgical*

Nursing, edition 4, p.1148). Special preparation emphasizes oral hygiene.

Postoperative care focuses on maintenance of a patent airway, including tracheostomy care and observing for signs of respiratory distress.

- Oral hygiene decreases the probability of infection, with the patient needing proper positioning to prevent aspiration (lying on the side or supine with the head turned to one side). The dressing should be observed for signs of hemorrhage or infection.
- Malnourishment delays wound healing; tube feedings may be started with surgery.
- The patient may need alternate forms of communication such as chalkboard or pad and pencil. Allow for personal verbalization of feelings regarding surgery. Obtain psychiatric referral for prolonged or severe depression.
- Facial disfigurement and other mutilating aspects of radical head and neck surgery may have a major long-term impact on the patient's body image and lifestyle, which may include learning to swallow again, altered physical appearance, taste and sensation changes, speech therapy, and reconstruction.

Patient Teaching
- Teach correct oral hygiene and dental care and encourage the patient to seek preventive dental care.
- Educate about predisposing factors.
- Instruct the patient to examine the mouth and to recognize danger signs of oral cancer. If any of these signs are present, the patient should be instructed to visit a physician. The danger signs are as follows:
  1. Unexplained pain or soreness in the mouth
  2. Unusual bleeding from the oral cavity
  3. Dysphagia
  4. Swelling or lump in the neck
  5. Any ulcerative lesion that does not heal within 2 to 3 weeks
- In the postoperative period, provide information about measures to help improve appearance, such as wearing clothes with high collars and wearing accessories that draw attention away from the neck.
- Answer questions honestly about body image and assure the patient of his/her self-worth.

The patient is often discharged with a tracheostomy and gastrostomy tube. The patient and family need to be taught how to manage these tubes and who to call if there are problems. Initially, home health care may be needed to evaluate the family or the patient's ability to perform self-care activities.

OSTEOARTHRITIS

Definition/Description

Osteoarthritis (OA), also known as degenerative joint disease (DJD), is a slowly progressive disorder of mobile joints, particularly weight-bearing articulations, and is characterized by degeneration of articular cartilage. The spectrum of disease severity is wide ranging—from annoying and uncomfortable symptoms to significantly disabling disease.

OA may occur as a primary idiopathic or secondary disorder. The cause of primary OA is unknown. Although both are influenced by multiple factors (e.g., metabolic, genetic, chemical), secondary OA has an identifiable precipitating event, such as previous trauma, infection, or congenital deformities, that is believed to predispose the person to later degenerative changes.

The most significant risk factor for OA is age. It is estimated that nearly one third of all adults have radiologic evidence of this disease, with an increasing incidence of 60% to 80% by age 60. Under 55 years of age, men and women are affected equally. In older individuals, hip OA is more common in men, whereas OA of the interphalangeal joints and the thumb base is more common in women.

Pathophysiology

Predisposing factors such as excessive use of or stress on a joint accelerate osteoarthritic changes, and genetic factors influence the development of Heberden's nodes. Other factors that influence the development of OA include congenital structural defects (e.g., Legg Calvé-Perthes disease), metabolic disturbances (e.g., diabetes mellitus), repeated intraarticular hemorrhage (e.g., hemophilia), neuropathic arthropathies, and inflammatory and septic arthritis.

Degenerative changes over time cause the normally smooth, white, translucent joint cartilage to become yellow and opaque, with rough surfaces and areas of *malacia* (softening). As the cartilage breaks down, fissures may appear and fragments of cartilage become loose. Secondary inflammation of the synovial membrane may follow.

Deterioration of cartilage is an active process. DNA synthesis, which is normally absent in adult articular cartilage, is active in OA tissue and appears to be directly proportional to disease severity.

Clinical Manifestations

Constitutional symptoms such as fatigue or fever are not present in OA. Other organ involvement is absent, which is an important difference between OA and inflammatory joint disorders such as rheumatoid arthritis (see Table 41).

Joints. Articular manifestations are related to the joint involved. The patient has pain on motion and weight-bearing that is generally relieved by rest. In advanced disease, sleep may be disrupted by night pain. Increasing pain is accompanied by progressive loss of function. Overall body coordination and posture may be affected as a result of the pain and loss of mobility. Advanced disease is complicated by gross deformity and *subluxation* (partial dislocation) caused by deterioration of cartilage, collapse of subchondral bone, and extensive bony overgrowth.

- Joints are usually affected asymmetrically. The joints most frequently involved are the distal and first interphalangeal joint(s) of the fingers, hips, knees, and lower lumbar and cervical vertebrae.

Nodules. *Heberden's nodes* are common, particularly in women with primary OA. These nodes are reactive bony overgrowths located at the distal interphalangeal joints. *Bouchard's nodes,* seen less commonly in OA, involve the proximal interphalangeal joints. Heberden's nodes and Bouchard's nodes may be seen with redness, swelling, tenderness, and aching. They often begin in one finger and spread to others. Although there is usually no significant loss of function, people are often distressed by the resulting disfigurement of their hands.

Hips. OA of the hips may be extremely disabling. Congenital or structural abnormalities are frequent causes. Sitting down is difficult, as is rising from a chair when the hips are lower than the knees. Eventually, loss of range of motion (ROM) is significant, with marked limitation of extension and internal rotation.

Knees. Softening of the posterior surface of the patella (chondromalacia patellae) is seen most commonly in young people. Degeneration of the weight-bearing surfaces of the femoral and tibial condyles is usually seen in older women and is associated with limitation of motion, crepitus, and flexion deformity.

Vertebral column. OA in the spine may produce localized symptoms of stiffness and pain. Herniation of the degenerating intervertebral disks causes muscle spasm or radicular pain.

Diagnostic Studies

- X-rays of involved joints show joint space narrowing, bony sclerosis, spur formation, and in some cases subluxation.
- Erythrocyte sedimentation rate (ESR) is normal except in instances of erosive OA, when moderate elevation may be noted.
- Synovial fluid aspirated from an involved joint may be increased in volume but is clear yellow and viscous. Fluid analysis reveals little or no sign of inflammation.

Table 41   Comparison of Rheumatoid Arthritis and Osteoarthritis

Parameter	Rheumatoid arthritis	Osteoarthritis
Age	Young and middle-aged	Usually >40 yr
Gender	Female more often than male	Same incidence
Weight	Weight loss	Usually overweight
Illness	Systemic manifestations	Local joint manifestations
Affected joints	PIPs, MCPs, MTPs, wrists, elbows, shoulders, knees, hips, cervical spine	DIPs, first CMCs, thumbs, first MTPs, knees, spine, hips
	Usually bilateral	Asymmetric, one or more joints
Effusions	Common	Uncommon
Nodules	Present	Heberden's nodes
Synovial fluid	Inflammatory	Noninflammatory
X-rays	Osteoporosis, narrowing, erosions	Osteophytes, subchondral cysts, sclerosis
Anemia	Common	Uncommon
Rheumatoid factor	Positive	Negative
Sedimentation rate	Elevated	Normal except in erosive osteoarthritis

CMC, Carpometacarpal; *DIP,* distal interphalangeal; *MCP,* metacarpophalangeal; *MTP,* metatarsophalangeal; *PIP,* proximal interphalangeal.

Therapeutic Management

There are no specific therapies for the management of OA. Therapy is aimed at pain control, prevention of progression and disability, and restoration of joint function. Once the diagnosis is confirmed, the patient should be assured that OA is likely to remain confined to a few joints and does not generally cause crippling. However, if joint destruction is extensive and pain is severe, surgery may be an option.

Pharmacologic Management

Aspirin is the most commonly used drug. It is generally prescribed in larger than usual doses and is given on a regular basis. In addition to relieving pain, aspirin reduces inflammation and consequently reduces swelling, stiffness, and possibly joint damage. Nonsteroidal antiinflammatory drugs (NSAIDs) are particularly beneficial for persons who are intolerant of aspirin or who do not respond adequately. Intraarticular injections of corticosteroids are used to treat a symptomatic flare. Systemic use of corticosteroids should be avoided because it may accelerate the disease process.

Nutritional Management

There is no specific diet except one that maintains optimal health. If a patient is overweight, a weight-reduction program becomes an important part of the total treatment plan. Body weight is magnified five times through the hips and three times through the knees. The additional strain of extra pounds can greatly increase pain and loss of function. In addition, heavy thighs lead to malalignment at the knee, increasing wear on the medial aspect.

Nursing Management

Goals

The patient with OA will balance rest and activity, use joint protection measures to improve activity tolerance, modify the home and work environment to include work-saving and joint-protecting assistive devices, use pharmacologic and nonpharmacologic pain management techniques to achieve satisfactory pain control, and perform ROM, muscle-strengthening, and aerobic exercise regularly.

Nursing Diagnoses

- Pain related to physical activity and lack of knowledge of pain self-management techniques
- Sleep pattern disturbance related to pain
- Impaired physical mobility related to weakness, stiffness, and/or pain on ambulation
- Self-care deficit related to joint deformity and pain with activity
- Altered nutrition: more than body requirements related to intake in excess of energy output

- Self-esteem disturbance related to changing social and work roles

Nursing Interventions

Prevention of primary OA is not possible; however, preventive education may include elimination of excessive strain on joints by reduction of occupational and recreational hazards and nutritional counseling for weight reduction. Community education may include proper body mechanics of lifting and good posture. Athletic instruction and physical fitness programs should include safety measures that protect and reduce trauma to the joint structures. Congenital conditions, such as Legg-Calvé-Perthes disease, that are known predisposing factors should be treated promptly.

The person is most troubled by pain, stiffness, limitation of function, and the frustration of coping with these physical difficulties on a daily basis. The older adult may believe that OA is an inevitable part of the aging process and that nothing can be done to ease the discomfort and related disability.

- The hospital or home health nurse should assist the patient with activities of daily living as necessary and help the patient plan rest periods during the day. The patient needs sufficient time to move stiff, painful joints, especially when arising in the morning or after any period of sustained inactivity. Proper body alignment should be maintained at all times.
- Safety measures in the home and work environment are important. These measures include removing scatter rugs, providing rails at stairs and bathtub, using night-lights, and wearing well-fitting supportive shoes. Assistive devices such as canes, walkers, elevated toilet seats, and grab bars reduce joint load and promote safety.
- Splints may be prescribed to rest and stabilize painful or inflamed joints. Soft collars and/or cervical traction may be used at home for cervical OA. Stiffness and pain of the hands can be relieved by warm water soaking, contrast baths, or paraffin. If swelling is more diffuse, stretch gloves can be worn at night to provide relief.
- Sexual counseling helps the patient and loved one to enjoy physical closeness by learning to adapt positions, alter timing, and increase awareness of the partner's needs.
- Nonpharmacologic techniques such as meditation, relaxation, and transcutaneous electric nerve stimulation (TENS) are particularly suited to chronic pain management. The nurse should be open to helping the patient and family develop creative new approaches to pain relief.
- The nurse assists the patient and family in overcoming feelings of helplessness and encourages active participation in managing chronic symptoms. The correct combination of joint pro-

tection, exercise (ROM, isotonic, and isometric), heat and cold therapy, and medication can restore self-esteem and improve physical functioning. Benefits exist with an aerobic exercise program such as walking or aquatics.

Patient Teaching

Teaching should include information about the nature and treatment of the disease, pain management, correct posture and body mechanics, correct use of assistive devices such as a cane or walker, principles of joint protection and energy conservation, and a therapeutic exercise program. Home management goals must be individualized to meet the patient's needs, and family and social supports should be included in goal setting and education.

OSTEOMALACIA

Definition/Description

Osteomalacia is an uncommon disorder of adult bone associated with vitamin D deficiency, which results in decalcification and softening of bone. This disease is the same as rickets in children except that the epiphyseal growth plates are closed in the adult.

- Vitamin D is required for absorption of calcium from the intestines. Insufficient vitamin D intake can interfere with the normal mineralization of bone, causing failure or insufficient calcification of bone, which results in bone softening and deformities.

Pathophysiology

Etiologic factors include lack of exposure to ultraviolet rays, GI malabsorption, chronic diarrhea, pregnancy, and kidney disease.

Clinical Manifestations

The most common clinical feature is persistent skeletal pain, especially while bearing weight. Other clinical manifestations include low back pain, progressive muscular weakness, weight loss, and progressive deformities of the spine (kyphosis) or extremities. Fractures are common and demonstrate delayed healing.

Diagnostic Studies

Laboratory findings include decreased serum calcium and phosphorus levels and elevated serum alkaline phosphatase. X-ray examination may demonstrate the effects of generalized bone demineralization, especially loss of calcium in the bones of the pelvis and the presence of associated bone deformity.

- Looser's transformation zones (ribbons of decalcification in bone that are seen on x-ray) are diagnostic of osteomalacia. Significant osteomalacia may exist without demonstrable x-ray changes.

Therapeutic Management

Therapeutic management is directed toward correction of the underlying cause. Vitamin D is usually supplemented, and the patient often shows a dramatic response. Calcium and phosphorus intake may also be supplemented.

Nursing Management

For nursing management, see Paget's Disease, therapeutic and nursing management, p. 436.

OSTEOMYELITIS

Definition/Description

Osteomyelitis is a bone infection caused by direct or indirect invasion by a microorganism. In children the long bones are most commonly affected, whereas in adults the vertebrae are more commonly affected. The course and virulence of osteomyelitis are influenced by the blood supply to the affected bone.

Pathophysiology

Direct-entry results from contamination associated with an open fracture or surgical implementation. *Indirect-entry* (hematogenous) results from a blood-borne infection from a distant site such as the teeth, infected tonsils, or furuncles. The most common infecting organism is *Staphylococcus aureus.*

After gaining entrance to the bone, the bacteria lodge in an area of bone (usually the metaphysis) in which circulation is slow. Bacteria grow, resulting in an increase in pressure, which eventually leads to ischemia and vascular compromise. Once ischemia occurs, the bone dies.

Sequestra, areas of devitalized bone, form havens for bacteria, and chronic osteomyelitis develops. The sequestra enlarge and serve as a source of bacteria for metastasis to other sites, including the lungs and brain. Unless resolved naturally or surgically, the necrotic sequestrum may develop a sinus tract, resulting in chronic wound drainage.

Clinical Manifestations

Chronic osteomyelitis can represent either a continuous persistent problem or a process of exacerbations and quiescence. It results from inadequately treated acute osteomyelitis. Pus accumulates, causing ischemia of the bone. Over time, granulation tissue turns to scar tissue. This avascular scar tissue provides an ideal site for bacterial growth and is impenetrable to antibiotics.

- A potentially fatal complication is the development of overwhelming sepsis from the spread of bacteria to other sites.
- Pathologic fractures may occur because of weakened, devitalized bone.
- Soft tissue and bone healing occur slowly in the presence of infection, and subsequent deformity of the extremity may develop.

Diagnostic Studies

- Wound culture determines the causative organism. A bone or tissue biopsy may also be necessary to determine the causative agent.
- Blood cultures are frequently positive, with an elevated leukocyte count and sedimentation rate also found.
- Radionuclide bone scans can establish the diagnosis within 24 to 72 hours. MRI may be used to help identify the boundaries of the infection.

Therapeutic Management

Vigorous antibiotic therapy is the treatment of choice for *acute osteomyelitis,* as long as ischemia has not yet occurred. Wound cultures should be taken before antibiotic therapy is initiated so that specific antibiotic therapy can be determined. If antibiotic therapy is not started early, surgical debridement and decompression are necessary to relieve pressure within the bone and prevent ischemia. Some type of immobilization for the affected part is usually indicated.

Treatment for *chronic osteomyelitis* includes surgical removal of poorly vascularized tissue and dead bone as well as extended use of antibiotics. After surgical debridement, the wound may be closed, and a suction irrigation system for removal of any devitalized tissues is inserted. Regional perfusion involving constant irrigation of the affected bone with antibiotics may be initiated. Ciprofloxacin (Cipro) is frequently used and has good bone penetration. Hyperbaric O_2 therapy may be used as an adjunctive therapy where available.

- Skin and bone grafting may be necessary if destruction is extensive. If infection and bone destruction are extensive, amputation of the extremity may be necessary to preserve life (see Amputation, p. 617).

Nursing Management

Goals

The patient with osteomyelitis will have satisfactory pain and fever control, have no transmission of infection to other areas of the body, not experience any complications associated with osteomyelitis, follow the treatment plan, and maintain a positive outlook on the disease outcome.

See the nursing care plan for the patient with osteomyelitis in Lewis/Collier/Heitkemper, *Medical-Surgical Nursing,* edition 4, p. 1872.

Nursing Diagnoses/Collaborative Problems

- Risk for infection transmission related to contaminated wound drainage
- Altered comfort: fever related to infection
- Pain related to inflammatory process secondary to infection
- Ineffective individual coping related to isolation, hospitalization, immobility, perceived powerlessness, and uncertain outcome
- Ineffective management of therapeutic regimen related to lack of knowledge regarding long-term management of osteomyelitis
- Impaired physical mobility related to limited use of affected extremity secondary to pain and edema
- Potential complication: pathologic fracture of involved bone related to presence of weakened necrotic bone

Nursing Interventions

Although there is no method of preventing osteomyelitis, patients with artificial implants such as a total joint replacement or a metallic bone implant should be educated about methods to prevent osteomyelitis. Some physicians recommend prophylactic doses of antibiotics for procedures such as tooth cleaning, colonoscopy, or vaginal examinations.

- The involved extremity should be handled carefully to avoid excessive manipulation, which increases pain and can cause a pathologic fracture.
- Soiled dressings should be handled carefully to prevent cross contamination of the wound or spread of the infection to other patients. When the dressing is changed, sterile technique is essential.
- Good body alignment and frequent position changes prevent complications associated with immobility and promote comfort. Foot drop can develop quickly in the lower extremity if the foot is not correctly supported. A splint is frequently applied to the involved extremity in an attempt to maintain immobilization, support, and comfort.

- The patient should be instructed to avoid any activities, such as exercise or heat application, that increase circulation and serve as stimuli to the spread of infection.
- For patients who are frightened and discouraged because of the serious nature of the disease, pain, and the length and cost of treatment, continued psychologic support is an integral part of nursing management.

Patient Teaching

- If at home, the patient and family must be instructed on the proper care and management of the venous access device for delivering antibiotics. They must also be taught how to administer antibiotics.
- If there is an open wound, dressing changes may be necessary. The patient may require supplies and instruction on the technique.

OSTEOPOROSIS

Definition/Description

Osteoporosis is a condition in which total bone mass is decreased. It is a crippling, painful bone disease that is the major cause of fractures in postmenopausal women and older adults in general. Osteoporosis is increasing in incidence because more people are surviving to an older age. At least 15 million persons in the United States have some degree of osteoporosis.

Risk factors for osteoporosis are female gender, increasing age, Caucasian race, oophorectomy, prolonged immobility, and insufficient dietary calcium. Increased risk is associated with cigarette smoking and alcoholism.

Pathophysiology

Osteoporosis is eight times more common in women than in men for several reasons: (1) women tend to have lower calcium intake than men throughout their lives; (2) women have less bone mass because of their generally smaller frame size; (3) resorption begins at an earlier age in women and is accelerated at menopause; (4) pregnancy and breast-feeding deplete a woman's skeletal reserve unless calcium intake is adequate; and (5) longevity increases the likelihood of osteoporosis, and women generally live longer than men.

- Specific diseases associated with osteoporosis include intestinal malabsorption, kidney disease, rheumatoid arthritis, advanced alcoholism, cirrhosis of the liver, and diabetes mellitus. Many agents are known to decrease calcium retention, including corticosteroids, aluminum-containing antacids, caffeine, and nicotine. A genetic marker, the vitamin D receptor gene has been linked to bone density.

Peak bone mass is determined by a combination of four major factors: genetic makeup, nutrition, exercise, and hormone function. From age 40 to menopause, women lose approximately 0.3% to 0.5% of their cortical bone per year; this accelerates immediately after menopause and then declines again after 8 to 10 years. When bone loss (resorption) exceeds bone formation and bones fracture under common, everyday stress, the condition is known as *osteoporosis*.

Clinical Manifestations

Osteoporosis occurs most commonly in the bones of the spine, hips, and wrists. Over time, wedging and fractures of the vertebrae produce gradual loss of height, and a humped back known as *dowager's hump* or *kyphosis*. The usual first signs are back pain or spontaneous fractures.

Diagnostic Studies

Osteoporosis often goes unnoticed because it cannot be detected by x-ray until more than 25% to 40% of calcium in the bone is lost. It is usually evident when the patient is 60 to 65 years of age.

- Serum calcium, phosphorus, and alkaline phosphatase levels remain normal, although alkaline phosphatase may be elevated after a fracture.

Therapeutic and Nursing Management

Management of patients includes calcium and vitamin D supplementation, estrogen replacement in postmenopausal women, and thiazide administration for renal calcium loss. If osteopenia is evident on bone densitometry, treatment with agents such as calcitonin or a bisphosphonate may be considered. Intermittent cyclical therapy with etidronate, which inhibits osteoclast-mediated bone resorption, significantly increases vertebral bone mass and decreases the rate of vertebral fracture in women with postmenopausal osteoporosis.

After menopause, estrogen replacement therapy is used to prevent osteoporosis. Estrogen attaches to specific receptors in bone cells, leading to decreased bone resorption. Estrogen replacement continues to have significant beneficial effects for 5 to 10 years after menopause.

Prevention of osteoporosis focuses on adequate calcium intake (1000 mg/day in premenopausal women and postmenopausal women taking estrogen, and 1500 mg/day in postmenopausal women who are not receiving supplemental estrogen) and regular exercise to strengthen bones. If dietary intake of calcium is inadequate, supplemental calcium should be taken. Calcium supplementation inhibits age-related bone loss; however, no new bone is formed.

The same measures used to prevent osteoporosis, such as weight-bearing exercise and adequate calcium intake, are also beneficial in treating osteoporosis. Although loss of bone cannot be significantly reversed, further loss can be prevented if a three-part program of estrogen replacement, exercise, and calcium is followed.

Efforts are made to keep patients with osteoporosis ambulatory to prevent further loss of bone mass as a result of immobility. Treatment also involves protecting areas of potential pathologic fractures; for example, a corset can be used to prevent vertebral collapse.

OTITIS MEDIA

Definition/Description

Otitis media is usually an acute childhood disease associated with colds, sore throats, and blockage of the eustachian tube. It is the most common problem of the middle ear. Untreated or repeated attacks of acute otitis media may lead to chronic otitis media. Chronic infection of the middle ear is more common in the person who experienced episodes of acute otitis media in early childhood.

Pathophysiology

Although most patients have mixed infections, bacteria are the predominant etiologic agents. Because the mucous membrane is continuous, both the middle ear and the air cells of the mastoid can be involved in the chronic infectious process. Organisms involved in chronic otitis media include *Staphylococcus aureus,* streptococci, *Proteus mirabilis, Pseudomonas aeruginosa, and Escherichia coli.*

Untreated conditions can result in eardrum perforation and the formation of a cholesteatoma, a cystic mass composed of epithelial cells and cholesterol. Enzymes produced by it may destroy adjacent bones, including ossicles. Additional complications of chronic otitis media include sensorineural deafness, facial weakness, lateral sinus thrombosis, brain or subdural abscess, and meningitis.

Clinical Manifestations

Acute otitis media. Pain, fever, malaise, headache, and reduced hearing are evident.

Chronic otitis media. Purulent, foul-smelling discharge, accompanied by hearing loss and occasionally by ear pain, nausea, and episodes of dizziness is evident. Additional complaints may include hearing loss as a result of ossicle destruction, tympanic membrane perforation, or accumulation of fluid in the middle ear space. Chronic otitis media is usually painless. However, if pain is present, it indicates fluid under pressure.

Diagnostic Studies
- Otoscopic examination for perforated eardrum
- Culture and sensitivity tests to identify the infectious agent
- X-rays, polytomography, or CT scan of temporal bone

Therapeutic Management
The aim of treatment is to rid the middle ear of infection. Systemic antibiotic therapy based on sensitivity testing is usually initiated. In addition, the patient with chronic infection may need to undergo frequent evacuation of drainage and debris in an outpatient setting. Antibiotic eardrops and 2% acetic acid drops are used to reduce infection. If there is recurrence, the patient may be treated with parenteral antibiotics.

One surgical procedure for acute otitis media is myringotomy, which involves an incision in the tympanum to release increased ear pressure and exudate. Another is tympanoplasty, which restores middle ear structure and function when chronic tympanic membrane perforation occurs.

Since the advent of antibiotics, the incidence of severe and prolonged infections of the middle ear have been greatly reduced. Prompt treatment of an episode of acute otitis media generally prevents spontaneous perforation of the tympanic membrane.

Nursing Management
Goals
The patient with otitis media should verbalize satisfaction with pain relief, identify factors that increase risk of injury, and postoperatively have adequate knowledge to take care of self and identify complications associated with untreated otitis media.

Nursing Diagnoses/Collaborative Problems
- Impaired verbal communication related to hearing loss
- Risk for injury related to decreased hearing acuity
- Pain related to surgical incision
- Potential complication: bleeding from operative site

Nursing Interventions
Following a tympanoplasty, postoperative care includes the following:
- Assess the degree of pain to plan appropriate intervention.

- Assess and monitor dizziness.
- Instruct the patient to avoid blowing the nose because this causes increased pressure in the eustachian tube and middle ear and could dislodge the graft to the tympanum. Coughing and sneezing can cause a similar disruption.
- Teach signs and symptoms of complications associated with tympanoplasty.
- Monitor the operative site for unusual bleeding and/or discharge.

OVARIAN CANCER

Definition/Description

Ovarian cancer is the most deadly gynecologic malignancy in the United States; most patients with ovarian cancer have advanced disease at diagnosis. This disease occurs commonly in women between the ages of 40 and 65 and has a high familial incidence.

Cancer of the ovary seems to be linked to multiparity, infertility, advanced age, long history of menstrual irregularities, and higher socioeconomic group. Breast-feeding, multiple pregnancies, oral contraceptives, and early age at first birth seem to reduce the risk of ovarian cancer.

Pathophysiology

From 80% to 85% of ovarian cancers are epithelial carcinomas. Germ cell tumors account for another 10%. Histologic grading is a very important prognostic determinant (see Cancer, p. 88).

Ovarian cancer has two patterns of metastasis: lymphatic and direct spread. Primary lymphatic drainage of the ovary is through the retroperitoneal nodes surrounding the renal hilum; secondary drainage is through the iliac lymphatics; and tertiary drainage is through the inguinal lymphatics. Ovarian cancer also metastasizes directly to the abdominal cavity, the diaphragm, and the omentum.

Clinical Manifestations

In its early stages ovarian cancer is asymptomatic. As the malignancy grows, a variety of symptoms, such as an increase in abdominal girth, bowel and bladder dysfunction, pain, menstrual irregularities, and ascites can occur.

Diagnostic Studies

CA-125 is a specific marker for ovarian cancer. It is useful both in detecting disease in its early stages and in following the response to treatment. CA-125 is positive in 80% of women with epithelial ovarian cancer with blood levels decreasing as the cancer cells decrease.

- Bimanual pelvic examination, ultrasonography, and laparoscopy remain the most reliable diagnostic tools.
- Ultrasound, CT scan, and/or laparoscopy are performed to establish the diagnosis and degree of metastasis.

Therapeutic Management

The usual treatment for stage I disease (limited to the ovaries) is a total abdominal hysterectomy and bilateral salpingo-oophorectomy, with removal of as much of the tumor as possible (i.e., tumor debulking). Ascitic fluid is submitted for cytologic study, and appropriate biopsies are performed to determine the stage of the disease. The addition of chemotherapy or the instillation of intraperitoneal radioisotopes is usually done for stage I disease (see Chemotherapy, p. 631).

The patient with stage II disease (limited to the true [minor] pelvis) may receive external abdominal and pelvic radiation, intraperitoneal radiation, or systemic combined chemotherapy after tumor-reducing surgery. After completion of systemic chemotherapy in patients who are clinically free of symptoms, a "second-look" surgical procedure is often performed to determine whether there is any evidence of disease. This option does not necessarily improve the outcome. If no disease is found, the chemotherapy is stopped, and the patient is monitored for recurrent disease.

Chemotherapy (e.g., cisplatin, carboplatin) is one of the mainstays of treatment for stage III (limited to the abdominal cavity) and stage IV (distant metastases) disease. Surgical debulking is often done in conjunction with chemotherapy for advanced disease. Intraperitoneal chemotherapy may be used for patients who have minimal residual disease after surgery.

- Irradiation and chemotherapy may be used to shrink the size of the tumor and to relieve pressure and pain.

Nursing Management

For nursing management, see Surgical Procedures Involving the Female Reproductive System, p. 677.

PAGET'S DISEASE

Definition/Description

Paget's disease (osteitis deformans) is a skeletal bone disorder in which there is excessive bone resorption followed by replacement of normal marrow by vascular fibrous connective tissue. It occurs most often after the fourth decade of life and most commonly in men. The cause of Paget's disease is unknown.

Pathophysiology

The disease is characterized by deformities of bone caused by unexplained abnormal remodeling and resorption of bone, fibrotic changes, and remodeling with structurally uneven bone. Regions of the skeleton commonly affected are the pelvis, long bones, spine, ribs, and cranium.

Clinical Manifestations

In mild forms of Paget's disease, patients may remain free of symptoms, and the disease may be discovered incidentally on x-ray.

- Initial manifestations are usually an insidious development of skeletal pain (which may progress to severe intractable pain), complaints of fatigue, and progressive development of bowlegs.
- Pathologic fracture is the most common complication and may be the first indication of the disease. Other complications include malignant osteosarcoma, chondrosarcoma, or fibrosarcoma.

Diagnostic Studies

Diagnostic studies reveal markedly elevated serum alkaline phosphatase levels in advanced forms of the disease. X-rays reveal that the normal contour of the affected bone is curved and the bone cortex is thickened, especially in weight-bearing bones and the cranium.

Therapeutic and Nursing Management

Therapeutic management is limited to symptomatic and supportive care and correction of secondary deformities by either surgical implementation or braces. Bone resorption, relief of acute symptoms, and lowering the serum alkaline phosphatase levels may be significantly influenced by the administration of calcitonin, which inhibits osteoclastic activity. Resistance to calcitonin therapy may occur after 2 years of use. Diphosphonates and their derivatives also inhibit the activity of Paget's disease.

- Radiation therapy and local surgical procedures such as periosteal stripping may be used for control of the patient's pain.

A firm mattress should be used to provide back support and to relieve pain. The patient may be required to wear a corset or light brace to relieve back pain and provide support when in the upright position. The patient should be proficient in the correct application of such devices and know how to examine areas of the skin regularly for friction damage.

- Activities such as lifting and twisting should be discouraged. Good body mechanics are essential.
- Analgesics and muscle relaxants may be administered to relieve pain.
- A properly balanced nutritional program is very important in the management of metabolic disorders of bone, especially pertaining to vitamin D, calcium, and protein, which are necessary to ensure the availability of the components for bone formation.

Because metabolic bone disorders increase the possibility of pathologic fractures, the nurse must use extreme caution when the patient is turned or moved. It is important to keep the patient as active as possible to retard demineralization of bone resulting from disuse or extended immobilization. A supervised exercise program is an essential part of the treatment program. If the patient's condition permits, ambulation without causing fatigue must be continued.

- Prevention measures such as patient education, use of an assistive device, and environmental changes should be actively pursued to prevent falls and subsequent fractures.

PANCREATITIS, ACUTE

Definition/Description

Acute pancreatitis is an acute inflammatory process of the pancreas with the degree of inflammation varying from mild edema to severe hemorrhagic necrosis. Some patients recover completely, others have recurring attacks, and chronic pancreatitis develops in others. Acute pancreatitis can be life-threatening.

Pathophysiology

Many factors can cause injury to the pancreas. The primary etiologic factors are biliary tract disease and alcoholism. Other causes of acute pancreatitis include trauma (postsurgical, abdominal); viral infections (mumps); penetrating duodenal ulcer; cysts; abscesses;

cystic fibrosis; certain drugs (corticosteroids, sulfonamides, non-steroidal antiinflammatory drugs [NSAIDs]); and metabolic disorders such as hyperparathyroidism and renal failure. In some cases the cause is not known.

The most common pathogenic mechanism is believed to be autodigestion of the pancreas. The etiologic factors cause injury to pancreatic cells or activation of the pancreatic enzymes in the pancreas rather than in the intestine.

The pathophysiologic involvement of acute pancreatitis ranges from edematous pancreatitis, which is mild and self-limiting, to necrotizing pancreatitis, in which the degree of necrosis correlates with the severity of manifestations.

Clinical Manifestations

Abdominal pain is the predominant symptom of acute pancreatitis. The pain is usually located in the left upper quadrant but may be in the midepigastrium. It commonly radiates to the back because of the retroperitoneal location of the pancreas. The pain has a sudden onset and is described as severe, deep, piercing, and continuous or steady. It is aggravated by eating and frequently has its onset when the patient is recumbent; it is not relieved by vomiting. The pain may be accompanied by flushing, cyanosis, and dyspnea. The patient may assume various positions involving flexion of the spine in an attempt to relieve the severe pain.

- Other manifestations include nausea and vomiting, low-grade fever, leukocytosis, hypotension, tachycardia, and jaundice. Abdominal tenderness with muscle guarding is common. Bowel sounds may be decreased or absent. The lungs are frequently involved, with crackles present.
- Intravascular damage from circulating trypsin may cause areas of cyanosis or greenish to yellow-brown discoloration of the abdominal wall. Other areas of ecchymoses are the flanks (*Grey Turner's spots* or *sign,* a bluish flank discoloration) and the periumbilical area (*Cullen's sign,* a bluish periumbilical discoloration).

Complications

Local complications of acute pancreatitis are pseudocyst and abscess.

- A pancreatic *pseudocyst* is a cavity continuous with or surrounding the outside of the pancreas. Symptoms are abdominal pain, palpable epigastric mass, nausea and vomiting, and anorexia. The serum amylase level frequently remains elevated. Pseudocysts usually resolve spontaneously within a few weeks, but they may burst, perforating the pancreas and causing peritonitis, or they may rupture into the stomach or duodenum.

- A pancreatic *abscess* is a large fluid-containing cavity within the pancreas. It results from extensive necrosis in the pancreas. It may become infected or perforate into adjacent organs. Manifestations include upper abdominal pain, abdominal mass, high fever, and leukocytosis. Pancreatic abscesses require prompt surgical drainage to prevent sepsis. Shock may occur because of hemorrhage into the pancreas or toxemia from the activated pancreatic enzymes.

Systemic complications of acute pancreatitis are pulmonary complications (pleural effusion, atelectasis, and pneumonia) and tetany resulting from hypocalcemia. When hypocalcemia occurs, it is a sign of severe disease. It is due in part to the combining of calcium and fatty acids during fat necrosis.

Diagnostic Studies

- Serum amylase, the most commonly used diagnostic measure, is elevated.
- Serum lipase and urinary amylase are elevated.
- Other laboratory abnormalities include hyperglycemia, hyperlipidemia, and hypocalcemia.
- Abdominal x-ray and ultrasound scan of the pancreas may also be performed.

Therapeutic Management

Objectives of therapeutic management of acute pancreatitis include relief of pain, prevention or alleviation of shock, reduction of pancreatic secretions, control of fluid and electrolyte imbalance, prevention or treatment of infections, and removal of the precipitating cause, if possible.

A primary consideration is the relief and control of pain. Meperidine (Demerol) is preferred because it causes less spasm of the smooth muscles of the ducts than morphine. It may be combined with an antispasmodic. If shock is present, blood volume replacements and expanders such as dextran or albumin may be given.

It is important to reduce or suppress pancreatic enzymes to decrease stimulation of the pancreas and allow it to rest. The patient is allowed to take nothing by mouth (NPO). NG suction may be used to reduce vomiting and gastric distention and to prevent gastric digestive juices from entering the duodenum. Certain drugs may also be used for this purpose.

- Inflamed and necrotic pancreatic tissue is a good medium for bacterial growth. Antibiotic therapy should be instituted early if infection occurs.
- Surgical intervention may be indicated when the diagnosis is uncertain and in patients who do not respond to conservative therapy. Surgery is necessary for an abscess, acute pseudocyst,

and severe peritonitis. Percutaneous drainage of a pseudocyst can be performed, and a drainage tube is left in place. Surgical treatment of associated biliary tract disease may be necessary.

Several different drugs may be used in the treatment of both acute and chronic pancreatitis (see Table 41-18 in Lewis/Collier/Heitkemper, *Medical-Surgical Nursing,* edition 4, p. 1290).

Nursing Management

Goals

The patient with acute pancreatitis will have relief of pain, return of fluid and electrolyte balance, minimal to no complications, and no recurrent attacks.

See the nursing care plan for the patient with acute pancreatitis in Lewis/Collier/Heitkemper, *Medical-Surgical Nursing,* edition 4, p. 1292.

Nursing Diagnoses/Collaborative Problems

- Pain related to distention of the pancreas, peritoneal irritation, obstruction of the biliary tract, and ineffective pain and comfort measures
- Fluid volume deficit related to nausea, vomiting, NG suction, and restricted oral intake
- Altered nutrition: less than body requirements related to anorexia, dietary restrictions, nausea, loss of nutrients from vomiting, and impaired digestion resulting in decreased use of nutrients
- Altered oral mucous membranes related to NG tube and NPO status
- Ineffective management of therapeutic regimen related to lack of knowledge of preventive measures, diet restrictions, and follow-up care
- Potential complication: shock related to destruction of blood vessel walls by proteolytic enzymes
- Potential complication: fluid and electrolyte imbalance related to loss of fluids into peritoneal cavity

Nursing Interventions

The nurse should encourage the early diagnosis and treatment of biliary tract disease such as cholelithiasis. The patient should be encouraged to eliminate alcohol intake, especially if there have been any previous episodes of pancreatitis. Attacks of pancreatitis become milder or disappear with the discontinuance of alcohol use.

Because abdominal pain is a prominent symptom of pancreatitis, a major focus of nursing care is the relief of pain. Giving the prescribed medications before the pain becomes too severe makes the medication more effective. Therefore it is helpful to ascertain how long the pain medication provides relief. Measures such as comfortable positioning, frequent changes in position, and relief of nausea and vomiting assist in reducing the restlessness that usually accompanies the pain.

- Some patients experience lessened pain by assuming positions that flex the trunk and draw the knees up to the abdomen. A side-lying position with the head elevated 45 degrees decreases tension on the abdomen and may help ease the pain. It is important to control pain and restlessness because they increase body metabolism and subsequent stimulation of pancreatic secretions.
- Nursing measures for the patient who is on NPO status or has an NG tube should include frequent oral and nasal care to relieve the dryness of the mouth and nose.
- Observation for electrolyte imbalances is important because frequent vomiting, along with gastric suction, may result in decreased chloride, sodium, and potassium levels. It is important to observe for symptoms of hypocalcemia such as tetany and numbness or tingling around the lips and in the fingers. The patient should be assessed for a positive Chvostek's or Trousseau's sign.
- Observation for fever and other manifestations of infection is important. Respiratory infections are common because of the retroperitoneal fluid raising the diaphragm, which causes the patient to take shallow, guarded abdominal breaths. Prevention of respiratory infections includes turning, coughing, deep breathing, and assuming a semi-Fowler's position.

Most patients will need home care follow-up. The patient may have lost physical reserve and muscle strength. Physical therapy may be needed. Continued care to prevent infection and detect any complications is important.

Patient Teaching

- Counseling regarding abstinence from alcohol is important to prevent future attacks of acute pancreatitis and the development of chronic pancreatitis.
- Beverages containing caffeine should not be consumed.
- Because smoking and stressful situations can overstimulate the pancreas, they should be avoided.
- Dietary teaching should include restriction of fats because they stimulate the pancreas. Carbohydrates are less stimulating to the pancreas, so they should be encouraged. The patient should be instructed to avoid crash dieting and bingeing since these can precipitate attacks.
- The patient and family should be given instructions regarding the recognition and reporting of symptoms of infection, diabetes mellitus, or steatorrhea (foul-smelling, frothy stools). These changes indicate possible destruction of pancreatic tissue.

P

- The nurse should make sure the patient fully understands the prescribed regimen. Each aspect must be explained. The importance of taking required medications and following the recommended diet should be stressed.

PANCREATITIS, CHRONIC

Definition/Description
Chronic pancreatitis is progressive destruction of the pancreas, with fibrotic replacement of pancreatic tissue. Strictures and calcifications may also occur in the pancreas. Chronic pancreatitis may follow acute pancreatitis, but it may also occur in the absence of any history of an acute condition. In the United States chronic pancreatitis is found almost exclusively in alcoholics.

Pathophysiology
Chronic obstructive pancreatitis is associated with biliary disease. The most common cause is inflammation of the sphincter of Oddi associated with cholelithiasis. Cancer of the ampulla of Vater, duodenum, or pancreas is another cause.

Chronic calcifying pancreatitis is associated with inflammation and sclerosis that mainly occurs in the head of the pancreas and around the pancreatic ducts. The ducts are obstructed with protein precipitates that block the pancreatic duct and eventually calcify. This is followed by fibrosis and glandular atrophy. Pseudocysts and abscesses commonly develop. This type of chronic pancreatitis, the most common form, is also called alcohol-induced pancreatitis.

Clinical Manifestations
As with acute pancreatitis, a major manifestation of chronic pancreatitis is abdominal pain. The patient may have episodes of acute pain, but it usually is chronic (recurrent attacks at intervals of months or years). The attacks may become more and more frequent until they are almost constant, or they may diminish as the pancreatic fibrosis develops. The pain is located in the same areas as in acute pancreatitis but is usually described as a heavy, gnawing feeling or sometimes as burning and cramplike. The pain is not relieved with food or antacids.

- Other manifestations are symptoms of pancreatic insufficiency, including malabsorption with weight loss, constipation, mild jaundice with dark urine, steatorrhea, and diabetes mellitus. The steatorrhea may become quite severe with voluminous, foul-smelling, fatty stools. Urine and stool may be frothy. Some abdominal tenderness may be noted.

Diagnostic Studies

- Secretin stimulation test is the most useful test in diagnosing chronic pancreatitis.
- Serum amylase, bilirubin, and alkaline phosphatase levels are elevated.
- Mild leukocytosis and elevated sedimentation rate are present.
- Hyperglycemia is noted.
- Fatty stools (steatorrhea) are found in fecal fat determination, with neutral fat indicative of maldigestion.
- Arteriography and x-rays may demonstrate fibrosis and calcification.

Therapeutic and Nursing Management

When the patient with chronic pancreatitis is experiencing an acute attack, the therapeutic management is identical to that for acute pancreatitis. At other times the focus is on prevention of further attacks, relief of pain, and control of pancreatic exocrine and endocrine insufficiency. It sometimes takes large frequent doses of analgesics to relieve the pain, and narcotic addiction may become a problem.

- Treatment of chronic pancreatitis sometimes requires surgery. When biliary disease is present or if an obstruction or pseudocyst develops, surgery may be indicated. Other operations performed are procedures to divert bile flow or relieve ductal obstruction.
- Total pancreas transplantation and islet cell transplantation are experimental techniques currently being studied in clinical trials to provide long-term replacement of endocrine function.

PANCREATIC CANCER

Definition/Description

Carcinoma of the pancreas is the fourth leading cause of death from cancer in the United States. It is more common in men and in African-Americans. The risk increases with age, with the peak incidence occurring between 65 and 79 years of age.

The prognosis for a patient with cancer of the pancreas is poor. Most patients die within 5 to 12 months of the initial diagnosis, and the 5-year survival rate is very low (3%).

Pathophysiology

The cause of pancreatic cancer is unknown. There may be some relationship between cancer, diabetes mellitus, and chronic pancreatitis. It is not clear whether the cancer follows these diseases or whether these diseases occur as a result of pancreatic cancer.

Major risk factors seem to be cigarette smoking, high consumption of fat and meat, diabetes mellitus, and exposure to chemicals such as benzidine and coke. Pancreatic cancer develops twice as frequently in persons with a history of heavy cigarette use (more than two packs a day) as in nonsmokers.

Clinical Manifestations

Common manifestations include abdominal pain (dull, aching), anorexia, rapid and progressive weight loss, nausea, and jaundice.

Pain is very common and is related to the location of malignancy. Extreme unrelenting pain is related to extension of the cancer into the retroperitoneal tissues and nerve plexuses. The pain is frequently located in the upper abdomen or left hypochondrium and frequently radiates to the back. It is commonly related to eating and also occurs at night.

Diagnostic Studies

Better diagnostic measures are needed for detection of pancreatic cancer since current methods detect only advanced stages.

- Cytologic examination of the pancreatic juice may reveal malignant cells.
- The secretin test frequently results in a decreased volume of pancreatic juice, with normal bicarbonate and enzyme production.
- Carcinoembryonic antigen (CEA) is elevated in advanced disease, with CA 19-9 an even more specific tumor marker.
- Endoscopic retrograde cholangiopancreatography (ERCP) shows obstruction or narrowing of the pancreatic ducts.
- CT scan identifies a solid tumor mass.

Therapeutic Management

Surgery provides the most effective treatment of cancer of the pancreas. The classic surgery is a radical pancreaticoduodenectomy or Whipple's procedure. This surgery entails resection of the proximal pancreas (proximal pancreatectomy), the adjoining duodenum (duodenectomy), the distal portion of the stomach (partial gastrectomy), and the distal segment of the common bile duct. An anastomosis of the pancreatic duct, common bile duct, and stomach to the jejunum is done.

Radiation therapy alters survival rates very little but is effective for pain relief. External radiation is usually used, but implantation of internal radiation seeds into the tumor has also been used. Chemotherapy has limited success.

- Adjuvant therapy, which uses surgical resection, radiation, and chemotherapy, is believed to be the most effective way to manage the almost always fatal cancer of the pancreas (see Radiation Therapy, p. 675, and Chemotherapy, p. 631).

Nursing Management

Because the patient with carcinoma of the pancreas has many of the same problems as the patient with pancreatitis, nursing care includes the same measures (see Pancreatitis, Acute, p. 437).

- The nurse should provide symptomatic and supportive nursing care. Medications and comfort measures to relieve pain should be provided before the patient reaches the peak of pain.
- Psychologic support is essential, especially during times of anxiety or depression, which seem to occur frequently.
- Adequate nutrition is an important part of the care plan. Frequent and supplemental feedings may be necessary. Measures to stimulate the appetite as much as possible and to overcome anorexia and nausea and vomiting should be included.
- Because bleeding can result from impaired vitamin K production, the nurse should assess for bleeding from body orifices and mucous membranes.
- A significant component of nursing care is helping the patient and family or significant others through the grieving process.

PARKINSON'S DISEASE

Definition/Description

Parkinsonism is a syndrome that consists of slowness in the initiation and execution of movement *(bradykinesia)*, increased muscle tonus *(rigidity)*, tremor, and impaired postural reflexes. Parkinson's disease is a form of parkinsonism. About 1% of the population over the age of 50 years is affected. The disease shows no gender, socioeconomic, or cultural preference. The average age of the patient with Parkinson's disease is 65 years. There is no apparent genetic cause and no known cure. The disease rarely occurs in African-Americans.

Many other disorders resemble this disease, including drug-induced parkinsonism, postencephalitic parkinsonism, and arteriosclerotic parkinsonism. The pathophysiology of these disorders, with the exception of drug-induced parkinsonism, is damage or loss of the dopamine-producing cells of the substantia nigra, which leads to depletion of dopamine in the basal ganglia. Dopamine influences the initiation, modulation, and completion of movement and regulates unconscious autonomic movements. In cases of drug-induced parkinsonism the dopamine receptors in the brain are blocked.

Pathophysiology

There are many causes of parkinsonism. Encephalitis lethargica, or type A encephalitis, has been associated with the onset of parkinsonism. Parkinson-like symptoms have also occurred after intoxication with a variety of chemicals, including carbon monoxide, manganese (among copper miners), and an analogue of meperidine (MPTP). Drug-induced parkinsonism can follow reserpine, methyldopa, haloperidol, and phenothiazine therapy. Most patients with parkinsonism have the degenerative or idiopathic form, for which the term *Parkinson's disease* is usually reserved.

The pathology of Parkinson's disease is associated with degeneration of the dopamine-producing neurons in the substantia nigra of the midbrain. In Parkinson's disease the levels of dopamine-synthesizing enzymes and metabolites are reduced, and postmortem analysis shows loss of normal melanin pigment in the substantia nigra and a loss of neurons. In addition, deficient amounts of γ-aminobutyric acid (GABA), serotonin, and norepinephrine have been found in basal ganglia and in the substantia nigra.

Clinical Manifestations

Onset is gradual and insidious, with a gradual progression and a prolonged course. In the beginning stages, only a mild tremor, slight limp, or a decreased arm swing may be evident. Later the patient may have a shuffling, propulsive gait with arms flexed and loss of postural reflexes. In some patients there may be a slight change in speech patterns.

Tremor, often the first sign, may be minimal initially, so the patient is the only one who notices it. Parkinsonian tremor is more prominent at rest and is aggravated by emotional stress or increased concentration. The hand tremor is described as "pill rolling" because the thumb and forefinger appear to move in a rotary fashion as if rolling a pill, coin, or other small object. Tremor can involve the diaphragm, tongue, lips, and jaw.

Rigidity, the second sign of the classic triad of symptoms, is increased resistance to passive motion when the limbs are moved through their range of motion. Parkinsonian rigidity is typified by a jerky quality, as if there were intermittent catches in the movement of a cogwheel, when the joint is moved. This is called *cogwheel rigidity.*

Bradykinesia is particularly evident in the loss of automatic movements, which is secondary to the physical and chemical alteration of the basal ganglia. In the unaffected patient, automatic movements are involuntary and occur subconsciously, including blinking of the eyelids, swinging of the arms while walking, swallowing of saliva, self-expression with facial and hand movements, and minor movement of postural adjustment.

In addition, the patient lacks spontaneous activity, which accounts for the stooped posture, masked facies ("deadpan" expression), drooling of saliva, and shuffling gait. There is difficulty initiating movement. Movements such as getting out of a chair cannot be executed unless they are consciously willed.

Complications

Many of the complications are caused by the decomposition and loss of spontaneity of movement.

- Swallowing may become very difficult (dysphagia) in severe cases, leading to malnutrition or aspiration. General debilitation may lead to pneumonia, urinary tract infections, and skin breakdown.
- Mobility is greatly decreased. The gait slows, and turning is especially difficult. The posture is that of the "old man" image, with the head and trunk bent forward and the legs constantly flexed. The lack of mobility may lead to constipation, ankle edema, and, more seriously, contractures.
- Orthostatic hypotension may occur and, along with the loss of postural reflexes, may result in falls or other injury.
- Bothersome complications include seborrhea, excessive sweating, conjunctivitis, insomnia, incontinence, and depression.
- Many of the apparent complications of Parkinson's disease are side effects of prolonged medication therapy, particularly levodopa. Dyskinesias (e.g., athetosis of the neck) and weakness and akinesia (total immobility) may cause problems.

Diagnostic Studies

Because there is no specific diagnostic test for Parkinson's disease, the diagnosis is based solely on the patient's history and the clinical features.

- A firm diagnosis can be made only when there are at least two of the three characteristic signs of the classic triad: tremor, rigidity, and bradykinesia. Although dementia occurs in up to 40% of patients with Parkinson's disease, intellectual impairment does not occur in the majority of patients.
- Ultimate confirmation of Parkinson's disease is a positive response to antiparkinson medication.

Therapeutic Management

Because there is no cure for Parkinson's disease, management is aimed at relieving symptoms. Antiparkinson drugs either enhance dopamine secretion or supply it (dopaminergic), or they antagonize or block the effects of the overactive cholinergic neurons. The only other treatment for Parkinson's disease is cryothalamectomy or stereotaxic thalamotomy for correction of severe unilateral tremor.

Surgical treatment is most effective in younger patients. Transplantation of fetal tissue into the caudate nucleus in an attempt to provide viable dopamine-producing cells to the brain holds promise.

Pharmacologic Management

Drug therapy is aimed at correcting an imbalance of neurotransmitters within the CNS.

- Levodopa with carbidopa (Sinemet) is often the first drug to be used. Levodopa is a precursor of dopamine and is converted to dopamine in the basal ganglia. Sinemet is the preferred drug because it contains carbidopa, an enzyme that breaks down levodopa before it reaches the brain. This results in more levodopa reaching the brain.
- Bromocriptine is a dopamine agonist in that it activates dopamine receptors.
- Anticholinergic drugs act by decreasing the activity of acetylcholine (ACh), thus providing balance between cholinergic and dopaminergic actions.
- Antihistamines (e.g., diphenhydramine [Benadryl]) with anticholinergic properties are sometimes used to relieve tremor and rigidity.
- The antiviral agent amantadine (Symmetrel) is also effective although its exact mechanism of action is not known. Amantadine promotes the release of dopamine from neurons.

Nutritional Management

Diet is of major importance to avoid malnutrition and constipation. Patients who have dysphagia and bradykinesia need appetizing foods that are easily chewed and swallowed. The diet should contain adequate roughage and fruit to avoid constipation. Ample time should be planned for eating to avoid frustration and encourage independence.

Nursing Management

Goals

The patient with Parkinson's disease will maximize neurologic function, maintain independence in activities of daily living for as long as possible, and optimize psychosocial well-being.

See the nursing care plan for the patient with Parkinson's disease in Lewis/Collier/Heitkemper, *Medical-Surgical Nursing,* edition 4, p. 1779.

Nursing Diagnoses

- Impaired physical mobility related to rigidity, tremor, bradykinesia, and akinesia
- Altered nutrition: less than body requirements related to dysphagia
- Constipation related to immobility

- Sleep pattern disturbance related to medication side effects (e.g., hallucinations), anxiety, rigidity, and muscle discomfort
- Impaired verbal and and written communication related to dysarthria and tremor or bradykinesia
- Self-care deficit related to parkinsonian symptoms

Nursing Interventions

- Promotion of physical exercise and a well-balanced diet are major concerns for nursing care. Exercise can limit the consequences of decreased mobility such as muscle atrophy, contractures, and constipation. Overall muscle tone as well as specific exercises to strengthen muscles involved with speaking and swallowing should be included.
- Because Parkinson's disease is a chronic degenerative disorder with no acute exacerbations, nurses should note that health teaching and nursing care are directed toward maintenance of good health, encouragement of independence, and avoidance of complications such as contractures.

Patient Teaching

Problems secondary to bradykinesia can be alleviated by relatively simple measures.

- Instructions for patients who tend to "freeze" while walking include (1) consciously thinking about stepping over imaginary lines on the floor, (2) dropping rice kernels and stepping over them, (3) rocking from side to side, (4) lifting the toes when stepping, (5) taking one step backward and two steps forward. The patient should be assessed for the possibility of levodopa overdose because it is a common cause of akinesia "freezing."
- Getting out of a chair can be facilitated by using an upright chair with arms and placing its back legs on small (2-inch) blocks.
- Other aspects of the environment can be altered. Rugs and excess furniture can be removed to avoid stumbling.
- Clothing can be simplified by the use of slip-on shoes and Velcro hook-and-loop fasteners or zippers on clothing instead of buttons and hooks. An elevated toilet seat can facilitate getting on and off the toilet.
- The nurse should work closely with the patient's family in exploring creative adaptations that allow the greatest amount of independence and self-care.

Pelvic Inflammatory Disease

Definition/Description

Pelvic inflammatory disease is an infectious condition of the pelvic cavity that may involve the fallopian tubes (salpingitis), ovaries (oophoritis), pelvic peritoneum, and pelvic vascular system. The infection can be acute, subacute, or chronic.

Pathophysiology

The most frequent causative organisms of pelvic inflammatory disease (PID) are *Neisseria gonorrhoeae* and *Chlamydia trachomatis.* These organisms, as well as mycoplasma, streptococci, and anaerobes, may gain entrance to the pelvic cavity during sexual intercourse or after abortion, pelvic surgery, or childbirth. Users of intrauterine devices (IUDs) or women with multiple sexual partners have an increased risk of developing the condition. PID is a common complication of gonorrhea and chlamydial infections.

Once introduced, the infection spreads by two typical routes.

- One route is along the uterine endometrium to the tubes and into the peritoneum. Salpingitis, pelvic peritonitis, or tuboovarian abscess may result. The second route is primarily through the uterine or cervical lymphatics, across the parametrium, to the tubes or ovaries.

Clinical Manifestations

The patient with *acute PID* seeks medical attention because of crampy or continuous bilateral lower abdominal pain.

- In acute cases movement or ambulation increases the pain. Irregular menstrual bleeding and vaginal discharge, occasionally greenish or brownish yellow and foul smelling, frequently accompany the pain. Dysuria, dyspareunia, fever, and chills may also be present. Nausea and vomiting are seen in advanced cases.

Women with *subacute* or *chronic PID* may have presenting symptoms of increased cramps with menses, irregular bleeding, and moderate pain with intercourse.

- Chronic PID can result if the acute phase of the condition is not treated, is treated inadequately, or does not respond to treatment. In long-term untreated cases, pelvic cellulitis and sometimes thrombophlebitis of the pelvic veins can occur.

Complications

Frequently the patient is rendered sterile as a result of adhesions and strictures that may develop in the fallopian tubes. Ectopic pregnancy may result when a tube is partially obstructed because the sperm may pass through the stricture but the fertilized ovum cannot reach the uterus. Pelvic and tubal ovarian abscesses may "leak" or rupture, resulting in pelvic or generalized peritonitis. As the circulation is flooded with bacterial endotoxins from the infected areas, septic shock may result.

Diagnostic Studies

A careful health history will often show the recent occurrence of an acute infection of the lower genital tract. The physical examination often reveals the presence of pain and tenderness in both lower abdominal quadrants. Movement of the pelvic organs during the vaginal examination increases the pain. Masses that are fixed and poorly defined may be found, indicating enlargement of the fallopian tubes or ovaries or abscess formation.

- Leukocyte count and erythrocyte sedimentation rate are elevated.
- Cultures for gonorrhea and chlamydia and Gram stains for other bacteria are done on secretions taken from the vagina, cervix, or cul-de-sac.
- Laparoscopy is used to view the reproductive organs and to obtain specimens from the tubal mucosa for culture studies.
- Vaginal ultrasonic examinations can aid in diagnosing abscesses.

Therapeutic Management

Risk factors, such as multiple sexual partners, sexual activity in female teenagers, low socioeconomic status, IUD contraception, previous PID, and contact with untreated male sexual partners, are considered when planning education for patients with PID.

Treatment of PID may be carried out on an outpatient basis or may require hospitalization. The patient is given a combination of antibiotics such as cefoxitin and doxycycline to provide broad coverage against the causative organisms. Instructions are given to avoid coitus and douching, restrict general activities, get adequate rest and nutrition, and return to the clinic for reevaluation in 48 to 72 hours if symptoms persist or increase.

If outpatient treatment is not successful or if the patient is acutely ill or in severe pain, admission to the hospital is indicated. Maximum doses of parenteral antibiotics are given. In some situations corticosteroids are administered to reduce inflammation and improve the chance for subsequent fertility. Analgesics to relieve pain and IV fluids to prevent dehydration are also prescribed.

Application of heat to the lower abdomen or sitz baths may be used to improve circulation and decrease pain. Bed rest in the semi-Fowler's position promotes drainage of the pelvic cavity by gravity and may prevent development of abscesses high in the abdomen. Sexual partners of women with PID should also be treated as possible sources of infection.

Indications for surgical intervention include the presence of abscesses with the potential for rupture and peritonitis, failure of the patient to respond to conservative management, and a history of frequent exacerbations. The abscess may be drained without laparotomy, or it may be necessary to remove the infected areas along with the uterus, tubes, and ovaries.

- The extent of disease, as well as the age and condition of the patient determine the degree of surgery. Childbearing function in young women is preserved whenever possible.

Nursing Management
Goals
The patient with PID will experience relief of symptoms, practice good perineal hygiene and safe sex, not become infertile as a result of the disease, and comply with the treatment regimen to prevent the disease from becoming chronic.

See the nursing care plan for the patient with pelvic inflammatory disease in Lewis/Collier/Heitkemper, *Medical-Surgical Nursing,* edition 4, p. 1607.

Nursing Diagnoses
- Anxiety related to imposed activity restrictions, perceived loss of control, and lack of knowledge of outcome on reproductive status and course of disease
- Acute pain related to infectious process
- Risk for infection transmission related to vaginal discharge and lack of knowledge of proper hygiene and appropriate sexual practices regarding precautionary measures
- Impaired skin integrity related to vaginal drainage

Nursing Interventions
Prevention, early recognition, and prompt treatment of vulvar, vaginal, and cervical infections can help prevent PID and its serious complications. If the nurse knows the factors that predispose a person to the development of PID, patients who are at risk can be identified and appropriate interventions planned.

- Gynecologic surgery, childbearing, and abortion may predispose the woman to infection. In these instances careful medical and surgical asepsis is imperative to prevent the introduction of organisms into the pelvis. The nurse should counsel the patient to seek medical attention for any unusual vaginal discharge or possible infection of the reproductive organs.
- The patient should be encouraged by the awareness that some discharges are not indicative of infection and that early diagnosis and treatment of an infection can prevent complications.

- Routine cultures for *N. gonorrhoeae* and chlamydia should be taken at the time a pelvic examination is being done on every sexually active woman.
- Women should be informed of the methods of preventing infection as well as the signs of infection in their partners.

During the acute phase of PID, frequent perineal cleansing is indicated to prevent the spread of the infection. The character, amount, color, and odor of the vaginal discharge are recorded. Excoriation of the vulva may occur from the vaginal discharge. An explanation of the need for limited activity (bed rest in a semi-Fowler's position) increases patient cooperation. The nurse should assess the patient's pain level and plan appropriate interventions such as heat to the lower abdomen, sitz baths, and administration of analgesics.

Efforts must be made to prevent the spread of infection to others. Proper handwashing with a germicidal soap and use of universal precautions when handling and disposing of soiled perineal pads are required. Disinfection of utensils, bedpans, and all items in direct contact with the patient is an additional measure used to contain the infection. The need for these precautions should be explained to the patient, and her participation in them should be encouraged.

The patient with chronic PID experiences chronic pelvic discomfort and requires repeated treatment. Her emotional response to the disease and the therapy should be assessed. The patient may feel well one day and develop distressing discomfort the next. She may become discouraged and depressed. The nurse should be aware of these feelings and provide the patient with emotional support and information about the course of the disease.

The patient may have guilt feelings about the problem, especially if it was associated with a sexually transmitted disease. She may also be concerned about the complications associated with PID, such as adhesions and strictures of the fallopian tubes, sterility, and the increased incidence of ectopic pregnancy. Discussions with the patient and significant others regarding these feelings and concerns can assist the patient to cope with them more effectively.

PEPTIC ULCER DISEASE

Definition/Description

Peptic ulcer disease is an erosion of the GI mucosa resulting from the digestive action of hydrochloric acid (HCl) and pepsin. Any portion of the GI tract that comes in contact with gastric secretions is susceptible to ulcer development, including the lower esophagus, stomach, duodenum, and the margin of a gastrojejunal anastomosis site after surgery.

Peptic ulcers can be classified as acute or chronic, depending on the degree of mucosal involvement, and gastric or duodenal, according to the location. Eighty percent of all peptic ulcers are duodenal.

- An *acute ulcer* is associated with superficial erosion and minimal inflammation. It is of short duration and resolves quickly when the cause is identified and removed.
- A *chronic ulcer* is of long duration, eroding through the muscular wall, with formation of fibrous tissue. It is continuously present for many months or intermittently throughout the person's lifetime. A chronic ulcer is at least four times as common as an acute ulcer.
- Gastric and duodenal ulcers, although defined as peptic ulcers, are distinctly different in etiology and incidence. (See Table 42 for a comparison of gastric and duodenal ulcers.)

Pathophysiology

Peptic ulcers develop only in the presence of an acid environment. Under specific circumstances the mucosal barrier can be impaired and back-diffusion of acid can occur. When the barrier is broken, HCl freely enters the mucosa, and injury to tissues occurs. This results in cellular destruction and inflammation. Histamine is released from damaged mucosa, resulting in vasodilatation and increased capillary permeability. A variety of agents are known to destroy the mucosal barrier. The critical pathologic process in gastric ulcer formation may not be the amount of acid that is secreted but the amount that is able to penetrate the mucosal barrier.

- *Helicobacter pylori* is a dominant factor in the promotion of peptic ulcer formation. This organism promotes gastric mucosal destruction (see Gastritis, p. 240).

Clinical Manifestations

It is common with gastric or duodenal ulcers to have no pain or other symptoms (gastric and duodenal mucosa do not have pain sensory fibers). When pain does occur with a duodenal ulcer, it is described as "burning" or "cramplike" and is most often located in the midepigastrium region beneath the xyphoid process. Pain associated with gastric ulcer is located high in the epigastrium and occurs spontaneously about 1 to 2 hours after meals. The pain is described as "burning" or "gaseous." The pain can occur when the stomach is empty or when food has been ingested. Some persons do not experience any pain until a serious complication such as hemorrhage or perforation occurs.

Complications

Three major complications of chronic peptic ulcers are hemorrhage, perforation, and gastric outlet obstruction. All are considered emergency situations and are initially treated conservatively. However, surgery may become necessary at any time during the course of therapy.

Hemorrhage is the most common complication. It develops from erosion of granulation tissue at the base of the ulcer during healing or from erosion of the ulcer through a major blood vessel. Duodenal ulcers account for a greater percentage of upper GI bleeding than gastric ulcers.

Perforation, the most lethal complication, occurs when the ulcer penetrates the serosal surface, with spillage of either gastric or duodenal contents into the peritoneal cavity. The size of the perforation is directly proportional to the length of time the patient has had the ulcer.

- Manifestations of perforation are sudden, with a dramatic onset, and include severe upper abdominal pain that quickly spreads throughout the abdomen. Symptoms also include shallow and rapid respirations and absent bowel sounds.

Gastric outlet obstruction may occur over time as a result of edema, inflammation, fibrous scar tissue, and pylorospasm associated with active ulcer formation. Symptoms include upper abdomen swelling, loud peristalsis, visible peristalic waves, vomiting, and constipation.

Diagnostic Studies

- Fiberoptic endoscopy is used to determine the degree of ulcer healing with treatment, obtain a tissue biopsy, and/or obtain specimens to test for *H. pylori.*
- Barium studies are used for the diagnosis of pyloric obstruction by recurrent ulcers.
- Exfoliative cytology differentiates between a benign and a malignant tumor.
- Gastric analysis determines the amount and composition of gastric secretions.
- Complete blood count (CBC), urinalysis, liver enzyme studies, serum amylase determination, and stool examination may be performed for further diagnostic information.

Therapeutic Management

The aim of treatment is to decrease gastric acidity, enhance mucosal defense mechanisms, and minimize harmful effects on the mucosa.

Conservative Management

The prescribed regimen consists of adequate rest, dietary interventions, medications, elimination of smoking, and long-term fol-

Table 42 Comparison of Gastric and Duodenal Ulcers

	Gastric ulcers	Duodenal ulcers
Lesion	Superficial; smooth margins; round, oval, or cone-shaped	Penetrating (associated with deformity of duodenal bulb from healing of recurrent ulcers)
Location of lesion	Predominantly antrum, also in body and fundus of stomach	First 1-2 cm of duodenum
Gastric secretion	Normal to decreased	Increased
Incidence	■ Greater in women	■ Greater in men, but increasing in women especially postmenopausal
	■ Peak age fifth to sixth decade	■ Peak age 35-45 yr
	■ More common in persons of lower socioeconomic status and in unskilled laborers	■ Associated with psychologic stress
	■ Increased with smoking, drug, and alcohol use	■ Increased with smoking, drug, and alcohol use

	■ Increased with incompetent pyloric sphincter ■ Increased with stress ulcers after severe burns, head trauma, and major surgery	■ Associated with other diseases (e.g., chronic obstructive pulmonary disease, pancreatic disease, hyperparathyroidism, Zollinger-Ellison syndrome, chronic renal failure)
Clinical manifestations	■ Burning or gaseous pressure in high left epigastrium and back and upper abdomen ■ Pain 1-2 hr after meals; if penetrating ulcer, aggravation of discomfort with food ■ Occasional nausea and vomiting, weight loss	■ Burning, cramping, pressurelike pain across midepigastrium and upper abdomen; back pain with posterior ulcers ■ Pain 2-4 hr after meals and midmorning, midafternoon, middle of night, periodic and episodic ■ Pain relief with antacids and food; occasional nausea and vomiting
Recurrence rate	High	High
Complications	Hemorrhage, perforation, outlet obstruction, intractability	Hemorrhage, perforation, obstruction

P

low-up care. Strict adherence to the prescribed regimen of drugs is mandatory because peptic ulcer recurrence is high without treatment. Drug therapy that includes the use of antacids, histamine H_2-receptor antagonists, antisecretory agents, and anticholinergics is often prescribed. Aspirin and nonsteroidal antiinflammatory drugs (NSAIDs) should be discontinued. The patient is placed on antibiotics to eradicate *H. pylori* infection.

Healing of a peptic ulcer requires many weeks of therapy. Pain disappears after 3 to 6 days, but ulcer healing is much slower. Complete healing may take 3 to 9 weeks, depending on the ulcer size and the treatment regimen employed.

Acute exacerbation of a peptic ulcer can usually be treated with the same regimen used for conservative management. Blood products may be given for bleeding. However, the situation is considered more serious because of the chronicity of the ulcer and possible complications of perforation, hemorrhage, and obstruction.

- One method of symptom relief is to keep the stomach empty for 24-48 hours by using a nasogastric (NG) tube and intermittent suctioning, with IV fluid and electrolyte infusions given.
- In perforation, the focus of therapy is to stop the spillage of gastric contents by use of an NG tube or surgery. Blood volume is replaced with antibiotics, and pain medication is also given.
- In gastric outlet obstruction, the aim of therapy is to decompress the stomach via an NG tube.

Nutritional Management

Nutritional management is individualized with the avoidance of foods that cause pain or discomfort. Protein is considered the best neutralizing food, but it also stimulates gastric secretions. Carbohydrates and fats are the least stimulating to HCl secretion, but they do not neutralize well. The patient must determine a suitable combination of these essential nutrients without causing undue distress to the ulcer.

Surgical Management

Many physicians believe that surgery is necessary after therapy has been tried and proved unsuccessful. The types of surgery to treat ulcers include partial gastrectomy, vagotomy, or pyloroplasty. Postoperative complications from surgery are dumping syndrome, postprandial hypoglycemia, and bile reflux gastritis.

- *Dumping syndrome* is the direct result of surgical removal of a large portion of the stomach and pyloric sphincter. These changes drastically reduce the reservoir capacity of the stomach. Onset of symptoms occurs at the end of a meal or within 15 to 30 minutes after eating. The patient usually describes feelings of generalized weakness, sweating, palpitations, and dizziness. Symptoms are self-limiting.

- *Postprandial hypoglycemia* is considered a variant of the dumping syndrome since it is the result of uncontrollable gastric emptying of a bolus of fluid high in carbohydrate into the small intestine, resulting in hyperglycemia. Symptoms are sweating, weakness, mental confusion, palpitations, and tachycardia. Treatment limits sugar intake, with small frequent meals recommended.
- The major symptom associated with *bile reflux gastritis* is continuous epigastric distress that increases after meals. Vomiting relieves distress but only temporarily. The administration of cholestyramine (Questran), either before or with meals, has met with considerable success.

Nursing Management
Goals
The patient with peptic ulcer disease will experience a reduction or absence of discomfort related to the disease, exhibit no signs of GI complications related to the ulcerative process, have complete healing of peptic ulcer, make appropriate lifestyle changes to prevent recurrence, and comply with prescribed therapeutic regimen.

See the nursing care plan for the patient with peptic ulcer disease in Lewis/Collier/Heitkemper, *Medical-Surgical Nursing,* edition 4, p. 1194.

Nursing Diagnoses/Collaborative Problems
- Pain related to gastric secretion, decreased mucosal protection, and ingestion of gastric irritants
- Ineffective management of therapeutic regimen related to lack of knowledge of long-term management of peptic ulcer disease and/or unwillingness to modify lifestyle
- Ineffective individual coping: depression and frustration related to exacerbation and possible complications of disease process
- Potential complication: perforation of GI mucosa secondary to impaired mucosal tissue integrity; hemorrhage secondary to eroded mucosal tissue.

Nursing Interventions
Very often during the acute phase all that is necessary for the patient's immediate recovery is to maintain NPO (nothing by mouth) status for a few days, have an NG tube inserted and connected to intermittent suction, and replace fluids intravenously. The rationale for this therapy must be conveyed to the anxious patient and family. Vital signs are taken frequently, with hematocrit and hemoglobin levels monitored so shock and perforation can be detected early.

After an acute exacerbation the patient is often more amenable to following the plan of care and open to suggestions for changes in lifestyle. Changes are difficult for most people and may be met with resistance. Teaching regarding complications and their manifestations is important.

Postoperative care of the patient after major abdominal surgery is similar to postoperative care after abdominal laparotomy (see Abdominal Pain, Acute, nursing management after laparotomy, p. 3). Additional considerations include:

- Gastric aspirate from an NG tube must be carefully observed for color, amount, and odor during immediate postoperative period.
- The patient must be observed for signs of decreased peristalsis and lower abdominal discomfort that may indicate impending intestinal obstruction.
- The patient is kept comfortable and free of pain by administration of prescribed medications and by frequent changes in position.
- The dressing is observed for signs of bleeding or odor and drainage indicative of an infection. Ambulation is encouraged and is increased daily after the first postoperative day.
- Because the patient is generally returning to the same home and work environment and because basic personality has not changed, there is always the danger of ulcer redevelopment, especially at the site of anastomosis. Adequate rest, nutrition, and avoidance of known stressors are keys to complete recovery.

Patient Teaching

General instructions for the newly diagnosed patient should cover aspects of the disease process itself, nutritional therapy, medication, possible changes in lifestyle, and regular follow-up care.

- Specifically, the patient must be well informed about each drug prescribed, why it is ordered, and the expected benefits.
- Stress reduction techniques should be taught to the patient because relaxation results in decreased acid production and reduction in pain.
- The need for long-term follow-up care must be stressed. Because successful treatment is frequently followed by recurrence of ulcer disease, the patient should be encouraged to seek immediate intervention if symptoms such as pain and discomfort recur or if blood is noted in stools or vomitus.

PERICARDITIS, ACUTE

Definition/Description

Pericarditis is a syndrome caused by inflammation of the pericardial sac (the pericardium). The pericardium provides lubrication to decrease friction during systolic and diastolic heart movements and assists in preventing excessive dilatation of the heart during diastole.

Pathophysiology

Acute pericarditis is most often idiopathic, with a variety of suspected viral causes. The coxsackievirus B group is the most commonly identified virus and tends to elicit pleuropericarditis in adults and myopericarditis in children. In addition to idiopathic or viral pericarditis, other causes of this syndrome include uremia, bacterial infection, acute myocardial infarction (MI), tuberculosis, neoplasm, and trauma.

Pericarditis in the patient with acute MI may be described as two distinct syndromes. Acute pericarditis immediately follows myocardial damage within the initial 48- to 72-hour period. Dressler's syndrome (late pericarditis) appears 2 to 4 weeks after infarction.

An inflammatory response is the characteristic pathologic finding in acute pericarditis. There is an influx of neutrophils, increased pericardial vascularity, and eventually fibrin deposition on the visceral pericardium.

Clinical Manifestations

Characteristic manifestations found in acute pericarditis include chest pain, dyspnea, and a pericardial friction rub.

- Intense pleuritic chest pain is generally sharpest over the left precordium or retrosternally, but it may radiate to the trapezius ridge and neck (mimicking angina) or sometimes to the epigastrium or the abdomen (mimicking abdominal or other noncardiac pathologic conditions). The pain is aggravated by lying supine, deep breathing, coughing, swallowing, and moving the trunk. It is eased by sitting up and leaning forward.
- Dyspnea is related to the patient's need to breathe in rapid, shallow breaths to avoid chest pain and may be aggravated by fever and anxiety.
- The *hallmark finding* is the pericardial friction rub. The rub is a scratching, grating, high-pitched sound believed to arise from friction between the roughened pericardial and epicardial surfaces. It is best heard with the stethoscope diaphragm firmly placed at the lower left sternal border of the chest. The pericardial friction rub does not radiate widely or vary in timing from the heart beat, but it may require frequent auscultation for identification because it may be elusive and transient. Timing the pericardial friction rub with the pulse (and not respirations) will help to distinguish it from a pleural rub.

Complications

Complications that may result from acute pericarditis are pericardial effusion and cardiac tamponade.

Pericardial effusion is generally a rapid accumulation of excess pericardial fluid that occurs in chest trauma. However, as in tuberculous pericarditis, a slowly developing effusion may result. Large effusions may compress adjoining structures. Pulmonary tissue compression can cause cough, dyspnea, and tachypnea. Phrenic nerve compression can induce hiccups, and compression of the recurrent laryngeal nerve may result in hoarseness. Heart sounds are generally distant and muffled, although BP is usually maintained by compensatory changes.

Cardiac tamponade develops as the pericardial effusion increases in size. Compensatory mechanisms ultimately fail to adjust to the decreased cardiac output. The patient with pericardial tamponade is often confused, agitated, and restless and has tachycardia and tachypnea, with a low-output state. The neck veins are usually markedly distended because of jugular venous pressure elevation, and a significant pulsus paradoxus is present. Pulsus paradoxus, an inspiratory drop in systolic BP >10 mm Hg, results because the normal inspiratory decline in systolic BP of <10 mm Hg is exaggerated in cardiac tamponade.

Diagnostic Studies

- Auscultation of the chest for pericardial friction rub
- ECG changes, which are key diagnostic clues
- Echocardiography to determine the presence of pericardial effusion or cardiac tamponade
- Pericardiocentesis and pericardial biopsy to determine the cause of pericarditis
- CT scan and nuclear scan of the heart

Therapeutic Management

Management of acute pericarditis is directed toward identification and treatment of the underlying problem. Antibiotics should be used to treat bacterial pericarditis. Corticosteroids are generally reserved for patients with pericarditis secondary to systemic lupus erythematosus, patients already taking corticosteroids for a rheumatologic or other immune system condition, or patients who do not respond to nonsteroidal antiinflammatory drugs. When necessary, prednisone is usually given in a tapering dosage schedule. Pain and inflammation are routinely treated with nonsteroidal antiinflammatory agents. High-dose salicylates (300 to 900 mg orally four times a day) or indomethacin (25 to 50 mg orally four times a day) are commonly used.

Pericardiocentesis is usually performed when acute cardiac tamponade has reduced the patient's systolic BP 30 mm Hg or more from the baseline. Hemodynamic support as the patient is prepared for the pericardiocentesis may include administration of volume expanders and inotropic agents.

Nursing Management

Management of the patient's pain and anxiety is a primary nursing consideration. Assessment of the amount, quality, and location of the pain is important, particularly in distinguishing the pain of acute MI (or reinfarction) from that of pericarditis. Careful nursing observations should be made regarding ischemic chest pain, which is generally located retrosternally in the left shoulder and arm with a pressurelike burning quality and is unaffected by posture. In contrast, pericarditic pain is usually located in the precordium, the left trapezius ridge, and has a sharp, pleuritic quality that changes with respirations. Relief from this pain is often obtained by leaning forward and is worsened by recumbency.

- Pain relief measures include maintaining the patient on bed rest with the head of the bed elevated to 45 degrees and providing a padded overbed table.
- Antiinflammatory medications help to alleviate the patient's pain. However, because of the potential for GI problems with the use of high doses of these medications, specific nursing interventions should include the administration of these drugs with food or milk, generally 30 minutes before or 2 hours after meals, and instruction to the patient to avoid any alcoholic beverages while taking the medications.
- Monitoring for signs and symptoms of tamponade and making preparations for possible pericardiocentesis are additional interventions.
- Anxiety-reducing measures for the patient include providing simple, complete explanations of all procedures performed. These explanations are particularly important for the patient during the time a diagnosis is being established and for the patient who has already experienced an acute MI and has pericarditis (Dressler's syndrome).

PERITONITIS

Definition/Description

Peritonitis is a localized or generalized inflammatory process of the peritoneum. It may appear in acute and chronic forms, and it may be caused by trauma or rupture of an organ containing chemical irritants or bacteria that are released into the peritoneal cavity (Table 43).

Pathophysiology

The response of the peritoneum to the leakage of GI contents is localization of the offending agent by attempting to "wall it off." If that attempt fails, peritonitis worsens. The tissue begins to swell, and fibrinous exudate develops. Adhesions may be formed. These adhesions may shrink and disappear when the infection is eliminated. Normally peritoneal injuries heal without formation of adhesions, unless other factors, such as infection, ischemia, or foreign substances, are present.

Clinical Manifestations

Abdominal pain is the most common symptom of peritonitis, followed by ascites.

- A universal sign is tenderness over the involved area. Rebound tenderness, muscular rigidity, and spasm are other major signs of irritation of the peritoneum.
- Abdominal distention, fever, tachycardia, tachypnea, nausea and vomiting, and altered bowel habits may also be present.

Complications of peritonitis include hypovolemic shock, septicemia, intraabdominal abscess formation, paralytic ileus, and organ failure.

Diagnostic Studies

- Complete blood count (CBC) to determine hemoconcentration and leukocytosis

Table 43	Causes of Peritonitis
Primary	**Secondary**
Blood-borne organisms	Appendicitis with rupture
Genital tract organisms	Blunt or penetrating trauma to abdominal organs
Cirrhosis with ascites	Diverticulitis with rupture
	Ischemic bowel disorders
	Obstruction in the GI tract
	Pancreatitis
	Perforated peptic ulcer
	Peritoneal dialysis
	Postoperative breakage of anastomosis

- Serum electrolytes
- Abdominal x-ray to show dilated loops of bowel consistent with paralytic ileus, free air if perforation, or air and fluid levels if GI obstruction present
- Abdominal paracentesis and culture of fluid
- CT scan or ultrasound to identify ascites or abcesses
- Peritoneoscopy in patients without ascites

Therapeutic Management

The goals of management are to identify and eliminate the cause, combat infection, and prevent complications. Patients with milder cases of peritonitis or those who are poor surgical risks may be managed nonsurgically. Treatment consists of antibiotics, nasogastric (NG) suction, analgesics, and IV fluid administration. Patients who require surgery need preoperative preparation. These patients may be placed on total parenteral nutrition (see Total Parenteral Nutrition, p. 679) because of increased nutritional requirements.

Nursing Management

Goals

The patient with peritonitis will have resolution of inflammation, relief of abdominal pain, freedom from complications (especially hypovolemic shock), and normal nutritional status.

Nursing Diagnoses/Collaborative Problems

- Abdominal pain related to inflammation of the peritoneum and abdominal distention
- Risk for fluid volume deficit related to collection of fluid in peritoneal cavity as a result of trauma, infection, or ischemia
- Altered nutrition: less than body requirements due to nausea and vomiting
- Anxiety related to uncertainty of cause or outcome of condition and pain
- Potential complication: hypovolemic shock related to loss of circulatory volume

Nursing Interventions

The patient with peritonitis is very ill and needs skilled supportive care. Monitoring for pain and response to analgesic therapy is necessary. The patient may be positioned with knees flexed to increase comfort. The nurse should provide rest and a quiet environment. Sedatives may be given to allay the patient's anxiety.

- Accurate monitoring of fluid intake and output and electrolyte status is necessary to determine replacement therapy. Vital signs are monitored frequently.
- Antiemetics may be administered to decrease nausea and vomiting and further fluid losses. The patient is on NPO (nothing by

mouth) status and may have an NG tube in place to decrease gastric distention.

- If the patient has an open-incision surgical procedure, drains are inserted to remove purulent drainage and excessive fluid. Postoperative care of the patient is similar to the care of the patient with an exploratory laparotomy (see Abdominal Pain, Acute, nursing management after laparotomy, p. 3).

PHARYNGITIS, ACUTE

Definition/Description

Acute pharyngitis is an acute infection of the pharynx caused by a bacteria, virus, or fungus. Acute follicular pharyngitis ("strep throat") results from streptococcal bacterial invasion. Gonorrhea and herpes simplex virus (HSV) may cause pharyngitis as a result of transmission during orogenital contact. Acquired immunodeficiency syndrome (AIDS) must be considered as a potential diagnosis in any at-risk patient who has symptoms of pharyngitis, tonsillitis, and cervical lymphadenopathy.

Clinical Manifestations

Symptoms of acute pharyngitis may range in severity from complaints of "scratchy throat" to pain so severe that swallowing is difficult.

- White irregular patches suggest infection with *Candida albicans,* commonly seen in the patient who is immunosuppressed or has AIDS.
- In viral infections the throat may appear mildly red.
- In strep throat the throat is typically an intense red-purple with patchy yellow exudate and localized lymphadenopathy.
- In diphtheria a gray-white false membrane, termed a pseudomembrane, is seen covering the oropharynx, nasopharynx, and laryngopharynx and sometimes extends to the trachea.

Diagnostic Studies

Cultures are done to establish the cause and direct appropriate management. Even with severe infection, cultures may be negative.

Therapeutic and Nursing Management

Goals of management are infection control, symptomatic relief, and prevention of secondary complications. Because cultures can be negative even when infection is present, the patient suspected of having strep throat is often treated with antibiotics. Candida infections are treated with nystatin, an antifungal antibiotic. Treatment for pharyngitis should continue until the symptoms are gone. The patient should be encouraged to increase fluid intake and to take cool, bland liquids and gelatin that will not irritate the pharynx. Citrus juices should be avoided because they irritate the mucous membranes.

PHEOCHROMOCYTOMA

P

Definition/Description

Pheochromocytoma, the most common disorder of the adrenal medulla, is characterized by a neoplasm that produces excessive catecholamines. Most of these tumors (95%) are benign and encapsulated. Pheochromocytoma can occur at any age and in either gender, but it is found most commonly in patients between the ages of 40 and 60.

Clinical Manifestations

The most striking clinical features of pheochromocytoma are severe episodic hypertension, severe pounding headache, and profuse sweating. Attacks of episodic hypertension result from sympathetic nervous system stimulation and are often accompanied by anxiety, palpitations, and profuse sweating.

Attacks may be provoked by exercise, hypoglycemia, sexual activity, emotional distress, hyperventilation, compression or palpation of the tumor, surgery, and major trauma. The duration of the attacks may vary from a few minutes to several hours.

- Additional symptoms may include vasomotor changes (e.g., pallor, facial flushing, pupil dilatation), orthostatic hypotension, and visual blurring.

Diagnostic Studies

Measurement of urinary metanephrines is the simplest and most reliable diagnostic test. Plasma catecholamines are also elevated. It is preferable to measure catecholamines during an "attack." CT scans and MRI are used for tumor localization.

Therapeutic Management

Treatment consists of surgical removal of the tumor. Before surgery the patient is hospitalized for treatment to correct hypovolemia and cardiovascular complications to decrease the risk of surgery. Sympathetic blocking agents (e.g., phenoxybenzamine [Dibenzyline], propranolol [Inderal]) are administered to reduce the BP and alleviate other symptoms of catecholamine excess.

- Preoperative and postoperative care is similar to that for any patient undergoing adrenalectomy except that BP fluctuations from catecholamine imbalances tend to be severe and need to be carefully monitored.
- Complete removal of the tumor cures the hypertension in 75% of the cases. In the rest, hypertension persists or returns but is usually well controlled by standard therapy (see Hypertension, p. 318).

PNEUMONIA

Definition/Description

Pneumonia is an acute inflammation of the lung parenchyma. Pneumonia can be caused by bacteria, viruses, Mycoplasma organisms, fungi, protozoa, chemicals, dust, gases, and a variety of other organisms and materials (Table 44). Pneumonia is usually classified according to the causative organism. Sometimes pneumonia is classified on the basis of areas and type of lung involvement (e.g., lobar, necrotizing, lobular, or interstitial).

Pathophysiology

Normally the airway distal to the larynx is sterile because of protective defense mechanisms. Pneumonia is more likely to result when defense mechanisms become incompetent or are overwhelmed by infectious agents. Risk factors for pneumonia are varied and include:

- Altered consciousness, which depresses cough and epiglottal reflexes
- Tracheal intubation, which interferes with the normal cough reflex and mucociliary mechanism
- Impaired mucociliary mechanism resulting from air pollution, cigarette smoking, viral upper respiratory tract infections, and normal aging changes
- Malnutrition in which the formation and function of lymphocytes and polymorphonuclear leukocytes are altered
- Certain diseases such as leukemia, alcoholism, and diabetes mellitus, which are associated with increased frequency of gram-negative bacilli in the oropharynx
- Altered oropharyngeal flora, which can occur secondary to antibiotic therapy

Clinical Manifestations and Complications

For the clinical manifestations and complications of pneumonia, see Table 44.

Diagnostic Studies

- Gram stain of sputum to identify the infecting organism
- Sputum culture and sensitivity test using transtracheal aspiration or bronchoscopy with aspiration if unable to obtain via cough or induced production of sputum
- Chest x-ray, which often shows a pattern characteristic of the infecting organism
- Arterial blood gases (ABGs) (if indicated), which reveal hypoxemia
- Complete blood count (CBC) count and white blood cell (WBC) count (leukocytosis usually found)
- Blood cultures to identify the infecting organism

Therapeutic Management

Prompt treatment with the appropriate antibiotic almost always cures bacterial and mycoplasma pneumonia. Currently, there is no effective treatment for viral pneumonia. Penicillin is the drug of choice for a number of bacterial pneumonias. Table 24-4 in Lewis/Collier/Heitkemper, *Medical-Surgical Nursing,* edition 4, p. 629, outlines major antimicrobial agents used in the treatment of pneumonia and respiratory infections.

In uncomplicated cases the patient responds to drug therapy within 1 to 2 days. Indications of improvement include decreased temperature, improved breathing, and reduced chest pain.

Supportive measures may also be used, including O_2 therapy, analgesics to relieve chest pain, and antipyretics such as aspirin or acetaminophen. During the acute febrile phase the patient's activity should be restricted, and rest should be encouraged and planned.

Pneumococcal vaccine is indicated primarily for the individual considered at high risk who (1) has chronic illnesses such as lung and heart disease and diabetes mellitus, (2) is recovering from a severe illness, (3) is 65 years of age or older, or (4) is in a nursing home or other long-term care facility. The current recommendation is that the vaccine is good for the person's lifetime. In the immunosuppressed individual at high risk for development of fatal pneumococcal infection, revaccination should be considered every 5 to 6 years.

Nursing Management

Goals

The patient with pneumonia will have clear breath sounds, normal breathing patterns, normal chest x-ray, and no complications related to pneumonia.

Table 44 Comparison of Types of Pneumonia

Causative agent	Characteristics	Clinical manifestations/complications
■ Pneumococcal pneumonia (*Streptococcus pneumoniae*)	URI usually preceding; incubation period of 1-3 days; peak incidence in winter and spring; nasopharyngeal carriers; persons with chronic heart or lung disease, diabetes mellitus, cirrhosis at risk	Abrupt onset; elevated temperature; tachypnea; chills and rigor; productive cough (often bloody, rusty, or green); nausea and vomiting; malaise; myalgia; pleuritic chest pain; pleural effusions; empyema; metastatic infection (meninges, joints, heart valves); bacteremia
■ Staphylococcal pneumonia (*Staphylococcus aureus*)	Acquisition via hematogenous route or via aspiration into lungs; nasopharyngeal carriers; risk factors of chronic lung disease, leukemia, other debilitating diseases; influenza infection often preceding (10-14 days earlier); drug abusers, diabetics, patients on long-term hemodialysis at risk as carriers; occurrence more frequent in hospitalized patients than persons in community; prolonged antibiotic therapy usually necessary; high mortality in chronically debilitated patients and newborns	Abrupt onset; chills; high fever; productive cough with sputum (often bloody and purulent); tachypnea; progressive dyspnea; pleuritic chest pain; empyema; pleural effusions

P

- Streptococcal pneumonia
  (*Streptococcus pyogenes*)

  Occurrence in military populations after influenza epidemics and sporadically in community; strep throat often associated; occurrence most frequent in winter; transmission to lung by inhalation or aspiration; destruction of lung tissue

  Fever (usually >39° C); chills; cough; pharyngitis; hemoptysis; pleuritic chest pain; dyspnea; myalgia; empyema; pleural effusions; bacteremia; pneumothorax

- Pseudomonas pneumonia
  (*Pseudomonas aeruginosa*)

  Most common gram-negative hospital-acquired pneumonia; predisposition from endotracheal intubation, suctioning, respiratory therapy equipment; high mortality in critically ill patients; persons with chronic lung disease, debilitating diseases, tracheostomies, cancer, and kidney transplants or those taking immunosuppressive drugs or broad-spectrum antibiotics at risk; high mortality

  High fever; cough; copious sputum; hypoxia; cyanosis; lung abscess

- Influenza pneumonia
  (*Haemophilus influenzae*)

  Increase in incidence; transmission to lung by endogenous aspiration; alcoholics and persons with chronic lung disease, recent viral infections, and immune deficiencies at risk; high mortality, especially in older adult patients

  Usual gradual onset; fever; chills; cough; purulent sputum; hemoptysis; sore throat; dyspnea; nausea and vomiting; pleuritic chest pain; pleural effusions; lung abscess (common); empyema (common)

Continued.

Table 44 Comparison of Types of Pneumonia—cont'd

Causative agent	Characteristics	Clinical manifestations/ complications
■ Legionnaires' disease (*Legionella pneumophila*)	Occurrence in outbreaks or sporadic transmission to lung from airborne organisms; proliferation of organisms in water reservoirs (e.g., air-conditioning cooling towers); cigarette smokers and persons with serious underlying diseases (e.g., chronic lung or heart conditions) at increased risk	Myalgia (initially); headache (initially); fever; chills; nonproductive cough; pleuritic chest pain; nausea and vomiting; diarrhea; mental confusion; respiratory failure (major complication)
■ Anaerobic streptococci, fusobacteria, *Bacteroides* species	Transmission to lung usually by aspiration of oropharyngeal secretions; persons with poor dental hygiene, periodontal disease, and history of altered consciousness at risk	Similar to pneumococcal pneumonia, except for insidious onset; foul-smelling sputum; necrotizing pneumonitis (aspiration induced); lung abscess; empyema
■ Influenza viruses; adenovirus; parainfluenza viruses; respiratory syncytial virus	Influenza A most common in civilian adults; responsible for about one half of all pneumonias; peak incidence in winter; transmission from person to person by respiratory droplets; usually self-limiting; symptomatic treatment; adverse effect on many respiratory defense mechanisms, predisposing patients to secondary bacterial pneumonia	Fever; chills; headache; myalgia; anorexia; sneezing; nasal congestion; cough (initially nonproductive)

See the nursing care plan for the patient with pneumonia in Lewis/Collier/Heitkemper, *Medical-Surgical Nursing,* edition 4, p. 631.

Nursing Diagnoses/Collaborative Problems

- Ineffective breathing pattern related to pneumonia, anxiety, and pain
- Ineffective airway clearance related to pain, positioning, fatigue, and thick secretions
- Pain related to pleuritis and ineffective pain management or comfort measures
- Altered nutrition: less than body requirements related to increased metabolism, fatigue, anorexia, nausea, and vomiting
- Activity intolerance related to fatigue, treatment regimen, interrupted sleep and wake cycle, hypoxia, and weakness
- Potential complication: hypoxemia related to impaired gas exchange in lungs
- Risk for altered health maintenance related to lack of knowledge regarding treatment regimen after discharge

Nursing Interventions

Interventions focus on preventing the occurrence of pneumonia. If possible, exposure to upper respiratory tract infections (URIs) should be avoided. If a URI occurs, it should be treated promptly with supportive measures (e.g., rest, fluids, antipyretics). If symptoms persist for more than 3 or 4 days, the person should obtain medical care. The individual at high risk for pneumonia (e.g., the chronically ill and older adult) should be encouraged to obtain both influenza and pneumococcal vaccines.

In the hospital the nursing role involves identifying the patient at risk and taking measures to prevent the development of pneumonia.

- The patient with altered consciousness should be placed in positions (e.g., side-lying, upright) that will prevent aspiration. The patient should be turned and repositioned at least every 2 hours to facilitate adequate lung expansion and to discourage pooling of secretions.
- The patient who has a feeding tube generally requires attention to positioning of the tube to prevent aspiration.
- The patient who has difficulty swallowing (e.g., stroke patient) needs assistance in eating, drinking, and taking medication to prevent aspiration.
- The gag reflex should be present in the individual who has had local anesthesia to the throat before administration of fluids or food.
- The patient who has recently had surgery and others who are immobile need assistance with turning, coughing, and deep-breathing.

- Overmedication with narcotics or sedatives, which can cause a depressed cough reflex, should be avoided.
- Strict medical asepsis and adherence to universal precautions should be practiced to reduce the incidence of nosocomial infections.

Patient Teaching

Teaching the individual to practice good health habits, such as proper diet and hygiene, adequate rest, and regular exercise, can help the person maintain natural resistance to infecting organisms.

- It is extremely important to emphasize the need to take all of the prescribed medication and to return for follow-up medical care and evaluation.
- Adequate rest is needed to maintain progress toward recovery and to prevent relapse. The patient needs to be told that it may be weeks before his/her usual vigor and sense of well-being are felt.
- The patient considered at high risk for pneumonia should be told about available vaccines and should discuss them with the health care worker.
- Deep-breathing and coughing exercises should be practiced for 6 to 8 weeks after the patient is discharged from the hospital.

PNEUMOTHORAX

Definition/Description

Pneumothorax is a complete or partial collapse of a lung as a result of an accumulation of air in the intrapleural space. This condition should be suspected after any blunt trauma to the chest wall occurs. A pneumothorax may be closed or open.

Pathophysiology

Closed pneumothorax has no associated external wound. The most common form is *spontaneous pneumothorax,* which is caused by rupture of small blebs on the visceral pleural space. The cause of blebs is unknown; there is a tendency for this condition to recur. Closed pneumothorax occurs most commonly in male cigarette smokers between 20 and 40 years of age.

- Other causes of closed pneumothorax include injury to the lungs from mechanical ventilation, insertion of a subclavian catheter, perforation of the esophagus, injury to the lungs from broken ribs (see Flail Chest, p. 226, and Fracture, Rib, p. 238), and ruptured blebs or bullae in the patient with chronic obstructive pulmonary disease (COPD).

Open pneumothorax occurs when air enters the pleural space through an opening in the chest wall. Examples include stab or gunshot wounds and surgical thoracotomies. A penetrating chest wound is often referred to as a *sucking chest wound.*

Tension pneumothorax may result from an open or closed pneumothorax or when chest tubes are clamped or become blocked after insertion for pneumothorax. In an open chest wound, a flap may act as a one-way valve; thus air can enter on inspiration but cannot escape. Intrathoracic pressure increases, the lung collapses, and the mediastinum shifts toward the unaffected side, which is subsequently compressed. As intrathoracic pressure increases, cardiac output is altered because there is decreased venous return and compression of the great vessels.

- Tension pneumothorax is a medical emergency because both respiratory and circulatory systems are affected.

Hemothorax involves accumulation of blood in the intrapleural space. It is frequently found in association with open pneumothorax and is then called a *hemopneumothorax.* Causes of hemothorax include chest trauma, lung malignancy, complication of anticoagulant therapy, and pulmonary embolus.

Clinical Manifestations

Symptoms of respiratory distress include shallow, rapid respirations; dyspnea; and air hunger.

- Chest pain and a cough with or without hemoptysis may be present.
- On auscultation there are no breath sounds over the affected area, and hyperresonance may be heard.

If a tension pneumothorax develops, severe respiratory distress, tachycardia, and cyanosis occur. The trachea and point of maximal impulse (PMI) shift to the unaffected side.

Therapeutic and Nursing Management

If the amount of air or fluid accumulated in the intrapleural space is minimal, no treatment may be needed because it will gradually be absorbed, or the pleural space can be aspirated with a large-bore needle. Needle aspiration is often a lifesaving measure.

- Open pneumothorax should be covered with a vented dressing. (A vented dressing is one secured on three sides with the fourth side left untaped.) This allows air to escape from the vent and decreases the likelihood of a tension pneumothorax developing. If the object that caused the open chest wound is still in place, it should not be removed until a physician is present.

The most common treatment for a pneumothorax and hemothorax is to insert a chest tube and connect it to water-seal drainage

(see Chest Tubes and Pleural Drainage, p. 637). Repeated spontaneous pneumothoraces may need to be treated surgically by a partial
pleurectomy or by application of an irritating agent such as tetracycline to the pleural surfaces via a catheter to promote adherence of
the pleurae to one another, a procedure called *pleurodesis* or *sclerosing*.

POLYCYSTIC RENAL DISEASE

Definition/Description

Polycystic renal disease is characterized by multiple renal cysts that
enlarge and destroy the surrounding tissue by compression. They
are filled with fluid and may contain blood or pus. The *childhood
form* of polycystic disease is a rare autosomal recessive disorder
that is often rapidly progressive. The *adult form* of polycystic disease is an autosomal dominant disorder that is latent for many years
and has clinical manifestations presenting when the patient is about
40 years of age. The cysts involve both kidneys and occur in both
men and women.

Clinical Manifestations

Symptoms appear when the cysts begin to enlarge. A common early
symptom of adult cystic disease is flank pain, which is either steady
and dull or abrupt in onset as well as episodic and colicky. On physical examination, palpable bilateral enlarged kidneys are often
found.
 - Other clinical manifestations include hematuria, urinary tract
   infection (UTI), and hypertension.
 - Usually the disease progresses to chronic renal failure.

Diagnostic Approach

Diagnosis is based on clinical manifestations, family history, intravenous pyelogram (IVP), ultrasound, and CT scan.

Therapeutic Management

There is no specific treatment for polycystic kidney disease. A major aim of treatment is to prevent UTIs or to treat them with appropriate antibiotics if they occur. Nephrectomy may be necessary if
pain, bleeding, or infection becomes a chronic, serious problem.
When the patient begins to experience progressive renal failure, the
therapeutic and nursing interventions are determined by the remaining renal function.

Nursing Management

Interventions are those used for management of end-stage renal disease (see Renal Failure, Chronic, p. 500). They include diet modification; fluid restriction; medications; assisting the patient in accepting the chronic disease process; and assisting the patient and the family in dealing with the altered body image, financial concerns, and other issues related to the hereditary nature of the disease.

P

POLYCYTHEMIA

Definition/Description

Polycythemia is the production and presence of an increased number of red blood cells (RBCs). The increase in erythrocytes can be so great that blood circulation is impaired as a result of increased blood viscosity (hyperviscosity) and volume (hypervolemia).

Pathophysiology

The two types of polycythemia are *primary polycythemia* or *polycythemia vera* and *secondary polycythemia* (Fig. 3). Their etiologies and pathogenesis differ, although their complications and clinical manifestations are similar.

Polycythemia vera is a neoplastic disease arising from a chromosomal mutation in a single pluripotent stem cell. Therefore not

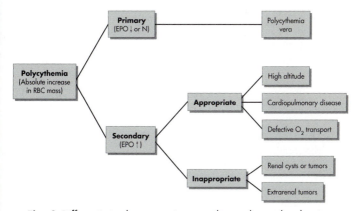

Fig. 3 Differentiating between primary and secondary polycythemia. *EPO,* Erythropoietin; *N,* normal; *RBC,* red blood cell.

only are erythrocytes involved but also granulocytes and platelets are, leading to an increased production of each of these blood cells. The disease develops insidiously and follows a chronic vacillating course. It usually first appears in patients over 50 years of age. Patients have enhanced blood viscosity and blood volume and congestion of organs and tissues with blood.

- The major cause of morbidity and mortality from polycythemia vera is thrombosis.

Secondary polycythemia is caused by hypoxia rather than a defect in the development of the RBC. Hypoxia stimulates erythropoietin production in the kidney, which in turn stimulates erythrocyte production. The need for O_2 may be caused by high altitude, pulmonary disease, cardiovascular disease, defective O_2 transport, or tissue hypoxia.

Clinical Manifestations

Clinical manifestations of polycythemia vera resulting from hypertension caused by hypervolemia and hyperviscosity include subjective complaints of headache, vertigo, dizziness, tinnitus, and visual disturbances.

Manifestations caused by blood vessel distention, impaired blood flow, thrombosis, and tissue hypoxia include angina, congestive heart failure (CHF), intermittent claudication, and thrombophlebitis.

- Generalized pruritus may be a striking symptom and is related to histamine release from an increased number of basophils and mast cells.
- Hemorrhage can be acute or catastrophic and may result in petechiae, ecchymoses, epistaxis, or GI bleeding.
- Hepatomegaly and splenomegaly from organ engorgement may contribute to patient complaints of satiety and fullness. The patient may also experience pain from a peptic ulcer caused by either increased gastric secretions or liver and spleen engorgement. *Plethora* (ruddy complexion) may also be present.
- Hyperuricemia is caused by the increase in cell destruction that accompanies excessive cell production. This problem may cause a secondary form of gout.

Diagnostic Studies

- Elevated hemoglobin, red blood cell (RBC) count, and white blood cell (WBC) count with basophilia
- Elevated platelets (thrombocytosis) and platelet dysfunction
- Elevated leukocyte alkaline phosphatase, uric acid, and vitamin B_{12} levels
- Bone marrow examination in polycythemia vera shows hypercellularity of RBCs, WBCs, and platelets

- Splenomegaly in 90% of patients with primary polycythemia but not in secondary polycythemia

Therapeutic Management

Treatment of polycythemia vera is directed toward reducing blood volume and viscosity as well as bone marrow activity. Phlebotomy may be done to diminish blood volume until the desired hematocrit level is achieved. The aim of phlebotomy is to reduce and keep the hematocrit to less than 45% to 48%. An individual managed with repeated phlebotomies eventually becomes iron deficient, although this effect is rarely symptomatic. Iron supplementation should be avoided.

- Hydration therapy is used to reduce the blood's viscosity.
- Myelosuppressive agents such as busulfan (Myleran), hydroxyurea (Hydrea), melphalan (Alkeran), and radioactive phosphorus may be given to inhibit bone marrow activity.
- Allopurinol may reduce the number of acute gouty attacks.
- Antiplatelet agents, such as aspirin and dipyridamole, used to prevent thrombotic complications are controversial because of increased irritation of the gastric mucosa, resulting in GI symptoms, including bleeding.

Nursing Management

Primary polycythemia vera is not preventable. However, because secondary polycythemia is generated by any source of hypoxia, problems may be prevented by maintaining adequate oxygenation. Therefore controlling chronic pulmonary disease and avoiding high altitudes may be important.

When acute exacerbations of polycythemia vera develop, the nurse has several responsibilities. Depending on the institution's policies, the nurse may either assist with or perform the phlebotomy.

- Fluid intake and output must be judiciously evaluated during hydration therapy to avoid fluid overload (which further complicates the circulatory congestion) and underhydration (which can cause the blood to become even more viscous).
- If myelosuppressive agents are used, the nurse must administer the drugs as ordered and observe the patient and teach him/her about the medication's side effects.
- Assessment of the patient's nutritional status and collaboration with the dietitian may be necessary to offset the inadequate food intake that can result from GI symptoms of fullness, pain, and dyspepsia.
- Activities must be instituted to decrease thrombus formation. Active or passive leg exercises (and ambulation when possible) should be initiated.

- Because of its chronic nature, polycythemia vera requires ongoing evaluation. Phlebotomy may need to be done every 2 to 3 months. The nurse must evaluate the patient for the development of complications.

PREGNANCY, ECTOPIC

Definition/Description

Ectopic pregnancy results from the implantation of the fertilized ovum anywhere outside the uterine cavity. The most frequent site is the fallopian tube, but the location may be ovarian, abdominal, or cervical. Risk factors for ectopic pregnancy are current intrauterine device (IUD) use, history of infertility, history of pelvic inflammatory disease (PID), and prior tubal surgery. However, approximately 50% of all ectopic pregnancies are not explained by these factors.

Pathophysiology

Any blockage of the tube or reduction of tubal peristalsis delays the passage of the zygote to the uterine cavity and can result in tubal fertilization. Although implantation occurs, the thin tubal wall can expand only minimally with growth of the gestational sac before it ruptures. Tubal pregnancy has been known to interfere with future reproductive ability because of strictures and scarring.

Clinical Manifestations

A woman may be asymptomatic and seek care because she missed her menses. However, the majority of women with tubal pregnancy exhibit subacute symptoms, which usually occur 6 to 8 weeks after the last normal menstrual period. Symptoms may range from menstrual irregularity, vaginal spotting (which occurs after fetal death and estrogen withdrawal), and crampy pain in the lower abdomen (due to tubal distention). Significant pelvic or abdominal tenderness may not be present on physical examination.

- The more dramatic presentation is a woman who has had intermittent abdominal cramping with an acute exacerbation. She may faint or feel faint with pain radiating into her shoulder. The referred pain to the shoulder results from intraabdominal bleeding.
- The profuse bleeding that occurs with a ruptured ectopic pregnancy is the reason it is one of the leading causes of maternal death. Hypovolemic shock may result, as manifested by its classic signs and symptoms (see Shock, p. 521).

Diagnostic Studies

Ectopic pregnancy generally represents a diagnostic challenge, not only because of its vague manifestations but also because of its similarity to a wide variety of other pelvic and abdominal disorders such as salpingitis, spontaneous abortion, rupture of a cyst, appendicitis, or peritonitis.

- Vaginal ultrasonography is used to determine the presence of an intrauterine gestational sac in early pregnancy.
- Serum radioimmunoassay for human chorionic gonadotropin (hCG) level is used as an indication of pregnancy.
- Culdocentesis (aspiration of the cul-de-sac) for unclotted blood or a laparoscopy is used to confirm the diagnosis when signs and symptoms are pronounced.

Therapeutic Management

Once a definitive diagnosis of ectopic pregnancy is made, surgery should proceed immediately. If the tube has ruptured, the patient may be given a blood transfusion and supplemental IV fluids to relieve shock and restore blood volume for surgery.

- A salpingectomy or salpingostomy may be done to remove the products of conception from an unruptured tubal pregnancy. Salpingectomy is more commonly performed, especially if the contralateral tube appears normal. All gross abdominal blood and clots are removed to prevent intraperitoneal adhesions.
- An alternative to surgery is drug-induced pregnancy termination with the use of a single intramuscular injection of methotrexate (MTX).

Nursing Management

Nursing care depends on the condition of the patient. Before a diagnosis has been confirmed, the nurse should be alert to signs of increasing pain and vaginal bleeding that may indicate that rupture of the tube has occurred. Vital signs are monitored closely, along with observation for signs of shock.

- Explanations and preparation for diagnostic procedures are given when appropriate. Preparation of the patient for abdominal surgery may follow rapidly.
- The patient's emotional status should be assessed. Reassurance and support for the surgery should be given to both the patient and her family.
- Postoperatively, the patient may express a fear of future ectopic pregnancies and have many questions about the impact of this experience on her future fertility.

PRESSURE ULCERS

Definition/Description

Pressure ulcers are caused by unrelieved tissue pressure. A pressure ulcer or sore results from continual tissue pressure or from tissue layers sliding over other tissue layers (shearing). The result is damage to the underlying tissues. Predisposing factors that may lead to the development of an ulcer include impaired circulation, anemia, contractures, immobility, incontinence, old age, and poor nutrition. More than 95% of all pressure ulcers occur over a bony prominence, primarily the pelvic girdle.

Clinical Manifestations

The four clinical stages of classification of pressure ulcers according to depth are the following:

Stage I: Nonblanchable erythema of intact skin

Stage II: Partial-thickness skin loss with a superficial abrasion or crater or a blister

Stage III: Full-thickness skin loss with damage down to, but not through, the fascia

Stage IV: Full-thickness skin loss with extensive destruction, tissue necrosis, or damage to the muscle or bone or to supporting structures

When eschar is present, accurate staging is not possible until the eschar has sloughed or the wound has been debrided. If a pressure ulcer becomes infected, signs of infection, such as leukocytosis and fever, may occur.

Therapeutic and Nursing Management

Once a pressure ulcer has developed, interventions are based on the grade and size of the ulcer and the presence of infection. Careful documentation should be made of the pressure ulcer size.

- A *stage I ulcer* usually heals completely once pressure on the affected area is relieved. The affected area should not be massaged and can be covered with an adhesive sterile transparent dressing. This dressing can be left in place the usual 1 to 2 weeks the ulcer takes to heal.
- A *stage II ulcer* is reversible if detected early. It is irrigated with a prescribed solution, and a transparent dressing with a pouch to collect exudate is applied. The dressing should be reapplied if the edges become loose. This ulcer takes 2 to 4 months to heal.
- A *stage III ulcer* is irrigated daily, and a transparent or hydrocolloidal dressing is applied. Both transparent and hydrocol-

loid dressings are contraindicated for an infected pressure ulcer or one with exposed muscles, tendons, or bones (stage IV).

- A *stage IV ulcer* is treated by debridement, IV fluids, and antibiotics. A wet-to-dry gauze dressing is applied daily after wound irrigation with a prescribed solution. Enzymes may be used to liquefy necrotic tissue. With the use of sterile technique, a saline-soaked gauze dressing is gently packed into the wound. Once the wound is clean, surgical debridement and reconstruction of the pressure ulcer site may be necessary. These ulcers may take months to years to heal.
- Adequate nutrition for healing is important since the patient is often debilitated and has a poor appetite. Necessary caloric intake can reach 4200 calories/day.

Patient Teaching

Emphasis is placed on educating the patient and care provider in preventing ulcer recurrence, including causative factors, use of pressure-reduction devices such as alternating pressure mattresses, lifting sheets and frequent repositioning, identification of early pressure ulcer signs, nutritional support, and care techniques for active ulcers.

PROSTATE CANCER

Definition/Description

Cancer of the prostate is the most common form of cancer in men. It is rarely found in men under 60 years of age. It is the second leading cause of cancer death in men (lung cancer is first). Because of the lack of symptoms, 75% of first-time patients over age 65 are diagnosed with late disease. A high-fat diet, family history, and/or environmental factors may be linked to prostate cancer.

Pathophysiology

Prostate cancer is an androgen-dependent adenocarcinoma. The tumor is slow growing and usually begins in the posterior or lateral portions of the prostate. Tumor is spread by three routes: direct extension, lymphatics, and bloodstream. Direct extension is by continuity to the seminal vesicles, urethral mucosa, bladder wall, and external sphincter. The cancer later spreads to the pelvic bones, head of the femur, lower lumbar spine, liver, and lungs.

Clinical Manifestations

Prostate cancer is asymptomatic in the early stages. Eventually the patient may have symptoms similar to those of benign prostatic hyperplasia, including dysuria, dribbling, frequency, hematuria, nocturia, and retention. On rectal examination, the prostate feels hard, enlarged (unilateral), and fixed.

- Pain in the lumbosacral area that radiates down to the hips or legs, when coupled with urinary symptoms, is strongly indicative of metastasis. As the cancer spreads to bone, the pain can become severe, especially in the back and legs because of spinal cord compression.

Diagnostic Studies

- Rectal examination with palpation of the prostate gland
- Prostate specific antigen (PSA) level determination; elevated levels are indicative of prostatic pathology, not necessarily cancer
- Prostatic acid phosphatase (PAP) levels monitored for elevation in advanced stages
- Transrectal ultrasound allowing visualization of the outer lobes of the prostate
- Biopsy, needle aspiration, or open biopsy when a suspicious lesion is located
- Bone scan to assess cancer spread

Therapeutic Management

Management of prostate cancer depends on the stage of the cancer. Prostate cancer is staged on the basis of tumor growth (see Table 52-5 in Lewis/Collier/Heitkemper, *Medical-Surgical Nursing,* edition 4, p. 1636). Surgery is the most accurate method of staging because the extent of tumor growth and lymph node involvement can be assessed most accurately by means of inspection during the operation and evaluation of the pathology reports.

- The decision about which treatment course to pursue is a joint one between the patient and physician based on a careful analysis of the facts and the patient's unique situation.

Surgical intervention is often the first line of treatment, particularly in the earlier stages of the disease. A transurethral resection of the prostate (TURP) or total prostatectomy may be the treatment, or the patient may be followed up carefully with annual rectal examinations and PSA testing.

- For patients with stage C tumor, the surgical procedure is usually a radical prostatectomy involving resection of the prostate gland, seminal vesicles, and part of the ampulla of the vas deferens.
- Surgery is usually not considered an option for stage D cancer, except to relieve obstruction, because metastasis outside the prostate has already occurred.

A nerve-sparing technique is sometimes used to prevent erectile dysfunction. This surgery is useful for patients in whom there is no lymph node involvement, no elevation of prostatic acid phosphatase levels, and no clinical evidence of extracapsular extension.

Surgical removal of the prostate, followed by orchiectomy (removal of the testes), removes the source of 90% of circulating androgens. Orchiectomy often provides rapid relief of bone pain and may induce sufficient shrinkage of the prostate to relieve urinary obstruction in later stages of disease when surgery is not an option.

Hormonal therapy is also used in the treatment of prostate cancer. Estrogen (e.g., diethylstilbestrol) treatment can be substituted for orchiectomy. It causes regression of the prostate size and metastatic bone lesions. Leuprolide (Lupron) and goserelin (Zoladex), agonists of luteinizing hormone-releasing hormone, block androgens at the pituitary level.

Other therapies include external beam radiation for the early stages and radiation therapy for disseminated prostate cancer (see Radiation Therapy, p. 675). Spot radiation can be extremely helpful in alleviating pain associated with isolated osseous metastasis.

Nursing Management
Goals
The patient with prostate cancer will be an active participant in the treatment plan, have satisfactory pain control, follow the therapeutic plan, accept the effect of the therapeutic plan on sexual function, and find a satisfactory way to achieve sexual expression.

Nursing Diagnoses
- Decisional conflict related to the numerous alternative treatment options
- Pain related to surgery, prostatic enlargement, bone metastasis, and bladder spasms
- Urinary retention related to obstruction of the prostate, blood clots, and loss of bladder tone
- Sexual dysfunction related to effects of treatment
- Anxiety related to uncertain outcome of disease process on life and lifestyle and effect of treatment on sexual functioning

Nursing Interventions
One of the most important roles for nurses in relation to prostate cancer is to encourage the patient to have an annual prostate examination to increase the chance of early detection. Men should have an annual rectal examination starting at the age of 40.

- The nurse needs to provide psychologic support for the patient and his family to help them cope with the diagnosis of cancer.
- Preoperative and postoperative phases of therapy are the same as for benign prostatic hyperplasia (see Benign Prostatic Hyperplasia, p. 64).
- Pain control is the primary nursing intervention for the terminally ill patient. Hospice care is often appropriate and most

beneficial to the patient and family. (Hospice care is discussed in Lewis/Collier/Heitkemper, *Medical-Surgical Nursing,* edition 4, p. 311.)

Patient Teaching

If the patient is discharged with an indwelling catheter in place, the nurse must teach appropriate catheter care. The patient should be instructed to clean the urethral meatus with soap and water once a day, maintain a high fluid intake, keep the collecting bag lower than the bladder at all times, keep the catheter securely anchored to the inner thigh or abdomen, and report any signs of bladder infection, such as bladder spasms, fever, or hematuria.

PULMONARY EMBOLISM

Definition/Description

Pulmonary embolism is a thrombotic occlusion of the pulmonary arterial system. The most common source of a thrombus is the deep leg veins. Pulmonary embolism is the most frequently encountered pulmonary illness in a general hospital and is responsible for more than 50,000 deaths annually in the United States.

Pathophysiology

Thrombi in deep veins can dislodge spontaneously. However, a more common mechanism is jarring of the thrombus by mechanical forces, such as sudden standing, and changes in the rate of blood flow, such as those that occur with the Valsalva maneuver. The thrombus breaks loose and travels as an embolus until it lodges in the pulmonary vasculature. The result of thromboembolic occlusion is complete or partial occlusion of the pulmonary arterial blood flow to parts of the lung. Thus the lung is ventilated but not perfused. As pressure increases in the pulmonary vasculature, pulmonary hypertension may result.

Clinical Manifestations

The severity of manifestations depends on the size of the embolus, and the size and number of blood vessels occluded. The most common manifestation is sudden onset of unexplained dyspnea, tachypnea, and/or tachycardia.

- Other manifestations are cough, chest pain, hemoptysis, crackles, fever, accentuation of the pulmonic heart sound, and sudden change in mental status as a result of hypoxemia.

Massive emboli may produce sudden collapse of the patient with shock, pallor, severe dyspnea, and crushing chest pain. However, some people with massive emboli do not have pain. The pulse is rapid and weak, the BP is low, and an ECG indicates right ventricular strain. When rapid obstruction of 50% or more of the pulmonary vascular bed occurs, acute cor pulmonale may result because the right ventricle can no longer pump blood into the lungs. Death occurs in more than 60% of people with massive emboli.

Medium-sized emboli often cause pleuritic chest pain accompanied by dyspnea, slight fever, and a productive cough with blood-streaked sputum. A physical examination may indicate tachycardia and a pleural friction rub.

Small emboli frequently are undetected or produce vague, transient symptoms. The exception to this is in the patient with underlying cardiopulmonary disease, in whom even small or medium-sized emboli may result in severe cardiopulmonary compromise.

Complications

Pulmonary infarction (death of lung tissue) occurs in less than 10% of patients with emboli. Infarction is more likely when (1) the occlusion is of a large or medium-sized pulmonary vessel (>2 mm in diameter), (2) insufficient collateral blood flow from the bronchial circulation exists, or (3) preexisting lung disease is present. Infarction results in alveolar necrosis and hemorrhage. Concomitant pleural effusion is frequently found.

Pulmonary hypertension occurs when more than 50% of the cross-sectional area of the normal pulmonary bed is compromised. Pulmonary hypertension also results from hypoxemia. As a single event, an embolus does not cause pulmonary hypertension unless it is massive. However, recurrent small to medium-sized emboli may result in chronic pulmonary hypertension. Pulmonary hypertension eventually results in dilatation and hypertrophy of the right ventricle. Depending on the degree of pulmonary hypertension and its rate of development, death may result rapidly or only mild or transient alterations may be produced.

Diagnostic Studies

- Continuous ECG monitoring is done, with dysrhythmia being the most common finding with pulmonary emboli.
- Lung scan (perfusion and ventilation) screens for embolism.
- Chest x-ray is not useful unless an infarction has occurred.
- Arterial blood gases (ABGs) are abnormal with pulmonary occlusion.
- Complete blood count (CBC) with differential is taken.
- Pulmonary angiography is a definitive test for embolism.
- Venous studies may diagnose deep vein thrombosis as the embolism source.

Therapeutic Management

Objectives of therapeutic treatment are to prevent further growth or multiplication of thrombi in the lower extremities, prevent embolization from the upper or lower extremities to the pulmonary arteries, and provide cardiopulmonary support if indicated. Supportive therapy for the patient's cardiopulmonary status varies according to the severity of the pulmonary embolism.

- Administration of O_2 by mask or cannula may be adequate for some patients. O_2 is given in a concentration determined by ABG analysis. In some situations endotracheal intubation and mechanical ventilation may be needed to maintain adequate oxygenation.
- Respiratory measures such as turning, coughing, and deep breathing are important to prevent or treat atelectasis.
- If shock is present, vasopressor agents may be necessary to support systemic circulation. If heart failure is present, digitalis and diuretics are used.

Pain resulting from pleural irritation or reduced coronary blood flow is treated with narcotics, usually morphine. Properly managed anticoagulant therapy is effective for many patients. Heparin and warfarin (Coumadin) are the drugs of choice. Anticoagulant therapy for thromboembolic conditions may not be indicated in the presence of blood dyscrasias, hepatic dysfunction causing alteration in the clotting mechanism, overt bleeding, a history of cerebrovascular accident, or neurologic conditions. Thrombolytic agents such as urokinase and streptokinase have been shown to dissolve pulmonary emboli within 24 to 48 hours. Both agents have been suggested for use in patients with massive emboli or in whom surgery is contraindicated.

If the degree of pulmonary arterial obstruction is severe (usually >50%) and the patient does not respond to conservative therapy, an immediate embolectomy may be indicated. Pulmonary embolectomy is possible; the need though is rare.

- To prevent further pulmonary embolization, surgical procedures appropriate for thrombophlebitis may be used (see Thrombophlebitis, p. 566). These procedures may include insertion of intracaval filter devices and extravascular vena cava interruption.

Nursing Management

Nursing measures aimed at prevention of pulmonary embolism parallel those for prophylaxis of thrombophlebitis (see Thrombophlebitis, p. 566).

The prognosis of a patient with pulmonary emboli is good if therapy is promptly instituted. The patient should be kept in bed in a semi-Fowler's position to facilitate breathing. A patent IV line should be maintained for medications and fluid therapy. O_2 should be administered as ordered. Careful monitoring of vital signs, ECG, blood gases, and lung sounds is critical to assess the patient's status.

- The patient is usually anxious because of pain, the inability to breathe, and fear of death. Carefully explaining the situation and providing emotional support and reassurance helps to relieve the patient's anxiety. During the acute phase someone should be with the patient as much as possible.
- Many patients with pulmonary emboli have been hospitalized for a primary problem such as sepsis, acute respiratory failure, or surgical intervention. Interventions should also focus on problems related to the primary disorder.

Patient Teaching

The patient requires much psychologic and emotional support. In addition to thromboembolic problems, he/she may have an underlying chronic illness requiring long-term treatment.

- To provide supportive therapy, the nurse must understand and differentiate between the various problems caused by the underlying disease and those related to thromboembolic disease.
- Long-term management is similar to that for the patient with thrombophlebitis (see Thrombophlebitis, p. 566).
- Discharge planning is aimed at limiting progression of the condition and preventing complications. The nurse must reinforce the need for the patient to return to the health care facility for regular follow-up examinations.

PULMONARY HYPERTENSION

Definition/Description

Pulmonary hypertension is elevated pulmonary pressure resulting from an increase in pulmonary vascular resistance to blood flow through small arteries and arterioles.

Pathophysiology

The increase in pulmonary vascular resistance may be anatomic or vasomotor. Reasons for an anatomic increase in vascular resistance include loss of capillaries as a result of alveolar wall damage (e.g., chronic obstructive pulmonary disease [COPD]), stiffening of the pulmonary vasculature (e.g., pulmonary fibrosis), and obstruction of blood flow (e.g., pulmonary emboli).

A vasomotor increase in pulmonary vascular resistance is found in conditions characterized by alveolar hypoxia and hypercapnia.

These conditions cause localized vasoconstriction and shunting of blood away from poorly ventilated alveoli.

- Alveolar hypoxia and hypercapnia can be caused by a wide variety of conditions, including pickwickian syndrome, kyphoscoliosis, and neuromuscular disease.

Pulmonary hypertension is almost always caused by pulmonary or cardiac disorders. However, *primary pulmonary hypertension* is not associated with either pulmonary or cardiac disease. A person with this disorder is typically a woman between the ages of 20 and 40. The basic cause of the problem is unknown. No definitive therapy is available, and the course is often one of continual downhill progression within several years of the onset of symptoms.

Clinical Manifestations

Common manifestations are dyspnea and weakness. These symptoms initially occur only when there is an increased cardiac output (e.g., during exercise or with fever) or during hypoxia (e.g., with pulmonary infection). Eventually the condition occurs even during rest.

- Pulmonary hypertension increases the workload of the right ventricle and causes right ventricular hypertrophy.

Therapeutic and Nursing Management

The primary management of pulmonary hypertension is directed at treating the underlying problem that precipitated the problem. Low-flow O_2 therapy is used to correct the hypoxemia and reduce vasoconstriction in chronic states of respiratory disorders. In acute stages (e.g., those resulting from pulmonary emboli) higher concentrations of O_2 may be required. Diuretics and a low-sodium diet will help to decrease the plasma volume and the load on the heart. Bronchodilator therapy is indicated if the underlying respiratory problem is due to an obstructive disorder.

- Continuous low-flow O_2 during sleep, exercise, and small frequent meals may allow the patient to feel better and be more active.
- Vasodilator therapy has been evaluated as a possible treatment and has been shown to produce sustained hemodynamic and symptomatic improvement in some patients.
- Anticoagulation has also been used with success.
- New approaches include the use of high-dose calcium channel blockers and continuous infusion of prostacyclin.
- When medical treatment fails, heart-lung or lung transplantation is an option for some patients.

PYELONEPHRITIS

Definition/Description

Pyelonephritis is an acute or chronic inflammatory process of the renal pelvis and parenchyma of the kidney.

Pathophysiology

The inflammatory process is generally caused by bacterial invasion from normal inhabitants of the intestinal tract (e.g., *Escherichia coli*). Pyelonephritis can develop via the ascending route from cystitis, with the infection usually starting in the renal medulla and then spreading to the adjacent cortex. The infected portion then heals by fibrosis and scarring. Repeated attacks of acute pyelonephritis in conjunction with preexisting factors such as bladder tumors, prostatic hyperplasia, urinary stones, vesicoureteral reflux, and neurogenic bladder can result in chronic pyelonephritis.

Chronic pyelonephritis is usually the end result of long-standing urinary tract infections (UTIs) with relapses and reinfections creating chronic inflammation and scarring. The level of renal functioning can vary in chronic pyelonephritis.

Clinical Manifestations

Acute pyelonephritis manifestations may vary from acute lassitude to the sudden onset of chills, fever, vomiting, malaise, flank pain, dysuria, costovertebral tenderness on the affected side, and frequent urination. Symptoms of cystitis may or may not be found (see Cystitis, p. 168). If bacteremia is present, the patient will have a high fever, elevated white blood cell (WBC) count, and may go into septic shock. Acute manifestations generally subside within a few days even without specific therapy, although bacteriuria and/or pyuria may persist.

Bacteremia (the presence of bacteria in the blood) can occur secondary to a UTI ascending to the kidney and can result in sepsis. The patient will have a high fever and elevated WBC count. Some patients develop septic shock syndrome as a result of endotoxins produced by gram-negative bacteria that are released in the blood (see Shock, p. 521).

Chronic pyelonephritis usually includes a history of recurrent acute infections that lead to progressive destruction of functioning nephrons. Chronic pyelonephritis may then progress to chronic renal failure (see Renal Failure, Chronic, p. 500).

Diagnostic Studies

- Urinalysis with culture, sensitivity, and Gram stain testing for detection of hematuria, red blood cells (RBCs), WBCs, pyuria, and bacteria
- Palpation for flank pain
- Blood culture if bacteremia is suspected
- Intravenous pyelogram (IVP), ultrasound, or CT scan to reveal structural abnormalities

Therapeutic Management

An essential principle of therapeutic management is to consider factors that may be contributing to infection. The acute management of mild symptoms includes bed rest, outpatient management or short hospital stay for IV antibiotics, administration of oral antibiotics (e.g., trimethoprim-sulfamethoxazole, fluoroquinolone) for 14 days, high fluid intake, and follow-up urine cultures. For more acutely occurring severe symptoms, management includes hospitalization, parenteral antibiotics (e.g., aminoglycosides [amikacin and gentamycin], cephalosporins [cefoxitin, cefoperazonel]), high fluid intake, and follow-up urine culture.

Nursing Management

Goals

The patient with pyelonephritis will have relief of pain, normal body temperature, no complications, and no recurrence of symptoms.

See the nursing care plan for the patient with an urinary tract infection in Lewis/Collier/Heitkemper, *Medical-Surgical Nursing,* edition 4, p. 1341.

Nursing Diagnoses

- Altered comfort: fever related to infection
- Pain related to dysuria, urgency, frequency, and bladder spasms secondary to inflammation of tissue trauma
- Altered patterns of urinary elimination: incontinence, dysuria, urgency, or nocturia related to UTI
- Risk for altered health maintenance related to lack of knowledge regarding prevention of recurrence and signs and symptoms of recurrence

Nursing Interventions

Measures for acute pyelonephritis are similiar to those for cystitis (see Cystitis, p. 168). Because the patient with structural abnormalities of the urinary tract is at high risk for infection, the need for regular medical care should be stressed. Interventions vary depending on the severity of symptoms. Bed rest is often indicated to increase patient comfort.

Patient Teaching

Emphasis should be placed on the (1) need to continue medications as prescribed, (2) need for a follow-up urine culture to ensure proper management, and (3) identification of recurrence of infection or relapse.

- In addition to antibiotic therapy, the patient should be encouraged to drink at least eight glasses of fluid every day. Increased fluid intake should be continued, even after the infection has been treated.
- The patient with frequent relapses or reinfections may be treated with long-term low-dose antibiotics. Understanding the rationale for therapy is important to enhance patient compliance.

REFRACTIVE ERRORS

Definition/Description

Refractive errors are the most common visual problems. This defect in vision prevents light rays from converging into a single focus on the retina. Types of refractive errors include:

- *Myopia* (nearsightedness), caused by light rays focusing in front of the retina
- *Hyperopia* (farsightedness), caused by light rays focusing behind the retina
- *Presbyopia,* the loss of accommodation as a result of age, with the crystalline lens becoming larger, firmer, and less elastic
- *Astigmatism,* associated with unequal corneal curvature in which incoming light rays are bent unequally
- *Aphakia,* the absence of the crystalline lens as a result of congenital defect or cataract extraction surgery

Clinical Manifestations

The major symptom is blurred vision. Additional complaints may include ocular discomfort, eye strain, or headaches.

Therapeutic Management

Management of refractive errors is correction, which may include eyeglasses, contact lenses, or keratorefractive surgery.

REITER'S SYNDROME

Definition/Description

Reiter's syndrome is a self-limiting disease associated with arthritis, urethritis, conjunctivitis, and mucocutaneous lesions. Although the exact etiology is unknown, Reiter's syndrome appears to be a reactive arthritis that appears after certain enteric (e.g., *Shigella*) or venereal (e.g., *Chlamydia trachomatis*) infections. The prognosis is favorable, with most patients recovering after 2 to 16 weeks.

- The disease usually affects males, and 85% of patients with Reiter's are positive for HLA-B27, which provides evidence for a genetic predisposition.

Clinical Manifestations

The arthritis of Reiter's syndrome tends to be asymmetric, frequently involving the weight-bearing joints of the lower extremities and sometimes the lower part of the back. Arthralgias usually begin 1 to 3 weeks after the appearance of the initial infection.

- The full attack may be accompanied by fever and other constitutional complaints, including anorexia, with considerable weight loss, and may prove highly debilitating. Soft-tissue manifestations commonly include Achilles tendinitis.

Therapeutic Management

Lesions heal without a trace, and many patients have a complete remission with full joint function. About one half of the patients have recurring acute attacks; others follow a chronic course, having continued synovitis and a progression of x-ray changes closely resembling those of ankylosing spondylitis. Progressive disease may result in major disability.

- Treatment is symptomatic. Joint inflammation is alleviated with nonsteroidal antiinflammatory drugs.

RENAL CELL CARCINOMA

Definition/Description

Renal cell carcinoma (adenocarcinoma) is the most common type of malignant kidney tumor. It is twice as common in men as in women and is typically discovered when the person is 50 to 70 years old. Risk factors include cigarette smoking, gender, family history, and exposure to cadmium.

Clinical Manifestations

There are no characteristic early symptoms. Generalized symptoms of weight loss, weakness, and anemia are the earliest manifestations. The classic manifestations of gross hematuria, flank pain, and a palpable mass are those of advanced disease. Local extension of renal cancer into the renal vein and vena cava is common. The most common sites of metastases include the lungs, liver, and long bones.

Diagnostic Studies

- Intravenous pyelogram (IVP) with nephrotomography to detect most masses
- Ultrasound to help differentiate between a tumor and a cyst
- Arteriography, percutaneous needle aspiration, CT scan, and MRI

Cancer Staging

The tumor, node, metastases (TNM) classification is used for renal cancer staging (see Table 12, p. 71). Robson's system for staging renal carcinoma is also used, as determined by limitation to the renal capsule (stage I) through the presence of distant metastases (stage IV).

Therapeutic Management

Treatment of choice is a radical nephrectomy, which is the removal of the kidney, adrenal gland, surrounding fascia, and part of the ureter and draining of the lymph nodes. Radiation therapy is used palliatively in inoperable cases and when there are metastases to bone or lungs (see Radiation Therapy, p. 675). At present, chemotherapy or hormonal therapy is not effective. Biologic response modifiers, including α-interferon, tumor necrosis factor (TNF), and interleukin-2, are under investigation for treatment of metastatic disease.

RENAL FAILURE, ACUTE

Definition/Description

Renal failure is severe impairment of or total lack of kidney function. Renal failure is classified as *acute* or *chronic*. Acute renal failure most commonly has a rapid onset. In contrast, chronic renal failure usually develops insidiously over time.

- Acute renal failure is characterized by a rapid decline in renal function with progressive *azotemia* (an accumulation of nitrogenous waste products such as blood urea nitrogen [BUN]) and increasing levels of serum creatinine.
- Acute renal failure is usually associated with a decrease in urinary output to <400 ml/day (oliguria), although it is possible to have normal or increased urinary output.
- Acute renal failure usually develops over hours or days. Most commonly, acute renal failure follows prolonged hypotension, hypovolemia, or contact with a nephrotoxic agent.

Pathophysiology

The etiology of acute renal failure is categorized according to pathogenesis into prerenal, intrarenal (or renal parenchyma), and postrenal causes.

- *Prerenal* causes consist of factors outside the kidneys that impair renal blood flow and lead to decreased glomerular perfusion and filtration. Prerenal disease can lead to intrarenal disease (tubular necrosis) if renal ischemia is prolonged. Prerenal causes are the most common, accounting for 50% to 70% of all cases of acute renal failure. Examples include hypovolemia, decreased cardiac output, and decreased peripheral vascular resistance.

- *Intrarenal* causes include conditions that lead to actual damage to renal tissue (parenchyma), resulting in malfunctioning nephrons. Primary renal diseases such as acute glomerulonephritis and acute pyelonephritis may lead to acute renal failure. More commonly the predisposing insult is acute tubular necrosis (ATN), which may be caused by ischemia, nephrotoxins, or myoglobin from necrotic muscle cells.
- *Postrenal* causes involve mechanical obstruction of urinary outflow. As the flow of urine is blocked, urine backs up into the renal pelvis, ultimately resulting in renal failure. The most common causes are prostate cancer, benign prostatic hyperplasia, calculi, trauma, and tumors. These causes are almost always treatable.

Clinical Manifestations

Clinically acute renal failure may progress through the phases of oliguria, diuresis, and recovery. In some situations the patient does not recover from acute renal failure, and chronic renal failure results.

The *oliguric phase* commonly is manifested by oliguria, which is caused by a reduction in the glomerular filtration rate (GFR). Oliguria usually occurs within 1 to 7 days of the causative event. Additional urinary changes include bloody urine with casts, red blood cells (RBCs), white blood cells (WBCs), specific gravity fixed at around 1.010, and urine osmolality at about 300 mOsm/L. This is the same specific gravity and osmolality as plasma.

- Fluid volume excess occurs when urinary output decreases. Neck veins become distended, pulse becomes more bounding, and edema and hypertension may develop. Fluid overload can lead to congestive heart failure, pulmonary edema, and pericardial and pleural effusions.
- Metabolic acidosis results when the kidneys cannot synthesize ammonia, which is needed for the excretion of hydrogen ions (H^+). The patient may develop Kussmaul's (rapid, deep) respirations to increase the excretion of carbon dioxide.
- Serum potassium levels increase and potassium levels may exceed 6 mEq/L (6 mmol/L). Treatment must be initiated immediately to prevent cardiac dysrhythmias.
- Nitrogenous product accumulation (azotemia) occurs with oliguria because BUN and creatinine levels are elevated.

The *diuretic phase* begins with a gradual increase in daily urine output of 1 to 3 L/day but may reach 3 to 5 L/day or more. In this phase the kidneys have recovered their ability to excrete wastes but not to concentrate urine. Uremia may still be severe. *Uremia* refers to the clinical situation in which azotemia progresses to a symptomatic state.

- The diuretic phase may last 1 to 3 weeks with the patient's acid-base, electrolyte, and waste-product parameters beginning to normalize near the end of this phase. Because of large losses of fluid and electrolytes, the patient must be monitored for hyponatremia, hypokalemia, and dehydration.

The *recovery phase* begins when GFR increases so that BUN and serum creatinine levels start to stabilize and then decrease. Although major improvements occur in the first 1 to 2 weeks of this phase, renal function can continue to improve for up to 12 months after acute renal failure.

- The outcome is influenced by the patient's overall health, the severity of renal failure, and the number and type of complications. Mortality from acute renal failure varies from 30% to 60%, depending on the cause. The most common cause of death is infection, with the incidence of infection highest in patients in whom surgery or traumatic injury contributed to renal failure.

Diagnostic Studies

- History is the most important tool for distinguishing the possible cause.
- Serum creatinine and BUN levels are elevated initially.
- Serum electrolytes, especially potassium, are altered.
- Urinalysis is done to assess sediment, casts, hematuria, pyuria, and/or crystals.
- Retrograde pyelogram, renal scan, and ultrasound are used.
- CT scan or MRI are also done.

Therapeutic Management

Because acute renal failure is potentially reversible, the primary goal of treatment is to maintain the patient in as normal a state as possible while the kidneys are repairing themselves. The precipitating cause is determined and corrected, if possible. Management is focused on controlling patient symptoms and preventing complications. This includes (1) correcting hypovolemia and maintaining cardiac output for adequate kidney perfusion, with a trend to initiate early and frequent dialysis (see Dialysis, p. 643), (2) monitoring fluid intake during the oliguric phase, (3) decreasing potassium levels, and (4) managing nutrition to decrease the body's catabolism of protein by providing carbohydrate and fat sources.

Nursing Management

Goals

The patient with acute renal failure will completely recover, have no residual loss of kidney function, be maintained in normal fluid and electrolyte balance, have decreased anxiety, and comply with and understand the need for careful follow-up care.

Nursing Diagnoses/Collaborative Problems

- Fluid volume excess related to renal failure and fluid retention
- Risk for infection related to invasive lines, uremic toxins, and altered immune responses secondary to renal failure
- Altered nutrition: less than body requirements related to altered metabolic state and dietary restrictions
- Fatigue related to anemia and uremic toxins
- Anxiety related to disease process, therapeutic interventions, and uncertainty of prognosis
- Potential complication: hyperkalemia related to decreased renal excretion of potassium
- Potential complication: dysrhythmias related to electrolyte imbalances
- Potential complication: metabolic acidosis related to inability of the kidneys to excrete hydrogen ions

Nursing Interventions

Prevention of acute renal failure is essential because of the high mortality. It is primarily directed toward (1) identifying and monitoring high-risk populations, (2) controlling industrial chemicals and nephrotoxic drugs, and (3) preventing prolonged episodes of hypotension and hypovolemia. In the hospital the patient at greatest risk for developing acute renal failure is the person who has experienced massive trauma, extensive burns, cardiac failure, or obstetric complications or who has a baseline renal insufficiency as a result of another chronic disease.

- These patients must be monitored carefully for intake and output, fluid and electrolyte balance, and possible blood transfusion reactions. Extrarenal losses of fluid from vomitus, diarrhea, and hemorrhage must be assessed and recorded.
- Prompt replacement of lost extracellular fluids will help prevent ischemic tubular damage associated with trauma, burns, and extensive surgery. Intake and output records and the patient's weight provide valuable indicators of fluid volume status.
- Aggressive diuretic therapy for the patient with fluid overload as a result of any cause can lead to inadequate renal vascular perfusion.

Acute intervention involves managing fluid and electrolyte balance during the oliguric and diuretic phases, including observing and recording accurate intake and output of fluids and daily weights.

- The nurse must be knowledgeable about common signs and symptoms that result from hypervolemia (in the oliguric phase) or hypovolemia (in the diuretic phase), hypernatremia or hyponatremia, hyperkalemia or hypokalemia, and other electrolyte imbalances that may occur in acute renal failure. Because infection is the leading cause of death in acute renal failure, meticulous aseptic technique is critical. The use of an indwelling catheter should be avoided.
- Respiratory complications, especially pneumonitis, can be prevented. Humidified O_2, intermittent positive-pressure breathing, turning, coughing, deep breathing, and ambulation are measures that the nurse can use to help the patient maintain adequate respiratory ventilation.
- Skin care and measures to prevent decubitus ulcers should be performed because the patient usually develops edema and experiences loss of muscle tone. Mouth care is important to prevent stomatitis.

Patient Teaching

Once kidney function has returned, follow-up care and regular evaluation of renal function should be emphasized.

- The patient should be taught the signs and symptoms of recurrent renal disease, especially the manifestations of fluid and electrolyte imbalances. Measures to prevent recurrence of acute renal failure must be addressed.
- The long-term convalescence of 3 to 12 months may cause social and financial hardships for the family, and appropriate counseling and referrals should be done.

RENAL FAILURE, CHRONIC

Definition/Description

Chronic renal failure is the progressive, irreversible destruction of both kidneys. The disease progresses until many nephrons are destroyed and replaced by nonfunctional scar tissue. Although there are many different causes of chronic renal failure, the end result is a systemic disease involving every body organ.

Pathophysiology

In the majority of cases the individual passes through the early stages of chronic renal failure without recognizing the disease state because the remaining nephrons hypertrophy to compensate. The prognosis and course of chronic renal failure are highly variable.

Although there are no distinct stages in chronic renal failure, disease progression may be divided into three stages:

1. *Diminished renal reserve:* This stage is characterized by normal blood urea nitrogen (BUN) and serum creatinine levels and an absence of symptoms.
2. *Renal insufficiency:* This stage occurs when the glomerular filtration rate (GFR) is about 25% of normal. BUN and serum creatinine levels are increased. Easy fatigue and weakness are common symptoms. As renal failure progresses, nocturia, polyuria, headaches, nausea, and pruritis may occur.
3. *End-stage renal disease (ESRD)* or *uremia:* The last stage occurs when GFR is <5% to 10% of normal or when creatinine clearances are less than 5 to 10 ml/min. It is at this stage that most patients are no longer able to carry out basic activities of daily living because of the progressive nature of the symptoms.

Clinical Manifestations

As renal function progressively deteriorates, every body system becomes involved. Manifestations are a result of retained substances, including urea, creatinine, hormones, and abnormal electrolyte concentrations. Manifestations of uremia vary among patients, according to the etiology of renal failure, comorbid conditions, age, and degree of compliance with the prescribed medical regimen.

Specific manifestations include:

- *Urinary system:* Polyuria, nocturia, fixed specific gravity at 1.010 with renal insufficiency followed by oliguria and anuria as renal failure progresses.
- *Metabolic disturbances:* BUN and creatinine levels increase; insulin resistance causes moderate hyperglycemia and hyperlipidemia.
- *Electrolyte and acid-base imbalances:* Hyperkalemia, sodium retention, and metabolic acidosis.
- *Hematologic system:* Anemia, bleeding tendencies, and infection.

Additional systemic signs include hypertension, peripheral edema, pulmonary edema, diarrhea, nausea and vomiting, constipation, peripheral neuropathy, osteomalacia, yellowish discoloration of skin, hypothyroidism, and personality changes.

Diagnostic Studies

- Renal scan, CT scan, and renal ultrasound may be able to identify renal disease.
- Hematocrit and hemoglobin level are decreased.
- BUN and serum creatinine are elevated.

- Serum electrolytes are abnormal.
- Urinalysis and urine culture are used.

Therapeutic Management

When a patient is diagnosed as having chronic renal insufficiency, conservative management is attempted before maintenance dialysis is begun (see Dialysis, p. 643). Every effort is made to detect and treat potentially reversible causes of renal failure (e.g., cardiac failure, dehydration, pyelonephritis, nephrotoxins, lower urinary tract obstruction). Conservative management is directed toward preserving existing renal function, treating symptoms, preventing complications, and providing for patient comfort. This primarily consists of pharmacologic and nutritional management and supportive care.

Pharmacologic therapy includes administration of erythropoietin, phosphate binders, antihypertensive medication, and measures to lower potassium. Dosages are adjusted for decreased renal function.

Nutritional therapy includes the restriction of protein, water, sodium, and potassium.

Nursing Management

Goals

The patient with chronic renal failure will demonstrate the knowledge and ability to comply with the therapeutic regimen, participate in decision making for the plan of care and future treatment modality, demonstrate effective coping strategies, and continue with activities of daily living within physiologic limitations.

See the nursing care plan for the patient with chronic renal failure in Lewis/Collier/Heitkemper, *Medical-Surgical Nursing,* edition 4, p. 1388.

Nursing Diagnoses

- Fluid volume excess related to an inability of the kidney to excrete fluid, excessive fluid intake, and elevated plasma sodium levels
- Anticipatory grieving related to loss of kidney function
- Risk for injury: fracture related to alterations in the absorption of calcium and excretion of phosphate and altered vitamin D metabolism
- Impaired skin integrity related to a decrease in oil and sweat gland activity, deposition of calcium-phosphate precipitates, capillary fragility, excess fluid, and neuropathy
- Risk for sexual dysfunction related to effects of uremia on reproductive and endocrine systems and the psychosocial impact of renal failure and its treatment

Nursing Interventions

If a patient has a history of renal disease, hypertension, or diabetes mellitus or a family history of renal disease, regular check-ups, including serum creatinine, BUN, and urinalysis, are essential.

- When a patient is prescribed potentially nephrotoxic drugs, it is important to monitor renal function with serum creatinine and BUN determinations.
- Individuals need to be instructed on maintaining adequate fluid intake each day (at least 2 L). Any changes in urine appearance (color, odor), frequency, or volume need to be reported to the health care provider. Routine urinalysis should be part of a physical examination.
- While the patient is being maintained on conservative management, the decision regarding future therapies, if any, should be made. This should be done before complications such as mental status changes, bleeding, progressive neuropathies, and persistent congestive heart failure occur.
- The patient and family need a clear explanation of what is involved in dialysis and transplantation.

Patient Teaching

It is important to educate the patient and family because they are responsible for diet, medications, and follow-up care.

- The patient should weigh daily, learn to take daily BP measurement, and be able to identify signs and symptoms of edema, hyperkalemia, and other electrolyte imbalances.
- The patient and family need to understand the importance of strict dietary adherence. The dietitian and nurse need to meet with the patient and family on a continuing basis to assist in diet planning. A diet history and consideration of cultural variations make diet planning and adherence more easily achieved goals.
- The patient needs a complete understanding of drugs, dosages, and common side effects. It may be helpful to make a list of medications and the time of administration that can be posted in the home in convenient locations. The patient needs to be instructed to avoid certain over-the-counter drugs, such as laxatives and antacids, that contain magnesium.

It is important that the patient be motivated to assume the primary role in management of the disease.

RETINAL DETACHMENT

Definition/Description

Retinal detachment is a separation of the sensory retina and the underlying pigment epithelium, with fluid accumulation between the two layers. Risk factors include high myopia, aphakia, proliferative diabetic retinopathy, and ocular trauma.

Pathophysiology

The most common cause of this condition is a retinal break, which is an interruption in the full thickness of the retinal tissue. Additional causes include retinal holes with spontaneous atrophic breaks and retinal tears in which the vitreous shrinks with aging and pulls on the retina.

Once there is a retinal break, liquid vitreous enters between the sensory and retinal pigment epithelium layers, causing detachment. Untreated retinal detachment leads to blindness in the involved eye.

Clinical Manifestations

Symptoms of a detached retina include photopsia ("light flashes"), floaters, or a ring in the vision field. Once the retina is detached, the patient complains of painless loss of peripheral or central vision.

Diagnostic Studies

- Visual acuity measurements are the first diagnostic procedure with the complaint of vision loss.
- Direct visualization of the retina is made through direct and indirect ophthalmoscopy or slit-lamp microscopy.
- Ultrasound may be useful in identifing a detachment if the cornea, lens, or vitreous humor are hazy or opaque.

Therapeutic Management

Retinal breaks are evaluated to determine if prophylactic laser photocoagulation or cryopexy is necessary to avoid retinal detachment. Some breaks will not progress to detachment, so the patient may be observed and given precise information about the warning signs of impending detachment and instructions to seek immediate evaluation if any of these signs occur. The general ophthalmologist will usually refer the patient with retinal detachment to a retinal specialist.

Retinal detachment treatment has two objectives: (1) to seal any retinal breaks and (2) to relieve inward retinal traction. Surgical treatment to seal breaks may include laser photocoagulation, cryopexy, and diathermy. Management of inward retinal traction involves scleral buckling, pneumatic retinopexy, and vitrectomy.

- Reattachment is successful in 90% of all cases, with visual prognosis dependent on the extent, length, and area of detachment.

Nursing Management
Goals
The patient with a retinal detachment will experience minimal anxiety throughout the event, be aware of reportable signs and symptoms if surgery is not indicated, and maintain an acceptable level of comfort postoperatively.

Nursing Diagnoses
- Pain related to surgical correction and unusual positioning
- Fear related to the possibility of permanent vision loss in the affected eye
- Self-care deficit syndrome related to imposed activity restrictions and visual deficits

Nursing Interventions
Retinal detachment is a situation with an urgent need for surgery. The patient needs emotional support, especially during the immediate preoperative period.

- For postoperative pain the nurse should administer prescribed pain medications and teach the patient to take the medication as necessary when discharged.
- Discharge planning is important, and the nurse should begin this process as early as possible because the patient may not be hospitalized for long.

Patient Teaching
- Instruct the patient with a high risk of retinal detachment about the signs of detachment.
- Promote the use of proper protective eyewear to help avoid retinal detachments related to trauma.
- Verify the prescribed level of activity with the patient's surgeon and help the patient plan for any necessary assistance related to activity restrictions.
- Postoperatively, teach the patient the signs of retinal detachment because the risk of detachment in the unaffected eye is approximately 10%.

RHEMATIC FEVER AND HEART DISEASE

Definition/Description

Rheumatic fever is an inflammatory disease of the heart, potentially involving all layers (endocardium, myocardium, and pericardium). The resulting damage to the heart from rheumatic fever is called rheumatic heart disease, a chronic condition characterized by scarring and deformity of the heart valves.

Pathophysiology

Rheumatic fever almost always occurs as a delayed sequela (usually 2 to 3 weeks) after a group A β-hemolytic streptococcal infection of the upper respiratory system, usually a pharyngeal infection. Acute rheumatic fever (ARF) affects the heart, joints, central nervous system (CNS), and skin because of an abnormal humoral and cell-mediated immune response to group A β-hemolytic streptococcal antigens. It is possible that these antigens cross-react with other tissues and bind to receptors on heart, muscle, joint, and brain cells, triggering immune and inflammatory responses.

About 40% of ARF episodes are marked by carditis, and all layers of the heart (endocardium, myocardium, and pericardium) may be involved.

- Rheumatic endocarditis is found primarily in the valves, with swelling and erosion of the valve leaflets. Vegetations form and create a fibrous thickening of the valve leaflets, fusion of commissures and chordae tendineae, and fibrosis of the papillary muscle. Stenosis and regurgitation may occur in valve leaflets.
- Myocardial involvement is characterized by *Aschoff's bodies,* which are nodules formed by a reaction to inflammation with accompanying swelling and fragmentation of collagen fibers.
- Rheumatic pericarditis affects the pericardium, which becomes thickened and covered with a fibrinous exudate.

The lesions of rheumatic fever are systemic, especially involving the connective tissue. The joints (polyarthritis), skin (subcutaneous nodules), CNS (chorea), and lungs (fibrinous pleurisy and rheumatic pneumonitis) can be involved in rheumatic fever.

Clinical Manifestations

The presence of two major criteria or one major and two minor criteria indicates a high probability of ARF (see Table 34-12 in Lewis/Collier/Heitkemper, *Medical-Surgical Nursing,* edition 4, p. 1018). Either combination must have evidence of an existing streptococcal infection.

Major criteria

- *Carditis* is the most important manifestation of ARF. Cardiac enlargement and congestive heart failure (CHF) occur secondary to myocarditis; pericarditis results in distant heart sounds, chest pain, pericardial friction rub, or signs of effusion.
- *Polyarthritis,* the most common finding in rheumatic fever, involves swelling, heat, redness, tenderness, and limitation of motion. The arthritis is migratory, affecting one joint and then moving to another.
- *Chorea (Sydenham's chorea)* is the major CNS manifestation. It is characterized by weakness, ataxia, and choreic movement that is spontaneous, rapid, and purposeless and tends to intensify with voluntary activity.
- *Erythema marginatum* lesions are a less common feature. The bright-pink maplike macular lesions occur mainly on the trunk or inner aspects of the upper arm and thigh but never on the face. The rash is nonpruritic and nonpainful and is neither indurated or raised. It is usually transitory (lasting for a few hours), may recur intermittently for months, and is exacerbated by heat (e.g., a warm bath).
- *Subcutaneous nodules* are firm, small, hard, painless swellings found most commonly over bony prominences (e.g., knees, elbows, spine, scapulae).

Minor criteria. Minor clinical manifestations, which are frequently present, are helpful in recognizing the disease. These include fever, arthralgia, prolonged P-R interval, and previous occurrence of rheumatic fever or rheumatic heart disease.

Diagnostic Studies

- Antistreptolysin O (ASO) titer is the most specific test to confirm group A streptococcal infection.
- A throat culture is usually negative at the onset of the disease.
- Erythrocyte sedimentation rate (ESR) is elevated.
- White blood cell (WBC) count is elevated.
- Chest radiography may show a CHF-induced enlarged heart.
- Echocardiogram may show valvular insufficiency, pericardial fluid, or thickening.
- ECG reveals a prolonged P-R interval with delayed atrioventricular conduction.

Therapeutic Management

No specific treatment will cure rheumatic fever. Management consists of drug therapy and supportive measures. Antibiotic therapy does not modify the course of the acute disease or the development of carditis. Penicillin eliminates residual group A β-hemolytic streptococci remaining in the tonsils and pharynx and prevents the spread of organisms to close contacts. Salicylates and corticosteroids are used in the management of ARF. Both are effective in controlling the fever and joint manifestations. Corticosteroids are used if severe carditis is present.

- The patient without carditis may be ambulatory as soon as acute symptoms have subsided and may return to normal activity when antiinflammatory therapy has been discontinued.
- When carditis is present, ambulation is postponed until CHF has been controlled with treatment. Full activities should not be resumed until antiinflammatory therapy has been discontinued.

Nursing Management
Goals
The patient with rheumatic fever will have no residual cardiac disease, resume daily activities without joint pain, and verbalize the ability to manage the disease.

See the nursing care plan for the patient with rheumatic fever and heart disease in Lewis/Collier/Heitkemper, *Medical-Surgical Nursing,* edition 4, p. 1021.

Nursing Diagnoses
- Activity intolerance related to arthralgia
- Risk for injury related to chorea
- Ineffective management of therapeutic regimen related to lack of knowledge concerning the need for long-term prophylactic antibiotic therapy and possible disease sequelae, lack of compliance, lack of resources

Nursing Interventions
Rheumatic fever is one of the few cardiovascular diseases that is preventable. Prevention is frequently classified as primary and secondary.

Primary prevention involves early detection and immediate treatment of group A β-hemolytic streptococcal pharyngitis. Adequate treatment of streptococcal pharyngitis prevents initial attacks of rheumatic fever. The nurse's role is to educate people in the community to seek medical attention for symptoms of streptococcal pharyngitis and emphasize the need for adequate treatment of a streptococcal sore throat.

Secondary prevention focuses on the use of prophylactic antibiotics to prevent recurrent rheumatic fever. A person who has had rheumatic fever is more susceptible to a second attack after a streptococcal infection. The best prevention is monthly injections of benzathine penicillin G.

- Prophylactic treatment should continue for life in individuals who had rheumatic carditis as children. Rheumatic fever without carditis after the age of 18 years may need only 5 years of prophylactic antibiotic therapy or may continue indefinitely in patients with frequent exposure to group A streptococcus.

The primary goals of acute intervention are control and eradication of the infecting organism; prevention of cardiac complications; relief of joint pain, fever, and other symptoms; and support of the patient psychologically and emotionally.

- The nurse should administer antibiotics as ordered and teach the patient that oral antibiotics require adherence to the full 10-day course of therapy. Precautions with respiratory secretions should be maintained for 24 hours after initiation of antibiotic therapy.
- Tepid sponge baths should be given to relieve fever, and antipyretics should be administered as prescribed. Oral fluids should be encouraged if the patient is able to swallow; IV fluids should be administered as prescribed.
- Promotion of optimal rest is essential to reduce cardiac workload and diminish the metabolic needs of the body. After acute symptoms have subsided, the patient without carditis should ambulate.
- Relief of joint pain is important. Painful joints should be positioned for comfort and proper alignment. Removal of covers from painful joints can be done with a bed cradle. Heat may be applied, and salicylates may be administered to relieve joint pain.
- Psychologic and emotional care can be more important than physical care. Any alteration in cardiac function may be perceived as a threat to the person's body image.

Patient Teaching
- The patient with a previous history of rheumatic fever should be taught about the disease process, possible sequelae, and the continual need for prophylactic antibiotics.
- The patient must be made aware of the high risk of recurrence if a streptococcal infection develops and should be informed about the risk of exposure to streptococcal infections from contact with school-age children, individuals in military service, and people in health care positions.
- Ongoing patient education and reinforcement should include encouragement of good nutrition and hygienic practices and emphasis on the importance of receiving adequate rest.
- The patient should be instructed in the use of prophylactic antibiotic therapy. The dosage of antibiotics used in maintenance prophylaxis is not adequate to prevent infective endocarditis when invasive procedures are performed. Additional prophylaxis is necessary if a patient with known rheumatic heart disease has dental or surgical procedures involving the upper respiratory, GI, or genitourinary tract.

R

- The patient should also be cautioned about the possibility of development of valvular heart disease. The nurse should teach the patient to seek medical attention if symptoms such as excessive fatigue, dizziness, palpitations, or dyspnea on exertion develop.

RHEUMATOID ARTHRITIS

Definition/Description

Rheumatoid arthritis is a chronic systemic disease characterized by recurrent inflammation of the diarthrodial joints and related structures. It is frequently accompanied by a variety of extraarticular manifestations, such as rheumatoid nodules, arteritis, neuropathy, scleritis, pericarditis, lymphadenopathy, and splenomegaly.

Rheumatoid arthritis (RA) is characterized by periods of remission and exacerbation. The course of the illness varies, ranging from episodes of illness separated by periods of remission to a more continuous progressive disease.

Of the approximately 6 million Americans who have RA, 75% are women. There are no geographic or racial predispositions. Although RA can occur at any age, it most often occurs in women of childbearing age.

Pathophysiology

The cause of RA remains unknown. Several etiologies are possible, including infection (e.g., Epstein-Barr virus, parvoviruses, mycobacteria) and autoimmunity. RA is characterized by the presence of autoantibodies (known as *rheumatoid factor*) against altered immunoglobulin G (IgG). These autoantibodies combine with the altered IgG to form immune complexes that deposit in the joints, blood vessels, pleura, and other places.

Certain familial factors may influence the expression of the disease. An increased prevalence of the human leukocyte antigen (HLA) HLA-DR4 occurs in 65% of persons with RA.

The pathogenesis of RA is more clearly understood than its etiology. If unarrested, the disease progresses through four stages.

First stage. The unknown etiologic factor initiates joint inflammation, or synovitis, with swelling of the synovial lining membrane and production of excess synovial fluid.

Second stage. Pannus (granulation inflammatory tissue) is formed at the juncture of the synovium and cartilage. This extends over the surface of the articular cartilage and eventually invades the joint capsule and subchondral bone.

Third stage. Tough fibrous connective tissue replaces pannus, occluding the joint space. Fibrous ankylosis results in decreased joint motion, malalignment, and deformity.

Fourth stage. As fibrous tissue calcifies, bony ankylosis may result in total joint immobilization.

Clinical Manifestations

RA typically develops insidiously. Nonspecific manifestations such as fatigue, anorexia, weight loss, and generalized stiffness may precede the onset of arthritic complaints. The stiffness becomes more localized after weeks to months. Some patients report a history of a precipitating stressful event such as infection, childbirth, surgery, or emotional upset.

Articular involvement is manifested by pain, limitation of motion, and signs of inflammation (heat, swelling, and tenderness). Joint symptoms are bilaterally symmetric and frequently affect the small joints of the hands and feet and the larger peripheral joints, including the wrists, knees, and hips.

- The patient characteristically has joint stiffness on arising in the morning and after periods of inactivity. Table 41, p. 423, compares the manifestations of RA and osteoarthritis.
- As disease activity progresses, inflammation and fibrosis of the joint capsule and supporting structures may lead to deformity and disability. Atrophy of muscles and destruction of tendons around the joint cause one articular surface to slip past the other (subluxation). Typical deformities of the hand include "ulnar drift," "swan neck," and boutonniere deformities.

Rheumatoid nodules, present in 25% of all people with RA, are the most common extraarticular finding. They appear subcutaneously as firm, nontender masses and are usually found on the olecranon bursae or along the extensor surface of the forearm. Nodules develop insidiously and can persist or regress spontaneously. They are usually not removed unless they are significantly disabling because of the high probability of recurrence. Nodules may also appear on the eye or lungs; these indicate active disease and a poor prognosis.

Vasculitis (inflammation of blood vessels) may be responsible for peripheral neuropathy, myopathy, cardiopulmonary involvement, and ischemic ulcerations of the skin. See Figure 60-5 in Lewis/Collier/Heitkemper, *Medical-Surgical Nursing,* edition 4, p. 1906.

Diagnostic Studies

Although no single laboratory test is conclusive, several findings are helpful in diagnosing RA in conjunction with the history and physical examination.

- Moderate anemia is common.

- The erythrocyte sedimentation rate (ESR) is elevated in 85% of patients and is useful in monitoring the response to therapy.
- Serum rheumatoid factor is present in titers >1:160 in nearly 80% of cases. Antinuclear antibody and lupus cell tests may be positive in a smaller percentage of patients.
- Synovial fluid analysis may show increased volume and turbidity but decreased viscosity. The white blood cell (WBC) count is elevated (often as high as 30,000/μL [30 × 10⁹/L]) and consists predominantly of polymorphonuclear leukocytes.
- Inflammatory changes in the synovium can be confirmed by tissue biopsy.
- X-ray findings (not specifically diagnostic) may reveal bone demineralization and soft-tissue swelling during early months of the disease. Later, narrowing of the joint space, destruction of articular cartilage, erosion, subluxation, and deformity are present. Malalignment and ankylosis occur in advanced disease.

Therapeutic Management

Management of RA begins with a comprehensive program of pharmacotherapy and education. Physical comfort is promoted with nonsteroidal antiinflammatory drugs (NSAIDs) and rest. The patient and family are educated about the disease process and home management strategies. Responsible compliance with medications includes correct administration, reporting of side effects, and frequent medical and laboratory follow-up visits. Physical therapy maintains joint motion and muscle strength. Occupational therapy develops upper extremity function and encourages joint protection through the use of splinting, pacing techniques, and assistive devices.

Pharmacologic Management

Aspirin and NSAIDS are commonly used. For patients with mild disease, hydroxychloroquine is often prescribed. Often a low dose of prednisone is given with or instead of hydroxychloroquine. Corticosteroid therapy can be used to achieve disease control. Intraarticular injections are administered for a flare in one or two joints. *Bridge therapy* (5 mg of the prescribed corticosteroid given orally for 4 to 6 weeks) is used until one of the longer-acting drugs, such as hydroxychloroquine, gold, or D-penicillamine, has been taken long enough to suppress disease activity. *Burst corticosteroid therapy* consists of high-dose (e.g., 60 mg) corticosteroid used for a severe articular flare, which is then quickly tapered in 10 to 14 days. *Pulse therapy* (Solu-Medrol, at dosages of no more than 1 g/day intravenously for 3 days) is used to achieve fast control of inflammation and results in fewer side effects over the long term as a result of the patient taking a smaller daily dose.

For patients with moderate to severe disease with symmetric joint involvement and a positive rheumatoid factor assay, a more aggressive drug regimen may be initiated. Methotrexate, usually the first drug of choice, has a rapid antiinflammatory effect and reduces clinical symptoms in days to weeks. Methotrexate therapy requires frequent laboratory follow-up. Gold therapy may be considered for patients who do not respond to methotrexate. Azathioprine or D-penicillamine may be used if the patient does not respond to either methotrexate or gold therapy.

Nutritional Management

There is no special diet; however, balanced nutrition is important. A sensible weight-loss program, consisting of balanced nutrition and exercise, will reduce stress on arthritic joints. Limited sodium intake may help minimize weight gain caused by sodium retention. The patient must be encouraged to continue a balanced diet and not to alter the corticosteroid dose or to stop therapy abruptly. Weight slowly adjusts to normal several months after the cessation of therapy.

R

Nursing Management

Goals

The patient with RA will have satisfactory pain relief, have minimal loss of functional ability of the affected joints, participate in the planning and carrying out of the therapeutic regimen, maintain a positive self-image, and perform self-care to the maximum amount possible.

Nursing Diagnoses

- Fatigue related to exacerbation of disease activity, anemia, drug side effects, muscle atrophy, sleep disturbance, or depression
- Pain related to joint inflammation, overuse of joint, and ineffective pain or comfort measures
- Impaired physical mobility related to joint pain, stiffness, and swelling
- Joint deformity related to disease activity, noncompliance, and lack of knowledge of contracture prevention
- Altered nutrition: less than body requirements related to fatigue, pain, treatment, or self-care deficit
- Altered family processes related to patient's inability to function secondary to chronic illness and treatment regimen
- Self-care deficit (partial to total) related to disease progression, weakness, and contracture
- Ineffective management of therapeutic regimen related to complexity of chronic health problems, pain, and fatigue
- Body image disturbance related to chronic disease activity, long-term treatment program, deformities, stiffness, and inability to perform usual activities

Nursing Interventions

Prevention of RA is not possible at this time. However, community education programs should include information concerning the symptoms of RA to promote early diagnosis and treatment. The primary objectives in management may be approached by a comprehensive program of daily antiinflammatory medication, rest, joint protection, therapeutic heat, exercise, and thorough patient and family education.

Nursing interventions begin with a careful assessment of physical needs (joint pain, swelling, range of motion [ROM], and general health status); psychosocial needs (family support, sexual satisfaction, emotional stress, financial constraints, vocation and career limitations); and environmental needs (transportation, home/work modifications).

- Suppression of inflammation is most effectively achieved through the administration of antiinflammatory and/or remittive agents. Education centers around the action and side effects of each drug and the importance of laboratory monitoring. The nurse must make the drug regimen as clear and simple as possible. High-dose IV corticosteroid therapy requires careful observation for changes in BP, peripheral edema, and signs of congestive heart failure.
- Nonpharmacologic relief of pain includes the use of therapeutic heat and cold, rest, relaxation techniques, biofeedback, transcutaneous electric nerve stimulation, and hypnosis.
- Lightweight splints are sometimes used to rest an inflamed joint and prevent deformity from muscle spasms and contractures. These splints should be removed, skin care given, ROM exercises performed, and splints reapplied as prescribed.
- Morning care and procedures should be planned around the patient's morning stiffness. Sitting or standing in a warm shower, sitting in a tub with warm towels around the shoulders, or soaking the hands in a basin of warm water may help to relieve joint stiffness and allow the patient to comfortably perform activities of daily living.
- Regularly scheduled rest periods alternated with activity throughout the day help relieve fatigue and pain and minimize excessive weight-bearing. The nurse should assist the patient in pacing activities and setting priorities on the basis of realistic goals.
- Good body alignment while resting is important. A firm mattress or bedboard should be used. Positions of extension should be encouraged, and positions of flexion should be avoided. Pillows should never be placed under the knees. A small flat pillow may be used under the head and shoulders. Splints and

casts may be helpful in maintaining proper alignment and promoting rest, especially when joint inflammation is present.

Protecting joints from stress is very important. Nursing interventions include helping the patient identify ways to modify tasks. Each patient needs to learn ways to accomplish routine activities that put less stress on the joints. The emphasis is on changing the way the task is done and on work-simplification techniques. Sample activities that protect small joints are listed in Table 60-8 in Lewis/Collier/Heitkemper, *Medical-Surgical Nursing,* edition 4, p. 1912.

- Patient independence may be increased by occupational therapy training with assistive devices that help simplify tasks, such as built-up utensils, buttonhooks, and raised toilet seats. A cane or a platform-wheeled walker offers support and relief of pain when walking.

Heat and cold therapy help to relieve stiffness, pain, and muscle spasm. Application of ice may be beneficial in an acute episode, and moist heat appears to offer better relief of chronic stiffness.

The nurse should reinforce patient compliance with an individualized exercise program and evaluate that the exercises are being done correctly. Gentle ROM exercises are usually done daily to keep the joints functional. The nurse needs to emphasize that usual daily activities do not provide adequate exercise to maintain joint motion.

Patient Teaching

Self-management and adherence to an individualized home program are contingent on a thorough understanding of RA, the nature and course of the disease, and the objectives of treatment. In addition, the patient's perception of the disease and value system must be considered.

- The nurse can help the patient recognize common fears and concerns faced by all people living with a chronic illness. Evaluation of the family support system is important. The patient is constantly threatened by problems of limited function and fatigue, loss of self-esteem, and fear of disability and deformity.
- Alterations in sexuality should be discussed. Financial planning may be necessary. Community resources such as a home care nurse, homemaker services, and vocational rehabilitation may be considered. Self-help groups are beneficial for some patients.

Seizure Disorders

Definition/Description

A seizure is a sudden alteration in normal brain activity that causes distinctive changes in behavior and body function. Seizures may accompany a variety of disorders, or they may occur spontaneously without any apparent cause.

- In the adult metabolic disturbances that cause seizures include acidosis, electrolyte imbalances, hypoglycemia, hypoxia, alcohol and barbiturate withdrawal, and dehydration.
- Extracranial disorders that can cause seizures include heart, lung, liver, and kidney disease, systemic lupus erythematosus, diabetes, hypertension, and septicemia.

Epilepsy connotes spontaneously recurring seizures. There are an estimated 1 to 2 million patients with epilepsy in the United States. Incidence rates are very high during the first year of life, decline through childhood and adolescence, plateau in middle age, and rise sharply again among the elderly.

Pathophysiology

The most common causes of epilepsy during the first 6 months of life are severe birth injury, congenital defects involving the central nervous system (CNS), infections, and inborn errors of metabolism. In individuals between 20 to 30 years of age, epilepsy usually occurs as a result of structural lesions, such as trauma, brain tumors, or vascular disease. After the age of 50, primary causes of epilepsy are cerebrovascular lesions and metastatic brain tumors. Three fourths of all cases cannot be attributed to a specific cause.

Seizures are paroxysmal uncontrolled electrical discharges of brain neurons that interrupt normal function. In recurring seizures (epilepsy) a group of abnormal neurons *(seizure focus)* seem to undergo spontaneous firing. This firing spreads by physiologic pathways to involve adjacent or distant areas of the brain. Often the brain area from which epileptic activity arises is found to have scar tissue *(gliosis)*. Scarring is thought to interfere with the normal chemical and structural environment of brain neurons, making them fire abnormally.

Clinical Manifestations

The preferred method of classifying seizures is the International Classification System (see Table 45). This system is based on the clinical and electroencephalographic (EEG) manifestations of seizures.

Table 45	International Classification of Epileptic Seizures

Generalized Seizures (Bilaterally Symmetrical and Without Local Onset)
Absence seizures, atypical absence seizures
Myoclonic seizures
Clonic seizures
Tonic seizures
Tonic-clonic seizures
Atonic seizures

Partial Seizures (Local Onset)
- Simple partial seizures (no impairment of consciousness)
  With motor symptoms
  With somatosensory or special sensory symptoms
  With autonomic symptoms
  With psychic symptoms
- Complex partial seizures (impairment of consciousness)
  Simple partial seizures with progression to impairment of consciousness
  With no other features
  With features of simple partial seizures
  With automatisms
  Impairment of consciousness at onset
  With no other features
  With features of simple partial seizures
  With automatisms

Unclassified Epileptic Seizures (Inadequate or Incomplete Data)

Modified from Commission on Classification and Terminology of the International League against Epilepsy: Proposal for revised clinical and electroencephalographic classification of epileptic seizures, *Epilepsia* 22:489, 1981.

Seizures are divided into two major classes, *generalized* and *partial*. Depending on the type, a seizure may progress through several phases, which include (1) a *prodromal* phase with warning signs that precede a seizure, (2) an *aural* phase with a sensory warning, (3) an *ictal* phase with full seizure, and (4) a *postictal* phase, which is the period of recovery after the seizure.

Generalized Seizures

Generalized seizures are characterized by bilateral synchronous epileptic discharge in the brain. Because the entire brain is affected at the onset of the seizures, there is no warning or aura. In most cases the patient loses consciousness for a few seconds to several minutes.

- *Clonic-tonic (grand mal) seizures* are the most common generalized seizures. This type of seizure is characterized by loss of consciousness and falling to the ground if upright, followed by stiffening of the body (tonic phase) for 10 to 20 seconds and subsequent jerking of the extremities (clonic phase) for another 30 to 40 seconds. Cyanosis, excessive salivation, tongue or cheek biting, and incontinence may accompany the seizure. In the postictal phase the patient usually has muscle soreness, is very tired, and may sleep for several hours. The patient has no memory of the seizure activity.

- *Typical absence (petit mal) seizures* usually occur in children and rarely continue beyond adolescence. The typical clinical manifestation is a brief staring spell that lasts only a few seconds. There may be an extremely brief loss of consciousness. When untreated, the seizures may occur up to 100 times a day. Absence seizures are often precipitated by hyperventilation and a sensation of flashing lights.

- *Atypical absence seizures* are another type of generalized seizure characterized by a staring spell. A brief warning, peculiar behavior during the seizure, and/or confusion after the seizure are also common.

Partial Seizures

Partial (focal) seizures begin in a specific region of the cortex, as indicated by the EEG and clinical manifestations. Partial seizures may be confined to one side of the brain and may remain partial or focal in nature, or they may spread to involve the entire brain, culminating in a generalized tonic-clonic seizure. Any tonic-clonic seizure preceded by an aura or warning is a partial seizure that generalizes secondarily.

- Partial seizures are further divided into those with simple motor or sensory phenomena and those with complex symptoms (also called *psychomotor* seizures). The terms *focal motor, focal sensory,* and *Jacksonian* have been used to describe seizures of the simple partial type.

Status epilepticus is the most serious complication. In this state seizures recur in rapid succession and the patient does not regain consciousness or normal function between seizures.

- Status epilepticus can involve any type of seizure. During repeated seizures the brain uses more energy than can be supplied. Neurons become exhausted and cease to function. Permanent brain damage may result.

- Tonic-clonic status epilepticus is most dangerous because it can cause ventilatory insufficiency, hypoxemia, cardiac dysrhythmias, and systemic acidosis, all of which can be fatal.

Diagnostic Studies

- Complete health history and physical examination to include birth and development history, significant illnesses and injuries, family history, history of febrile seizures, and comprehensive neurologic assessment
- Seizure history to include precipitating factors, antecedent events, and seizure description (including onset, duration, frequency, postictal state)
- Complete blood count (CBC), urinalysis, electrolytes, blood urea nitrogen, fasting blood glucose
- Lumbar puncture
- CT scan and EEG

Therapeutic Management

Most seizures do not require professional emergency medical care because they are self-limiting and rarely cause bodily injury. However, if status epilepticus occurs, if significant bodily harm occurs, or if the event is a first-time seizure, medical care should be sought immediately. Table 56-7 in Lewis/Collier/Heitkemper, *Medical-Surgical Nursing,* edition 4, p. 1760, summarizes emergency care of the patient with a generalized tonic-clonic seizure.

Epilepsy is treated primarily with antiepileptic medication. Therapy is aimed at preventing seizures since cure is not possible. Medications generally act by stabilizing nerve cell membranes and preventing spread of the epileptic discharge. Alternative therapies for epilepsy are surgical removal of the epileptic focus and biofeedback or operant conditioning in selected cases.

Surgery may be considered to control intractable seizures, prevent cerebral degeneration from repeated seizures, and improve quality of life.

Pharmacologic Management

The primary goal of antiepileptic drug therapy is to obtain maximum seizure control with a minimum of toxic side effects. The principle of drug management is to begin with a single drug and increase the dosage until the seizures are controlled or toxic side effects occur.

- The primary drugs for treatment of generalized tonic-clonic and partial seizures may include phenytoin (Dilantin), carbamazepine (Tegretol), and phenobarbital. The primary drugs for treatment of absence, akinetic, and myoclonic seizures may include ethosuximide (Zarontin), divalproex sodium (Depakote), and clonazepam (Klonopin). Two new antiepileptic drugs are felbamate (Felbatol) and gabapentin (Neurontin).

Nursing Management

Goals

The patient with seizures will be free from injury during a seizure, have optimal mental and physical functioning while taking antiepileptic medication, and have satisfactory psychosocial functioning.

Nursing Diagnoses

- Ineffective airway clearance related to tracheobronchial obstruction
- Ineffective individual coping related to perceived loss of control, denial of diagnosis, or misconceptions regarding disease
- Ineffective breathing pattern related to neuromuscular impairment secondary to prolonged tonic phase of seizure or during postictal period
- Impaired verbal communication related to transient aphasia secondary to postictal state
- Self-concept disturbances related to diagnosis of epilepsy
- Ineffective management of therapeutic regimen related to lack of knowledge about management of epilepsy
- Risk for injury related to seizure activity and subsequent impaired physical mobility secondary to postictal weakness or paralysis

Nursing Interventions

Children with fever should be treated quickly to avoid high temperatures, which may cause seizures. The patient with epilepsy should practice good general health habits (e.g., maintaining a proper diet, getting adequate rest, exercising). The patient should be helped to identify events or situations that precipitate seizures and should be given suggestions for avoiding them or handling them better.

The nurse caring for a hospitalized epileptic patient or a patient who has had seizures should focus on observation and treatment of the seizure, education, and psychosocial intervention.

- When a seizure occurs, the nurse should carefully observe and record details of the event because the diagnosis and subsequent treatment depend on the seizure description.
- Assessment of the postictal period should include a detailed description of the level of consciousness, vital signs, memory loss, muscle soreness, speech disorders (aphasia, dysarthria), weakness or paralysis, sleep period, and the duration of each sign or symptom.
- During the seizure it is important to maintain a patent airway. This may involve supporting and protecting the head, turning the patient to the side, loosening constrictive clothing, or easing the patient to the floor if sitting in a chair. After the seizure the patient may require suctioning and O_2.

- A seizure can be a frightening experience for the patient and for others who may witness it. The nurse should assess the patient's level of understanding and provide information about how and why the event occurred.

Patient Teaching

Prevention of recurring seizures is the major goal in the treatment of epilepsy. Because epilepsy cannot be cured, medication must be taken regularly and continuously, often for a lifetime.

- The nurse should ensure that the patient knows the specifics of the medication regimen and what to do if a dose is missed.
- The patient should be cautioned not to adjust the medication amount or schedule without professional guidance because this can increase the seizure frequency and can even cause status epilepticus.
- The patient should be encouraged to report any medication side effects and to keep regular appointments with the health care provider.
- The nurse should teach family members and significant others the first-aid treatment of tonic-clonic seizures.
- The nurse should provide psychosocial support for the patient by providing education and helping to identify coping mechanisms.

SHOCK

Definition/Description

Shock is a clinical syndrome resulting in decreased blood flow to body tissues, which causes cellular dysfunction and eventual organ failure. Regardless of cause, the end result is inadequate supply of O_2 and nutrients to body cells attributable to impaired tissue perfusion.

Pathophysiology

Shock is a dynamic event in which several different processes may be occurring at the same time. A patient may progress toward death or normal homeostatic functioning over a widely varying period of time. The shock syndrome can be divided into the following four stages:

1. *Initial stage:* Cellular changes start to occur as tissue perfusion decreases and anaerobic metabolism increases.
2. *Compensatory stage:* In this potentially reversible stage a variety of compensatory mechanisms maintain adequate perfusion.

3. *Progressive stage:* Compensatory mechanisms are ineffective and fail to maintain vital organ perfusion.
4. *Irreversible or refractory stage:* Compensatory mechanisms are nonfunctioning, resulting in cellular necrosis and multiple organ dysfunction. Death is imminent.

Complications of shock include infection, acute tubular necrosis (ATN), acute respiratory distress syndrome (ARDS), and disseminated intravascular coagulation (DIC).

Classification of Shock

This classification of shock is based on a consideration of defects in the three primary mechanisms responsible for adequate circulation: (1) vascular tone *(distributive shock),* (2) ability of the heart to act as a pump *(cardiogenic shock),* and (3) intravascular volume *(hypovolemic shock).* Patients may have more than one form of shock simultaneously. Table 46 presents the classification and precipitation factors of the three main types of shock.

- *Distributive shock* includes neurogenic, septic, and anaphylactic shock. In distributive shock relative hypovolemia occurs when vasodilatation increases the vascular space size. This results in altered distribution of blood volume rather than actual volume loss.
- *Cardiogenic shock* is referred to as "pump failure," with the major cause being myocardial infarction. Cardiogenic shock can also occur in blood flow obstruction with cardiac tamponade, pulmonary embolism, and tension pneumothorax. In this type of shock the heart can no longer pump blood efficiently to all parts of the body. There is no decreased intravascular volume or vasodilatation of the vascular space.
- *Hypovolemic shock* can occur with hemorrhage (most common cause), burns, loss of GI fluid, or diabetic ketoacidosis. An actual loss of intravascular fluid volume can be attributable to either external fluid loss or internal fluid shifts from the intravascular space to the interstitial or intracellular spaces. Loss of fluid results eventually in inadequate tissue perfusion. There is no decrease in the pumping ability of the heart.

Clinical Manifestations

According to shock syndrome stages:
1. *Initial stage:* No signs or symptoms are present.
2. *Compensatory stage:* Subtle symptoms that are often overlooked include sensorium changes (restlessness, irritability); slight heart rate increase and increased respirations; decreased urine output; thirst; and cool, pale extremities (except in septic shock—extremities are warm and dry).

Table 46   **Classification and Precipitating Factors of Shock**

Distributive Shock
Neurogenic shock
   Injury and disease to spinal cord
   Spinal anesthesia, deep general anesthesia, or epidural block
   Vasomotor center depression (e.g., severe pain, drugs, hypoglycemia, emotional stress)

Septic shock
   Infection (e.g., urinary tract, respiratory tract, postpartum, caused by invasive procedures [especially urologic procedures] and indwelling lines and catheters)
   Compromised patients, including older adults, patients with chronic disease (e.g., diabetes, cancer, acquired immunodeficiency syndrome), patients receiving immunosuppressive therapy, malnourished or debilitated patients

Anaphylactic shock
   Drugs (especially penicillin)
   Insect bites/stings
   Contrast media
   Blood transfusions
   Anesthetic agents
   Foods
   Vaccines

Cardiogenic Shock
   Myocardial infarction (most common cause)
   Dysrhythmias
   Severe congestive heart failure
   Cardiomyopathy
   Obstructive causes (pericardial tamponade, pericardial diseases, tension pneumothorax, acute valvular damage, pulmonary embolism)

Hypovolemic Shock
External fluid losses
   Hemorrhage (most common cause)
   Burns
   Excessive use of diuretics
   Loss of GI fluid (vomiting, diarrhea, nasogastric suctioning)
   Diabetes insipidus
   Diabetic ketoacidosis
Internal fluid shifts
   Interstitial blood pooling (ascites, peritonitis, bowel obstruction)
   Internal bleeding (fracture of long bones, ruptured spleen, femoral arterial punctures or catheters in patients undergoing anticoagulant therapy)

S

3. *Progressive stage:* Listlessness; confusion; falling BP and narrowed pulse pressure; tachycardia; shallow increased respirations; a further decrease in urine output; hypothermia; cold, pale, and clammy skin; and thirst with dry lips and mucosa.
4. *Irreversible or refractory stage:* All organ systems affected with decompensation are evident; unconscious and unresponsive to stimuli, systolic BP falling with diastolic BP approaching zero; cardiac dysrhythmias; pulse weak and heart rate slow; Cheyne-Stokes respirations; intestinal sepsis; renal ischemia with minimal urine output; hypothermia; and cyanosis.

Diagnostic Studies

- History—if possible, to identify the cause of shock
- Physical examination—observe for shock manifestations, especially overall central nervous system function
- Blood studies—may include complete blood count (CBC), disseminated intravascular coagulation (DIC) screen, erythrocyte sedimentation rate (ESR), blood urea nitrogen (BUN), glucose, electrolytes, arterial blood gases (ABGs), lactate, blood cultures, and liver enzymes
- Placement of central venous pressure (CVP) or pulmonary artery (PA) catheter, as indicated
- Chest x-ray
- Twelve-lead ECG and cardiac monitor
  See Table 7-4 in Lewis/Collier/Heitkemper, *Medical-Surgical Nursing,* edition 4, p. 127, for further information.
  Table 47 presents the hemodynamic effects of shock.

Therapeutic Management

The critical factor in management is early recognition and treatment. Prompt intervention can alter the shock process and prevent the development of the irreversible refractory stage and death. Successful management depends on the ability to (1) identify the patient at high risk for shock, (2) diagnose shock syndrome swiftly and accurately, (3) control or alleviate the primary cause, and (4) implement appropriate therapeutic measures to correct pathologic changes and enhance tissue perfusion.

Whenever possible, the patient in shock should be treated in an intensive care unit and receive continuous ECG monitoring. A general goal is to keep the mean arterial BP >60 mm Hg. Overall areas of focus include:

- O_2 and ventilatory assistance (see Intubation, Endotracheal, p. 657; Oxygen Therapy, p. 669; and Mechanical Ventilation, p. 662)
- Supine positioning with legs elevated at an angle of 45 degrees (after neck and spine injuries have been ruled out)

Table 47   Hemodynamic Effects of Shock

Type of shock	Cardiac output	Central venous pressure	Systemic vascular resistance	Pulmonary artery pressure	Pulmonary capillary wedge pressure
Hypovolemic	↓	↓	↑	↓	↓
Cardiogenic	↓	↑ or N	↑	↑	↑
Anaphylactic	↑ or N	↓	↓	↓ or N	↓ or N
Septic	↑ or N	↓	↓	↓	↓
Neurogenic	↓	↓	↓	↓	↓

N, Normal.

- Fluid replacement
- Maintenance of fluid and electrolyte balance and acid-base balance
- Monitoring and treating cardiac dysrhythmias (see Dysrhythmias, p. 200)

Additionally, each type of shock has specific additional management, including pharmacologic drugs, whose primary purpose is to correct poor tissue perfusion. (See Table 7-5 in Lewis/Collier/Heitkemper, *Medical-Surgical Nursing*, edition 4, p. 128.)

Nursing Management
Goals
The patient with hypovolemic shock will have adequate tissue perfusion, normal BP, and no complications related to shock.

See nursing care plan for the patient in hypovolemic shock in Lewis/Collier/Heitkemper, *Medical-Surgical Nursing*, edition 4, p. 136.

Nursing Diagnoses/Collaborative Problems
- Decreased cardiac output related to hypovolemia
- Fear and anxiety related to severity of condition
- Potential complication: organ ischemia related to decreased tissue perfusion: neurologic, renal, gastrointestinal, respiratory and/or peripheral vascular

Nursing Interventions
It is important to prevent shock. To prevent shock, the nurse must first identify persons who are at risk. In general, the very old, the very young, and persons with chronic debilitating diseases are at increased risk. More specifically, any person who sustains surgical or accidental trauma is at risk of shock resulting from hemorrhage, spinal cord injury, and burn injuries. Specific examples of persons at high risk for shock include a person with diabetes mellitus whose disease is not well controlled or who does not adhere to therapy, a person with an acute myocardial infarction, and a person with a severe allergy to such substances as drugs, shellfish, and insect bites.

Prevention of shock can include interventions such as early mobilization of spinal cord injuries (to prevent neurogenic shock), careful monitoring of fluid balance (to prevent hypovolemic shock), and monitoring the patient at risk for sepsis for signs of infection.

When shock develops, it is important to monitor the patient's ongoing physical and emotional status to detect subtle changes in condition, plan and implement nursing interventions and therapy, evaluate the patient's response to therapy, and provide emotional support to the patient and significant others.

Nursing responsibilities also include judging when it is necessary to alert other health team members to changes in the patient's status that may require reevaluation of treatment. Ongoing reassessment of the patient's condition is important.

Communication with the patient is important and includes:
- It is important to talk to the patient, even if he/she is intubated or appears comatose.
- The patient needs simple explanations of procedures before they are carried out and information regarding the current plan of care and rationale.
- If the patient asks questions about progress and prognosis, simple and honest answers should be given.

SJÖGREN'S SYNDROME

Definition/Description
Sjögren's syndrome is characterized by autoantibodies to two protein ribonucleic acid (RNA) complexes termed SS-A/Ro and SS-B/La. Manifestations are caused by inflammation and dysfunction of the exocrine glands, particularly the salivary and lacrimal glands. More than 90% of the patients are women, and half have rheumatoid arthritis or another connective tissue disease.

Clinical Manifestations
Decreased tearing leads to a "gritty" sensation in the eyes, burning, and photosensitivity.
- Dry mouth produces buccal membrane fissures, dysphagia, and frequent dental caries.
- Dry nasal and respiratory passages are common and can result in a cough. Often the parotid glands are enlarged.
- Other exocrine glands may also be affected; for example, vaginal dryness may lead to dyspareunia.

Diagnostic Studies
- Histologic study reveals lymphocyte infiltration of the salivary and lacrimal glands, but the disease may become more generalized and involve the lymph nodes, bone marrow, and visceral organs (pseudolymphoma). Extraglandular proliferation may become malignant (e.g., lymphoma).
- Rheumatoid and antinuclear factors are present in the majority of patients.
- Anemia, leukopenia, hypergammaglobulinemia, and elevated erythrocyte sedimentation rate (ESR) are usually found.
- Ophthalmologic examination (Schirmer test), salivary flow rates, and lower lip biopsy of minor salivary glands are used to confirm the diagnosis.

Therapeutic Management

Treatment is symptomatic, including (1) artificial tears instillation as often as necessary to maintain adequate hydration and lubrication, (2) surgical punctal occlusion, and (3) increased fluids with meals. Dental hygiene is important.

- Increased humidity at home may reduce respiratory infections. Vaginal lubrication with a water-soluble product such as K-Y jelly may increase comfort during sexual intercourse.
- Corticosteroids and immunosuppressive drugs are indicated for treatment of pseudolymphoma.

SPINAL CORD INJURY

Definition/Description

Spinal cord injuries are classified by mechanism, level, or degree. The major mechanisms of injury are flexion, hyperextension, flexion-rotation, extension-rotation, or compression. The level of injury may be cervical, thoracic, or lumbar. Cervical and lumbar injuries are most common because these levels are associated with the greatest flexibility and movement.

The degree of spinal cord involvement may be either complete or incomplete (partial).

- *Complete cord* involvement (transection) results in flaccid paralysis and total loss of sensory and motor function below the level of the lesion (injury). If the cervical cord is involved, paralysis of all four extremities, particularly the hands and forearms, occurs and results in quadriplegia. If the thoracic or lumbar cord is damaged, the result is paraplegia.
- *Incomplete cord* lesion involvement (partial transection) results in a mixed loss of voluntary motor activity and sensation and leaves some tracts intact. The degree of sensory and motor loss varies, depending on the level of the lesion, and reflects the specific nerve tracts damaged and those spared.

The at-risk population for spinal cord injury is primarily young adult males between the ages of 15 and 30 years and those who are impulsive or risk takers in daily living. A history of numerous injuries before the spinal cord injury is common. The causes of spinal cord injury include motor vehicle accidents, falls, acts of violence, and sports injuries. The resulting spinal cord injury can be due to cord compression by bone displacement, interruption of blood supply to the cord, or traction resulting from pulling on the cord.

Pathophysiology

Penetrating trauma, such as gunshot and stab wounds, can result in tearing and transection. Complete cord dissolution in severe trauma is related to autodestruction of the cord.

Shortly after the injury hemorrhagic areas in the center of the spinal cord (gray matter) are grossly visible within 1 hour. Within 4 hours there may be an infarction in the gray matter. Hemorrhage, edema, and metabolites act together to produce ischemia, which progresses to necrotic destruction of the cord. By 24 hours permanent damage has occurred because of edema secondary to the inflammatory response.

Hemorrhagic necrosis causes the lesion to be complete after 48 hours, and any function of nerves that arise in and pass through this level is lost. Because additional edema extends the level of injury beyond the immediate level of destruction for 72 hours to 1 week, the exact extent of injury cannot be determined before that time.

In addition to discrete damage at the trauma site, the entire cord below the level of the lesion fails to function, resulting in *spinal shock* characterized by hypotension, bradycardia, and warm, dry extremities. Loss of sympathetic innervation causes peripheral vasodilatation, venous pooling, and decreased cardiac output. These effects are generally associated with a cervical or high thoracic injury. With spinal shock there is also flaccid paralysis below the level of injury. This affects musculoskeletal, bowel, and bladder function.

- Spinal shock generally lasts for 7 to 10 days after onset but can last from weeks to months. Indications that spinal shock has ended include spasticity, reflex emptying of the bladder, and hyperreflexia.

Clinical Manifestations

Manifestations of spinal cord injury are related to the level and degree of injury. The patient with an incomplete lesion may demonstrate a mixture of symptoms. The higher the injury, the more serious are the sequelae because of the proximity of the cervical cord to the medulla and brainstem. Movement and rehabilitation potential related to specific locations of the spinal cord injury are described in Table 57-3 in Lewis/Collier/Heitkemper, *Medical-Surgical Nursing,* edition 4, p. 1803). In general, sensory function closely parallels motor function at all levels.

- Accidents that cause spinal cord trauma can also result in head injury. The patient should be assessed for signs of concussion and increased intracranial pressure. In addition, a careful assessment for musculoskeletal injuries and trauma to the internal organs should be performed. Urinary output is examined for hematuria, which is also indicative of internal injuries.

Complications

Respiratory system. Cervical injury or fracture above the level of C4 presents with a total loss of respiratory muscle function. Mechanical ventilation is required to keep the patient alive.

Cardiovascular system. Any cord transection above the level of T5 markedly decreases the influence of the sympathetic nervous system. Bradycardia occurs as a result of the opposed effect of the parasympathetic nervous system on the heart, and vasodilatation results in hypotension. Close cardiac monitoring is necessary.

Urinary system. Retention is common in acute spinal cord injuries and spinal shock. While the patient is in spinal shock the bladder is atonic and will become overdistended. An indwelling catheter is inserted to drain the bladder.

Gastrointestinal system. If the cord transection has occurred above the level of T5, primary problems are related to hypomotility. Decreased GI motor activity will contribute to the development of a paralytic ileus and gastric distention. A nasogastric tube for intermittent suctioning may relieve the gastric distention.

Integumentary system. A major consequence of the lack of movement is tissue breakdown in the area of denervation, which can occur quickly and lead to major infection or sepsis. A certain degree of muscle atrophy occurs during the flaccid paralytic state, whereas contractures tend to occur during the spastic state.

Peripheral vascular problems. Deep-vein thrombosis (DVT) is a common problem accompanying spinal cord injury. Pulmonary embolism is one of the leading causes of death in patients with spinal cord injury. Techniques for assessment of DVT include Doppler examination, impedance plethysmography, and measuring leg and thigh girth.

Autonomic dysreflexia. Also known as hyperreflexia, autonomic dysreflexia is a massive uncompensated cardiovascular reaction mediated by the sympathetic division of the autonomic nervous system. It occurs in response to visceral stimulation once spinal shock is resolved in patients with spinal cord lesions above T7.

- This condition is a life-threatening situation that requires immediate resolution. If resolution does not occur, the condition can lead to status epilepticus, stroke, and even death.
- The most common precipitating cause is a distended bladder or rectum, although any sensory stimulation may cause autonomic dysreflexia.
- Manifestations include hypertension (up to 300 mm Hg systolic), blurred vision, throbbing headache, marked diaphoresis above the level of the lesion, bradycardia (30 to 40 beats/min), piloerection (erection of body hair), nasal congestion, and nausea. It is important that when a patient with a spinal cord injury complains of a headache that the BP be measured.

Diagnostic Studies

- Complete neurologic examination for evaluation of the degree of deficit and establishment of the level and degree of injury
- Arterial blood gases (ABGs)
- Electrolytes, glucose, hemoglobin, and hematocrit levels
- Urinalysis
- Anteroposterior, lateral, and odontoid spinal x-ray studies to document injury
- CT scan and MRI
- Myelography and electromyography (EMG)

Therapeutic Management

After stabilization at the accident scene, the person should be transferred to a medical facility. Respiratory, cardiac, urinary, and GI function are monitored closely. The patient may go directly to surgery after initial immobilization and stabilization or to the intensive care unit for monitoring and management.

Surgical Management

Surgery is necessary when there is continued compression of the spinal cord by extrinsic forces. Surgery stabilizes the spinal column. In general, accepted criteria for early surgery include (1) evidence of cord compression, (2) progressive neurologic deficit, (3) compound fracture of the vertebra, (4) bony fragments that may dislodge and penetrate the cord, (5) penetrating wounds of the spinal cord or surrounding structures, and (6) a bone fragment in the spinal cord.

- More common surgical procedures include decompression laminectomy by anterior cervical and thoracic approaches with fusion, posterior laminectomy with the use of acrylic wire mesh and fusion, and insertion of stabilizing rods (e.g., Harrington rods for the correction and stabilization of thoracic deformities). (Specific surgical and nursing interventions for these techniques are discussed in Lewis/Collier/Heitkemper, *Medical-Surgical Nursing,* edition 4, p. 1886.)

Pharmacologic Management

Vasopressor agents employed in the acute phase are useful adjuvants to treatment. Dopamine is the drug of choice. Methylprednisolone produces a number of effects that may account for the overall improvement noted in the patient with the spinal cord injury, including reduction of posttraumatic spinal cord ischemia, improvement of energy balance, improvement of nerve impulse conduction, and decrease in the release of free fatty acids from spinal cord tissues.

- Pharmacologic agents are used to treat specific autonomic dysfunctions, such as GI hyperactivity, bleeding, bradycardia, orthostatic hypotension, inadequate emptying of the bladder, and autonomic dysreflexia.

Nursing Management
Goals
The patient with a spinal cord injury will maintain an optimal level of neurologic functioning, have minimal or no complications of immobility, and return to home and the community at an optimal level of functioning.

See the nursing care plan for the patient with spinal cord injury in Lewis/Collier/Heitkemper, *Medical-Surgical Nursing,* edition 4, p. 1807.

Nursing Diagnoses
- Impaired physical mobility related to spinal cord injury, vertebral column instability, or forced immobilization by traction
- Impaired skin integrity related to immobility and poor tissue perfusion
- Constipation related to the injury, inadequate fluid intake, diet low in roughage, and immobility
- Altered patterns of urinary elimination: retention related to injury and limited fluid intake
- Self-care deficit: total related to paralysis
- Risk for dysreflexia related to reflex stimulation of sympathetic nervous system secondary to loss of automatic control after resolution of spinal shock
- Altered nutrition: less than body requirements related to paralytic ileus, need for increased intake of nutrients, and inability to eat independently
- Sexual dysfunction related to inability to achieve erection or perceive pelvic sensations and lack of knowledge of alternate means of achieving sexual satisfaction
- Risk for injury related to sensory deficit and lack of self-protective abilities
- Body image disturbance related to quadriplegia
- Altered family processes related to change in function of ill family member

Nursing Interventions
High cervical injury due to flexion-rotation is the most complex spinal cord injury and will be discussed in this section. Interventions for this type of injury can be modified for patients with less severe problems.

Immobilization. Proper immobilization of the neck involves maintenance of a neutral or extension position. The body should always be correctly aligned and turning should be performed so that the patient is moved as a unit to prevent movement of the spine. For cervical injuries skeletal traction is usually provided by Crutchfield, Gardner-Wells, or other skull tongs.

- Infection at the sites of tong insertion is a potential problem. Preventive care includes cleansing the sites twice a day with normal saline solution and applying an antibiotic ointment that acts as a mechanical barrier to the bacteria.

- Meticulous skin care is critical because decreased sensation and circulation make the patient particularly susceptible to skin breakdown. Patients should be removed from backboards as soon as possible and cervical collars must be properly fitted or replaced with other forms of immobilization to prevent coccygeal and occipital area skin breakdown.

Respiratory problems. If the patient is exhausted from labored breathing or if ABGs deteriorate (indicating inadequate oxygenation), endotracheal intubation or tracheostomy and mechanical ventilation should be initiated. (See Intubation, Endotracheal, p. 657; Tracheostomy, p. 682; and Mechanical Ventilation, p. 662) Respiratory arrest is a possibility that requires careful monitoring and prompt action if it occurs. Pneumonia and atelectasis are potential problems because of the loss of vital capacity.

- The nurse should regularly assess breath sounds, ABGs, tidal volume, vital capacity, skin color, breathing patterns (especially the use of accessory muscles), subjective comments about the ability to breathe, and the amount and color of sputum.
- In addition to monitoring activities, the nurse can intervene in maintaining ventilation by administration of O_2 until the ABGs stabilize, chest physiotherapy and quad-assist coughing, incentive spirometry, and tracheal suctioning.

Cardiovascular problems. If bradycardia is symptomatic, an anticholinergic medication such as atropine is administered. A temporary pacemaker may be inserted in some instances (see Pacemakers, p. 671). Hypotension is managed with a vasopressor agent such as dopamine and by fluid replacement.

- Elastic compression gradient stockings can be used to prevent thromboemboli and to promote venous return.
- The nurse should also perform range-of-motion (ROM) exercises and heel-cord stretching regularly. The thighs and calves of the legs should be assessed every shift for signs of deep-vein thrombosis.
- The nurse also needs to monitor the patient for indications of hypovolemic shock secondary to hemorrhage.

Fluid and nutritional maintenance. During the first 48 to 72 hours after the injury, the GI tract may stop functioning (paralytic ileus) and a nasogastric tube must be inserted.

- Once bowel sounds are present or flatus is passed, oral food and fluids can gradually be introduced. Because of severe catabolism, a high-protein, high-caloric diet is necessary for energy and tissue repair.
- In patients with high cervical cord injuries, swallowing must be evaluated before oral feedings are started. If the patient is

unable to resume eating within 3 to 4 days, total parenteral nutrition may be started to provide nutritional support.

Bowel and bladder management. An indwelling catheter is usually inserted as soon as possible after injury. Its patency must be ensured by irrigation and frequent inspection. Strict aseptic technique for catheter care is essential to avoid introducing infection.

- Urinary tract infections are a common problem. A large fluid intake and the liberal use of juices such as cranberry, grape, and apple can be used to prevent infections.
- Suppositories are used in combination with a laxative to assist in bowel evacuation. Enemas are used only if absolutely necessary because they can overdistend the rectum.

Temperature control. Because there is no vasoconstriction, piloerection, or heat loss through perspiration below the level of injury, temperature control is largely external to the patient. The nurse needs to monitor the environment closely to maintain an appropriate temperature.

Sensory deprivation. The nurse must compensate for the patient's absent sensations to prevent sensory deprivation. This is done by stimulating the patient above the level of injury. Conversation, music, strong aromas, and interesting flavors should be a part of nursing care. Prism glasses are provided so that the patient can read and watch television. Every effort should be made to prevent the patient from withdrawing from the environment.

Reflexes. Penile erections can occur from a variety of stimuli, causing embarrassment and discomfort. Spasms ranging from mild twitches to convulsive movements below the level of the lesion may also occur. They can be relieved with the use of warm baths, whirlpool treatments, antispasmodics, and muscle relaxants. Peak spasticity occurs after 2 years; if the spasticity is severe, destruction of the reflexes (cordotomy) may be necessary. This procedure compromises retraining and should only be done as a last resort.

Physiologic and psychologic rehabilitation is complex and involved. Many of the problems identified in the acute period become chronic and continue throughout life. Rehabilitation focuses on refined retraining of physiologic processes.

- Braces, electronic wheelchairs, and mechanical devices are used to maximize the patient's remaining function.
- The patient with a high cervical spinal cord injury has increased mobility with phrenic nerve stimulators or electronic diaphragmatic pacemakers.

If the patient can be successfully guided through the acute period, the patient's life can be fuller and richer than previously believed possible. Unfortunately, some individuals may not have such a positive future outlook. The nurse has a pivotal role in the coordinated efforts of the health team to influence a positive outcome.

SPINAL CORD TUMORS

Definition/Description

Tumors that affect the spinal cord account for 0.5% to 1% of all neoplasms. These tumors are classified as primary (arising from some component of cord, dura, nerves, or vessels), secondary (due to intraspinal extension from the vertebrae, neck, or thoracic abdominal tumors), and metastatic (from primary growths in the breast, prostate, lung, kidney, and other sites).

- Spinal cord tumors are further classified as extradural, intradural extramedullary, and intradural intramedullary tumors (see Table 57-11 in Lewis/Collier/Heitkemper, *Medical-Surgical Nursing,* edition 4, p. 1819).
- Neurofibromas, meningiomas, gliomas, and hemangiomas are the most frequently occurring neoplasms.

Because many of these tumors are slow growing, their symptoms stem from the mechanical effects of slow compression and irritation of nerve roots, displacement of the cord, and/or gradual obstruction of the vascular supply. Slowness of growth does not cause autodestruction as in traumatic lesions. Therefore complete functional restoration is possible when the tumor is removed, except with intradural intramedullary tumors.

Clinical Manifestations

The most common early symptom of a spinal cord tumor outside the cord is pain in the back with radiation of pain simulating intercostal neuralgia, angina, or herpes zoster. The location of the pain depends on the level of compression. The pain generally worsens with activity, coughing, straining, and lying down.

- Sensory disruption is manifested by coldness, numbness, and tingling in an extremity or in several extremities, slowly progressing upward until it reaches the level of the lesion.
- Impaired sensation of pain, temperature, and light touch precedes a deficit in vibration and position sense that may progress to complete anesthesia.
- Motor weakness accompanies sensory disturbances and consists of slowly increasing clumsiness, weakness, and spasticity.
- Bladder disturbances are marked by urgency with difficulty in starting the flow and progressing to retention with overflow incontinence.

Manifestations of an intradural spinal tumor develop as progressive damage to the long spinal tracts occurs, producing paralysis, sensory loss, and bladder dysfunction. Pain can be severe as a result of compression of spinal roots or vertebrae.

Diagnostic Studies

Diagnosis of extradural tumors is made through routine spinal x-rays, whereas intradural and intramedullary tumors require myelography for detection. Cerebrospinal fluid analysis may reveal tumor cells.

Therapeutic and Nursing Management

Compression of the spinal cord is an emergency. Relief of the ischemia related to the compression is the goal of therapy. Corticosteroids are generally prescribed immediately to relieve tumor-related edema. Dexamethasone is usually used, often in large doses (up to 100 mg initially).

Treatment for nearly all spinal cord tumors is surgical removal. The exception is the metastatic tumor that is sensitive to radiation and has caused only minimal neurologic deficits in the patient. In general, tumors of the extradural or intradural-extramedullary group can be completely removed surgically. The cord is decompressed after removal of the tumor by a laminectomy.

- Radiation therapy after surgery is frequently done. Chemotherapy has also been used in conjunction with radiation therapy (see Radiation Therapy, p. 675, and Chemotherapy, p. 631).

Relief of pain and return of function are the ultimate goals of treatment.

- Nurses need to be aware of the neurologic status of the patient before and after treatment. Ensuring that the patient receives pain medication as needed is an important nursing responsibility. Depending on the amount of neurologic dysfunction exhibited, the patient may need to be cared for as though recovering from a spinal cord injury (see Spinal Cord Injury, p. 528).

SPLEEN DISORDERS

Definition/Description

The spleen performs many functions and is affected by many illnesses. There are many different causes of splenomegaly, including hemolytic anemia, infection, cirrhosis, congestive heart failure, and polycythemia vera. The term *hypersplenism* refers to the occurrence of splenomegaly and peripheral cytopenias (anemia, leukopenia, thrombocytopenia).

- The degree of splenic enlargement varies with the disease. For example, massive splenic enlargement occurs with chronic myelocytic leukemia and thalassemia major, whereas mild splenic enlargement is associated with congestive heart failure and systemic lupus erythematosus. When the spleen enlarges, its normal filtering and sequestering capacity increases. Consequently, there is often a reduction in the number of circulating blood cells.

Clinical Manifestations

A slight to moderate enlargement of the spleen is usually asymptomatic and is commonly found during a routine examination of the abdomen. Massive splenomegaly can be tolerated, but patients may complain of abdominal discomfort and early satiety. Other techniques to assess spleen size include Tc-colloid liver-spleen scan, CT scan, and ultrasound scan.

Therapeutic Management

Management of an enlarged spleen may involve a *splenectomy*. Spleen removal can have a dramatic effect in increasing red blood cell (RBC), white blood cell (WBC), and platelet counts. Another major indication for splenectomy is splenic rupture. The spleen may rupture from trauma, inadvertent tearing during other surgical procedures, and diseases such as mononucleosis.

Nursing Management

Nursing responsibilities for patients with spleen disorders vary depending on the nature of the problem.

- Splenomegaly may be painful and may require analgesic administration; care in moving, turning, and positioning; and evaluation of lung expansion since spleen enlargement may impair diaphragmatic excursion.
- If anemia, thrombocytopenia, or leukopenia develops from splenic enlargement, nursing measures must be instituted to support the patient and prevent life-threatening complications.
- Postsplenectomy patients are especially vulnerable to infection. A younger patient is at significantly greater risk than an older patient, but the risk is present for all ages. Postsplenectomy patients are highly susceptible to infection from encapsulated organisms such as pneumococcus. This complication is prevented by immunization with polyvalent pneumococcal vaccine (e.g., Pneumovax).

SPRUE

Definition/Description

Two closely related malabsorption conditions are *nontropical sprue* and *tropical sprue*. Tropical and nontropical sprue are found in adults. Nontropical sprue is most commonly referred to as *celiac sprue* (especially in children) but is also called *adult celiac disease* and *gluten-induced enteropathy*.

In celiac disease there is marked atrophy and flattening of the villi. As a result, absorption within the small intestine is reduced. The proposed reason for the injury to the villi is a hypersensitivity response initiated by gluten and gliadin (a breakdown product of gluten). Gluten is a protein found in wheat, rye, barley, and oats. The hypersensitivity leads to an inflammatory response of the mucosa.

Tropical sprue is a chronic disorder acquired in endemic tropical areas. The exact cause is unknown, but the disorder has been linked to an infectious agent. Folate deficiency is also believed to play a role in the development of this disease. Clinically tropical sprue resembles nontropical sprue.

Clinical Manifestations

Patients may become symptomatic at any age with celiac sprue, but the incidence peaks in childhood when gluten is first introduced and then during the fourth and fifth decades.

- Symptoms include steatorrhea (bulky, foul-smelling, yellow-gray, greasy stools with putty-like consistency), diarrhea, weight loss, abdominal distention, and excessive flatulence. There may also be signs of multiple vitamin deficiencies (e.g., glossitis, cheilosis).

Diagnostic Studies

Diagnosis of sprue may be made by stool content analyses or intestinal biopsy. Barium enema may demonstrate abnormalities including obliteration of intestinal folds.

Therapeutic Management

Treatment of sprue syndrome is based on the underlying cause.

- In nontropical sprue a gluten-free diet usually leads to clinical recovery. Wheat, barley, oats, and rye products should be avoided. Soybean flours may be used. For those patients who are unresponsive to dietary exclusion therapy (gluten-free diet), corticosteroids may be used.

- Tropical sprue is treated with broad-spectrum antibiotics (e.g., tetracycline) in conjunction with folic acid therapy. The patient who responds to this therapy and achieves a remission is usually maintained on folic acid.

STOMACH (GASTRIC) CANCER

Definition/Description
The rate of stomach (gastric) cancer has been steadily declining in the United States since the 1930s. The disease is the sixth leading cause of cancer mortality in the United States. Stomach cancer is typically at an advanced stage when diagnosed and is not amenable to surgical resection.

Pathophysiology
Many factors have been implicated in gastric cancer. It is believed that a diet of smoked, highly salted, or spiced foods may have a carcinogenic effect. A genetic etiology has also been postulated. In addition, persons with blood group A have a greater incidence of gastric cancer than does the general population. Other predisposing factors are atrophic gastritis, pernicious anemia, and benign gastric polyps.

Tumors located at the cardia and fundus are associated with a poor prognosis. These tumors typically infiltrate rapidly to the surrounding tissue, regional lymph nodes, and liver. Patients with tumor growth along the lesser curvature have a better survival rate.

- Tumor growth is insidious and follows a pattern of continuous infiltration. Cancer of the stomach may spread by direct extension along the mucosal surface and may infiltrate through the gastric wall.
- Once the stomach wall has been penetrated by tumor growth, adjacent organs and structures that may become involved are the esophagus, duodenum, omentum, liver, and pancreas.
- Distant metastasis is facilitated by rich lymphatic plexuses in the stomach wall.
- Evidence of spread to the peritoneal cavity is manifested by ascites and by spread to the ovaries.

Clinical Manifestations
Manifestations can be categorized by the signs and symptoms of anemia, peptic ulcer disease, or indigestion.

- Anemia occurs with chronic blood loss as the lesion erodes the stomach mucosa. Signs include paleness, fatigue, weakness, and positive occult stools.
- Symptoms associated with peptic ulcer disease (pain and discomfort) also occur.
- Indigestion signs include vague epigastric fullness with early satiety after meals. Signs may also include weight loss, dysphagia, and constipation.

Diagnostic Studies
- Hemoglobin and hematocrit determine anemia and its severity.
- Stool examination is done for occult or gross bleeding.
- Exfoliative cytologic examination from washings obtained with gastric analysis demonstrates malignancy (false readings are sometimes obtained).
- An adjunctive diagnostic tool is carcinoembryonic antigen (CEA).
- Further studies may include upper GI barium tests and fiberoptic endoscopy and biopsy.

Therapeutic Management
The treatment of choice is surgical removal of the tumor. Surgical procedures performed are similar to those used for peptic ulcer disease (see Peptic Ulcer Disease, p. 453).
- Preoperative management focuses on correction of nutritional deficits, packed red blood cell (RBC) transfusions for treatment of anemia, and replacement of blood volume.

Complete cure is decreased considerably when lymph nodes are involved. Chemotherapy and radiation may be used if surgical cure is not feasible (see Chemotherapy, p. 631, and Radiation Therapy, p. 675).
- Chemotherapy is not very successful when used as the primary mode of treatment. Gastric tumor radiosensitivity is low, making radiation of little value except for treating obstruction.

Nursing Management
Goals
The patient with gastric cancer will experience minimal discomfort, achieve optimal nutritional status, and maintain a degree of spiritual and psychologic well-being appropriate to the disease stage.
Nursing Diagnoses
- Altered nutrition: less than body requirements related to inability to ingest, digest, or absorb nutrients
- Activity intolerance related to generalized weakness, abdominal discomfort, and nutritional deficits

- Anxiety related to lack of knowledge of diagnostic tests, unknown diagnostic outcome, disease process, and therapeutic regimen
- Pain related to underlying disease process and side effects of surgery, chemotherapy, or radiation therapy
- Anticipatory grieving related to perceived unfavorable diagnosis and impending death

Nursing Interventions

The nursing role in early detection of stomach cancer is focused primarily on identification of the patient at risk (e.g., pernicious anemia).

When diagnostic tests confirm the presence of malignancy, the nurse must give emotional and physical support, provide information, clarify test results, and maintain a positive attitude with respect to the patient's immediate recovery and long-term survival.

- Preoperative teaching plan is very similar to that for peptic ulcer disease surgery (see Peptic Ulcer Disease, p. 453).

Postoperative care generally includes close observation for signs of fluid leakage at the site of anastomosis as evidenced by an elevation in temperature and increasing dyspnea.

- The nurse should observe for manifestations of dumping syndrome and postprandial hypoglycemia, which may occur with total gastrectomy.
- Because most radiation therapy and chemotherapy are completed on an outpatient basis, the nurse should assess the patient's knowledge of radiation, care of skin, need for good nutrition and fluid intake during therapy, and appropriate use of antiemetic drugs (see Radiation Therapy, p. 675, and Chemotherapy, p. 631).

Patient Teaching

Before discharge, instruction should be given to the patient about relief of pain, including comfort measures and judicious use of analgesics. Additional considerations include:

- Wound care, if needed, must be taught to the primary caregiver in the home situation.
- Dressings, special equipment, or special services may be required for the patient's continued care at home.
- A list of community agencies available for assistance should be provided.
- Long-term follow-up must be stressed to the patient.
- The patient must be encouraged to comply with the prescribed dietary and medication regimens, keep appointments for chemotherapy or administration of radiation treatments, and keep the physician informed of any changes in the patient's physical condition.

Syndrome of Inappropriate Antidiuretic Hormone

Definition/Description
The syndrome of inappropriate antidiuretic hormone (SIADH) occurs when antidiuretic hormone (ADH) is released in amounts far in excess of those indicated by the plasma osmotic pressure. SIADH is associated with diseases that affect osmoreceptors in the hypothalamus.

- SIADH is characterized by fluid retention, serum hypoosmolality, dilutional hyponatremia, hypochloremia, concentrated urine in the presence of intravascular volume depletion, and normal renal function.

Pathophysiology
SIADH has various causes. Ectopic ADH production by carcinomas is not a primary pituitary disorder, but it has manifestations similar to such a disorder. Bronchogenic carcinoma is the most common ADH-secreting tumor.

- Pulmonary conditions such as pneumonia, tuberculosis, lung abscess, and positive-pressure breathing have been associated with SIADH.
- The syndrome is also associated with such diverse conditions as trauma (most frequently head trauma), meningitis, subarachnoid hemorrhage, peripheral neuropathy, delirium tremens, Addison's disease, psychoses, vomiting, stress, and the use of many medications.

The excess ADH increases renal tubular permeability and reabsorption of water into the circulation. Consequently, extracellular fluid volume expands, plasma osmolality declines, the glomerular filtration rate rises, and sodium levels decline.

Clinical Manifestations
Problems related to SIADH include low urinary output and weight gain without edema. As plasma osmolality and serum sodium levels continue to decline, cerebral edema may occur, leading to lethargy, anorexia, confusion, headache, convulsions, and coma. Other effects of hyponatremia include muscle cramps and weakness.

- The serum osmolality is much lower than the urine osmolality, indicating the inappropriate excretion of concentrated urine in the presence of highly dilute serum.
- Associated manifestations correlate with the serum sodium level. Initially, thirst, dyspnea on exertion, fatigue, and dulled sensorium may be evident. As the serum sodium levels fall,

symptoms become more severe and include vomiting, abdominal cramps, muscle twitching, and convulsions.

Therapeutic Management

The treatment goal is to restore normal fluid volume and osmolality. Fluids may be restricted to 800 to 1000 ml/day. If fluid restriction alone does not improve the symptoms, 3% to 5% (hypertonic) saline solution may be administered intravenously. A diuretic such as furosemide may be used to promote diuresis if cardiac symptoms develop. Because furosemide increases potassium excretion, potassium supplements may be needed.

- SIADH tends to be self-limiting when caused by head trauma or drugs. It is chronic when associated with tumors or metabolic diseases. Treatment of the underlying cause or discontinuing the causal medication is indicated to improve the clinical course.
- In chronic symptomatic SIADH, demeclocycline (Declomycin), a tetracycline that causes nephrogenic diabetes insipidus, is useful. This drug blocks the action of ADH at the level of the distal and collecting tubules, regardless of the ADH source.
- Other therapeutic measures in long-term management include furosemide and the use of urea, an osmotic diuretic.

Nursing Management

Careful nursing assessment of patients who have had surgery or those susceptible to the syndrome can help in the early detection of SIADH. The nurse should be alert for low urinary output with a high specific gravity, a sudden weight gain, or a serum sodium decline. If a patient has SIADH, nursing measures include:

- Restriction of total fluid intake to no more than 1000 ml/day and restriction of oral intake until normalization of serum sodium (if appropriate)
- Positioning the head of the bed flat or with no more than 10° of elevation to enhance venous return to the heart and to increase left atrial filling pressure, reducing ADH release
- Positioning the siderails up because of potential alterations in mental status
- Turning of the patient every 2 hours, proper positioning, range-of-motion exercise, and massage (if patient bedridden)
- Use of seizure precautions such as padded siderails, accessible padded tongue blade, and dim lighting
- Assistance with ambulation
- Provision of frequent oral hygiene

When SIADH is chronic, patients must learn to self-manage their treatment regimens.

- Fluids are restricted to 800 to 1000 ml/day. Sucking on hard candy or ice chips can help decrease thirst. The patient may be treated with a diuretic to remove excess fluid volume.
- The diet should be supplemented with sodium and potassium, especially if diuretics are prescribed. Salts of these electrolytes must be well diluted to prevent GI irritation or damage. They are best taken at mealtime to allow mixing with and dilution by food.
- Patients should be taught the symptoms of fluid and electrolyte imbalances, especially those involving sodium and potassium, so that they can monitor their responses to treatment. If a patient is to be treated with demeclocycline, the need for close follow-up care should be stressed because of the nephrotoxic side effects and the potential for fungal infections associated with this drug.

SYPHILIS

Definition/Description

Syphilis ranks third among communicable diseases reported in the United States. Between 1984 and 1990 the number of reported cases of primary and secondary syphilis in the United States more than doubled to over 50,000 cases, the highest level since the early 1950s. An increasing incidence among minority populations accounted for the greater part of this increase.

Pathophysiology

The causative organism of syphilis is *Treponema pallidum,* a spirochete. It is extremely fragile and is easily destroyed by drying, heating, or washing. The organism is thought to enter the body through very small breaks in the skin or mucous membranes. Its entry is facilitated by the minor abrasions that often occur during sexual intercourse.

- Not all people who are exposed to syphilis acquire the disease; about one third become infected after intercourse with an infected person.
- In addition to sexual contact, syphilis may be spread through contact with infectious lesions and sharing of needles among drug addicts.
- Congenital syphilis is transmitted from an infected mother to the fetus in utero.
- The incubation period for syphilis ranges from 10 to 90 days but is usually considered to be 3 weeks. Immunity to reinfec-

tion may develop if the disease is not eradicated during the primary stage.

Syphilis is a disease of the blood vessels. The tissue reaction to the presence of *T. pallidum* multiplying in the lymphatics and perivascular spaces is characterized by dilatation and swelling of the capillaries and proliferation of the endothelium and a perivascular infiltration of lymphocytes, giant cells, and fibroblasts, with the formation of new blood vessels.

- Scar tissue formation is the method of healing of syphilis. The severity and extent of the damage varies.

There is an association between syphilis and human immunodeficiency virus (HIV) infection. Persons at highest risk for acquiring syphilis are also at high risk for acquiring HIV. Often both infections are present in the same person. Therefore the evaluation of all patients with syphilis should include serologic testing for HIV with the patient's consent.

Clinical Manifestations

Syphilis presents a variety of signs and symptoms that can mimic a number of less serious diseases. Consequently, it is more difficult to recognize syphilis than other venereal diseases. If it is not treated, specific clinical stages are characteristic of the disease progression.

- In the *primary stage* chancres, which are painless indurated lesions found on the penis, vulva, and lips and in the mouth, vagina, and rectum, are seen at the site of bacterial invasion. *T. pallidum* multiplies in the epithelium, producing a granulomatous tissue reaction (chancre).
- *Secondary syphilis* is systemic. During this stage blood-borne bacteria spread to all major organ systems. Manifestations characteristic of the secondary stage include cutaneous eruptions, *alopecia* (hair loss), and generalized adenopathy. The cutaneous eruptions include a bilateral, symmetric rash usually involving the palms and soles; mucous patches in the mouth, tongue, or cervix; and *condylomalata* (moist papules) in the anal and genital area.
- *Latent syphilis* follows the secondary stage and is a period during which the immune system is able to suppress the infection. There are no signs or symptoms of syphilis during this time.
- *Late syphilis* (also called tertiary syphilis) is the most severe stage of the disease. Because antibiotics can cure syphilis, manifestations of late syphilis are rare. However, when it does occur, it is responsible for significant morbidity and mortality. *Gummas* (destructive skin, bone, and soft tissue lesions associated with late syphilis) are probably caused by a severe hypersensitivity reaction to the microorganism. Within the cardiovascular system late syphilis may cause aneurysms, heart valve

insufficiency, and heart failure. Within the central nervous system (CNS), the presence of *T. pallidum* in cerebrospinal fluid (CSF) may cause manifestations of neurosyphilis.

Complications

Complications occur in late syphilis. The gummas of benign late syphilis may produce irreparable damage to bone, liver, or skin but seldom result in death.

- In cardiovascular syphilis the resulting aneurysm may press on structures such as intercostal nerves, resulting in pain. Scarring of the aortic valve results in aortic valve insufficiency and, eventually, heart failure.
- *Neurosyphilis* (general paresis) is responsible for degeneration of the brain with mental deterioration. Problems related to sensory nerve involvement are a result of *tabes dorsalis* (progressive locomotor ataxia). There may be sudden attacks of pain anywhere in the body; loss of vision and position sense in the feet and legs can also occur. Walking may become even more difficult as joint stability is lost.

Diagnostic Studies

- Dark-field microscopy confirms the diagnosis with the presence of spirochetes from tissue scrapings of primary or secondary lesions.
- Nontreponemal or treponemal serologic testing for detection of specific antitreponemal antibodies is usually positive 10 to 14 days after chancre appearance.
- Testing for other sexually transmitted diseases (STDs) (HIV, gonorrhea, chlamydia) should be done.

Therapeutic and Nursing Management

Therapeutic management is aimed at eradication of all syphilitic organisms. However, treatment cannot reverse damage already present in the late stage of the disease.

- Parenteral penicillin remains the treatment of choice for all stages of syphilis. To date, there is no evidence to suggest a decrease in the effectiveness of penicillin against *T. pallidum.* Table 50-5 in Lewis/Collier/Heitkemper, *Medical-Surgical Nursing,* edition 4, p. 1571, describes therapy for the various stages of syphilis and is in accordance with U. S. Public Health Service recommendations. All stages of syphilis should be treated.
- Appropriate antibiotic treatment of maternal syphilis before the eighteenth week of pregnancy prevents infection of the fetus. Appropriate treatment after 18 weeks of pregnancy cures both mother and fetus because the antibiotics can cross the placen-

tal barrier. Treatment administered in the second half of pregnancy may pose a risk of premature labor.
- All patients with neurosyphilis must be carefully followed up with periodic serologic testing, clinical evaluation at 6-month intervals, and repeat CSF examinations for at least 3 years.

Systemic Lupus Erythematosus

Definition/Description

Systemic lupus erythematosus (SLE) is a chronic multisystem inflammatory disease of connective tissue that often involves the skin, joints, serous membranes (pleura, pericardium), kidney, hematologic system, and central nervous system (CNS). SLE is characterized by its variability within and among persons, with a chronic unpredictable course of exacerbations of disease activity alternating with periods of remission. Females have a higher incidence of SLE (about 5:1) than males. The disease is observed three times more often in African-American than in Caucasian women.

Pathophysiology

The exact etiology of SLE is unknown. However, factors implicated include genetic predisposition, sex hormones, race, environmental factors (e.g., ultraviolet radiation, drugs, chemicals), viruses and infections, stress, and immunologic abnormalities. SLE is a disorder of immune regulation.
- Hormones are known to play a role in the etiology of SLE. The disease often worsens during pregnancy and the immediate postpartum period. Healthy women are more immunologically reactive than healthy men because estrogens enhance immune reactivity. Onset or exacerbation of disease symptoms sometimes occurs after the onset of menarche, with the use of oral contraceptives, and during and after pregnancy.

The pathologic features relate to autoimmune reactions directed against constituents of the cell nucleus, particularly deoxyribonucleic acid (DNA). In SLE autoantibodies are produced against nuclear antigens (DNA, histones, ribonucleoproteins, and nucleolar factors), cytoplasmic antigens (ribosomal and cardiolipin), and blood cell surface antigens (white blood cells [WBCs], red blood cells [RBCs], platelets, and granulocytes).
- Accumulation of antigen-antibody (immune) complexes within the blood vessel walls and subsequent complement activation leads to a condition called lupus vasculitis. The ensuing ischemia within the blood vessel walls gradually leads to the thick-

ening of the internal cell lining, fibrinoid degeneration, and thrombus formation.

Clinical Manifestations

There is no characteristic pattern of progressive organ involvement; nor is it predictable which systems may become affected. General constitutional complaints including fever, weight loss, arthralgia, and excessive fatigue may precede an exacerbation of disease activity.

Dermatologic manifestations. The most common feature is an erythematous rash that can occur on the face, neck, and extremities. The classic butterfly rash, which is distributed across the bridge of the nose and cheeks, may appear as discoid (coinlike) lesions or as a diffuse maculopapular rash; it may occur anywhere on the body but is most frequently seen on the face and chest.

- Exposure to sunlight and to other sources of ultraviolet radiation can cause a severe skin reaction and may precipitate a flare-up of disease activity in persons who are photosensitive. Ulcers of the oral or nasopharyngeal membranes may occur. Transient diffuse or patchy hair loss (alopecia) is common, with or without underlying scalp lesions.

Musculoskeletal problems. Polyarthralgia with morning stiffness is often the patient's first complaint and may precede the onset of multisystem disease by many years. Arthritis occurs in 95% of all patients with SLE at some time in the disease course. Joint symptoms are typically migratory, producing pain without objective signs of inflammation.

- Lupus-related arthritis is generally nonerosive, but it may cause deformities such as swan neck, ulnar deviation, and subluxation with hyperlaxity of the joints.

Cardiopulmonary problems. Pericarditis may be present and is usually associated with myocardial disease. Patients treated with corticosteroids have a higher incidence of atherosclerosis. Pleurisy with or without effusion is seen in many patients at some time during the illness, and pulmonary function studies are generally abnormal. Raynaud's phenomenon may occur. Cardiovascular involvement is an ominous sign of advanced disease and contributes significantly to morbidity and mortality.

Renal problems. Clinical evidence of renal involvement is present in nearly one half of all patients and includes microscopic hematuria, excessive cellular casts in the urine sediment, proteinuria, and elevation of serum creatinine level. Kidney involvement varies in degree but may eventually end in renal failure. Nearly all patients with SLE show renal histologic abnormalities in renal biopsy studies or autopsy results. Nephritis is the leading cause of death in SLE.

Central nervous system problems. CNS involvement ranks close behind kidney disease and infection as a leading cause of death in SLE. Seizures are the most common neurologic manifestation and they may be of the grand mal, petit mal, or psychomotor type and are generally controlled by corticosteroids or anticonvulsant therapy.

- Organic brain syndrome may result from the deposition of immune complexes within brain tissue. It is characterized by disordered thought processes, disorientation, memory deficits, and psychiatric symptoms such as severe depression and psychosis. Recovery is expected although some residual impairment may result. Occasionally a cerebrovascular accident (stroke) or aseptic meningitis may be attributable to SLE.

Hematologic problems. The formation of antibodies against blood cells such as erythrocytes, leukocytes, thrombocytes, and coagulation factors is one of the most common features. Anemia, mild leukopenia, and thrombocytopenia are often present. Some patients show a tendency to bleed, whereas others show a tendency toward blood clots. In addition, patients have positive antinuclear antibodies (ANA).

Infection. Patients appear to have increased susceptibility to infections, possibly related to defects in their ability to phagocytize invading bacteria, deficiencies in production of antibodies, and the immunosuppressive effect of many antiinflammatory drugs. Pneumonia is the most common infection.

Diagnostic Studies

Diagnosis is based on the history, physical examination, and laboratory findings.

- Elevated erythrocyte sedimentation rate (ESR), increased γ-globulin levels, anemia, decreased WBC and platelet counts
- ECG or chest x-ray may show pericarditis or pleural effusion; urine sediment abnormalities (cellular casts, proteinuria), reduced serum complement, and tissue specimens demonstrating changes compatible with SLE are other confirmatory findings.

Autoantibodies directed against nuclear antigens (ANA) have been detected in 99% of persons with SLE. Although extremely sensitive, the presence of ANA is not specific for SLE because it is present in 5% of normal persons and 38% of all persons more than 60 years of age. Anti-double-stranded DNA is found most commonly in SLE and rarely seen in other rheumatic diseases. Anti-Sm antibody, an antibody to the Smith nuclear antigen, is a definitive serologic marker for SLE and is not demonstrated in other rheumatic diseases.

Therapeutic Management

Corticosteroids remain the mainstay for treatment of severe illness. Their use should be reserved for acute generalized exacerbation or serious organ involvement, although a reduced maintenance dosage is sometimes used. Immunosuppressive drugs may be used for symptoms that are resistant to corticosteroid therapy. The efficacy of treatment is most appropriately monitored by serial serum complement levels and anti-DNA titers.

An improving prognosis of SLE may be the result of earlier diagnosis, prompt recognition of serious organ involvement, and better therapeutic regimens. Survival is influenced by several factors, including age, race, gender, socioeconomic status, accompanying morbid conditions, and severity of disease.

Pharmacologic Management

Aspirin or other nonsteroidal antiinflammatory drugs (NSAIDs) may reduce mild symptoms such as fever and arthritic complaints. Antimalarial drugs such as hydroxychloroquine sulfate (Plaquenil) may be used to improve skin problems. Topical steroid preparations and intralesional steroid injections are effective treatments for skin lesions. Corticosteroids are used for acute generalized exacerbations and for treatment of serious organ involvement, including hematologic abnormalities. As clinical and laboratory values improve, dosages are gradually tapered. Immunosuppressive drug therapy such as azathioprine (Imuran) and cyclophosphamide (Cytoxan) is occasionally used in life-threatening situations for symptoms unresponsive to more conservative treatment.

Nursing Management

Goals

The patient with SLE will have satisfactory pain relief, comply with the therapeutic regimen to achieve maximum symptom management, avoid activities that induce disease exacerbation, and maintain a positive self-image.

See the nursing care plan for the patient with systemic lupus erythematosus in Lewis/Collier/Heitkemper, *Medical-Surgical Nursing,* edition 4, p. 1923.

Nursing Diagnoses

- Pain related to disease process and inadequate comfort measures
- Impaired skin integrity related to photosensitivity, skin rash, and alopecia
- Body image disturbance related to change in physical appearance
- Fatigue related to disease process
- Activity intolerance related to arthralgia, weakness, and fatigue

- Altered nutrition: less than body requirements related to anorexia, fatigue, oral ulcerations, and immunosuppressive therapy
- Ineffective management of therapeutic regimen related to lack of knowledge of long-term management of disease

Nursing Interventions

Prevention of SLE is not possible at this time. Education of health professionals and the community may promote a clearer understanding of the disease and earlier diagnosis and treatment.

During an exacerbation patients may become abruptly and dramatically ill. Nursing intervention includes accurately recording the severity of symptoms and documenting the response to therapy. Fever pattern, joint inflammation, limitation of motion, location and degree of discomfort, and fatigability should be specifically assessed.

- The patient's weight and fluid intake and output should be monitored because of the fluid-retention effect of steroids and the possibility of renal failure. Careful collection of a 24-hour urine specimen for protein may be required. The nurse should observe for signs of bleeding that result from drug therapy, such as pallor, skin bruising, petechiae, or tarry stools.
- Careful assessment of neurologic status includes observation for visual disturbances, headaches, personality changes, and forgetfulness. Psychosis may indicate CNS disease or may be the effect of corticosteroid therapy. Irritation of the nerves of the extremities (peripheral neuropathy) may produce numbness, tingling, and weakness of the hands and feet. Less frequently a stroke may result.
- The nurse must explain the nature of the disease and modes of therapy and prepare the patient for numerous diagnostic procedures. Emotional support for the patient and family is essential.

Patient Teaching

The patient must understand that even perfect adherence to the treatment plan is not a guarantee against exacerbation because the disease course is unpredictable. Patient and family education should include the following:

- Education on the disease process
- Names of medications and actions, side effects, dosage, and administration
- Energy-conservation and pacing techniques
- Daily heat and exercise program (for arthralgia)
- Avoidance of physical and emotional stress, overexposure to ultraviolet light, and unnecessary exposure to infection
- Regular medical and laboratory follow-up
- Referral resources to community and health care agencies

The nurse should counsel the patient and family that SLE has a good prognosis for the majority of persons. Many young couples require pregnancy and sexual counseling. Pacing techniques and relaxation therapy can help keep the patient actively involved. Daily planning should include recreational and occupational activities.

SYSTEMIC SCLEROSIS (SCLERODERMA)

Definition/Description

Systemic sclerosis (SS) or scleroderma is a disorder of connective tissue characterized by fibrotic, degenerative, and occasionally inflammatory changes in the skin, blood vessels, synovium, skeletal muscle, and internal organs. Skin thickening and tightening are the cardinal features. The disease may range from a diffuse cutaneous thickening with rapidly progressive and fatal visceral involvement to a more benign variant called *CREST* syndrome (*c*alcinosis, *R*aynaud's phenomenon, *e*sophageal hypomotility, *s*clerodactyly [skin change of the fingers], and *t*elangiectasia [macule-like angioma on the skin]).

SS affects women three times more frequently than men, with the female/male ratio increasing to 15:1 during the childbearing years. Although symptoms may begin at any time, the usual age at onset is between 30 and 50 years.

Pathophysiology

The exact cause of SS remains unclear. Collagen is overproduced and disrupts the normal functioning of internal organs, such as the lungs, kidney, heart, and GI tract. Widespread systemic disease may be the result of primary vessel injury or immune dysregulation. Disruption of the cell is followed by platelet aggregation, myointimal cell proliferation, and fibrosis.

Clinical Manifestations

Raynaud's phenomenon (paroxysmal vasospasm of the digits) occurs in most patients with SS and is the most common initial complaint in CREST syndrome. Raynaud's phenomenon may precede the onset of systemic disease by months, years, or even decades.

- Symmetric painless swelling or thickening of the skin of the fingers and hands may progress to diffuse scleroderma of the trunk. In CREST syndrome skin thickening is generally limited to the fingers and face. The skin loses elasticity and becomes taut and shiny, producing the typical expressionless facies with tightly pursed lips.

- Flexion contractures and atrophy of soft tissue may give the hands a clawlike appearance. Polyarthralgias and morning stiffness may be early symptoms.

Esophageal hypomotility causes frequent reflux of gastric acid, causing heartburn, and substernal dysphagia for solid foods. If swallowing becomes difficult, the patient often decreases food intake and loses weight. GI complaints may also include abdominal distention, diarrhea, malodorous floating stools (malabsorption syndrome) as a result of small-bowel disease, and constipation.

- Lung involvement includes pleural thickening and pulmonary fibrosis and pulmonary function abnormalities. Pulmonary hypertension is seen almost exclusively in CREST syndrome.
- Primary heart disease consists of pericarditis, pericardial effusion, and cardiac dysrhythmias. Myocardial fibrosis resulting in congestive failure occurs most frequently in those persons with diffuse SS.
- Renal disease is a major cause of death in SS. Malignant arterial hypertension associated with rapidly progressive and irreversible renal insufficiency is often present.

Diagnostic Studies

- The erythrocyte sedimentation rate (ESR) may be mildly elevated with hypergammaglobinemia.
- Antinuclear antibody (ANA) titers are elevated with autoantibody Scl-70 seen in diffuse SS.
- Nail-bed capillary microscopy shows capillary loop dilatation with limited disease and dilatation with avascular areas in patients with diffuse disease.
- If renal involvement is present, urinalysis may show proteinuria, microscopic hematuria, and casts.
- X-ray evidence of subcutaneous calcification, digital tuft resorption, distal esophageal hypomotility, and/or bilateral pulmonary fibrosis are diagnostic of SS.
- Pulmonary function studies reveal decreased vital capacity.
- Skin biopsy shows dermal collagen thickening, condensation, or homogenization.

Therapeutic Management

Management of SS offers no specific treatment with long-term effects. It is directed toward attempts to prevent or treat secondary complications of involved organs. Various drugs such as antiinflammatory agents, D-penicillamine, and colchicine have been used with varying degrees of success.

Physical therapy helps maintain joint mobility and preserve muscle strength. Occupational therapy assists the patient in maintaining functional abilities. Gastroesophageal reflux may be treated by antacids and periodic dilatation of the esophagus. Raynaud's phenomenon may be temporarily relieved by thoracic sympathectomy.

Pharmacologic Management

No specific drugs or combination of drugs have been proved effective as treatment for SS. Corticosteroids are generally reserved for patients with myositis or overlap syndromes (e.g., mixed connective tissue disease). Penicillamine (Cuprimine) increases the solubility of dermal collagen, and may cause thinning of the skin, but has many side effects. Colchicine is being used to inhibit the accumulation of collagen, but evidence is still insufficient to prove its therapeutic worth.

Supportive measures include oral vasodilating drugs and intraarterial injections of reserpine. Calcium channel blockers (nifedipine, diltiazem) are the treatment of choice for Raynaud's phenomenon. Infected ulcers of the fingertips may be treated by soaking with hyaluronidase and using bacterial antibiotic ointment. Joint symptoms may be relieved by aspirin and other nonsteroidal antiinflammatory drugs (NSAIDs). Antacids may be useful for heartburn. Tetracycline and other broad-spectrum antibiotics may improve intestinal malabsorption. Combinations of antihypertensive medications, including hydralazine, minoxidil, captopril, propranolol, and methyldopa, have been used in the treatment of hypertension and renal failure.

Nursing Management

Because prevention is not possible, nursing interventions often begin during hospitalization for diagnostic purposes. Emotional stress and a cold environment may aggravate Raynaud's phenomenon. Patients with SS should not have fingerstick blood testing done because of compromised circulation and poor digital healing. The nurse may help the patient to resolve feelings of helplessness by providing information about the illness and encouraging active participation in planning care.

- The hands and feet should be protected from cold exposure and possible burns or cuts that might heal slowly. Smoking should be avoided because of its vasoconstricting effect. Lotions may help to alleviate skin dryness and cracking but must be rubbed in for an unusually long time because of the thickness of the skin.
- Dysphagia may be reduced by eating small frequent meals, chewing carefully and slowly, and drinking fluids. Heartburn may be minimized by using antacids 45 to 60 minutes after each meal and by sitting upright for 30 to 45 minutes after eating. Using additional pillows or raising the head of the bed may help reduce nocturnal gastroesophageal reflux.

- Job modifications are often necessary because stair climbing, typing, writing, and cold exposure may pose particular problems.
- Some people need to wear gloves to protect fingertip ulcers and to provide extra warmth. Sensitive areas on fingertips resulting from ulcers or calcinosis may require padded utensils or special assistive devices to reduce discomfort.
- Daily oral hygiene must be emphasized, or neglect may lead to increased tooth and gingival problems.
- Psychologic support reduces stress and may positively influence the peripheral motor response. Biofeedback training and relaxation techniques may be used to reduce tension, improve sleeping habits, and raise digital temperature. Obvious changes in the face and hands lead to poor self-image and loss of mobility and function.

The patient must actively carry out therapeutic exercises at home. The nurse should reinforce heat therapy, the use of assistive devices, and organization of activities to preserve strength and reduce disability. Sexual dysfunction resulting from body changes, pain, muscular weakness, limited mobility, decreased self-esteem, and decreased vaginal secretions may require sensitive counseling by the nurse.

TESTICULAR CANCER

Definition/Description

Testicular tumors make up about 0.7% of all forms of cancer in men, with a peak incidence between 20 and 40 years of age. Testicular tumors are much more common in males who have had undescended testicles (cryptorchidism).

- Other predisposing factors include a history of mumps, orchitis, inguinal hernia in childhood, and testicular cancer in the contralateral testis.
- The etiology of testicular neoplasms is unknown. Testicular tumors may develop from the cellular components of the testis or from the embryonal precursors (germinal tumors). Nongerminal tumors are rare and usually benign and can occur at any age. Germinal tumors are almost always malignant.

Clinical Manifestations

Germinal tumors may have a slow or rapid onset, depending on the type.

- The patient may notice a lump in his scrotum, scrotal swelling, and a feeling of heaviness. The scrotal mass is usually nontender and firm and cannot be transilluminated.
- Manifestations associated with metastasis to other systems include back pain, dyspnea, hemoptysis, dysphagia, alterations in vision or mental status, and seizures.

Diagnostic Studies

Palpation of the scrotal contents is the first step in diagnosing testicular cancer. Additional tests that aid in diagnosis include a testicular sonogram and MRI.

- Once the diagnosis of a testicular neoplasm is suspected, a blood sample should be set aside before orchiectomy, for subsequent determination of the tumor marker glycoproteins α-fetoprotein (AFP) and human chorionic gonadotropin (hCG).
- Following orchiectomy, tumor staging is done on the biopsy specimen. Testicular cancer is histologically classified as seminoma and nonseminoma. After diagnosis and staging, AFP and hCG will continue to be monitored, if appropriate, to detect metastases and to assess response to therapy.

Therapeutic and Nursing Management

As with many forms of cancer, survival of the patient is closely associated with early recognition of the tumor. The scrotum is easily examined, and beginning tumors are usually palpable. Every male between the ages of 20 and 40 years should be taught and encouraged to perform a monthly testicular self-examination for the purpose of detecting testicular tumors or other scrotal abnormalities such as varicoceles. (For an illustration of testicular self-examination, see Figure 52-5 in Lewis/Collier/Heitkemper, *Medical-Surgical Nursing,* edition 4, p. 1642.)

- The patient may indicate some reluctance to examine his own genitals. With encouragement the patient can learn this simple procedure. He should be encouraged to do self-examinations frequently until he is comfortable with the procedure. The scrotum should be examined once a month. (See the guidelines for scrotal self-examination in Lewis/Collier/Heitkemper, *Medical-Surgical Nursing,* edition 4, p. 1642.)

Therapeutic management of testicular cancer involves surgical removal of the affected testis, cord, and resection of the regional and paraaortic lymph nodes.

- A high radical inguinal orchiectomy is the usual treatment to prevent local recurrence and metastases to the inguinal lymphatics.
- Radiation of the remaining lymph nodes and single or multiple chemotherapeutic agent regimens such as bleomycin, vincristine, cisplatin, and vinblastine are also used after surgery, depending on the histologic findings and disease stage.

The prognosis for patients with testicular cancer has improved, and 75% of affected patients obtain complete remission of the disease if it is detected in the early stages.

- All patients with testicular cancer, regardless of pathology or stage, require meticulous follow-up and monthly physical examinations, chest radiography, CT scan, and assessment of hCG and AFP (if appropriate). The goal is to detect relapse when the tumor burden is minimal.
- The man with testicular cancer should have the opportunity to discuss fertility and sperm banking during the preoperative period.

TETANUS

Definition/Description

Tetanus is an extremely severe polyradiculitis and polyneuritis affecting the spinal and cranial nerves. It results from the effects of a potent neurotoxin released by the anaerobic bacillus *Clostridium tetani.* The toxin interferes with the function of the reflex arc by blocking inhibitory transmitters at the presynaptic sites in the spinal cord and brainstem. The spores of the bacillus are present in soil, garden mold, and manure.

Pathophysiology

C. tetani enters the body through a traumatic or suppurative wound that provides an appropriate low-O_2 environment for the organisms to mature and produce toxin.

- Other possible sources include dental infection, injections of heroin, human and animal bites, frostbite, compound fractures, and gunshot wounds.
- The incubation period is usually 7 days but can range from 1 to 54 days, with symptoms frequently appearing after the original wound is healed. In general, the longer the incubation period, the milder the illness and the better the prognosis.

Clinical Manifestations

Manifestations of generalized tetanus include a feeling of stiffness in the jaw *(lockjaw)* or neck, slight fever, and other symptoms of general infection. Generalized tonic spasms occur because of the lack of reciprocal innervation.

- As the disease progresses, the neck muscles, back, abdomen, and extremities become progressively rigid. In severe forms continuous tonic convulsions may occur with *opisthotonos* (extreme arching of the back and retraction of the head). Laryngeal and respiratory spasms cause apnea and anoxia.
- Additional effects are manifested by overstimulation of the sympathetic nervous system, including profuse diaphoresis, labile hypertension, episodic tachycardia, hyperthermia, and dysrhythmias. The slightest noise, jarring motion, or bright light can set off the convulsion. These convulsions are agonizingly painful.
- Death is usually attributable to asphyxia or heart failure, the result of constantly recurring spasms.
- Residual injury, such as vertebral fracture, muscular contraction, and brain damage secondary to hypoxia may remain.

Therapeutic Management

The management of tetanus includes administration of tetanus toxoid booster (Td) and tetanus immune globulin (TIG) before the onset of symptoms to neutralize circulating toxins. Because of laryngospasm, a tracheostomy is usually performed early and the patient is maintained on mechanical ventilation. Any recognized wound should be debrided; an abscess should be drained.

- Serum electrolytes, complete blood cell count (CBC), albumin, clotting factors, glucose, and arterial blood gases (ABGs) are monitored. Cardiac function is monitored by ECG and auscultation.
- Control of spasms is essential and is managed by deep sedation, usually with diazepam (Valium), barbiturates, or chlorpromazine (Thorazine).
- If sedation does not control seizures, skeletal muscle–paralyzing drugs such as D-tubocurarine (curare) are used.
- Pain is relieved by means of codeine or meperidine, often with the addition of promethazine (Phenergan).

Nutrition is maintained through parenteral or nasogastric feeding. Those who recover have a long convalescence that includes extensive physiotherapy.

Nursing Management

Health teaching is aimed at ensuring tetanus prophylaxis, which is the most important factor influencing the incidence of this disease.

- The patient should be taught that immediate, thorough cleansing of all wounds with soap and water is important in the prevention of tetanus.
- If an open wound occurs and the patient has not been immunized within 10 years, the primary care provider should be contacted so that a tetanus booster can be given.

Acute intervention is aimed at supportive care based on the treatment of clinical manifestations. The patient should be placed in a quiet, darkened room insulated against noise. Judicious sedation should be given.

- Nursing care should be administered with the utmost caution to avoid triggering spasms. For example, the nurse should avoid unnecessary touching, use firm touching when necessary, avoid the use of linens to cover the patient, and maintain a slightly higher than normal ambient temperature.
- Nursing care related to tracheostomy and mechanical ventilation is given as appropriate.
- An indwelling bladder catheter may be used to prevent bladder distention and urinary reflux in the presence of spasms in the muscles of the pelvic floor.
- Attention must also be given to skin care.
- The patient needs emotional support during the acute phase because the fear of death is real. The family also needs support and explanations.

THALASSEMIA

Definition/Description

Thalassemia is a disease of inadequate production of normal hemoglobin. Hemolysis also occurs in thalassemia, but insufficient production of normal hemoglobin is the predominant problem.

- In contrast to iron-deficiency anemia in which heme synthesis is the problem, thalassemia involves a problem with the globin protein. Therefore the basic defect of thalassemia is abnormal hemoglobin synthesis.

Pathophysiology

Thalassemias are a group of autosomal recessive genetic disorders commonly found in members of ethnic groups whose origins are near the Mediterranean Sea. An individual with thalassemia may have a heterozygous or homozygous form of the disease.

- A person who is heterozygous has one thalassemic gene and one normal gene. They are said to have *thalassemia minor* or *thalassemic trait,* which is a mild form of the disease.
- A homozygous person has two thalassemic genes, causing a severe condition known as *thalassemia major.*

Clinical Manifestations

The patient with thalassemia minor is frequently asymptomatic because of adjustment to the gradually acquired chronic state of anemia. Occasionally, splenomegaly may develop, and mild jaundice may occur if malformed erythrocytes are rapidly hemolyzed.

- The person who has thalassemia major is pale and displays other general symptoms of anemia (see Anemia, p. 22). In addition, the person has marked splenomegaly, hepatomegaly, and jaundice from red blood cell (RBC) hemolysis. Chronic bone marrow hyperplasia leads to expansion of the marrow space. This may cause thickening of the cranium and maxillary cavity, leading to an appearance resembling Down syndrome.
- Thalassemia major is a life-threatening disease in which growth, both physical and mental, is often retarded.

Therapeutic Management

The laboratory abnormalities of thalassemia major are summarized in the section on Anemia (p. 22).

- The patient with thalassemia minor requires no treatment because the body adapts to the reduction of normal hemoglobin.
- The patient with thalassemia major is usually treated with blood transfusions and chelation therapy (therapy to reduce

iron overloading that can occur with chronic transfusion therapy). Medication and diet therapy are not effective in treating thalassemia. Transfusions are administered to keep the hemoglobin level at about 10 g/dl (100 g/L). This level is low enough to foster the patient's own erythropoiesis without enlarging the spleen.

- Because RBCs are sequestered in the enlarged spleen, thalassemia may be treated by splenectomy. However, even with therapeutic management, the person with thalassemia major will gradually progress to a fatal outcome because of the effects of chronic iron overload on the heart.

Thromboangiitis Obliterans (Buerger's Disease)

Definition/Description

Thromboangiitis obliterans (Buerger's disease) is an inflammatory thrombotic disorder of the medium-sized arteries and veins of the upper or lower extremities. Occlusion of the vessels occurs with the development of collateral circulation around areas of obstruction. The disorder, generally asymmetric, occurs predominantly in men between 25 and 40 years of age who smoke. A familial tendency has been observed.

- The basic cause is not known. There is a direct relationship to cigarette smoking: the disease occurs only in smokers, and when smoking is stopped the disease improves. Unlike atherosclerosis, lipid accumulation does not occur in the vessel media.

Clinical Manifestations

The symptom complex of Buerger's disease is often confused with that of atherosclerotic occlusive disease.

- The patient may have intermittent claudication. The development of pain at rest is a premonitory sign of gangrene and may develop in advanced stages of the disease process.
- Other signs and symptoms may include color and temperature changes in the affected limb or limbs, paresthesia, thrombophlebitis, and cold sensitivity. Painful ulceration and gangrene may necessitate an amputation of individual digits.

Therapeutic Management

Treatment includes avoidance of trauma to the extremity and complete cessation of smoking. Patients are often told that they have a choice between their cigarettes and their legs; they cannot have both. Supportive psychotherapy and pharmacologic treatment of underlying anxiety disorders are sometimes helpful in assisting the patient to stop smoking.

- The disorder is difficult to treat. Anticoagulants and vasodilator therapy have met with little success. Amputation, generally below the knee, may be necessary in advanced cases.

THROMBOCYTOPENIC PURPURA

Definition/Description

Immune thrombocytopenic purpura (ITP), the most common acquired thrombocytopenia, is a syndrome of abnormal destruction of circulating platelets. It was originally termed *idiopathic thrombocytopenic purpura* because its cause was unknown; however, it is now believed that ITP is an autoimmune disease.

- In ITP platelets are coated with antibodies. Although these platelets function normally, when they reach the spleen the antibody-coated platelets are recognized as foreign and are destroyed by macrophages.
- Platelets normally survive 8 to 10 days, but in ITP survival is only 1 to 3 days.
- Acute ITP is seen predominantly in children after a viral illness. Chronic ITP occurs most commonly in women between 20 and 40 years of age. Chronic ITP has a gradual onset and transient remissions occur.

Thrombotic thrombocytopenia purpura (TTP) is an uncommon syndrome characterized by microangiopathic hemolytic anemia, thrombocytopenia, neurologic abnormalities, fever (in the absence of infection), and renal abnormalities.

- The disease is associated with enhanced agglutination of platelets, which form microthrombi that deposit in arterioles and capillaries. The cause of the platelet agglutination is unknown.
- TTP is seen primarily in adults between the ages of 20 and 50 years, with a slight female predominance. The syndrome is occasionally precipitated by the use of estrogen or by pregnancy.
- TTP is a true medical emergency because bleeding and clotting occur simultaneously.

Clinical Manifestations

Although there are different etiologies, the clinical manifestations of thrombocytopenia are similar.

- Thrombocytopenia is most commonly manifested by the appearance of small, flat, pinpoint red or reddish-brown microhemorrhages known as *petechiae*. When the platelet count is low, red blood cells (RBCs) may leak from the blood vessels and cause petechiae.
- When petechiae are numerous, the resulting reddish skin bruise is known as *purpura*.
- Larger purplish lesions caused by hemorrhage are called *ecchymoses*. Ecchymoses may be flat or raised; on occasion pain and tenderness are present.
- Prolonged bleeding after routine procedures, such as venipuncture or intramuscular injection, may also indicate thrombocytopenia. Because the bleeding may be internal, the nurse must also be aware of manifestations that reflect this type of blood loss, including weakness, fainting, dizziness, tachycardia, abdominal pain, and hypotension.

The major complication of thrombocytopenia is hemorrhage. The hemorrhage may be insidious or acute and internal or external. It may occur in any area of the body, including joints, retina, and brain. Cerebral hemorrhage may be fatal. Insidious hemorrhage may first be detected by discovering the anemia that accompanies blood loss.

Diagnostic Studies

- Platelet count is decreased; below $20,000/\mu L$ ($20 \times 10^9/L$) spontaneous life-threatening hemorrhage may occur.
- Bleeding time is prolonged.
- Bone marrow aspirate and biopsy specimen may show normal or increased megakarocytes. These studies are done to rule out leukemia, aplastic anemia, and other myeloproliferative disorders.
- Hematocrit and hemoglobin levels reflect anemia.

Therapeutic Management

Immune thrombocytopenic purpura. Multiple therapies are used to manage the patient with ITP.

- Corticosteroids are used to treat ITP because of their ability to suppress the phagocytic response of splenic macrophages. This alters the spleen's recognition of platelets and increases the platelet's life span. In addition, corticosteroids depress autoimmune antibody formation. Corticosteroids also reduce capillary fragility and bleeding time.
- Treatment may also include high doses of IV immunoglobulin in the patient who is unresponsive to corticosteroids or splenectomy. The immunoglobulin works by competing with the antiplatelet antibodies for macrophage receptors. IV immuno-

globulin effectively raises the platelet count, but the beneficial effects are temporary.

- Danazol, an attenuated androgen, has been used with success in some patients. Immunosuppressive therapy used in refractory cases includes vincristine, vinblastine, azathioprine, and cyclophosphamide.

- Splenectomy is indicated if patients do not respond to prednisone initially or require unacceptably high doses to maintain an adequate platelet count. Approximately 80% of patients benefit from splenectomy, which results in a complete or partial remission.

- Platelet transfusions may be used to increase platelet counts in cases of life-threatening hemorrhage. Platelets should not be administered prophylactically because of the possibility of antibody formation.

- Aspirin and aspirin-containing compounds should be avoided in patients with thrombocytopenia.

Thrombotic thrombocytopenic purpura. TTP is treated with emergency plasma infusion and/or plasmapheresis. The mechanism for the therapeutic response is not fully understood. Treatment should be continued daily until the patient is in complete remission. Splenectomy, corticosteroids, and dextran (antiplatelet agent) have also been used with success.

Nursing Management

Goals

The patient with thrombocytopenia will have no gross or occult bleeding, maintain vascular integrity, and manage home care to prevent any complications related to an increased risk for bleeding.

See the nursing care plan for the patient with thrombocytopenia in Lewis/Collier/Heitkemper, *Medical-Surgical Nursing,* edition 4, p. 798.

Nursing Diagnoses

- Risk for altered cardiopulmonary, cerebral, or renal tissue perfusion related to acute or chronic blood loss
- Risk for altered oral mucous membrane related to treatment, disease, or blood-filled bullae
- Risk for impaired tissue integrity related to interventions and tissue sensitivity to trauma
- Ineffective management of therapeutic regimen related to lack of knowledge of disease process, activity, nutrition, and medication

Nursing Interventions

It is important for the nurse to discourage excessive use of over-the-counter (OTC) medications known to be possible causes of acquired thrombocytopenia. Many medications contain aspirin. Aspirin reduces platelet adhesiveness, thus potentially contributing to thrombocytopenia.

- It is also important for the nurse to encourage persons to have a complete medical evaluation if manifestations of bleeding tendencies (e.g., prolonged epistaxis, petechiae) develop. In addition, the nurse must be observant for early signs of thrombocytopenia in patients receiving cancer chemotherapy drugs.

During acute episodes of thrombocytopenia, the goal is to prevent or control hemorrhage. In the patient with thrombocytopenia, bleeding is usually from superficial sites; deep bleeding (into muscles, joints, abdomen) usually occurs only when clotting factors are diminished. It is important to emphasize that a seemingly minor nosebleed may lead to hemorrhage in a patient with severe thrombocytopenia.

- In a woman with thrombocytopenia, menstrual blood loss may exceed the usual amount and duration. Counting sanitary napkins used during menses is another important intervention to detect excess blood loss.
- The proper administration of platelet transfusions is an important nursing responsibility. Platelet concentrates, derived from fresh whole blood, can increase the platelet level effectively.
- The patient with either ITP or acquired thrombocytopenia should have planned periodic medical evaluations to assess the patient's status and to intercede in situations in which exacerbations and bleeding are likely to occur.

Patient Teaching

- Teach the patient about the disease process, medication, and activity and dietary recommendations to decrease anxiety and prevent complications.
- Discuss the complications and signs that should be reported, such as trauma prevention, need for high fluid intake, medication management, and need for periods of rest and exercise so the patient will be knowledgeable and able to manage his/her own care or direct others in care.
- Provide opportunities for the patient to verbalize concerns because discussing these with a supportive other decreases anxiety.
- Foster care decisions and planning by patient to increase the patient's sense of control and self-esteem.

THROMBOPHLEBITIS

Definition/Description

Thrombophlebitis is the formation of a thrombus (clot) in association with inflammation of the vein.

- The terms *phlebothrombosis* and *phlebitis* have been used to indicate whether the predominant process is thrombus formation or inflammation. In general, the preferred term is *thrombophlebitis* because both clots and inflammation are usually present. The initiating event is usually thrombus formation. Thrombophlebitis is classified as either *superficial* or *deep*.
- Superficial thrombophlebitis is often of minor significance and is treated with elevation, antiinflammatory agents, and warm compresses.
- Deep-vein thrombophlebitis is of greater significance and can result in embolization of thrombi from deep veins to lungs. This can be fatal and, at the least, results in prolonged hospitalization.

Pathophysiology

The three important factors (Virchow's triad) in the etiology of thrombophlebitis are (1) stasis of venous flow, (2) damage of endothelium (inner lining of the vein), and (3) hypercoagulability of blood. The patient who is at high risk for development of thrombophlebitis has predisposing conditions related to any of these three factors.

Venous stasis occurs if venous valves are dysfunctional or if muscles of the extremities are inactive.

- Venous stasis occurs in people who are obese, have congestive heart failure (CHF), have been on long trips without regular exercise, or are immobile for long periods (e.g., with spinal cord injuries or fractured hips). Also at risk are pregnant women and women in the postpartum period.

Damage of the endothelium is caused by trauma or external pressure. This occurs any time a venipuncture is performed. Damaged endothelium has decreased fibrinolytic properties, which facilitates thrombus development.

- Increased endothelial damage is sustained when patients undergoing IV therapy are receiving high-dose antibiotics, potassium, chemotherapeutic agents, or hypertonic solutions such as contrast media.
- Other factors predisposing to endothelial inflammation and damage include presence of an IV catheter in the same site for longer than 48 hours, use of contaminated IV equipment, a

fracture that causes damage to blood vessels, diabetes, blood pooling, burns, and any unusual physical exertion that results in muscular strain.

Hypercoagulability of the blood, which occurs in many hematologic disorders (e.g., polycythemia, severe anemias, and various malignancies) contributes to thrombophlebitis. A patient with systemic infections in which endotoxins are released also has hypercoagulability. In addition, hypercoagulability seems to be the contributing factor in idiopathic thrombophlebitis.

- The patient who takes oral contraceptives (especially those containing estrogen) is at increased risk for thromboembolic disease. Women who take contraceptives and smoke double their risk because of the constricting effect of nicotine on the blood vessel wall. Smoking may also cause hypercoagulability.

Thrombus formation results from the adherence of red blood cells (RBCs), white blood cells (WBCs), platelets, and fibrin. A frequent site of thrombus formation is the valve cusps of veins, where venous stasis allows accumulation of blood products.

- As the thrombus enlarges, increased amounts of blood cells and fibrin collect behind it, producing a larger clot with a "tail" that eventually occludes the lumen of the vein.
- If a thrombus only partially occludes the vein and blood flow continues, the thrombus becomes covered by endothelial cells and the thrombotic process stops.
- If the thrombus does not become detached, it undergoes lysis or becomes firmly organized and adherent within 24 to 48 hours. The organized thrombi may detach and then give rise to emboli.
- Turbulence of blood flow past the thrombus is a major factor contributing to its detachment from the vein wall. These emboli generally flow through the venous circulation, back to the heart, and into the pulmonary circulation.

Clinical Manifestations

Manifestations of thrombophlebitis vary according to the size and location of the thrombus and the adequacy of collateral circulation around the obstructive process.

- The patient with *superficial thrombophlebitis* may have a palpable, firm, subcutaneous cordlike vein with the area surrounding the vein tender to touch, reddened, and warm. A mild systemic temperature elevation and leukocytosis may be present. Edema of the extremity may or may not occur. The most common cause of superficial thrombophlebitis in the legs is related to varicose veins.

- The patient with *deep thrombophlebitis* may have no symptoms or have unilateral leg edema, pain, warm skin, and a temperature >100.4° F (38° C). If the calf is involved, tenderness may be present on palpation. *Homans' sign,* pain on dorsiflexion of foot when leg is raised, is a classic but unreliable sign because it is not specific for deep-vein thrombosis.

Complications

The most serious complications of thrombophlebitis are *pulmonary embolism, chronic venous insufficiency,* and *phlegmasia cerulea dolens.* Pulmonary embolism is the most feared complication of thrombophlebitis because of its lethal potential (see Pulmonary Embolism, p. 486).

- Chronic venous insufficiency, a common complication resulting from recurrent thrombophlebitis, results in valvular destruction, allowing retrograde flow of blood. Persistent edema, increased pigmentation, secondary varicosities, ulceration, and cyanosis of the limb when it is placed in a dependent position may develop in a person with this complication. Signs and symptoms of chronic venous insufficiency often do not develop for many years after deep thrombophlebitis.
- Phlegmasia cerulea dolens (swollen, blue, painful leg) may develop with severe thrombophlebitis of the lower extremities. It appears as a sudden massive swelling and an intense bluish discoloration of the extremity. Gangrene may occur as a result of arterial occlusion resulting from obstruction of venous outflow.

Diagnostic Studies

- Coagulation studies (platelet count, bleeding time, prothrombin time [PT], partial thromboplastin time [PTT]) may be elevated with blood dyscrasias.
- Duplex scanning is the most widely used test for deep-vein thrombosis.
- Plethysmography records abnormal findings with slow venous outflow.
- Venous Doppler evaluation is used to determine venous flow.
- MRI detects deep leg vein thrombosis.
- Venogram (phlebogram) can determine the location of a clot.

Therapeutic Management

The patient with superficial thrombophlebitis is usually kept in bed with elevation of the affected extremity until tenderness has subsided, usually for 5 to 7 days. Warm, moist heat may be used to relieve pain and treat inflammation. Mild oral analgesics (e.g., aspirin, codeine) are used to relieve pain. Nonsteroidal antiinflammatory agents (e.g., ibuprofen) are used to treat the inflammatory process and accompanying pain.

- Anticoagulant therapy is usually not indicated for superficial thrombophlebitis but is routinely used for deep-vein thrombophlebitis. The goals of anticoagulation therapy are to prevent propagation of clot, development of a new thrombus, and embolization. Anticoagulation therapy does not dissolve the clot. Lysis of clot begins spontaneously through the body's intrinsic fibrinolytic system. Heparin, administered by continuous IV infusion after an initial bolus dose, is given for up to 10 days and is followed by oral anticoagulants for 3 to 6 months.
- Bed rest with feet elevated above the level of heart is indicated until therapeutic levels of anticoagulation are achieved and the edema subsides.
- If edema is present when the patient becomes ambulatory, graduated compression elastic stockings are recommended. Use of compression gradient stockings is recommended for several months to support vein walls and valves and decrease pain on ambulation from swelling.

Most patients are treated conservatively, but a small percentage require surgical intervention. The primary indication for surgery is to prevent pulmonary emboli. Surgical procedures include venous thrombectomy (rarely performed) and inferior vena cava interruption. Venous thrombectomy involves removal of an occluding clot through an incision in the vein. This procedure is done to prevent pulmonary embolism and chronic venous insufficiency.

Nursing Management

Goals

The patient with thrombophlebitis will have relief of pain, decreased edema, no skin ulceration, and no evidence of pulmonary emboli.

See the nursing care plan for the patient with thrombophlebitis in Lewis/Collier/Heitkemper, *Medical-Surgical Nursing,* edition 4, p. 1060.

Nursing Diagnoses/Collaborative Problems

- Pain related to edema secondary to impaired circulation in extremities
- Altered health maintenance related to lack of knowledge about the disorder and its treatment
- Risk for impaired skin integrity related to alteration in peripheral tissue perfusion and possible valvular destruction
- Potential complication: hemorrhage related to anticoagulant medications
- Potential complication: pulmonary embolism related to dehydration, immobility, and embolization of thrombus

Nursing Interventions

Prophylactic measures to prevent thrombus formation include early ambulation and leg exercises postoperatively, use of elastic compression gradient stockings, avoidance of dehydration, and low-dose anticoagulant therapy. Heparin (5000 units subcutaneously every 8 to 12 hours) or oral anticoagulants are often recommended for the high-risk patient who is predisposed to thrombus formation.

- Another preventive measure is to avoid prolonged standing or sitting in a motionless, leg-dependent position. Frequent knee flexion, ankle rotation, and active walking should be done during long periods of sitting or standing, especially on long trips.
- The patient should be taught the importance of not smoking and to perform deep breathing and range-of-motion exercises. In addition, identify patients at high risk for deep-vein thrombophlebitis and institute appropriate preventive measures.

Acute care is directed toward reduction of inflammation and prevention of emboli formation.

- Intervention for superficial thrombophlebitis involves the use of warm moist packs or soaks, elevation of affected extremity, removal of an IV catheter if present, and provision of analgesia to minimize pain and inflammation.
- Intervention for deep-vein thrombophlebitis involves IV and oral anticoagulation, 5 to 7 days of bed rest with elevation of the affected extremity, and use of elastic support (elastic bandages or compression gradient stockings) to promote venous return.

While the patient is receiving anticoagulation therapy, closely observe for any indication of bleeding, including epistaxis and bleeding gingiva.

- Urine should be assessed for gross or microscopic hematuria. A smoky appearance to the urine is sometimes noted if blood is present.
- Particular attention should be paid to the protection of skin areas that may be traumatized. Surgical incisions should be closely observed for evidence of bleeding.
- Stools should be tested to determine the presence of occult blood from the GI tract.
- Mental status changes, especially in the older patient, should be assessed as a possible indication of cerebral bleeding.
- Hemoglobin and hematocrit levels should be monitored when the patient is receiving anticoagulant drugs. Medication doses are titrated according to the results of clotting studies. The nurse should first check the results of clotting studies before administering either heparin or coumarin. The antidote for heparin is protamine sulfate, and vitamin K is used as the antidote

for coumarin. These drugs must be immediately available if hemorrhage occurs.

Patient Teaching

Discharge teaching should stress the avoidance of contraceptives for the patient with recurrent thrombophlebitis, the hazards of smoking, the importance of compression gradient stockings, and the need to avoid constrictive girdles or garters.

- Exercise programs should be developed with an emphasis on swimming and wading, which are particularly beneficial because of gentle, even pressure of the water. A balanced program of rest and exercise, along with proper posture and avoiding long periods of sitting, improves arterial filling and venous return. The older patient should be taught safety precautions to prevent falls.
- Dietary considerations for the overweight patient are aimed at limiting caloric intake so that the desired weight can be attained. Fat intake should be reduced if lipid or triglyceride levels are above normal for the patient's age. Sodium may be limited if edema is present. A well-balanced diet is important because calcium, vitamin E, and vitamin K all play active roles in clotting.
- Review with the patient any medications currently being taken that may interfere with anticoagulant therapy.
- If the patient is discharged while receiving anticoagulant medication, both the patient and family need careful explanations of its dosage, actions, and side effects, as well as the importance of routine blood tests and need to report symptoms to the health care provider.

TOXIC SHOCK SYNDROME

Definition/Description

Toxic shock syndrome (TSS) is an acute condition caused by the toxin of a local infection of *Staphylococcus aureus,* which can develop into a systemic infection. TSS usually occurs in women who are menstruating and using tampons or who have chronic vaginal infections.

- TSS typically begins suddenly with high fever, vomiting, and profuse watery diarrhea. Within 48 hours, hypotensive shock and a characteristic rash develop. In the recovery phase there is a desquamation of varying skin surfaces.

There is no definitive test for TSS. However, cervical-vaginal isolates of *S. aureus* have been present 90% of the time with TSS.

- Once diagnosed by presumptive signs, prompt treatment with antistaphylococcal β-lactamase–resistant antibiotics and fluid replacement therapy is initiated.

Because TSS has been linked to the use of tampons during menstruation, it is recommended that superabsorbent tampons not be used. They provide a favorable milieu for bacterial growth because they can absorb a large amount of menstrual blood and may be left in place longer than other tampons.

- The nurse should advise patients to alternate tampons with sanitary napkins, using the latter at night. When tampons are used, they should be changed several times a day and inserted carefully to avoid abrasions.
- Good handwashing techniques should always be used.
- Women who have had TSS are at risk of recurrence and should be instructed not to use tampons until *S. aureus* is no longer present in the vaginal flora.

TRIGEMINAL NEURALGIA

Definition/Description

Trigeminal neuralgia (tic douloureux) is a relatively common cranial nerve disorder. It is more frequently seen in women than in men and usually begins in the fifth or sixth decade of life. Although this condition is considered benign, the severity of the pain and the disruption of lifestyle can result in almost total physical and psychologic dysfunction or even suicide.

Pathophysiology

The trigeminal nerve is the fifth cranial nerve (CN V) and has both motor and sensory branches. Only the sensory branches are involved in trigeminal neuralgia, primarily the maxillary and mandibular branches.

- Although no specific cause has been identified, nerve compression by tortuous arteries of the posterior fossa blood vessels, demyelinating plaques, herpesvirus infection, infection of teeth and jaw, and brainstem infarct have been suggested as initiating pathologic events.
- The effectiveness of antiepileptic drug therapy in shortening or suppressing the duration of an attack suggests a similar cell membrane defect as in epilepsy.

Clinical Manifestations

The classic feature of trigeminal neuralgia is an abrupt onset of paroxysms of excruciating pain described as burning, knifelike, or a lightning-like shock in the lips, upper or lower gums, cheek, forehead, or side of the nose.

- Intense pain, twitching, grimacing, and frequent blinking and tearing of the eye occur during the acute attack (giving rise to the term *tic*).
- The attacks are usually brief, lasting seconds to 2 or 3 minutes, and are generally unilateral.
- Recurrences are unpredictable; they may occur several times a day or weeks or months apart. After the refractory (pain-free) period, a phenomenon known as *clustering* can occur that is characterized by a cycle of pain and refractoriness that continues for hours.

The painful episodes are usually initiated by a triggering mechanism of light cutaneous stimulation at a specific point *(trigger zones)* along the distribution of the nerve branches.

- Precipitating stimuli include chewing, tooth brushing, a hot or cold blast of air on the face, washing the face, yawning, or even talking. Touch and tickle seem to predominate as causative triggers rather than pain or changes in temperature.
- As a result, the patient may not eat properly, neglect hygienic practices, wear a cloth over the face, and withdraw from interaction with other individuals. The patient may sleep excessively as a means of coping with the pain.

Diagnostic Studies

- Brain scan, CT scan, MRI
- Audiologic evaluation
- Electromyography
- Spinal tap
- Arteriography and posterior myelography

Therapeutic Management

The goal of treatment is relief of pain either medically or surgically.

- The majority of patients obtain adequate relief through antiepileptic drugs such as diphenylhydantoin (Dilantin) and carbamazepine (Tegretol). These drugs may prevent an acute attack or promote a remission of symptoms, although the mechanism by which they work is not known. Unfortunately, these drugs may lose their effectiveness and are not a permanent solution.
- Nerve blocking with local anesthetics is another treatment possibility. Local nerve blocking results in complete anesthesia of the area supplied by the injected branches. Relief of pain is only temporary, lasting from 6 to 18 months.

- Biofeedback is another strategy for pain management. For patients who are alert enough to understand the simple equipment and who can learn to use the feedback to regulate one physiologic parameter such as heart rate, biofeedback offers an innovative approach to the control of the pain. In addition to controlling their pain, patients also experience a strong sense of personal control by mastering the technique and altering certain body functions.

Surgical Management

If a conservative approach is not effective, surgical therapy is available. Percutaneous radiofrequency rhizotomy (electrocoagulation) and *microvascular decompression* afford the greatest relief of pain.

- *Percutaneous radiofrequency rhizotomy* consists of placing a needle into the trigeminal rootlets adjacent to the pons and destroying the area by means of a radiofrequency current. This can result in anesthesia of the face, although some degree of sensation may be retained and/or trigeminal motor weakness may develop. This procedure is easily performed with minimal risk to the patient.
- *Glycerol rhizotomy* has become more popular in the last 10 years and is preferred over percutaneous radiofrequency rhizotomy. Glycerol rhizotomy consists of an injection of glycerol through the foramen ovale into the trigeminal cistern. Glycerol rhizotomy is a more benign procedure with less sensory loss and fewer sensory aberrations than radiofrequency rhizotomy and with comparable or better pain relief.
- *Microvascular decompression* of the trigeminal nerve is accomplished by displacing and repositioning blood vessels that appear to be compressing the nerve at the root-entry zone where it exits the pons. This procedure relieves pain without residual sensory loss but is potentially dangerous, as is any surgery near the brainstem. Microvascular decompression may be poorly tolerated in older adults because manipulation of the brainstem may result in BP fluctuations. Such fluctuations can be dangerous if the cardiovascular system is already compromised.

Nursing Management

Goals

The patient with trigeminal neuralgia will be free of pain, maintain adequate nutritional and oral hygiene status, have minimal to no anxiety, and return to normal or previous socialization and occupational activities.

Nursing Diagnoses

- Pain related to inflammation or compression of the trigeminal nerve
- Altered nutrition: less than body requirements related to fear of eating
- Anxiety related to uncertainty of timing and initiating event of pain and uncertainty regarding effectiveness of pain-relieving factors
- Risk for altered oral mucous membranes related to unwillingness to practice oral hygiene measures secondary to potential for initiating pain
- Social isolation related to anxiety over pain attacks and desire to maintain a nonstimulating environment

Nursing Interventions

Pain relief is primarily obtained by the administration of the recommended drug therapy.

- The nurse should monitor the patient's response to therapy and note any side effects. Strong narcotics such as morphine should be used cautiously because of the potential for addiction over time. Moderate use of propoxyphene (Darvon) or pentazocine (Talwin) is acceptable.
- Alternative pain-relief measures, such as biofeedback, should be explored for the patient who is not a surgical candidate and whose pain is not controlled by other therapeutic measures.
- Careful assessment of pain, including history, pain relief, and drug dependency, can assist in selecting appropriate interventions.

Environmental management is essential during an acute period to lessen triggering stimuli. The room should be kept at an even, moderate temperature and free of drafts. A private room is preferred during an acute period.

- The nurse must use care to avoid touching the patient's face or jarring the bed. Many patients prefer to carry out their own care, fearing that they will be inadvertently injured by someone else.

The nurse should instruct the patient about the importance of nutrition, hygiene, and oral care, ensuring understanding if previous neglect is apparent.

- The nurse should provide lukewarm water and soft cloths or cotton saturated with solutions not requiring rinsing for cleansing the face. A small, very soft–bristled toothbrush or a warm mouthwash assist in promoting oral care.
- Hygiene activities are best carried out when analgesia is at its peak.

The patient will probably not engage in extensive conversation during the acute period. Alternative communication methods such as paper and pencil should be provided.

Food should be high in protein and calories and easy to chew. It should be served lukewarm and offered frequently. When oral intake is markedly reduced and the patient's nutritional status is compromised, a nasogastric tube is inserted on the unaffected side for nasogastric feedings.

For the patient who has had surgery, the postoperative pain should be compared with the preoperative level. The corneal reflex, extraocular muscles, hearing, sensation, and facial nerve function are evaluated frequently. General postoperative nursing care after a craniotomy is appropriate if intracranial surgery is performed.

- After a radiofrequency percutaneous electrocoagulation procedure, an ice pack is applied to the jaw on the operative side for 3 to 5 hours. To avoid injuring the mouth, the patient should not chew on the operative side until sensation has returned.

Patient Teaching

Regular follow-up care should be planned. The patient needs instruction regarding the dosage and side effects of medications.

- Although relief of pain may be complete, the patient should be encouraged to keep environmental stimuli to a moderate level and to use stress-reduction methods.
- Herpes simplex infection (cold sores) can occur from manipulation of the gasserian ganglion. Treatment consists of topical antiviral agents such as acyclovir.

Long-term management after surgical intervention depends on the residual effects of the procedure.

- If anesthesia is present or the corneal reflex is altered, the patient should be taught to (1) chew on the unaffected side, (2) avoid hot foods or beverages that can burn the mucous membranes, (3) check the oral cavity after meals to remove food particles, (4) practice meticulous oral hygiene and continue with semiannual dental visits, (5) protect the face against extremes of temperature, (6) use an electric razor, and (7) wear a protective eye shield.
- The patient may have developed protective practices to prevent pain and may need counseling or psychiatric assistance in the readjustment, especially in reestablishing personal relationships.

TUBERCULOSIS

Definition/Description

Tuberculosis (TB) is a bacterial disease transmitted by *Mycobacterium tuberculosis.* It usually involves the lungs but can also occur in the kidneys, bones, joints, reproductive tracts, lymph nodes, or meninges; or it can be disseminated throughout the body.

- With the introduction of chemotherapy in the late 1940s and early 1950s, there was a dramatic decrease in the prevalence of TB. Today 10 to 15 million people are infected with or harbor the tubercle bacillus; the majority of these individuals have healed or dormant TB. There are approximately 26,000 cases a year of new active TB with approximately 10% of these cases representing relapses.
- These statistics indicate that TB, in spite of being potentially curable and preventable, is still a major public health problem in the United States.
- The major factors that have contributed to the resurgence of TB have been (1) the emergence of multidrug-resistant strains of *M. tuberculosis* and (2) epidemic proportions of TB among patients who are HIV infected.

Pathophysiology

M. tuberculosis, a gram-positive, acid-fast bacillus, is usually spread via airborne droplet nuclei, which are produced when the infected individual coughs, sneezes, or speaks.

- Once released into a room, organisms are dispersed and can be inhaled. Brief exposure to a few tubercle bacilli rarely causes infection.
- TB is not highly infectious, and transmission usually requires close, frequent, or prolonged exposure. The disease cannot be spread by hands, books, glasses, dishes, or other fomites.

When bacilli are inhaled, they pass down the bronchial system and implant themselves on respiratory bronchioles or alveoli. The lower parts of the lungs are usually the site of initial bacterial implantation.

- After implantation, bacilli multiply with no initial resistance from the host.
- While a cellular immune response is being activated, bacilli can be spread through lymphatic channels to regional lymph nodes and via the thoracic duct to circulating blood.

A characteristic tissue reaction called an *epithelioid cell granuloma* results after the cellular immune system is activated. This granuloma (also called an *epithelioid cell tubercle*) is a result of the fusion of infiltrating macrophages. This reaction usually takes 10 to 20 days.

Healing of the primary lesion takes place by resolution, fibrosis, and calcification.

- When a tuberculous lesion regresses and heals, the infection enters a latent period in which it may persist without producing clinical illness. The infection may remain dormant for life, or it may develop into clinical disease if persisting organisms begin to multiply rapidly.
- If the initial immune response is not adequate, control of the organisms is not maintained and clinical disease results. Certain individuals are at a higher risk for clinical disease, including those who are immunosuppressed or have diabetes mellitus.
- Approximately 5% of individuals are incapable of containing the initial infective process.

Classification of TB according to the American Lung Association is presented in Table 48.

Clinical Manifestations

In the early stages of TB the person is usually free of symptoms. Many cases are found incidentally when routine chest x-rays are taken, especially in older adults.

- Systemic manifestations may initially consist of fatigue, malaise, anorexia, weight loss, low-grade fevers (especially in the late afternoon), and night sweats. Weight loss may not be excessive until late in the disease. Irregular menses may be present in premenopausal women.

A characteristic pulmonary manifestation is a cough that becomes frequent and produces mucoid or mucopurulent sputum. Chest pain characterized as dull or tight may also be present. Hemoptysis is not a common finding and is associated with more advanced cases.

- Sometimes TB has more acute, sudden manifestations; the patient has high fever, chills, generalized flulike symptoms, pleuritic pain, and a productive cough.
- The HIV-infected patient with TB often has atypical physical examinations and chest x-ray findings. Classical signs such as fever, cough, and weight loss may be attributed to *Pneumocystis carinii* pneumonia or other HIV-associated opportunistic diseases.

Complications

If a necrotic lesion erodes through a blood vessel, large numbers of organisms invade the bloodstream and spread to all body organs. This is called *miliary* or *hematogenous TB*.

Table 48	Classification of Tuberculosis

Class 0
No TB exposure; not infected (no history of exposure, negative tuberculin skin test)

Class 1
TB exposure; no evidence of infection (history of exposure; negative tuberculin skin test)

Class 2
TB infection without disease (significant reaction to tuberculin skin test, negative bacteriologic studies, no x-ray findings compatible with tuberculosis, no clinical evidence of tuberculosis)

Class 3
TB infection with clinically active disease (positive bacteriologic studies or both a significant reaction to tuberculin skin test and clinical or x-ray evidence of current disease)

Class 4
No current disease (history of previous episode of TB or abnormal, stable x-ray findings in a person with significant reaction to tuberculin skin test; negative bacteriologic studies if done; no clinical or x-ray evidence of current disease)

Class 5
TB suspect (diagnosis pending); person should not be in this classification for more than 3 mo

Modified from American Thoracic Society: *Diagnostic standards and classification of tuberculosis,* New York, 1990, *American Review of Respiratory Disease* 142:725, 1990.

- The patient may be either acutely ill with fever, dyspnea, and cyanosis or chronically ill with systemic manifestations of weight loss, fever, and GI disturbance.
- Hepatomegaly, splenomegaly, and generalized lymphadenopathy may also be present.

Pleural effusion may occur and is caused by the release of gaseous material into the pleural space. The bacteria-containing material triggers an inflammatory reaction and a pleural exudate of protein-rich fluid. Clinical manifestations include localized pleuritic pain on deep inspiration.

Acute pneumonia may result when large amounts of tubercle bacilli are discharged from the liquefied necrotic lesion into the lungs or lymph nodes.

- Clinical manifestations are similar to those of bacterial pneumonia, including chills, fever, productive cough, pleuritic pain, and leukocytosis.

Diagnostic Studies

- Tuberculin skin test: a positive reaction indicates TB infection
- Chest x-ray: diagnosis cannot be based solely on x-ray; other diseases may mimic TB
- Bacteriologic studies: (1) sputum smear—positive for acid-fast bacillus (AFB); (2) sputum culture—detects mycobacterium

Therapeutic Management

Most patients with TB are treated on an outpatient basis, and many can continue to work and maintain their lifestyles with few changes. Hospitalization may be used for diagnostic evaluation, the severely ill or debilitated, and those who experience adverse drug reactions or treatment failures.

Pharmacologic Management

The mainstay of TB treatment is pharmacologic. Drug therapy is used to treat an individual with clinical disease and to prevent disease in an infected person. In view of the growing prevalence of multidrug-resistant TB, the patient with active TB should be managed aggressively. Treatment of TB usually consists of a combination of at least three drugs. The reason for combination therapy is to increase the therapeutic effectiveness and decrease the development of *M. tuberculosis*–resistant strains.

- The four primary drugs used are isoniazid, rifampin, streptomycin, and ethambutol. A new combination drug, Rifamate, consists of 150 mg of isoniazid and 300 mg of rifampin.
- Other drugs are primarily used for treatment of resistant strains or if the patient develops toxicity to the primary drugs.
- An important reason for follow-up care in the patient with TB is to ensure adherence to the treatment regimen. Noncompliance is a major factor in the emergence of multidrug resistance and treatment failures.

Pharmacologic management can be used to prevent TB infection from developing into clinical disease. Isoniazid prophylaxis is recommended for all adult tuberculin reactors who have additional risk factors for active TB such as immunosuppression or diabetes mellitus.

Nursing Management

Goals

The patient with tuberculosis will comply with the therapeutic regimen, have no recurrence of disease, have normal pulmonary function, and take appropriate measures to prevent the spread of the disease.

Nursing Diagnoses

- Ineffective breathing pattern related to decreased lung capacity
- Altered nutrition: less than body requirements related to chronic poor appetite, fatigue, and productive cough
- Risk for noncompliance related to lack of knowledge of disease process, lack of motivation, and long-term treatment
- Altered health maintenance related to lack of knowledge about disease process and therapeutic regimen
- Activity intolerance related to fatigue, decreased nutritional status, and chronic febrile episodes

Nursing Interventions

The public health nurse and clinical nurse have especially important responsibilities including the following:

- Selective screening programs can be used in known high-risk groups for early detection of TB.
- Chest x-rays are used to assess for the presence of TB in persons with a positive tuberculin skin test.
- Contacts of the individual who has TB need to be identified. These contacts should be assessed for the possibility of infection and the need for chemoprophylactic treatment.
- When an individual has respiratory symptoms such as cough, dyspnea, or productive sputum, especially if accompanied by night sweats and unexplained weight loss, the nurse should assess for the presence of TB.

If hospitalization is needed:

- Respiratory isolation is indicated until the patient has been undergoing adequate drug therapy for at least 2 weeks and has shown a clinical response to therapy.
- Masks are of limited value unless they are made of a fabric designed to filter out droplet nuclei. Any mask used needs to be molded to fit tightly around the nose and mouth.

Follow-up care, including bacteriologic studies and chest x-ray, is generally indicated during the subsequent 12 months after the medication regimen is completed.

Patient Teaching

- In the hospital the patient should be taught to cover the nose and mouth with paper tissue every time he/she coughs, sneezes, or produces sputum. Masks are necessary only during face-to-face contacts; it is preferable for the patient to wear the mask.

- The patient should be educated so that the need for dedication to the prescribed medication regimen is fully understood. The patient should be reassured that TB can be cured if the regimen is followed.
- Because approximately 5% of individuals experience relapses, the patient should be taught to recognize symptoms that indicate recurrence of TB. If these symptoms occur, immediate medical attention should be sought.
- The patient also needs to be instructed about factors that could reactivate TB, such as immunosuppression and malignancy.

Ulcerative Colitis

Definition/Description
Ulcerative colitis is characterized by inflammation and ulceration of the colon and rectum. It may occur at any age but peaks between the ages of 15 and 40 years. Ulcerative colitis affects both sexes but has a higher incidence in women. It is more common in Jewish and upper middle-class urban populations.

Pathophysiology
The inflammation of ulcerative colitis is diffuse and involves the mucosa and submucosa with alternate periods of exacerbations and remissions (see Crohn's Disease, Table 24, p. 158). The disease usually begins in the rectum and sigmoid colon and spreads up the colon in a continuous pattern.

- The mucosa of the colon is hyperemic and edematous in the affected area. Multiple abscesses develop in the intestinal glands. As the disease advances, the abscesses break through the crypts into the submucosa, leaving ulcerations. These ulcerations also destroy mucosal epithelium, causing bleeding and diarrhea.

Loss of fluid and electrolytes occurs because of decreased mucosal surface area for absorption. Breakdown of cells results in protein loss through the stool. Areas of inflamed mucosa can form pseudopolyps. Granulation tissue develops, and the musculature becomes thickened, shortening the colon.

Clinical Manifestations
Ulcerative colitis may appear as an acute fulminating crisis or, more commonly, as a chronic disorder with mild to severe acute exacerbations that occur at unpredictable intervals over many years.

- The major symptoms are bloody diarrhea and abdominal pain. Pain may vary from the mild lower-abdominal cramping associated with diarrhea to the severe constant abdominal pain associated with acute perforations.
- With *mild disease* diarrhea may consist of semiformed stools containing little blood. The patient may have no other systemic manifestations.
- In *moderate disease* there is increased stool output (4 to 5 stools/day), increased bleeding, and systemic symptoms, including fever, malaise, and anorexia.
- In *severe fulminating disease* diarrhea is bloody, contains mucus, and occurs 10 to 20 times a day. In addition, fever, weight loss >10% of total body weight, anemia, tachycardia, and de-

U

hydration are present. Toxic megacolon and perforation may ensue.

Complications may be classified as intestinal or extraintestinal. *Intestinal complications* include hemorrhage, strictures, perforation, toxic megacolon, and colonic dilatation. *Extraintestinal complications* may be directly related to the colitis and small intestine pathology (malabsorption). Colitis-related complications are associated with active inflammation and can involve the joints, skin, mouth, and eyes. Skin lesions such as erythema nodosum and pyoderma gangrenosum are among the most frequently seen extraintestinal manifestations. Uveitis is the most common eye problem.

- A patient who has had ulcerative colitis for more than 10 years is at greater risk for colon cancer.

Diagnostic Studies

- Complete blood cell count (CBC) shows anemia from blood loss.
- White blood cell (WBC) count is elevated in toxic megacolon or perforation.
- Serum electrolyte decreases from diarrhea and vomiting include sodium, potassium, chloride, bicarbonate, and magnesium.
- Stool is examined for blood; culture and sensitivity are done.
- Hypoalbuminemia with severe disease may be caused by protein loss from the bowel.
- Fiberoptic colonoscopy is used to view the large intestine and sigmoidoscopy to view the rectum, sigmoid colon, and descending colon.
- Barium enema (double-contrast) may show areas of granular inflammation and ulcerations.

Therapeutic Management

Goals of treatment are to rest the bowel, control inflammation and infection, correct malnutrition, alleviate stress, and provide symptomatic relief using drug therapy.

- Drug therapy is an important aspect of treatment. Sulfasalazine (Azulfidine) is the principal drug used. It is effective in the maintenance of clinical remission and in the treatment of mild to moderately severe attacks. Corticosteroids are usually indicated for acute exacerbations. Hospitalization is indicated if the patient fails to respond to corticosteroid therapy, if fever or abdominal pain develops, or if complications are suspected.
- Immunosuppressive drugs (e.g., 6-mercaptopurine [6-MP]) are used in severe cases of ulcerative colitis when a patient has failed to respond to the usual medications and before surgery is considered.

Surgical Management

Surgery is indicated if the patient fails to respond to treatment; exacerbations are frequent and debilitating; massive bleeding, perforation, strictures, obstruction, or changes that suggest dysplasia occur; or carcinoma develops.

- Surgical procedures include (1) total proctocolectomy with permanent ileostomy, (2) total proctocolectomy with continent ileostomy (Kock pouch), and (3) total colectomy with rectal mucosal stripping and ileoanal reservoir. See Lewis/Collier/Heitkemper, *Medical-Surgical Nursing,* edition 4, p. 1226, for descriptions of these procedures and the nursing care plan for the patient with a colostomy or ileostomy, p. 1228.

Nutritional Management

An important component in the treatment of ulcerative colitis is diet. The dietitian is an important member of the team and should be consulted regarding dietary recommendations.

- The goals of diet management are to provide adequate nutrition without exacerbating symptoms, to correct and prevent malnutrition, to replace fluid and electrolyte losses, and to prevent weight loss. The diet for each patient must be individualized.

Nursing Management

Goals

The patient with ulcerative colitis will experience a decrease in the number and severity of acute exacerbations, maintain normal fluid and electrolyte balance, be free from pain or discomfort, comply with medical regimens, and maintain nutritional balance.

See the nursing care plan for the patient with ulcerative colitis in Lewis/Collier/Heitkemper, *Medical-Surgical Nursing,* edition 4, p.1232.

Nursing Diagnoses

- Diarrhea related to irritated bowel and intestinal hyperactivity
- Sleep pattern disturbance related to frequent stools
- Impaired skin integrity of perianal area related to diarrhea, immobility, and altered nutritional status
- Ineffective individual coping related to chronic disease, lifestyle changes, stress, and chronic pain
- Ineffective management of therapeutic regimen related to lack of knowledge of course of disease, appropriate lifestyle adjustments, and nutritional and pharmacologic interventions
- Anxiety related to possible social embarrassment, unfamiliar environment, diagnostic tests, and treatment
- Altered nutrition: less than body requirements related to decreased nutrient intake, increased nutrient loss through diarrhea, and decreased intestinal absorption

U

Nursing Interventions

During the acute phase, attention is focused on hemodynamic stability, pain control, fluid and electrolyte balance, and nutritional support. Accurate intake and output records need to be maintained, with the number and appearance of stools also monitored. Nursing care of the patient with ulcerative colitis is directed toward an intensive therapeutic and supportive program.

- Emotional support is important because the patient may feel insecure, dependent, and sensitive. It is important that the nurse establish a good working relationship and encourage the patient to talk about self and daily activities. An explanation of all procedures and treatments is necessary and may allay some apprehension.

- Bed rest may be ordered if the patient has a severe exacerbation. Nursing interventions to prevent complications of immobility should be instituted. A sedative or tranquilizer may be prescribed to ensure rest. The nurse should allow the patient extra time to eat.

- Rest is important because patients may lose sleep as a result of frequent episodes of diarrhea and abdominal pain. Nutritional deficiencies and anemia leave the patient feeling weak and listless. Activities should be scheduled around rest periods.

- Until diarrhea is controlled, the patient must be kept clean, dry, and free of odor. A bedpan and wipes should be kept within reach of the patient. The bedpan should be emptied as soon as possible. A deodorizer should be placed in the room. Antidiarrheal agents should be administered as ordered. If the patient has continuous diarrhea, the enterostomal therapy nurse or therapist may give helpful suggestions.

- Meticulous perianal skin care using plain water (no harsh soap) is necessary to treat and prevent skin breakdown. Dibucaine (Nupercainal), witch hazel, or other soothing compresses and/or prescribed ointment and sitz baths may reduce irritation and relieve discomfort of the anus.

URETHRITIS

Definition/Description

Urethritis is an inflammation of the urethra. It is often difficult to diagnose. Causes of urethritis include a bacterial or viral infection, *Trichomonas* and monilial infection (especially in women), chlamydia, and gonorrhea (especially in men).

Clinical Manifestations

The clinical manifestations of urethritis may be the same as those of cystitis (see Cystitis, p. 168).

- The female urethra may be extremely tender, or there may be a discharge, especially in men. Inflammatory changes may make recovery of bacteria difficult because they become entrapped in urethral tissue and do not appear in the urine.
- Urethritis may coexist with cystitis. Cultures on split urine collections or any urethral discharge may confirm a diagnosis of urethral infection.

Therapeutic Management

Treatment is based on identifying and treating the cause and providing symptomatic relief.

- Sulfamethoxazole with trimethoprim or nitrofurantoin are examples of medications used for bacterial infections. Tinidazol, nimorazol, or metronidazol may be used for *Trichomonas*. Medications such as nystatin (Mycostatin) may be prescribed for monilial infections. In chlamydial infections, doxycycline may be used.
- Women with negative urine cultures and no pyuria do not usually respond to antibiotics. Hot sitz baths without perfumed bath oil or bath salts may relieve the symptoms.

Patient Teaching

Patient teaching should include avoiding the use of vaginal deodorant sprays, properly cleansing the perineal area after bowel movements and urination, and avoiding sexual intercourse until symptoms subside.

• • •

See Cystitis, p. 168, for further management of urinary tract infections.

URINARY INCONTINENCE AND RETENTION

Definition/Description

Urinary incontinence or the involuntary loss of urine affects an estimated 10 million people in the United States. Incontinence involves physical (infection, pressure sores, perineal rashes), psychosocial (embarrassment, isolation, depression), and economic costs. However minor the problem, incontinence can cause severe psychologic distress.

- Incontinence is not an inevitable consequence of aging. In most cases among older adults, it can be significantly improved or corrected.

Retention is the inability to urinate in spite of the presence of urine in the bladder. Both incontinence and retention may occur in the same person.

Pathophysiology

Urinary incontinence can result from anything that interferes with bladder or urethral sphincter control.

- Causes may be transient such as confusion or depression, infection, medications, or restricted mobility.
- Congenital disorders that produce incontinence include exstrophy of the bladder, epispadias, spina bifida with myelomeningocele, and ectopic ureteral orifice.
- Acquired disorders include stress, overflow, urge, and reflex incontinence. For a complete description of urinary incontinence, see Table 43-13 in Lewis/Collier/Heitkemper, *Medical-Surgical Nursing,* edition 4, p. 1359.

Retention may be associated with incontinence but can also be independent of incontinence. Drugs that may cause retention include (1) antihypertensives (methyldopa [Aldomet], hydralazine [Apresoline]), (2) antiparkinsonian drugs (levodopa), (3) antihistamines, (4) anticholinergics (atropine), (5) antispasmodics (belladonna), (6) sedatives, and (7) anesthesia (especially spinal anesthesia).

- Postoperative urinary retention is not uncommon and is related to preoperative medication, anesthesia, supine position after surgery, and low fluid intake. Postoperative retention may also be related to the effects of surgical manipulation of the bladder nerves.
- Another cause of retention is urethral obstruction, which may be caused by congenital urethral stenosis, benign prostatic hyperplasia, fecal impaction, or tumors (involving bladder outlet).
- Psychologic problems may also contribute to urinary retention. Psychogenic urinary retention is found more commonly in women than in men.

Diagnostic Studies

- Intravenous pyelogram (IVP) and cystoscopy (including urethroscopy)
- Urodynamic studies to assess sphincter, perineal, and muscle activity
- Catheterization for residual urine

Therapeutic Management

Treatment should correct the factors responsible for incontinence or retention, if possible. It includes behavioral techniques, medications, electrostimulation, and surgery.

Surgical approaches vary, depending on the underlying problem.

- A transurethral resection of the prostate is used to treat benign prostatic hyperplasia.
- Urethral strictures are dilated.
- Several surgical procedures help correct anatomic malpositions of the bladder neck and urethra that cause female stress incontinence, including the Marshall-Marchetti procedure and the Pereyra procedure.
- Injection of urethral bulking agents, such as teflon or collagen, and implantation of a prosthetic urethral sphincter, are also done for stress incontinence in selected patients.

Pharmacologic Management

Vaginal or oral estrogen replacement is often prescribed for postmenopausal women to restore urethral suppleness.

- Anticholinergic agents such as oxybutynin (Ditropan) and dicyclomine hydrochloride (Bentyl) are used to treat hyperreflexic bladders by suppressing the unwanted contractions that occur when the bladder has only a small volume of urine.
- Parasympathomimetics (cholinergics) such as bethanechol (Urecholine) and neostigmine (Prostigmin) are used to treat flaccid bladders by stimulating bladder contractions.
- Imipramine and calcium channel blockers (nifedipine) reduce detrusor contractions and improve continence. Side effects from these drugs are common, especially in older patients.

U

Nursing Management

The nurse must recognize both the physical and the emotional problems that accompany incontinence. The patient's dignity, privacy, and feelings of self-worth must be maintained or enhanced. Most persons suffering from incontinence can be helped with proper diagnosis and modern therapeutic approaches.

- A patient with stress incontinence can be taught to do pelvic floor (perineal) muscle exercises (Kegel exercises). Consistency and persistence are necessary for success, and exercise regimens need to be individualized. Vaginal cones or biofeedback may help patients to identify the correct pelvic muscles, avoid using the incorrect muscles, and realize progress in regaining continence.

The nurse has a major responsibility to help patients with incontinence problems in a variety of settings.

- In the hospital nursing measures aimed at maintaining urinary continence include identifying transient causes and assessing

the patient for signs of bladder infection, fecal impaction, or
bladder distention. The nurse should offer the urinal or bedpan
or help the patient to the bathroom every 2 hours or at scheduled times.

Assuming the usual position for urination (standing for the man
and sitting and leaning forward for the woman) or using relaxation
techniques often helps a patient to urinate successfully, particularly
in unfamiliar settings.

- Applying pressure over the bladder area (Credé's maneuver)
  may be helpful when bladder outlet obstruction is not a problem. The nurse should be sure the patient has privacy and is not
  rushed when trying to urinate.
- Techniques to stimulate urination include running water in the
  sink, placing the patient's hands in water, and pouring warm
  water over the perineum.

Fluid restriction, incontinence pads, and keeping a urinal in place
at all times are only temporary measures to reduce the occurrence or
effects of incontinence. Long-term use of these measures discourages continence and can lead to dehydration and skin problems.

- The patient should be taught that incontinence is not a normal
  part of aging and can be eliminated or controlled in most cases.
- If bladder retraining cannot be achieved, external appliances or
  intermittent self-catheterization may be indicated.

URINARY TRACT CALCULI

Definition/Description

Each year an estimated 500,000 people in the United States have
nephrolithiasis (kidney stone disease), and 1% to 5% experience a
kidney stone at some time during their lives. Many of these people
require hospitalization. The term *calculus* refers to the stones and
lithiasis refers to stone formation.

- Except for *struvite* (an infected stone), which is more common
  in women, stone disorders are more common in men. The majority of patients are between 20 and 55 years of age.
- There are five major categories of stones: calcium phosphate,
  calcium oxalate, uric acid, cystine, and struvite (magnesium
  ammonium phosphate). Stone composition may be mixed, although calcium stones are the most common.
- The incidence is also higher in persons with a family history
  of stone formation. Recurrence of stones can occur in up to
  80% of patients.

Pathophysiology

Many factors are involved in the incidence and type of stone formation, including metabolic, dietary, genetic, climatic, lifestyle, and occupational influences. Many theories have been proposed to explain the formation of stones in the urinary tract.

- Crystals, when in a supersaturated concentration, can precipitate and unite to form a stone. Keeping urine dilute and free-flowing reduces the risk of recurrent stone formation in many individuals.
- Urinary pH, solute load, and inhibitors in the urine affect the formation of stones. The higher the pH, the less soluble are calcium and phosphate. The lower the pH, the less soluble are uric acid and cystine.

Other important factors in the development of stones include obstruction with urinary stasis and urinary infection with urea-splitting bacteria (e.g., *Proteus, Klebsiella, Pseudomonas,* and some species of staphylococci). These bacteria cause the urine to become alkaline and contribute to the formation of calcium-magnesium-ammonium phosphate stones (struvite or triple phosphate stones).

- Infected stones, when entrapped in the kidney, may assume a staghorn configuration as they enlarge. Infected stones are common in patients with an external urinary diversion, long-term indwelling catheter, neurogenic bladder, or urinary retention.

Clinical Manifestations

Urinary stones cause clinical manifestations when they cause obstruction to urinary flow.

- Symptoms include hematuria, abdominal or flank pain, and renal colic.
- The type of pain is determined by the location of the stone. If the stone is nonobstructing, pain may be absent. If it produces obstruction in a calyx or at the ureteropelvic junction (UPJ), the patient may experience dull costovertebral flank pain or even colic. Pain resulting from the passage of a calculus down the ureter is intense and colicky. The patient may be in mild shock, with cool, moist skin. As a stone nears the ureterovesical junction (UVJ), pain will be felt in the lateral flank and sometimes down into the testicles, labia, or groin.
- Other clinical manifestations include the presence of urinary infection accompanied by fever, vomiting, nausea, and chills.

Diagnostic Studies

- BUN and serum creatinine to assess renal function
- CT scan to differentiate a nonopaque stone from a tumor
- Urine and serum levels of substances involved in stone formation (e.g., calcium, phosphate, oxalate, uric acid)

- Urine pH for uric acid stones (tendency for acidic pH) and renal tubular necrosis (tendency for alkaline pH)
- X-rays of kidneys, ureters, and bladder (KUB) with tomograms to determine location, size, and number of radiopaque stones
- Intravenous pyelogram (IVP) or retrograde pyelogram to further localize degree and site of obstruction and confirm the presence of nonradiopaque stones (uric acid, cystine).

Therapeutic Management

Evaluation and management of a patient with nephrolithiasis consist of two concurrent approaches.

- The *first approach* is directed toward management of the acute attack. This involves treating the symptoms of pain, infection, or obstruction. At frequent intervals, narcotics are typically required for relief of renal colic pain. A high fluid intake (e.g., 3 to 4 L/day) is recommended to produce enough urine output to assist stone movement through the urinary tract. About 90% of stones pass spontaneously. However, stones more than 4 mm in size are unlikely to pass through the ureter.
- The *second approach* is directed toward evaluation of the etiology of the stone formation and prevention of further development of stones. Information to be obtained from the patient includes family history of stone formation, geographic residence, nutritional assessment including the intake of vitamins A and D, activity pattern (active or sedentary), history of periods of prolonged illness with immobilization or dehydration, and any history of disease or surgery involving the GI or genitourinary (GU) tract.

Indications for surgical, endoscopic, or lithotripsy stone removal include:

- Stones too large for spontaneous passage, associated with bacteriuria or symptomatic infection, causing impaired renal function, persistent pain, nausea, or ileus
- Inability of the patient to be treated medically
- Patient with solitary kidney

If the stone is located in the bladder, a *transurethral litholapaxy* may be performed. In this operation an instrument is inserted into the bladder via the urethra, and the stone is crushed and then washed out with irrigating solution. Small stones in the distal ureter may be removed transurethrally with instruments (baskets) that snare the stone.

- If extraction is not successful or if the stone is above the manipulation range in the ureter, *lithotripsy* (stone crushing) or open surgery is indicated.

Lithotripsy techniques include percutaneous ultrasonic lithotripsy, electrohydraulic lithotripsy, laser lithotripsy, and extracorporeal shock-wave lithotripsy. Extracorporeal shock wave lithotripsy and laser lithotripsy are the most common.

- In *laser lithotripsy* probes are used to fragment lower ureteral and large bladder stones. The medium used, a coumarin-based pulsed dye, works on a wavelength that fragments stones but does not injure the surrounding tissue.

- In *extracorporeal shock-wave lithotripsy,* a noninvasive procedure, the patient is anesthetized (spinal or general) and usually submerged in a water bath. Fluoroscopy or ultrasound is then used to focus the lithotripter on the affected kidney, and a high-voltage spark generator produces high-energy acoustic shock waves that shatter the stone without damaging the surrounding tissues. The stone is broken down into fine sand, which is excreted into the patient's urine within a few days after the procedure.

Hematuria is common after lithotripsy procedures. A self-retaining ureteral stent is often placed after the procedure to promote passage of this sand and to prevent obstruction caused by *steinstrasse* (a buildup of sand in the ureter). The stent is removed 1 to 2 weeks after lithotripsy. A primary advantage of these techniques compared with open surgery is the decrease in the length of hospitalization and the patient's earlier return to normal activities.

There is a small group of patients who need open surgical procedures, such as very obese patients or those with complex abnormalities in the calyces or at the UPJ. The type of open surgery needed depends on the location of the stone.

- A *nephrolithotomy* is an incision into the kidney to remove a stone. A *pyelolithotomy* is an incision into the renal pelvis to remove a stone. If the stone is located in the ureter, a *ureterolithotomy* is performed. A *cystotomy* may be indicated for bladder calculi. For open surgery on the kidney or ureter, a flank incision directly below the diaphragm and across the side is usually the preferred surgical approach.

Pharmacologic Management

Various medications are prescribed, depending on the specific problem underlying stone formation. Some examples are thiazides, sodium cellulose phosphate, allopurinol, and potassium citrate. These medications prevent stone formation in various ways, including altering urine pH, preventing excessive urinary excretion of a substance, or correcting a primary disease (e.g. hyperparathyroidism).

Treatment of struvite stones requires control of infection. This may be difficult if the stone remains in place.

- In addition to antibiotics, acetohydroxamic acid may be used. Acetohydroxamic acid, an inhibitor of the chemical action caused by the persistent bacteria, can be used effectively to retard struvite stone formation. If the infection cannot be controlled, the stone may need to be removed surgically.

Nutritional Management

A high fluid intake (at least 3000 ml/day) is recommended after an episode of urolithiasis to produce a urine output of at least 2 L/day.

- High urine output prevents supersaturation of minerals (i.e., dilutes the concentration) and flushes them out before they have a chance to precipitate.
- Increasing the fluid intake is especially important for those who live in a dry climate, perform physical exercise, have a family history of stone formation, or work in an occupation that requires outdoor work that can lead to dehydration.

Dietary intervention may be important in the management of urolithiasis.

- Recent research suggests that high dietary calcium, which was previously thought to contribute to kidney stones, may actually lower the risk by reducing the urinary excretion of oxalate, a common factor in many stones.
- Initial nutritional management should include limiting oxalate-rich foods and thereby reducing oxalate excretion. Foods high in purine, calcium, and oxalate are presented in Table 43-9 in Lewis/Collier/Heitkemper, *Medical-Surgical Nursing,* edition 4, p. 1350.

Nursing Management

Goals

The patient with urinary tract calculi will have relief of pain, no urinary tract obstruction, and an understanding of measures to prevent further recurrence of stones.

See the nursing care plan for the patient with acute urinary calculus, p. 1344, and the patient following lithotripsy, p. 1352, in Lewis/Collier/Heitkemper, *Medical-Surgical Nursing,* edition 4.

Nursing Diagnoses/Collaborative Problems

- Pain related to irritation of stone obstruction of urine flow and inadequate pain control or comfort measures
- Ineffective management of therapeutic regimen related to lack of knowledge about prevention of recurrence, diet, fluid requirements, and symptoms of recurrence
- Anxiety related to uncertain outcome and lack of knowledge regarding possible surgery
- Potential complication: urinary obstruction related to presence of stone in path of urine flow

Following lithotripsy

- Pain related to trauma and inflammation and inadequate pain control or comfort measures as manifested by complaints of pain
- Altered pattern of urinary elimination: decreased output and hematuria related to trauma or blockage of ureters or urethra
- Risk for infection related to introduction of bacteria following manipulation of the urinary tract
- Risk for recurrence of lithiasis related to lack of knowledge regarding prevention of recurrence

Nursing Interventions

Preventive measures are especially important for the person who is on bed rest or is relatively immobile for a prolonged time.

- It is important to maintain a high fluid intake and to prevent urinary stasis by turning the patient every 2 hours and helping the patient to sit or stand if possible.
- In the acute phase it is important to retrieve the stone if passed. All urine voided by the patient should be strained through gauze or a special urine strainer in an effort to detect the stone. Encouraging fluids and ambulation help the stone pass down the urinary tract.
- Narcotics will be required for renal colic because the pain is excruciating. Pain management and patient comfort are primary nursing responsibilities.

Stones that do not pass spontaneously must be removed. The nursing care of a patient following lithotripsy is discussed in the nursing care plan for the patient following lithotripsy in Lewis/Collier/Heitkemper, *Medical-Surgical Nursing,* edition 4, p. 1352.

Patient Teaching

Stone formation can be prevented, and the recurrence rate can be greatly reduced. After the acute phase it is important for the nurse to teach the patient ways to prevent recurrence.

- Dietary restriction of oxalate is important for patients who have calcium-oxalate stones. Diets that restrict purines may be helpful to patients at risk of developing uric acid stones.
- Follow-up care includes monitoring the patient's compliance with fluid and dietary recommendations.
- Periodic urine cultures may be indicated. Testing the pH of the urine is important, especially to assess the effectiveness of acidifying or alkalinizing agents.
- It is important to emphasize the need to avoid inadvertent dehydration from excessive exercise and to increase fluid needs during illness.

Urinary Tract Infection

Definition/Description

Urinary tract infections (UTIs) are the second most common bacterial disease. The most common cause is microbial invasion of the tissues of the urinary tract, most often by *Escherichia coli*.

- Bacterial counts of 10^5 organisms or more generally indicate a UTI. However, bacterial counts as low as 10^2 to 10^3 in a person with symptoms are indicative of UTI.
- Viral, fungal, and parasitic infections are not as common, but they are seen most frequently in the patient who is immunosuppressed, has diabetes mellitus, or has taken courses of antibiotics.

Classification

Infections may be broadly classified as upper and lower UTIs based on the patient's symptoms. Terminology may specifically delineate the site of inflammation or infection. Examples of terms are *pyelonephritis* (involvement of kidney and kidney pelvis) or *cystitis* (involvement of bladder).

- It may be difficult to determine the specific location of a UTI. A patient may have a simultaneous infection in both the upper and lower urinary tract, an infection of adjacent organs causing urinary infection–like symptoms, or no symptoms at all.

Determining whether a UTI is complicated or uncomplicated will be a significant factor in establishing the treatment plan.

- Uncomplicated infections are those that occur in an otherwise normal urinary tract.
- Complicated infections include the coexisting presence of obstruction, stones, or catheters, when diabetes or neurologic diseases exist, or when an infection is a recurrent one. The individual with a complicated infection is often at highest risk of renal damage.

Only about one-fourth of individuals who develop acute infection go on to develop recurrent UTI.

- Recurrent UTIs can be classified as *relapses* (recurrence with the same strain of bacteria from within the urinary tract that occurs within 1 to 2 weeks of stopping antibiotic therapy) or *reinfections* (recurrence with a new strain from outside the urinary tract).

Pathophysiology

The following risk factors may predispose a patient to infection:

- Renal scarring from previous infections

- Diminished ureteral peristalsis during pregnancy
- Urinary retention for any reason
- Presence of a foreign body such as a urinary catheter
- Vesicoureteral reflux of urine in a retrograde direction from the bladder toward the kidney
- Humoral or cellular immune deficiency in an otherwise normal urinary tract
- Female gender—shorter urethra that is in proximity to the vagina and rectum
- Presence of calculi
- Clinical disorder such as neurogenic bladder

The organisms that usually cause UTIs are introduced via the ascending route from the urethra. Other less common routes are via the bloodstream or lymphatic system. Most infections are due to gram-negative aerobic bacilli normally found in the GI tract.

- A common factor contributing to ascending infection is urologic instrumentation (e.g., catheterization and cystoscopic examinations). Instrumentation allows bacteria normally present at the opening of the urethra to enter the urethra or bladder.
- Sexual intercourse promotes milking of bacteria from the vagina and perineum and may cause minor urethral trauma that predisposes women to UTIs.
- Rarely do UTIs result from a hematogenous route, where bloodborne bacteria secondarily invade the kidneys, ureters, or bladder from elsewhere in the body.

An important source of UTIs is hospital-acquired, or *nosocomial,* infection. The cause is often *E. coli* and, less frequently, *Pseudomonas* organisms. Urologic instrumentation is the most common predisposing factor. UTIs account for about 40% of all nosocomial infections, and about 80% of these infections result from catheterization.

- The occurrence of UTIs is often related to the presence of abnormalities of the urinary tract, such as strictures and obstructions. An untreated UTI can lead to chronic pyelonephritis and a progressive decrease in renal function. If no abnormality exists, uncomplicated pyelonephritis rarely leads to progressive renal damage and renal failure.

For further information on UTIs, including manifestations, diagnostic studies, and management, see Cystitis, p. 168, Pyelonephritis, p. 491, and Urethritis, p. 586.

VAGINAL CANCER

Cancer of the vagina is rare. The most common type of vaginal cancer is squamous cell carcinoma. The most common presenting symptoms include abnormal bleeding, discharge, pain, urinary frequency, constipation, and tenesmus.

- An association between intrauterine exposure to diethylstilbestrol and clear cell adenocarcinoma of the vagina has been established.

Treatment of vaginal cancer depends on the type of cells involved, stage of the disease, size of the tumor, and location of the tumor.

- Squamous cell carcinomas can be treated with both surgery and radiation. Surgery is the preferred treatment in younger women. A radical hysterectomy, with partial vaginectomy and pelvic lymphadenectomy, is usually effective (see Surgical Procedures Involving the Female Reproductive System, p. 677). Both internal and external radiation is used, but proximity to the bladder and rectum is a concern with this therapy (see Radiation Therapy, p. 675).
- Vaginal cancer may spread locally, as well as by the lymphatic or hematogenous routes. Metastasis to regional pelvic nodes occurs, particularly in higher-stage tumors. Chemotherapy with multiagents has been used to treat metastatic disease (see Chemotherapy, p. 631).

Nursing care of the patient with vaginal cancer requires expert and sensitive care. Often the surgery is extensive, painful, and mutilating. Vaginal sexual activity may not be possible without vaginal reconstruction.

- Important points for the nurse to discuss with the patient with vaginal cancer include (1) the possible impact of surgery and radiation on vaginal sex; (2) potential problems such as dyspareunia and decreased libido (caused by radiation therapy); (3) the effect of surgery or radiation on her feelings about her sexuality and personhood; and (4) the need to continue regular health follow-up to detect metastasis if it occurs.

Vaginal, Cervical, and Vulvar Infections

Definition/Description

Infection and inflammation of the vagina, cervix, and vulva tend to occur when the natural defenses of the acid vaginal secretions (maintained by sufficient estrogen levels) and the presence of *Lactobacillus* are disrupted. A woman's resistance may also be decreased as a result of aging, poor nutrition, and the use of drugs that alter the mucosa.

Pathophysiology

Organisms gain entrance to these areas through contaminated hands, clothing, douche nozzles, and during intercourse, surgery, and childbirth. Table 49 presents the etiology, clinical manifestations, diagnostic methods, and therapeutic management of common inflammations and infections of the lower genital tract.

- Most lower genital tract infections are transmitted through sexual contact. Vulvar infections, such as herpes and genital warts, and vaginal infections, such as trichomoniasis and chlamydial cervicitis are common gynecologic conditions. Other lower genital tract infections include human papillomavirus and gonorrhea.
- Drugs such as oral contraceptives, antibiotics, and corticosteroids may produce changes in the vaginal discharge, which can trigger an overgrowth of the organisms present. For example, *Candida albicans* may be present in small numbers in the vagina. An overgrowth of this organism causes monilial or yeast vaginitis.

Clinical Manifestations

Common problems include yeast vaginitis, pelvic inflammatory disease, cervical abnormalities, and herpes infection (see Table 49).

Therapeutic and Nursing Management

A variety of treatment measures are prescribed for vaginal, cervical, and vulvar infections. Vaginal suppositories, ointments, and creams are often used when infection occurs. Instructions in their use are best given with the aid of a model of the pelvis. The importance of hand washing before and after their insertion should be stressed.

- If the infection is a sexually transmitted disease, the woman should be counseled and offered HIV testing. The partner should be examined and treated as well. Because treatment

Table 49 Infections of the Lower Genital Tract

Infection/etiology	Clinical manifestations/diagnostic methods	Treatment/management
■ **Bacterial vaginitis:** *Escherichia coli* and *Staphylococcus aureus*	Vulvar irritation, heavy yellowish discharge; microscopic examination—many WBCs; Gram stain—short rods or cocci	Triple sulfa vaginal cream; vinegar douche; sitz bath for vulvitis
■ **Monilial vaginitis:** *Candida albicans* (fungus)	Commonly found in mouth, GI tract, and vagina; pruritus, thick white curdy discharge; KOH microscopic examination—pseudohyphae; pH 4.0-4.7	Monistat, Gyne-Lotrimin, Myclex (available over the counter); available in cream or suppository
■ **Trichomoniasis:** *Trichomonas vaginalis* protozoa); sexually transmitted	Pruritus, frothy greenish or gray discharge; hemorrhagic spots on cervix or vaginal walls; saline microscopic examination—swimming trichimonads; pH 5.0-7.0.	Flagyl 2 g orally in single dose for patient and partner

Bacterial vaginosis: *Gardnerella vaginalis;* sexually transmitted	Watery discharge with fishy odor; may or may not have other symptoms; saline microscopic examination—epithelial cells; pH 5.0-5.5	Generic (Flagyl) 500 mg orally or clindamycin (Cleocin) 300 mg orally bid for 7 days; examine and treat partner
Cervicitis: *Chlamydia trachomatis, Neisseria gonorrhoeae, Staphylococcus aureus;* sexually transmitted	Mucopurulent discharge with postcoital spotting from cervical inflammation; culture for chlamydia and gonorrhea	Doxycycline 100 mg for 7 days or tetracycline 500 mg for 7 days; examine and treat partner
Severe recurrent vaginitis: Most often *Candida albicans;* may be first indication of HIV infection	All women unresponsive to first-line treatment should be counseled and offered HIV testing	Drug appropriate to opportunistic organism

HIV, Human immunodeficiency virus; *WBCs,* white blood cells.

measures are usually carried out by the patient, her understanding of them and her ability to perform the treatment correctly must be assessed.

- Heat in the form of a sitz bath, perineal irrigation, and douche is often prescribed to reduce inflammation, promote healing, and provide comfort.
- Scratching, excessive moisture (including too frequent bathing), and tight clothing should be avoided. The wearing of underpants or pantyhose with a cotton crotch is advocated. Chafing, increased heat and moisture, and interference with normal ventilation promote favorable conditions for the growth of fungal, protozoan, and bacterial agents.
- Cleanliness after urinating and defecating should be stressed. It may be necessary to review the importance of using daily health and hygienic practices with some patients. Instructions to seek care when symptoms arise should also be given.

When reinfection occurs readily, the possibility of a symptom-free male carrier or the presence of undiagnosed diabetes mellitus or HIV infection should be investigated. A review of the prescribed treatment measures for possible misunderstandings and a check on compliance with drug therapy may also be indicated.

- If the patient has cauterization or cryosurgery for chronic cervicitis, specific instructions are necessary. These instructions are similar to those following a dilatation and curettage (D & C). Cryosurgery involves the freezing and removal of abnormal cervical tissue through the use of a probe and liquid nitrogen. The treatment is quick and almost painless. The patient will have a watery discharge for 2 weeks. Topical antiseptic creams may be prescribed during the 7- to 8-week healing period.

Patient Teaching

Women need to know what situations increase the risk of vaginal, cervical, and vulvar infections.

- Douching more than once every week or two, for example, can be harmful because it destroys the vagina's balance of naturally occurring organisms.

It is important that the nurse be well informed about inflammation and infection of the genitals and sexually transmitted diseases (STDs) and to pass that information on to the patient without making assumptions about the patient's lifestyle.

- Without adequate information treatment may fail, resulting in an infection that may be recurrent (such as herpes) or impaired fertility, if the patient develops pelvic inflammatory disease.

- The nurse plays a vital role in providing information about the type of infection diagnosed, its treatment, and how to prevent its recurrence.

VALVULAR HEART DISEASE

Definition/Description

The types of valvular heart disease are defined according to the valve(s) affected and the two types of functional alterations, *stenosis* and *regurgitation*.

- The pressure on either side of an open valve is normally equal. However, in a stenotic valve the valve orifice is restricted, impeding forward flow of blood and creating a pressure gradient difference across an open valve. The degree of stenosis is reflected in the pressure gradient differences (i.e., the higher the gradient, the greater the stenosis).
- In regurgitation (also called *valvular incompetence* or *insufficiency*) incomplete closure of valve leaflets results in backward flow of blood.

Valvular disorders occur in children and adolescents primarily from congenital conditions such as tricuspid atresia, pulmonary stenosis, and aortic stenosis. Rheumatic heart disease is a common cause of adult valvular disease.

Mitral Stenosis

Pathophysiology. The majority of adult cases of mitral stenosis result from rheumatic heart disease. Less common causes include congenital mitral stenosis, rheumatoid arthritis, and systemic lupus erythematosus.

- Rheumatic endocarditis causes scarring of valve leaflets and chordae tendineae. Contractures develop with adhesions between commissures (the junctional areas) of the two leaflets.
- The stenotic mitral valve assumes a funnel shape because of thickening and shortening of structures composing the mitral valve. Flow obstruction increases left atrial pressure and volume, resulting in increased pressure in the pulmonary vasculature.

Clinical Manifestations

- Dyspnea, sometimes accompanied by hemoptysis, is the primary symptom of mitral stenosis because of reduced lung compliance.
- Palpitations from atrial fibrillation and fatigue may also be present. Auscultatory findings generally include a loud or accentuated first heart sound; an opening snap (best heard at apex

V

with a stethoscope diaphragm); and a low-pitched, rumbling diastolic murmur (best heard at apex with a stethoscope bell).

- Less frequently, patients with mitral stenosis may have hoarseness (from atrial enlargement), chest pain (from decreased cardiac output), seizures (from emboli), or cerebrovascular accident (from emboli).

Mitral Regurgitation

Pathophysiology. Mitral valve patency depends on the integrity of mitral leaflets, chordae tendineae, papillary muscles, left atrium, and left ventricle. An anatomic or functional abnormality of any of these structures can result in regurgitation.

- Causes of chronic and acute mitral regurgitation are numerous and may be inflammatory, degenerative, infective, structural, or congenital in nature. The majority of cases may be attributed to chronic rheumatic heart disease, mitral valve prolapse, and infectious endocarditis.
- In chronic mitral regurgitation, volume overload on the left ventricle and atrium and on the pulmonary bed is created by the backward flow of blood from the left ventricle into the left atrium during ventricular systole, resulting in varying degrees of left atrial enlargement and left ventricular dilatation.
- Acute mitral regurgitation does not result in dilatation of the left atrium or left ventricle. Without dilatation to accommodate regurgitant volume, pulmonary vascular pressures rise, ultimately causing pulmonary edema.

Clinical manifestations. The clinical course of mitral regurgitation is determined by the nature of its onset.

- The clinical picture in acute mitral regurgitation is that of pulmonary edema and shock. Patients will have thready peripheral pulses and cool, clammy extremities. Auscultatory findings of a new systolic murmur may be obscured by a low cardiac output state.
- Patients with chronic mitral regurgitation may remain asymptomatic for many years until the development of some degree of left ventricular failure.
- Initial symptoms include weakness, fatigue, and dyspnea that gradually progress to orthopnea, paroxysmal nocturnal dyspnea, and peripheral edema. Patients with chronic mitral regurgitation have brisk carotid pulses. Auscultatory findings reflect accentuated left ventricular filling leading to an audible third heart sound (S_3), even in the absence of left ventricular dysfunction.

Mitral Valve Prolapse

Pathophysiology. Mitral valve prolapse (MVP) occurs when the mitral valve leaflets extend beyond the atrioventricular junction and into the left atrium during ventricular systole.

- Etiology of mitral valve prolapse is unknown but is related to diverse pathogenic mechanisms. Mitral valve prolapse can occur in the presence of redundant mitral valve leaflets, enlarged mitral annulus, and abnormally contracting left ventricular wall segments.
- MVP is the most common form of valvular heart disease in the United States. MVP has been noted in all ages but is most common in women of childbearing age.
- There is an increased familial incidence in some patients, suggesting an autosomal dominant pattern of inheritance.

Clinical manifestations. MVP encompasses a broad spectrum of severity. Most patients are asymptomatic and remain so for their entire lives. The course of MVP is generally benign and manageable unless some severe problems associated with mitral regurgitation are present.

- A characteristic of MVP is a murmur from insufficiency that gets more intense through systole. This could be a late or holosystolic murmur.
- Another major sign is one or more clicks usually heard in midsystole to late systole (between first heart sound [S_1] and second heart sound [S_2] and less frequently in early systole. MVP does not alter S_1 or S_2 heart sounds.
- Dysrhythmias, ventricular premature contractions, and ventricular tachycardia may cause palpitations, lightheadedness, and dizziness.
- Infective endocarditis may occur in patients with mitral regurgitation associated with MVP.
- Patients may or may not have chest pain. If episodes of chest pain occur, the episodes tend to occur in clusters, especially during periods of emotional stress. The chest pain may occasionally be accompanied by dyspnea, palpitations, and syncope.

Aortic Stenosis

Pathophysiology. Congenitally abnormal stenotic aortic valves are generally discovered in childhood, adolescence, or young adulthood. A patient seen later in life usually has aortic stenosis from traumatic heart disease, calcific degeneration of a bicuspid valve, or senile calcific degeneration of a normal valve.

- Aortic stenosis results in obstruction to flow from the left ventricle to the aorta during systole. The effect is concentric left-ventricular hypertrophy and increased myocardial O_2 consumption because of increased myocardial mass.
- As the disease course progresses and compensatory mechanisms fail, reduced cardiac output leads to pulmonary hypertension.

Clinical manifestations. Symptoms of aortic stenosis generally develop when the valve orifice becomes approximately one third its normal size. Classically they include angina pectoris, syncope, and heart failure.

- Prognosis is poor for a patient with symptoms and whose valve obstruction is not relieved.
- Auscultatory findings of aortic stenosis typically reveal a normal or soft first heart sound (S_1), a prominent fourth heart sound (S_4), and a systolic, crescendo-decrescendo murmur that ends before the second heart sound (S_2).

Aortic Regurgitation

Pathophysiology. Aortic regurgitation may be the result of a primary disease of the aortic valve leaflets, the aortic root, or both.

- Acute aortic regurgitation is caused by bacterial endocarditis, trauma, or aortic dissection and constitutes a life-threatening emergency.
- Chronic aortic regurgitation is generally the result of rheumatic heart disease, a congenital bicuspid aortic valve, syphilis, or chronic arthritic conditions such as ankylosing spondylitis or Reiter's syndrome.
- The basic physiologic consequence of aortic regurgitation is retrograde blood flow from the ascending aorta into the left ventricle, resulting in volume overload.
- Myocardial contractility eventually declines, and blood volumes increase in the left atrium and pulmonary vasculature. Ultimately, pulmonary hypertension and right ventricular failure develop.

Clinical manifestations. Patients with acute aortic regurgitation have sudden clinical manifestations of cardiovascular collapse.

- The left ventricle is exposed to aortic pressure during diastole and the patient develops weakness, severe dyspnea, and hypotension that generally constitutes a medical emergency.
- Patients with chronic, severe aortic regurgitation have pulses that are water-hammer or collapsing type, with abrupt distention during systole and quick collapse during diastole *(Corrigan's pulse)*.
- Auscultatory findings may include a soft or absent S_1, presence of an S_3 or S_4, and a soft, decrescendo, high-pitched diastolic murmur. A systolic ejection murmur may also be heard; and the *Austin-Flint murmur,* a low-frequency diastolic rumble similar to that of mitral stenosis, may be auscultated.
- The patient with chronic aortic regurgitation generally remains asymptomatic for years and is seen with exertional dyspnea, orthopnea, and paroxysmal nocturnal dyspnea only after considerable myocardial dysfunction has occurred.
- A nocturnal angina accompanied by diaphoresis and abdominal discomfort may be present.

Diagnostic Studies for Valvular Heart Disease

- Chest x-ray reveals heart size, alterations in pulmonary circulation, and valve calcification.
- ECG shows variation in heart rate, rhythm, and possible ischemia or chamber enlargement.
- Echocardiography provides information on valve structure and function and on chamber enlargement.
- Cardiac catheterization detects chamber pressure changes and pressure gradients across the valves.

Therapeutic Management of Valvular Heart Disease

An important aspect of conservative management is prevention of recurrent rheumatic fever and infective endocarditis. Treatment of valvular heart disease depends on the valve involved and severity of the disease. It focuses on preventing exacerbations of heart failure, acute pulmonary edema, thromboembolism, and recurrent endocarditis. If manifestations of congestive heart failure (CHF) develop, digitalis, diuretics, and a low-sodium diet are recommended.

- Anticoagulant therapy is used to prevent and treat systemic or pulmonary embolization, and it is also used as a prophylactic measure in patients with atrial fibrillation.
- Dysrhythmias, especially atrial dysrhythmias, are common with valvular heart disease and are treated with digitalis, antidysrhythmic drugs, or electric cardioversion. ß-adrenergic blocking drugs may be used to slow ventricular rate in patients with atrial fibrillation.
- Oral nitrates may be prescribed for patients with aortic valvular disease because the resulting peripheral vasodilatation reduces blood volume returning to the heart and subsequently decreases the pressure gradient between aorta and left ventricle, allowing the ventricle to pump more effectively. In addition, nitrates improve coronary artery perfusion and reduce myocardial O_2 consumption.

An alternative treatment for some patients with valvular heart disease is the *percutaneous transluminal balloon valvuloplasty (PTBV)* procedure. Balloon valvuloplasty has been used for pulmonic, aortic, and mitral stenosis. The procedure, performed in the cardiac catheterization laboratory, involves threading a balloon-tipped catheter from the femoral artery to the stenotic valve so that the balloon may be inflated in an attempt to separate the valve leaflets.

- The PTBV procedure is generally indicated for older adult patients and patients who are poor surgical candidates.
- Complications and postprocedural care requirements are obviously lessened for those undergoing PTBV versus valve replacement, but long-term results of PTBV have not been determined.

Surgical Management

The type of surgery used for a particular patient depends on the valves involved, valvular pathology, severity of disease, and the patient's clinical condition. All types of valve surgery are palliative, not curative. Therefore patients will require lifelong health care.

- Valve repair is becoming the surgical procedure of choice. Reparative or reconstructive procedures are often used in mitral or tricuspid valvular heart disease. Repair of these valves has a lower operative mortality than replacement.

- *Mitral commissurotomy (valvulotomy)* is the procedure of choice for patients with pure mitral stenosis. The less precise *closed* method (without cardiopulmonary bypass) of commissurotomy has generally been replaced by the *open* method in the United States, Canada, and Western Europe. The closed mitral commissurotomy is generally performed in developing nations.

- Further repair or reconstruction of the valve may be necessary and can be achieved by *annuloplasty,* a procedure also used in cases of mitral or tricuspid regurgitation. Annuloplasty entails reconstruction of valve leaflets and the annulus, with or without aid of prosthetic rings (e.g., a Carpentier ring).

- Open surgical *valvuloplasty* involves repair of the valve or suturing of torn leaflets. It is primarily performed to treat mitral regurgitation or tricuspid regurgitation. The main advantage of a reparative procedure is that it avoids the risks associated with valve replacement. The disadvantage is that it may not be possible to establish total valve competence.

Prosthetic valves.   Valvular replacement may be required for mitral, aortic, tricuspid, and occasionally, pulmonic disease. The surgical treatment of choice for combined aortic stenosis and aortic regurgitation is valvular replacement.

- The two categories of prosthetic valves are *mechanical* and *biologic* (tissue) valves. Mechanical valves are made of combinations of metal alloys, pyrolite carbon, and Dacron. Biologic valves are constructed from bovine, porcine, and human cardiac tissue. Mechanical prosthetic valves are more durable and last longer than biologic tissue valves but have an increased risk of thromboembolism, which necessitates the use of long-term anticoagulant therapy. Biologic valves offer the patient freedom from anticoagulant therapy as a result of their low thrombogenicity. However, their durability is limited by the tendency for early calcification, tissue degeneration, and stiffening of leaflets.

- Long-term anticoagulation is recommended for all patients with mechanical prostheses and for patients with biologic tissue valves who are in atrial fibrillation. Some patients with biologic tissue valves or prosthetic rings may require anticoagulation during the first few months after surgery.

- Choice of a valvular prosthesis depends on many factors. For example, if a patient cannot take anticoagulant therapy (e.g., women of childbearing age), a biologic valve may be considered. A mechanical valve may be considered for a younger patient because it is more durable and lasts longer. For patients over the age of 65 the importance of durability is less of an issue, but the risks of noncompliance or hemorrhage from anticoagulants may be greater.

Nursing Management
Goals
The patient with valvular heart disease will have normal cardiac function, improved activity tolerance, and an understanding of the disease process and preventive measures.

See the nursing care plan for the patient with valvular heart disease in Lewis/Collier/Heitkemper, *Medical-Surgical Nursing,* edition 4, p. 1032.

Nursing Diagnoses/Collaborative Problems
- Activity intolerance related to insufficient oxygenation secondary to decreased cardiac output
- Ineffective management of therapeutic regimen related to lack of knowledge about disease process, signs and symptoms of congestive heart failure and infective endocarditis, and prevention and treatment strategies
- Pain related to decreased coronary blood flow and increased myocardial oxygen demand secondary to decreased cardiac output
- Sleep pattern disturbance related to pulmonary congestion
- Potential complication: decreased cardiac output
- Potential complication: hypervolemia related to cardiac failure
- Potential complication: systemic and pulmonary emboli

Nursing Interventions
Prevention of acquired rheumatic valvular disease is achieved by diagnosing and treating streptococcal infection and providing prophylactic antibiotics for patients with a history of rheumatic fever. Patients at risk for endocarditis must also be treated with prophylactic antibiotics.

- The patient must adhere to recommended therapies. The individual with a history of rheumatic fever, endocarditis, or congenital heart disease should know the symptoms suggestive of valvular heart disease so that early medical treatment may be obtained.

A patient with progressive valvular heart disease may require hospitalization or outpatient care for management of CHF, endocarditis, embolic disease, or dysrhythmias. CHF is the most common reason for ongoing medical care.

The role of the nurse is to implement and evaluate the effectiveness of therapeutic management.

- Activity should be designed after considering the patient's limitations. An appropriate exercise plan can increase cardiac tolerance. However, activities that regularly produce fatigue and dyspnea should be restricted, and an explanation should be provided to the patient.
- Smoking should be discouraged.
- The patient should be assisted in planning activities of daily living, with an emphasis on conserving energy, setting priorities, and taking planned rest periods. Referral to a vocational counselor may be necessary if the patient has a physically or emotionally demanding job.
- Auscultatory assessment of the heart should be performed to monitor the effectiveness of digitalis, ß-adrenergic blocking agents, and antidysrhythmic drugs.
- The patient should be instructed to wear a medical-alert bracelet.
- The patient must understand the importance of prophylactic antibiotic therapy to prevent endocarditis.

Patient Teaching

- Explain the nature and cause of the disease process to ensure that the patient has an adequate knowledge base on which to make decisions.
- Teach the signs and symptoms of heart failure and infective endocarditis to ensure early reporting and treatment of complications.
- Teach the need to avoid all invasive surgical or diagnostic procedures that may predispose to bacteremia until prophylactic antibiotics are given. Explain the importance of notifying the dentist, urologist, and gynecologist of valvular disease so prophylactic antibiotic treatment can be initiated.
- Explain the need for good oral hygiene and avoidance of fatigue to decrease the opportunity for infection.
- Discourage smoking to prevent an increased cardiac workload.
- Discuss prescribed medications, including dosage, purpose, and side effects, to promote safe and accurate self-medication.
- Monitor urinary output and daily weight when diuretics are prescribed. The patient's diet should be nutritionally well balanced, with sodium restriction to prevent fluid retention.
- Help the patient with a valvular disorder achieve and maintain an optimal level of health.
- In the patient who is undergoing anticoagulation therapy after surgery for valve replacement, check the prothrombin time reg-

ularly (usually monthly) to assess adequacy of therapy and to prevent side effects.

The patient needs to realize that valve surgery is not a cure and that regular follow-up examinations by the health care provider will be required. The nurse also needs to teach the patient about when to seek medical care. Any manifestations of infection or CHF, any signs of bleeding, and any planned invasive or dental procedures require that the patient notify the health care provider.

VARICOSE VEINS

Definition/Description

Varicose veins, or varicosities, are dilated, tortuous subcutaneous veins most frequently found in the saphenous system. They may be small and innocuous or large and bulging.

- *Primary* varicosities are those in which the superficial veins are dilated and the valves may or may not be rendered incompetent. The condition tends to be familial, is characteristically found bilaterally, and is probably caused by congenital weakness of veins.
- *Secondary* varicosities result from previous thrombophlebitis of deep femoral veins, with subsequent valvular incompetence. Secondary varicose veins may also occur in the esophagus as varices, in the anorectal area as hemorrhoids, and as abnormal arteriovenous connections (also known as *fistulas* and *malformations*).

Pathophysiology

The basic cause of varicose veins is unknown. Increased venous pressure may be caused by congenital weakness of vein structure, obesity, pregnancy, venous obstruction resulting from thrombosis or extrinsic pressure by tumors, or occupations that require prolonged standing.

- As veins enlarge, valves are stretched and become incompetent, allowing blood flow to be reversed. As back pressure increases and the venous pump (muscle movement that squeezes venous blood back toward heart) fails, further venous distention results.
- Increased venous pressure is transmitted to the capillary bed, and edema develops.

Clinical Manifestations

Discomfort from varicose veins varies dramatically among people and tends to be worsened by superficial thrombophlebitis. The most common symptom is an ache or pain after prolonged standing, which is relieved by walking or by elevating the limb. Some patients feel pressure or a cramplike sensation. Swelling may accompany the discomfort. Nocturnal leg cramps, especially in the calf area, may occur.

- Superficial thrombophlebitis is a serious consequence of varicose veins and may occur either spontaneously or after trauma, surgical procedures, or pregnancy. Rupture of varicose veins may occur because of weakening of the vessel wall. Ulceration as a result of skin infections or trauma may also develop.

Diagnostic Studies

- Duplex ultrasound can be used to detect obstruction and reflux in the venous system.

Therapeutic Management

Treatment is usually not indicated if varicose veins are only a cosmetic problem. If incompetency of the venous system develops, management involves rest with the feet elevated, the wearing of elastic compression gradient hose, and walking exercise.

Injection sclerotherapy is used in the treatment of unsightly superficial varicosities. Direct IV injection of a sclerosing agent (e.g., Sotradecol) reduces inflammation and results in eventual thrombosis of the vein. This procedure can be performed safely in an office setting and causes minimal discomfort. After injection the leg is wrapped with an elastic bandage for 24 to 72 hours to maintain pressure over the vein. Local tenderness subsides within 2 to 3 weeks, and eventually the thrombosed vein disappears. After injection the patient should be advised to wear compression stockings to help prevent development of further varicosities.

Surgical intervention for varicose veins involves ligation of the entire vein (usually saphenous) and dissection and removal of its incompetent tributaries. Surgical intervention is indicated when chronic venous insufficiency cannot be prevented or controlled with therapy. Recurrent thrombophlebitis in varicose veins is another indication for surgery.

Nursing Management

Prevention is a key factor related to varicose veins. The patient should be instructed to avoid sitting or standing for long periods of time, maintain ideal body weight, take precautions against injury to extremities, and avoid wearing constrictive clothing.

After *vein ligation surgery,* the nurse should encourage deep breathing, which helps promote venous return to the right side of the heart. The extremities should initially be checked hourly for color, movement, sensation, temperature, presence of edema, and pedal pulses. Bruising and discoloration are considered normal.

- Elevation of the extremities at a 15-degree angle is encouraged (except for periods of ambulation) to prevent development of venous stasis and edema. Elastic compression gradient stockings are also used and should be removed once every 8 hours for short periods and reapplied.

Long-term management of varicose veins is directed toward improving circulation, relieving discomfort, improving cosmetic appearance, and avoiding complications such as superficial thrombophlebitis and ulceration. Varicose veins can recur in other veins after surgery.

Patient Teaching

- The patient should be taught proper care of lower extremities, including cleanliness and use of individually fitted elastic hose. He/she should also be instructed to put on hose while still lying down just before arising in the morning.
- The importance of periodic positioning of legs above the heart should be stressed. The overweight patient will need assistance with weight reduction.
- The patient whose employment requires prolonged periods of standing or sitting should be encouraged to change position as frequently as possible.
- A pregnant patient with varicosities needs appropriate teaching as prescribed by the health care provider.

V

VULVAR CANCER

Cancer of the vulva is relatively rare, occurring mainly among women over 50 years of age, with a peak incidence over age 70. The malignancy is visible and accessible, making early diagnosis more likely.

- Although the exact cause is not known, cancer of the vulva may follow leukoplakia (irregular white patches on vulvar mucosa that produce intense pruritus) or other conditions causing chronic irritation of the area.
- The patient may initially experience pruritus, soreness of the vulva, unusual odor, discharge, or bleeding but tends to ignore these symptoms. Edema of the vulva and pelvic lymphadenopathy develop as the disease progresses.

- Diagnosis of vulvar cancer is done by means of pelvic examination and biopsy.

Treatment for vulvar cancer is vulvectomy. The extent of the surgery depends on the size and site of the malignancy. If it is in situ, a simple vulvectomy (surgical excision of the vulva) is done. If the cancer is invasive, a radical vulvectomy with superficial and deep lymph node dissection is indicated.

PART TWO

Treatments and Procedures

AMPUTATION

Description

The clinical features that indicate the need for an amputation depend on the underlying diseases or traumas. Common indications for amputation include circulatory impairment resulting from a peripheral vascular disorder, traumatic and thermal injuries, malignant tumors, uncontrolled or widespread infection of the extremity, and congenital disorders.

These conditions may manifest as loss of sensation, inadequate circulation, pallor, sweating, and local or systemic infection. Although pain is often present, it is not usually the primary reason for an amputation. The underlying problem dictates whether the amputation is performed as elective or emergency surgery.

- The goal of amputation surgery is to preserve extremity length and function while removing all infected or ischemic tissue. This improves the possibility of good prosthetic, cosmetic, and functional satisfaction.

Types of Amputation

The type of amputation depends on the reason for the surgery.

- A *closed amputation* is performed to create a weight-bearing stump; an anterior skin flap with dissected soft-tissue padding covers the bone stump. Special care is necessary to prevent the accumulation of drainage, which can produce pressure and harbor infection.
- *Disarticulation* is an amputation performed through a joint. A Symes amputation is a form of disarticulation at the ankle.
- An *open amputation* leaves a stump surface that is not covered with skin. This type of surgery is generally indicated for control of actual or potential infection. The wound is usually closed later by a second surgical procedure or closed by skin traction surrounding the stump. This type of amputation is often referred to as a *guillotine amputation.*

Nursing Management

Most lower-limb amputations result from peripheral vascular disease, and most upper-limb amputations result from severe trauma. Control of causative illnesses such as peripheral vascular disease, diabetes mellitus, chronic osteomyelitis, and skin ulcers can eliminate or delay the need for amputation.

- The patient with these problems must be taught to carefully examine the lower extremities daily for signs of potential problems. If the patient cannot assume this responsibility, a family member should be instructed on the procedure. The patient and family should be instructed to report to the health care provider problems such as change in skin color or temperature, decrease or absence of sensation, tingling, pain, or the presence of a lesion.

The nurse must recognize the tremendous psychologic and social implications of an amputation for the patient.

- The disruption in body image caused by an amputation often causes a patient to go through psychologic stages similar to the grieving process of death. Allowing the patient to go through a period of depression and recognizing it as a normal consequence of the amputation may do much to aid the patient's acceptance of the amputation. The patient's family must also be helped to work through the process to arrive at a realistic and positive attitude about the future.

Preoperative Care

Before surgery the nurse should reinforce information that the patient and family have received about the reasons for the amputation, the proposed prosthesis, and the mobility training program. In addition to the usual preoperative instructions, the patient undergoing an amputation has special education needs.

- To meet these needs, the nurse must know the level of amputation, the type of postsurgical dressing to be applied, and the type of prosthesis planned.
- The patient should receive instruction in the performance of upper extremity exercises such as push-ups in bed or the wheelchair to promote arm strength.

Patients should be warned that they may feel as though their amputated limbs are still present after surgery. This *phantom sensation* (a sensation of aching, tingling, or itching of the amputated limb) usually disappears but may cause patients grave concern unless they are forewarned. If pain was present in the affected limb preoperatively, the patient may experience *phantom limb pain* postoperatively. The patient may have feelings of coldness and heaviness or cramping, shooting, burning, or crushing pain.

- Often the patient may be extremely anxious about this pain because the patient knows the limb is gone but still feels pain in it. Usually, phantom limb pain goes away in time although it can become chronic.

Postoperative Care

Prevention or detection of complications are important nursing responsibilities during the postoperative period. Careful monitoring of the patient's vital signs and dressing can alert the nurse to hemorrhage in the operative area. Careful attention to sterile technique during dressing changes reduces the potential for wound infection and subsequent interruption of rehabilitation.

- If an immediate postoperative prosthesis has been applied, the nurse must monitor vital signs carefully because the surgical site is heavily covered and may not be visible.
- A surgical tourniquet must always be available for emergency use. If hemorrhage occurs, the surgeon should be notified immediately and efforts to control the hemorrhage should begin at once.

The surgeon must decide the type of prosthetic fitting that will be used after surgery.

- An *immediate prosthetic fitting,* often called the *immediate postsurgical fitting* or the *immediate postoperative fitting,* is done in the operating room after the amputation. The main advantages of this device are reduction of edema and the psychologic benefit of early ambulation. A disadvantage is the inability to directly visualize the surgical site.
- The *delayed prosthetic fitting* may be the best choice for certain patients. Patients who have had amputations above the knee or below the elbow, older adults, debilitated individuals, and those with infection usually have delayed prosthetic fittings. A temporary prosthesis may be used for partial weight bearing once the sutures are removed.

Not all patients are candidates for a prosthesis. It is important that the surgeon discuss ambulation possibilities frankly with the patient and family. The seriously ill or debilitated patient may not have the energy required to use a prosthesis. Mobility with a wheelchair may be the most realistic goal for this type of patient.

Flexion contractures may delay the rehabilitation process. The most common and debilitating contracture is hip flexion. To prevent flexion contractures, patients should avoid sitting in a chair with the hips flexed or having pillows under the surgical extremity for long intervals.

Patient Teaching

As the patient's overall condition improves, the nurse begins instruction in the principles and techniques of transferring from bed to chair and back. Active exercises and conditioning are essential in developing ambulation skills.

- Active range-of-motion exercises of all joints should be started as soon after surgery as the patient's pain level and medical status permit.
- Crutch walking is started as soon as the patient is physically able. If a patient has an immediate postsurgical fitting, orders related to weight bearing must be carefully followed to avoid disruption of the skin flap and delay of the training process.

Before discharge the patient and family need careful instruction related to stump care, ambulation, prevention of contractures, recognition of complications, exercise, and follow-up care. Table 50 outlines appropriate stump care.

Table 50	Patient Instruction for Stump Care

- Inspect the stump daily for signs of skin irritation, especially redness.
- Discontinue use of the prosthesis if an irritation develops. Have the area checked before resuming use of the prosthesis.
- Wash thoroughly each night with warm water and a bacterio-static soap. Rinse thoroughly and dry gently. Expose the stump to air for 20 min.
- Do not use any substance such as lotions, alcohol, powders, or oil unless prescribed by the physician.
- If a stump sock is worn, wear only the one supplied by the prosthetist. Change daily. Launder in a mild soap, squeeze, and lay flat to dry.

BLOOD TRANSFUSION THERAPY

Description

Traditionally, the term *blood transfusion* meant the administration of whole blood. Blood transfusion now has a broader meaning because of the ability to administer specific components of blood such as platelets, red blood cells (RBCs), or plasma.

Many therapeutic and surgical procedures depend on blood product support. However, blood component therapy only temporarily supports the patient until the underlying problem is resolved. Because transfusions are not free from hazards, they should be used only if necessary.

- Nurses must be careful to avoid developing a complacent attitude about this common but potentially dangerous therapy.

Administration Procedure

Blood components can be safely administered through any gauge needle into a free-flowing IV line. Larger-gauge needles (i.e., 19-gauge) may be preferred if rapid transfusion is desired. The blood administration tubing with a filter should have a stopcock or other means to develop a closed system, with blood open to one port and isotonic saline solution infusing through the other.

- Dextrose solutions or lactated Ringer's should not be used because they induce red blood cell hemolysis. No other additives (including medications) should be given through the same tubing as the blood unless the tubing is cleared with saline solution.

When the blood or blood components have been obtained from the blood bank, positive identification of the donor blood and recipient must be made.

- Improper product-to-patient identification causes 90% of transfusion reactions, thus placing a great responsibility on nursing personnel to carry out the identification procedure appropriately.

The nurse should follow the policy and procedures at the place of employment.

- The blood should be administered as soon as it is brought to the patient. It should not be refrigerated on the nursing unit. If the blood is not used right away, it should be returned to the blood bank.
- During the first 15 minutes of blood infusion the nurse should stay with the patient. If there are any unwanted reactions, they are most likely to occur at this time.
- The rate of infusion during this period should be no more than 2 ml/min. Blood should not be infused quickly unless an emergency exists. Rapid infusion of cold blood may cause the patient to become chilled. If rapid replacement of large amounts of blood is necessary, a blood-warming device should be used.
- After the first 15 minutes the rate of infusion is governed by the clinical condition of the patient and the product being infused. Most patients not in danger of fluid overload can tolerate the infusion of one unit of packed cells over 2 hours.
- The transfusion should not take more than 4 hours to administer. Blood remaining after 4 hours should not be infused because of the length of time it has been removed from refrigeration.

Blood Transfusion Reactions

If a transfusion reaction occurs, the following steps should be taken: (1) stop the transfusion, (2) maintain a patent IV line with saline solution, (3) notify the blood bank and the physician immediately, (4) recheck identifying tags and numbers, (5) monitor vital signs and urine output, (6) treat symptoms according to physician order, (7) save the blood bag and tubing and send them to the blood bank for examination, (8) complete transfusion reaction reports, (9) collect required blood and urine specimens at intervals stipulated by hospital policy to evaluate for hemolysis, and (10) document on transfusion reaction form and patient chart. The blood bank and laboratory are responsible for identifying the type of reaction.

The complications of transfusion therapy may be significant and necessitate judicious evaluation of the patient. Blood transfusion reactions can be classified as acute or delayed (see Tables 28-37 and 28-38 in Lewis/Collier/Heitkemper, *Medical-Surgical Nursing,* edition 4, pp. 826 and 827, respectively).

- Acute reactions include hemolysis, febrile reactions, allergic reactions, and circulatory overload.
- Delayed reactions include delayed hemolysis, infection (such as hepatitis B and C, human immunodeficiency virus, and malaria), iron overload, and graft-versus-host disease.

Autotransfusion

Autotransfusion, or autologous transfusion, consists of removing whole blood from a person and transfusing that blood into the same person.

- The problems of incompatibility, allergic reactions, and transmission of disease can be avoided. There are various reasons and methods of autotransfusion. These include the following types:
- *Autologous donation* or *elective phlebotomy (predeposit transfusion):* A person donates blood before a planned surgical procedure. The blood can be frozen and stored for up to 3 years. Usually the blood is stored without being frozen and is given to the person within a few weeks of donation.
- *Autotransfusion:* A newer method for replacing blood volume involves safely and aseptically collecting, filtering, and returning the patient's own blood that was lost during a major surgical procedure or from a traumatic injury. This system was originally developed in response to patient's concerns over the safety of blood from blood products. However, today it provides an important way to safely replace volume and stabilize bleeding patients. Collection devices can be attached to drains after chest or orthopedic procedures. Sometimes the collection device is a component of the drainage system.

CARDIOPULMONARY RESUSCITATION

Description

Cardiopulmonary resuscitation (CPR) is the process of externally supporting the circulation and respiration of a person who has a cardiac arrest. Resuscitation measures are divided into two components, basic cardiac life support (BCLS) and advanced cardiac life support (ACLS). The American Heart Association establishes standards for CPR.

Basic Cardiac Life Support

BCLS involves using CPR to externally support circulation and ventilation for a patient with cardiac or respiratory arrest. Artificial respiration (mouth-to-mouth, mouth-to-mask, mouth-to-nose, mouth-to-stoma) and external chest compression substitute for spontaneous breathing and circulation.

- The major objective of performing CPR is to provide oxygen to the brain, heart, and other vital organs until appropriate therapeutic management and resuscitation efforts involving advanced life support methods can be initiated or until resuscitation efforts are ordered to be stopped.

Rapid intervention is the key to success and is critical in preventing death of brain cells. CPR must be initiated within 4 to 6 minutes of cardiac or pulmonary arrest because brain cells begin to die *(brain death)* within 6 minutes of anoxia. National standards for knowledge and technique must be met for personnel to be certified to deliver CPR. Assessment of the victim must be stressed in teaching CPR. Each of the broad areas—**A**irway, **B**reathing, and **C**irculation (the ABCs of CPR)—should be reviewed (see Lewis/Collier/Heitkemper, *Medical-Surgical Nursing,* edition 4, pp. 993 and 996-997).

- Rescue breathing and chest compressions are combined for an effective resuscitation effort of the victim of cardiopulmonary arrest. When there is one rescuer, the rate of compression should be 80 to 100 compressions per minute with a compression-ventilation ratio of 15 compressions to 2 ventilations (Table 51). The compression rate for two-rescuer CPR is 80 to 100 per minute, with a compression-ventilation ratio of 5:1 (Table 52).
- The victim's condition must be assessed during CPR to determine the effectiveness of compressions and to determine whether the victim has resumed spontaneous circulation and breathing. The pulse should be checked by the ventilating rescuer during compressions to assess effectiveness of compressions in two-rescuer CPR. Chest compressions are stopped for 5 seconds at the end of the first minute and every few minutes thereafter to determine whether the victim has resumed spontaneous breathing and circulation.
- The goal of CPR is the return of spontaneous breathing and circulation, but it is rarely achieved without more definitive therapy with ACLS.

Advanced Cardiac Life Support

ACLS involves a systematic treatment approach in cardiac emergencies. ACLS includes (1) basic life support (BLS), (2) use of adjunctive equipment and special techniques for establishing and

Text continued on p. 628.

Table 51   Adult One-Rescuer CPR

Step	Objective	Critical performance
1. Airway	Assessment: determine unresponsiveness.	Tap or gently shake shoulder.
		Shout "Are you OK?"
	Call for help.	Call out "Help!"
	Position the victim.	Turn on back as unit, if necessary, supporting head and neck (4-10 sec).
	Open the airway.	Use head-tilt-chin-lift maneuver.
2. Breathing	Assessment: Determine cessation of breathing.	Maintain open airway.
		With ear over mouth, observe chest: look, listen, feel for breathing (3-5 sec).
	Ventilate twice.	Maintain open airway.
		Seal mouth and nose properly.
		Ventilate two times at 1-1.5 sec/inflation.
		Observe chest rise (adequate ventilation volume).
		Allow deflation between breaths.
3. Circulation	Assessment: Determine absence of pulse.	Feel for carotid pulse on near side of victim (5-10 sec).
		Maintain head-tilt with other hand.
	Activate EMS system.	If someone responded to call for help, send person to activate EMS system.
		Total time, step 1—Activate EMS system: 15-35 sec.

	Begin chest compressions.	Kneel by victim's shoulders.
		Make landmark check before hands are placed.
		Maintain proper hand position throughout.
		Keep shoulders over victim's sternum.
		Maintain equal compression and relaxation.
		Compress 1.5-2 in.
		Keep hands on sternum during upstroke.
		Wait for complete chest relaxation on upstroke.
		Say any helpful mnemonic (e.g., one-and-two-and-three-and . . .).
		Remember that compression rate is 80-100/min (15/9-11sec).
4. Compression-ventilation cycles	Do four cycles of 15 compressions and two ventilations.	Maintain proper compression-ventilation ratio of 15 compressions to two ventilations per cycle.
		Observe chest rise: 1-1.5 sec/inflation; four cycles/52-73 sec.
5. Reassessment	Determine absence of pulse.	Feel for carotid pulse (5 sec). If there is no pulse, go to step 6.
6. Continuation of CPR	Ventilate two times.	Ventilate two times.
		Observe chest rise: 1-1.5 sec/inflation.
	Resume compression-ventilation cycles.	Feel for carotid pulse every few min.

Modified from *Healthcare provider's manual for basic life support*, Dallas, 1993, American Heart Association.
CPR, Cardiopulmonary resuscitation; *EMS*, emergency medical services.

Table 52 **Adult Two-Rescuer CPR**

Step	Objective	Critical performance
1. Airway	One rescuer (ventilator):	
	Assessment: Determine unresponsiveness.	Tap or gently shake shoulder. Shout "Are you OK?"
	Position the victim.	Turn on back if necessary (4-10 sec).
	Open the airway.	Use a proper technique to open airway.
2. Breathing	Assessment: Determine cessation of breathing.	Look, listen, and feel for breath (3-5 sec).
	Ventilate twice.	Observe chest rise: 1-1.5 sec/inflation.
3. Circulation	Assessment: Determine absence of pulse.	Feel for carotid pulse (5-10 sec).
	State assessment results.	Say "No pulse."
	Other rescuer (compressor):	When another rescuer comes, first rescuer asks if EMS has been activated.
	Get into position for compressions.	Put hands, shoulders in correct position.
	Locate landmark notch.	Check landmark.

4. Compression-ventilation cycles	Compressor: Begin chest compressions.	Correct ratio compressions-ventilations is 5:1. Compression rate is 80-100/min (5 compressions/3-4 sec). Say any helpful mnemonic.
	Ventilator: Ventilate after every fifth compression and check compression effectiveness.	Stop compressing for each ventilation. Ventilate once (1-1.5 sec/inflation). Check pulse occasionally to assess compressions.
	(Minimum of 10 cycles)	
5. Calling for switch	Compressor: Call for switch when tired.	(Time for 10 cycles: 40-53 sec) Give clear signal to change roles. Compressor completes fifth compression. Ventilator completes ventilation after fifth compression.
6. Switching	Simultaneously switch: Ventilator: Move to chest.	Become compressor. Get into position for compressions. Locate landmark notch.
	Compressor: Move to head.	Become ventilator. Check carotid pulse (5 sec). Say "No pulse." Ventilate once (1-1.5 sec/inflation).
7. Continuation of CPR	Resume compression-ventilation cycles.	Repeat step 4.

Modified from *Healthcare provider's manual for basic life support,* Dallas, 1993, American Heart Association.

maintaining effective ventilation and circulation, (3) ECG monitoring and dysrhythmia recognition, (4) establishment and maintenance of IV access, (5) therapies for emergency treatment of patient with cardiac or respiratory arrest (including stabilization in postarrest phase), and (6) treatment of patients with suspected acute myocardial infarction (MI).

- The principle of early defibrillation has been emphasized in national emergency medical care organizations. With the invention of the automated external defibrillator (AED), which is simple to use and available throughout communities, more trained rescuers are available to provide early defibrillation. The importance of early, effective BLS and defibrillation before entrance into the ACLS system cannot be overemphasized.
- Drugs used in ACLS include oxygen therapy, IV fluids, morphine sulfate, and drugs used to control heart rate and rhythm and those used to improve cardiac output and BP (see Table 33-17 in Lewis/Collier/Heitkemper, *Medical-Surgical Nursing,* edition 4, p. 998).

Nursing Role During a Code

- There is a potential for a "code" or cardiopulmonary arrest situation in any clinical setting. The nurse should be well prepared to participate in resuscitation of a patient. The nurse must be familiar with code protocols, emergency equipment in the crash cart, and keep current with BCLS and ACLS skills.
- It is important for the nurse to be familiar with crash cart location and contents on the clinical unit. Most crash carts contain all necessary emergency supplies. Ideally, all crash carts in an individual clinic or hospital should be organized in the same fashion.

CASTS

Types of Casts

Immobilization of an acute fracture or soft-tissue injury can be accomplished by a variety of casts.

- The *sugar-tong splint* is typically used for acute wrist injuries. Multiple layers of plaster splints are applied to the padded forearm. The splinting material is wrapped with either elastic bandage or bias stocking. The major advantage of the sugar-tong cast is avoidance of the circumferential effects of a nonelastic cylinder.

- The *short arm cast* is frequently used for the treatment of stable wrist or metacarpal fractures. An aluminum finger splint can be fabricated into the short arm cast for treatment of phalangeal injuries. This cast provides wrist immobilization and permits unrestricted elbow motion.
- The *long arm cast* is commonly used for stable forearm or elbow fractures and unstable wrist fractures. It is similar to the short arm cast but extends to the proximal humerus, restricting motion in the wrist and elbow. When a sling is used, the nurse must ensure that the axillary region is well padded to prevent skin maceration associated with direct skin-to-skin contact.
- The *body jacket cast* is frequently used for immobilization and support for stable spine injuries of the thoracic or lumbar spine. This cast is applied around the chest and abdomen and extends from above the nipple line to the pubis.
- The *hip spica cast* is commonly used in treating femoral fractures. The purpose of the hip spica cast is to immobilize the affected extremity and the trunk securely. It includes two separate casts joined together: (1) the body jacket and (2) the long leg cast. The location of the femoral fracture will determine whether the unaffected extremity will have to be immobilized to restrict rotation of the pelvis and possible hip motion on the side of the femur fracture.
- Injuries to the lower extremity are frequently immobilized by either a *long leg cast* or a *short leg cast*. The usual indications for applying a long leg cast are an unstable ankle fracture, soft-tissue injuries, a fractured tibia, or knee injuries. The cast usually extends from the base of the toes to the groin and gluteal crease. The short leg cast can be used for a variety of conditions but is usually used for stable ankle and foot injuries.

Types of Cast Material

Plaster of Paris is wrapped and molded around the affected part after immersion in water. It is anhydrous calcium sulfate embedded in a gauze roll. The strength of the cast is determined by the number of layers of plaster bandage and the technique of application. As the cast dries, it recrystallizes and hardens. Heat is generated during the drying process. Increased edema from increased circulation may occur as a result of heat produced by the drying cast. After the cast is completely dry, it is strong and firm and can withstand stresses.

- The plaster is hard within 15 minutes, so the patient can move around without problems. However, it is not strong enough for weight bearing until it is dry (after about 24 to 48 hours).

| **Table 53** | **Patient Instructions for Cast Care** |

Do Not
    Get cast wet*
    Remove any padding
    Insert any foreign object inside cast
    Bear weight on new cast for 48 hr
    Cover cast with plastic for prolonged periods

Do
    Check with physician before getting cast wet
    Dry cast thoroughly after exposure to water†
      Blot dry with towel
      Use hair dryer on low setting until cast is thoroughly
        dry
    Elevate extremity above level of heart for first 48 hr
    Move joints above and below cast regularly
    Apply ice directly over fracture site for first 24 hr
      (avoid getting cast wet by keeping ice in plastic bag and
      protecting cast with cloth)
    Report signs of possible problems to health care provider
      Increasing pain
      Swelling associated with pain and discoloration of
        toes or fingers
      Pain during motion
      Burning or tingling under cast
    Keep appointment to have fracture and cast checked

*Plaster of Paris cast.
†Synthetic cast.

Thermolabile plastic (Orthoplast) and *thermoplastic resins* (Hexcelite) are molded after being heated in warm water. Polyurethane, which is formed from polyester and cotton fabric impregnated with a chemical, is water activated by immersing in cool water to start the chemical process.

- Casts made of this fiberglass tape are frequently used because they are lightweight and relatively waterproof and support earlier mobilization. They are appropriate in cases in which severe edema is not present or when multiple cast changes are not anticipated.

Cast Care

Immediately after a cast is applied, there is a short period of exothermic reaction during which heat is released from the plaster. The patient should be alerted to this occurrence because it can increase edema. A fresh cast should never be covered with a blanket, because air cannot circulate and heat builds up in the cast.

- The drying process is usually complete within 24 to 72 hours. During the drying period the cast should not be subjected to any wetness, soiling, or abnormal stresses that can cause weakening or a break in the cast.
- The cast should be carefully handled by the palms of the hands rather than with the fingertips to avoid indentations that will dry and become potential pressure areas.

Regardless of the type of material of which it is made, a cast can interfere with circulation and nerve function from being applied too tightly or because of excessive edema after application. Frequent neurovascular assessments of the immobilized extremity are critical.

- Elevation of the extremity above the level of the heart to promote venous return and applications of ice to control or prevent edema are measures frequently used during the initial phase of immobilization.
- The nurse should instruct the patient to exercise the joints above and below the cast.
- Pulling out cast padding and scratching or placing foreign objects inside the cast is forbidden because it predisposes the patient to skin breakdown and infection within the cast.

Patient instructions for cast care are presented in Table 53.

CHEMOTHERAPY

Description

Chemotherapy is a systemic treatment modality for cancer that uses chemicals (drugs). It is primarily used in the treatment of solid tumors, leukemia, and lymphomas. The principle of chemotherapy is to interrupt the cycle of cellular replication and proliferation.

- The two major types of chemotherapeutic drugs, cell-cycle nonspecific and cell-cycle specific, are often administered together. The aim of this combination approach is to promote a better tumor kill response by using agents that disrupt cellular replication and proliferation by different mechanisms.

Goals of Chemotherapy

The goal of chemotherapy is to reduce the number of cancer cells present in the primary tumor site(s) and also, if present, in metastatic tumor site(s). Several factors will determine the response of cancer cells to chemotherapy:

1. *Mitotic rate of tissue from which tumor arises.* The more rapid the mitotic rate, the greater the response to chemotherapy.
2. *Size of tumor.* The smaller the number of cancer cells, the greater the response to chemotherapy.
3. *Age of tumor.* The younger the tumor, the greater the response to chemotherapy. Younger tumors have a greater percentage of proliferating cells.
4. *Location of tumor.* Certain anatomic sites provide a protected environment from the effects of chemotherapy. For example, only a few drugs (nitrosoureas and bleomycin) cross the blood-brain barrier.
5. *Presence of resistant tumor cells.* Mutation of cancer cells within the tumor mass can result in variant cells that are resistant to chemotherapy.
6. *Physiologic and psychologic status of host.* A state of optimum health and a positive attitude will allow the patient to better withstand aggressive chemotherapy.

One method to prevent the existence of drug-resistant tumor cells is the use of high-dose chemotherapy. The aim of this approach is to maximize drug effects at the cellular level before the problem of resistance occurs.

Types of Chemotherapy

Chemotherapy drugs can be classified according to their mechanism of action (Table 54).

Administration of Chemotherapy

Chemotherapy is most commonly administered by oral or IV routes. A vascular access device allows for chemotherapy to be administered via the large vessels (venous or arterial) and also permits frequent, continuous or intermittent treatment with multiple punctures for vascular access. Types of these devices include Silastic right atrial catheters, implanted infusion ports, and infusion (external and implanted) pumps.

- Regional chemotherapy delivers the drug right to the tumor site. Examples of this type of administration include intraarterial, intraperitoneal, and intrathecal (intraventricular) chemotherapy.

Table 54   Classification of Chemotherapeutic Drugs

Mechanisms of action	Examples
Alkylating Agents ***Cell-cycle nonspecific*** ▪ Damage DNA by causing breaks in double-strand helix (similar to effect of radiation therapy); if repair does not occur, cells will die immediately or when they attempt to divide. ▪ Have heavy metal effect on DNA. ▪ Suppress mitosis at interphase.	Mechlorethamine (nitrogen mustard), cyclophosphamide (Cytoxan), chlorambucil (Leukeran), melphalan (Alkeran), triethylene thiophosphoramide (Thiotepa), busulfan (Myleran), dacarbazine (DTIC) Cisplatin (Platinol), carboplatin (JM-8, CBDCA) Procarbazine (Matulane, Natulan)
Antimetabolites ***Cell-cycle specific*** ▪ Interfere with synthesis of DNA by mimicking certain essential cellular metabolites that cell incorporates into synthesis of DNA; cells will die immediately.	Methotrexate (Amethopterin), cytosine arabinoside (Ara-C, Cytosar), 5-fluorouracil (5-FU), 6-mercaptopurine (6-MP), thioguanine (6-TG), floxuridine (FUDR), vidarabine (Vira-A)
Antitumor Antibiotics ***Cell-cycle nonspecific*** ▪ Modify function of DNA and interfere with transcription of RNA; cells will die immediately or when they attempt to divide.	Doxorubicin (Adriamycin), bleomycin (Blenoxane), mitomycin (Mutamycin), daunorubicin (Daunomycin), actinomycin D, plicamycin (Mithracin)

Continued.

Table 54 Classification of Chemotherapeutic Drugs—cont'd

Mechanisms of action	Examples
Plant Alkaloids	
Cell-cycle specific	
■ Interrupt cellular replication in mitosis at metaphase; cells will die immediately.	Vinblastine (Velban), vincristine (Oncovin), etoposide (Ve Pesid), taxol, vindesine
Nitrosureas	
Cell-cycle nonspecific	
■ Have similar effect to alkylating agents and also block specific enzymes needed for synthesis of purine; cells will die immediately or when they attempt to divide.	Carmustine (BCNU), lomustine (CCNU), semustine (Methyl CCNU), streptozotocin (STZ)
Corticosteroids	
Cell-cycle nonspecific	
■ Disrupt cell membrane and inhibit synthesis of protein; decrease circulating lymphocytes; inhibit mitosis; depress immune system; increase feeling of well-being.	Prednisone (Merticorten), dexamethasone (Decadron)

Hormones

Cell-cycle nonspecific

- Stimulate process of cellular differentiation; metastatic lesions are less able to survive in unfavorable environment; decrease process of cellular proliferation.

  Androgens (testosterone, fluoxymesterone [Halotestine]), estrogens (diethylstilbestrol), progestins (Provera, Delalutin, Megace)

Miscellaneous

- Destroy exogenous supply of L-asparagine, which is needed for cellular proliferation; normal cells can synthesize but cannot be synthesized by cancer cells.

  L-Asparaginase (Elspar)

- Have effect on DNA similar to alkylating agents; also block incorporation of thymidine into DNA.

  Hydroxyurea (Hydrea)

- Antiestrogens are used in breast cancer.

  Tamoxifen (Nolvadex)

- Antiadrenal drug blocks adrenal steroid production.

  Aminoglutethimide (Cytadren)

DNA, Deoxyribonucleic acid; *RNA,* ribonucleic acid.

Effects of Chemotherapy

The effects of chemotherapy are caused by (1) destruction of cells that have a rapid rate of cellular proliferation, (2) response of the body to products of cellular destruction (cellular waste products in circulation may cause fatigue, anorexia, and taste alterations), and (3) specific drug toxicities.

The adverse effects of these drugs can be classified as acute, delayed, or chronic. *Acute toxicity* includes vomiting, allergic reactions, and dysrhythmias. *Delayed effects* include mucositis, alopecia, and bone marrow depression. Mucositis can result in mouth sores, gastritis, and diarrhea. *Chronic toxicities* involve damage to organs such as the heart, liver, kidneys, and lungs. An extensive listing of side effects and problems caused by chemotherapy and radiation therapy is provided in Lewis/Collier/Heitkemper, *Medical-Surgical Nursing,* edition 4, Table 12-15, p. 283.

Nursing Management

One of the most important responsibilities of the nurse is that of differentiating between toxic effects of the drug and progression of the malignant process. The nurse also needs to differentiate between tolerable side effects and acute toxic effects of chemotherapeutic agents. Nausea and vomiting are expected and controllable side effects of many drugs. However, if paresthesia occurs with the use of vincristine or signs of heart failure appear with the use of doxorubicin, these serious reactions need to be reported to the physician so that drug dosages can be modified or discontinued.

- Some toxicities associated with chemotherapy may not be reversible. For example, ototoxicity may be an irreversible effect of cisplatin therapy, especially at higher doses. Periodic testing of hearing may be necessary to monitor for this toxicity.
- Results of laboratory studies of the patient who is receiving chemotherapy should be monitored. Particular attention should be given to the white blood cell (WBC), platelet, and red blood cell (RBC) counts.
- If the WBC count falls to less than 2000/μL (2×10^9/L), the drug regimen may need to be modified or discontinued. Every measure possible needs to be taken to prevent infections in a patient with leukopenia. If the platelet count falls to less than 50,000/μL (50 $\times$ 10^9/L), the patient must be assessed for any signs of bleeding, and measures should be taken to prevent bleeding. Platelet transfusions may be necessary.

Patient Teaching

Education of the patient is an extremely important part of the nurse's role related to chemotherapy. To decrease the fear and anxiety often associated with chemotherapy, patients must be taught what to expect during a course of treatment.

- The patient's attitude toward treatment should be explored so that any misconceptions or fears can be discussed.
- The patient needs to be told of the possible side effects of chemotherapy that may be experienced during treatment. This may be a discouraging revelation.
- The patient should also be informed that supportive care (e.g., antiemetics and antidiarrheals) will be provided as needed.

Many emotions are experienced and expressed when hair loss occurs, including anger, grief, embarrassment, and fear. For some persons, the loss of hair is one of the most stressful events experienced during the course of the illness.

- Alopecia caused by chemotherapeutic agents is usually reversible. The degree and duration of hair loss depend on the dose of the chemotherapeutic agent, the duration of the treatment, and the nutritional status of the patient.
- Sometimes the hair begins to grow back while the patient is still receiving chemotherapeutic agents, but generally the hair cells do not grow back until the agents are discontinued. Often the new hair has a different color and texture than the hair that was lost.

CHEST TUBES AND PLEURAL DRAINAGE

Description

Chest tubes are inserted into the pleural space to remove air and fluid from the pleural space and to restore normal intrapleural pressure so that the lungs can reexpand.

Chest Tube Insertion

Chest tubes can be inserted in the emergency department (ED), at the patient's bedside, or in the operating room (OR), depending on the situation. In the OR chest tubes are inserted via a thoracotomy incision. In the ED or at the bedside the patient is placed in a sitting position or is lying down with the affected side elevated.

- The area is prepared with antiseptic solution, and the site is infiltrated with a local anesthetic agent. After a small incision is made, one or two chest tubes are inserted into the pleural space.
- As shown in Fig. 4, one catheter is placed anteriorly through the second intercostal space to remove air; the other is placed

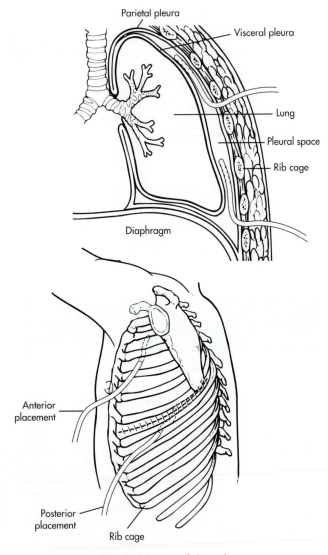

Fig. 4 Placement of chest tubes.

posteriorly through the eighth or ninth intercostal space to drain fluid and blood.

- Tubes are sutured to the chest wall, and the puncture wound is covered with an airtight dressing.
- After the tubes are in place in the pleural space, they are connected to drainage tubing and pleural drainage. Each tube may be connected to a separate drainage system and suction. More commonly a Y connector is used to attach both chest tubes to the same drainage system.

Pleural Drainage

Most pleural drainage systems have three basic compartments, each with its own separate function. The three compartments were bottles in early drainage systems and were known as the *three-bottle system* (see Fig. 5).

- The first compartment, or *collection chamber,* receives fluid and air from the chest cavity. The air in the chamber is vented to the second compartment called the *water-seal chamber,* which acts as a one-way valve. Air enters from collection chamber through a connector that enters under water in the second compartment. The air bubbles up through the water, and

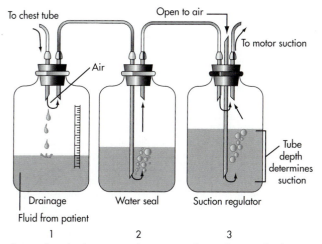

Fig. 5 Three-bottle water-seal suction. *Bottle 1* is drainage bottle. Vertical piece of tape should be applied to outer surface of drainage bottle. Time and fluid level should be marked hourly on tape. *Bottle 2* is water-seal bottle. *Bottle 3* is suction control bottle. Length of glass tube below water surface determines amount of suction.

no air can reenter the collection chamber because of the water seal.

- A third compartment, which is used to apply controlled suction to the system, is called the *suction control chamber.*
- Removal of air from the pleural space is facilitated during periods when the patient's intrathoracic pressure is increased, such as during exhalation, coughing, or sneezing. As a result, more air bubbles are noted in the water-seal chamber during these activities.
- A lack of bubbling during exhalation or coughing may indicate a blockage in the chest tube (e.g., kinking, clotting) or expansion of the lung with no further air in the pleural space.

Nursing Management

General guidelines for nursing care include the following:

- Keep all tubing as straight as possible and coiled loosely. Do not let the patient lie on it.
- Keep all connections between chest tubes, drainage tubing, and drainage collector tight. Taping at connections and at top of bottle helps prevent air leaks.
- Keep water seal and suction control chamber at appropriate water levels by adding sterile water as needed because water loss by evaporation may occur.
- Place piece of tape on outside of drainage bottle. Time of measurement and fluid level should be marked according to prescribed orders. Any change in quantity or characteristics of drainage should be reported to physician.
- Observe for air bubbles in the water-seal chamber and fluctuations in glass tube or chest tubes. Air should be bubbling out from the glass tube. If no fluctuations are observed (rising with inspiration and falling with expiration in spontaneously breathing patient; opposite occurs during positive-pressure mechanical ventilation), drainage system is blocked or lungs are reexpanded. If bubbling increases, there may be an air leak.
- Check for bubbling in water seal. Normally, this is intermittent. When bubbling is continuous and constant, the nurse may determine the source of the air leak by momentarily clamping the tubing at successively distal points away from the patient until the bubbling ceases. Retaping tubing connections or replacing drainage apparatus may be necessary to prevent the air leak.
- Monitor the patient's clinical status. Vital signs should be taken frequently, lungs auscultated, and the chest wall observed for any abnormal chest movements.
- Never elevate the drainage system to the level of the patient's chest because this will cause fluid to drain back into the lungs.

Secure bottles to metal drainage stand or racks. Drainage bottles should not be emptied unless they are in danger of overflowing.

- Encourage the patient to cough and breathe deeply periodically to facilitate lung expansion.
- Check the position of the bottle or drainage system. If the bottle is overturned and the water seal is disrupted, return to an upright position and encourage the patient to take a few deep breaths, followed by forced exhalations and cough maneuvers.

Milking and stripping of chest tubes may briefly increase the amount of negative pressure applied to the pleural space. Increased negative pressure should enhance evacuation of fluid in the chest tubes and prevent development of clots and obstruction from stagnation of fluids.

- Although further study is still needed to evaluate the effects of routine stripping of pleural and mediastinal tubes, present practice advocates the use of these procedures when there is bloody drainage or when fluid in the collection bottle tends to clot.
- When chest tubes are used for air collection alone, stripping and milking is not usually performed.
- The nurse should keep in mind that these procedures can cause the patient to experience pain and that dislodgement of the tube may occur if the tube is not stabilized above the area that is being stripped.

Clamping of chest tubes is no longer advocated as routine clinical practice unless they become disconnected or momentarily to change drainage apparatus and to check for air leaks. The danger of a rapid accumulation of air in the pleural space causing tension pneumothorax is far greater than that of a small amount of atmospheric air entering the pleural space.

Chest tubes are removed when the lungs are reexpanded and fluid drainage has ceased. The patient with chest tubes may have daily chest x-rays to follow the course of lung reexpansion.

- The tube is removed by cutting the sutures; applying a sterile petroleum jelly gauze dressing; having the patient take a deep breath, exhaling, and bearing down (Valsalva maneuver); and then the tube is removed. Sometimes pain medication is given before chest tube removal.
- The site is covered with an airtight dressing, the pleura seals itself off, and the wound is healed in several days. The wound should be observed for drainage, and the dressing should be reinforced if necessary.
- The patient should be observed for any manifestations of respiratory distress, which may signify a recurrent or new pneumothorax.

Coronary Artery Bypass Graft Surgery

Description
A coronary artery bypass graft (CABG) operation consists of the construction of new conduits (vessels to transport blood) when the coronary arteries are obstructed.

- This procedure provides blood flow beyond the stenosis so that the myocardium distal to the obstruction continues to receive blood flow.

Procedure
This procedure usually involves a graft from the saphenous vein or the internal mammary artery (IMA) for aortocoronary bypass. In the former procedure the saphenous vein from one of the patient's legs is removed and reversed (so that the valves will not obstruct the blood flow).

- Saphenous veins used as grafts develop diffuse intimal hyperplasia, which contributes to ultimate stenosis and occlusions of the graft. The use of aspirin (325 mg po daily) improves vein graft patency and is used postoperatively in these patients.
- Because the patency rate of the IMA is higher than that of saphenous veins, the IMA may prove to be a better conduit for improving long-term prognosis. Use of the left IMA, which is left attached to its origin from its left subclavian artery, is mobilized from the chest wall and anastomosed to the coronary artery distal to the stenosis. The right IMA may also be used in a similar fashion.

If a patient has had a previous CABG with saphenous vein grafts or the IMA and at the time of reoperation has no conduits to harvest, the gastroepiploic artery or inferior epigastric artery may be used.

- These arteries are excellent conduits. However, use of these arteries requires the additional need for a laparotomy.
- This increases the length of surgery, and wound complications at the harvest site are not uncommon, especially in an obese or diabetic patient.
- Because of the number of patients requiring reoperation, the use of alternative arteries and veins will become increasingly common.

Nursing Management
CABG remains a palliative treatment for coronary artery disease (CAD) and not a cure. It does provide the patient with improved outcomes, quality of life, and survival.

- The number of older adults who are candidates for CABG has increased, and they have become a subpopulation of patients who have specialized needs before and after surgery.

Results of coronary revascularization are less favorable for women than men. Coronary artery disease is the leading cause of death among women. The severity of the clinical variables in women, including a more severe angina and poorer congestive heart failure (CHF) score (despite a better ejection fraction), and the smaller mean diameter of the coronary vessels in women are all considered possible causes of their increased risk of CABG. The mortality rate of women undergoing CABG is often double that of men the same age.

Nursing care involves caring for two surgical sites: the chest and the leg.

- The care of the leg wound is similar to the postoperative care after the stripping of varicose veins (see Varicose Veins, p. 611; also see nursing management of varicose veins in Lewis/Collier/Heitkemper, *Medical-Surgical Nursing,* edition 4, p. 1062).
- The management of the chest wound, which involves a thoracotomy, is similar to that of other chest surgeries. (The nursing management is presented in the nursing care plan for the patient after thoracotomy in Lewis/Collier/Heitkemper, *Medical-Surgical Nursing,* edition 4, p. 669. The overall management of the patient requiring cardiac surgery is presented on p. 958 of the same text.)

DIALYSIS

Description

Dialysis is a technique in which substances move from the blood through a semipermeable membrane and into a dialysis solution (dialysate). Dialysis is used to correct fluid and electrolyte imbalances and to remove waste products in renal failure. Dialysis can also be used to treat drug overdoses.

The two methods of dialysis are *peritoneal dialysis* (PD) and *hemodialysis* (HD). (See Table 55, which compares peritoneal dialysis and hemodialysis.)

- In PD the peritoneal membrane is used as the semipermeable membrane.
- In HD an artificial membrane (usually made of cellulose-based or synthetic materials) is used as the semipermeable membrane that is in contact with the patient's blood.

Table 55   Comparison of Peritoneal Dialysis and Hemodialysis

Peritoneal dialysis		Hemodialysis	
Advantages	**Disadvantages**	**Advantages**	**Disadvantages**
Immediate initiation in almost any hospital	Bacterial or chemical peritonitis	Rapid fluid removal	Vascular access problems
Portable system with CAPD	Protein loss into dialysate	Rapid removal of urea and creatinine	Dietary and fluid restrictions
Fewer dietary restrictions	Exit-site and tunnel infections	Effective potassium removal	Heparinization necessary
Relatively short training time	Self-image problems with catheter placement	Less protein loss	Extensive equipment necessary
Usable in patient with vascular access problems	Hyperglycemia	Lowering of serum triglycerides	Disequilibrium and hypotension during dialysis
Less cardiovascular stress	Aggravated hyperlipidemia		Added blood loss that contributes to anemia
Preferable for diabetic patients	Surgery for catheter placement		Specially trained personnel necessary
	Contraindication in patients with multiple abdominal surgeries or trauma		

CAPD, Continuous ambulatory peritoneal dialysis.

Dialysis is begun when a patient in renal failure can no longer be adequately managed conservatively.

- A general guideline is to start dialysis when glomerular filtration rate (GFR) (or creatinine clearance) is less than 5 to 10 ml/min. However, this criterion varies widely in different clinical situations, and the physician determines when to start dialysis on an individual basis. Certain uremic complications, including encephalopathy, uncontrollable hyperkalemia, pericarditis, and accelerated hypertension, indicate a need for immediate dialysis.

Peritoneal Dialysis

In recent years the use of PD to treat both acute and chronic renal failure has increased considerably. The large surface area of the peritoneum makes it a good semipermeable membrane for performing clinical dialysis.

Peritoneal Catheters

Peritoneal access is obtained by inserting a catheter through the anterior abdominal wall (Fig. 6). The prototype of the catheter that is used was developed by Tenckhoff in 1968 and is made of silicone rubber tubing. Other types of catheters for chronic PD are variations

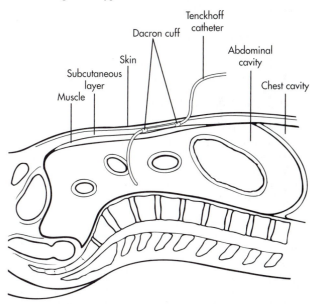

Fig. 6 Tenckhoff catheter in peritoneal dialysis.

of the Tenckhoff catheter, including the Toronto-Western, Purdue-Column Disc, and Gore-Tex catheters.

- The tip of the catheter rests in the peritoneal cavity and has many perforations spaced throughout the distal end of the tubing to allow fluid to flow in and out of the catheter.

The technique of catheter placement varies; it is usually done by surgery so placement is visualized and complications minimized.

- Before the start of PD, it is preferable to allow a waiting period of 7 to 14 days for proper sealing of catheter and tissue ingrowth. However, some centers start dialysis 5 to 7 days after catheter insertion. About 2 to 4 weeks after catheter implantation the exit site should be clean, dry, and free of redness and tenderness.
- Once the catheter incision site is healed (usually 4 to 6 weeks), the patient may shower and then pat the catheter and exit site dry.
- Daily catheter care includes cleansing with antibacterial soap, application of an antiseptic solution, or a sterile dressing, as well as examination of the catheter site for signs of infection.
- The patient receiving dialysis at home will receive about four exchanges per day. An acutely ill hospitalized patient may receive 12 to 24 exchanges per day.

Peritoneal Dialysis Procedure

The three phases of the peritoneal dialysis cycle are *inflow* (fill), *dwell* (equilibration), and *drain*. (The three phases are called an *exchange*.)

- During inflow a prescribed amount of solution, usually 2 L, is infused over about 10 minutes. The flow rate may be decreased if the patient becomes uncomfortable. After the solution has been infused, the inflow clamp is closed before air enters the tubing.
- During the dwell phase, or equilibration, diffusion and osmosis occur between the patient's blood and peritoneal cavity. The duration of dwell time can last 20 to 30 minutes to 8 or more hours, depending on the method of PD.
- Drain time takes 15 to 30 minutes and may be facilitated by gently massaging the abdomen or changing the patient's position.

The cycle starts again with infusion of another 2 L of solution. For manual PD a period of about 30 to 50 minutes is required to complete an exchange.

Complications of Peritoneal Dialysis

Complications of peritoneal dialysis include exit site infection, peritonitis, abdominal pain, hernias, lower back problems, bleeding, protein loss, pulmonary complications, and encapsulating sclerosing peritonitis. For a discussion of complications, see Lewis/Collier/Heitkemper, *Medical-Surgical Nursing*, edition 4, p. 1396.

Clinically, the patient on PD does at least as well as the patient on HD and sometimes better. There are fewer dietary restrictions, and greater mobility is possible than with conventional HD.

- The major disadvantage is the possibility of developing peritonitis. As further improvements in techniques are made (e.g., improved connecting and sterilizing devices, in-line filters, improved catheters), the incidence of peritonitis is decreasing.
- PD is especially indicated for the individual who has vascular access problems and responds poorly to the hemodynamic stresses of HD (e.g., older adult patient with diabetes and cardiovascular disease). The diabetic patient with end-stage renal disease (ESRD) does better on PD than on HD.

Hemodialysis

Vascular Access

In hemodialysis vascular access is needed for the high blood flow required to perform HD (see Fig. 7).

- An arteriovenous fistula is created in the forearm or thigh by a side-to-side, end-to-side, or end-to-end anastomosis between an artery (usually radial or ulnar) and a vein (usually cephalic). The fistula provides for arterial blood flow through the vein. The increased pressure of the arterial blood flow through the vein makes the vein dilate and become tough, making it accessible for repeated venipuncture and allowing it to handle high blood flows required for HD. The vein is accessed using two large-gauge needles.
- Grafts used for vascular access are made of synthetic materials (PTFE, polytetrafluoroethylene/Teflon) and form a "bridge" between the arterial and venous blood supplies. Grafts are surgically anastomosed between an artery (usually brachial) and a vein (usually antecubital). The graft, like the fistula, is under the skin and accessed with two large-gauge needles. Because grafts are made of manmade materials, they can become infected easily and are thrombogenic.
- In some situations when temporary vascular access is required, percutaneous cannulation of the subclavian, internal jugular, or femoral vein is used.

Dialyzers

The dialyzer is usually a hollow fiber tube that contains thousands of parallel fibers packed in a cylinder. The fibers are the semipermeable membrane made of cellulose-based or other synthetic materials.

- The blood is pumped through the fibers, and dialysis fluid bathes the outside of them with dialysis and ultrafiltration occurring through the pores of the semipermeable membrane.

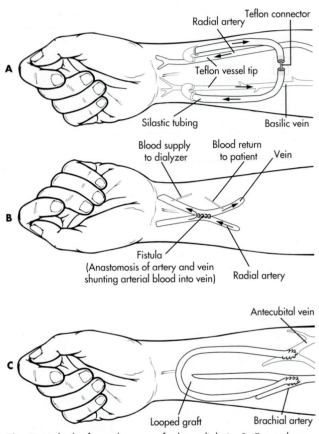

Fig. 7 Methods of vascular access for hemodialysis. **A,** External cannula or shunt. **B,** Internal arteriovenous fistula. **C,** Looped graft in forearm.

- Most chronic dialysis units now reprocess and reuse the dialyzers for the same patient after cleaning and subsequent disinfection. With reuse the dialyzers become more biocompatible so that there are fewer side effects from blood-membrane interactions during the dialysis procedure.

Dialysis Procedure

To initiate chronic dialysis two needles are placed in the fistula or graft. The needle closest to the fistula is used to obtain "arterial" blood from the patient and send it to the dialyzer with the assistance of a blood pump. The dialyzer is usually primed with saline solution. The saline solution is infused into the patient as blood fills the dialyzer circuit. Heparin is added to the blood as it flows into the dialyzer to prevent clotting.

- Once the blood enters the extracorporeal circuit, it is propelled through the dialyzer by a blood pump at a flow rate of 200 to 500 ml/min, while the dialysate (warmed to body temperature) circulates in the opposite direction at a rate of 300 to 900 ml/min.
- Blood is returned from the dialyzer to the patient through the "venous" line through the second needle.

In addition to the dialyzer, there is a dialysate delivery and monitoring system. This system pumps the dialysate through the dialyzer countercurrent to the blood flow. Adjustments can be made for ultrafiltration by creating a positive pressure in the blood side or a negative pressure on the dialysate side or by a combination of both. The dialysis system has an alarm system to warn of blood leaking into the dialysate or air leaking into the blood; alterations in dialysate temperature, concentration, or pressure; and extremes in BP readings.

- Dialysis is terminated by flushing the dialyzer with saline solution to return all blood to the patient. The needles are then removed from the patient, and firm pressure is applied to the venipuncture sites until the bleeding stops.

Complications of Hemodialysis

Complications of hemodialysis include (1) disequilibrium syndrome with rapid changes in extracellular fluid composition, (2) hypotension from rapid vascular volume removal, (3) muscle cramps resulting from rapid removal of sodium and water and loss of blood from dialyzer or with patient who has clotting problems, (4) hepatitis from blood transfusions, and (6) sepsis at the vascular access site,

HD is still an imperfect technique in treating ESRD. It cannot replace the metabolic and hormonal functions of the kidneys. HD can relieve most of the symptoms of chronic renal failure and, if started early, can prevent certain complications. However, it does not alter the accelerated atherosclerosis.

HEIMLICH MANEUVER

The management of a foreign body obstruction of the airway depends on whether the person is conscious or unconscious. Table 56 outlines the actions involved in basic life support and explains how to perform them.

Table 56 Management of Foreign Body Airway Obstruction

Action	Helpful hints
Conscious Adult	
1. Determine if victim is able to speak or cough.	Rescuer can ask "Are you choking?" Victim may be using universal distress signal of choking: clutching neck between thumb and index finger.
2. Abdominal thrust: perform Heimlich maneuver until foreign body is expelled or victim becomes unconscious (see Fig. 8).	Stand behind victim and wrap arms around victim's waist. Press fist into abdomen with quick inward and upward thrusts.
3. Chest thrust: for victims who are in advanced pregnancy or who are obese.	Chest thrusts: stand behind victim and place arms under victim's armpits to encircle chest. Press with quick backward thrusts.

Victim Is or Becomes Unconscious

1. Activate EMS.
   Call 911.

2. Check for foreign body obstruction.
   Sweep deeply into mouth with hooked finger to remove foreign body (see Fig. 9).

3. Attempt rescue breathing.
   Open airway. Try to give two breaths. If needed, reposition head and try again.

4. If airway is obstructed, perform Heimlich maneuver.
   Kneel astride victim's thighs. Place heel of one hand on victim's abdomen in midline slightly above navel and well below tip of xyphoid. Place second hand on top of first. Press into abdomen with quick upward thrusts.

5. Repeat sequence until successful.
   Alternate these maneuvers in rapid sequence: finger sweep, rescue breathing attempt, and abdominal thrusts.

Modified from Basic life support heart saver guide: a student handbook for CPR and first aid for choking, Dallas, 1993, American Heart Association.
EMS, Emergency medical services.

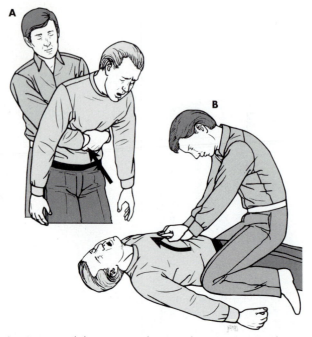

Fig. 8 A, Heimlich maneuver administered to conscious (standing) victim of foreign body airway obstruction. **B,** Heimlich maneuver administered to unconscious (lying) victim of foreign body airway obstruction—astride position.

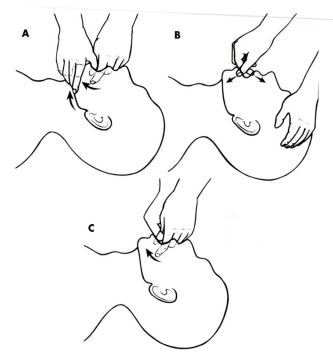

Fig. 9 A, Finger sweep maneuver administered to unconscious victim of foreign body airway obstruction. With victim's head up, rescuer opens victim's mouth by grasping both tongue and lower jaw between thumb and fingers and lifting (tongue-jaw lift). This action draws tongue from back of throat and away from foreign body. Obstruction may be partially relieved by this maneuver. **B,** Crossed-finger technique for opening airway. If rescuer is unable to open victim's mouth with tongue-jaw lift, crossed-finger technique may be used. Rescuer opens mouth by crossing index finger and thumb and pushing teeth apart. **C,** Index finger of rescuer's available hand is inserted along inside of cheek and deeply into throat to base of tongue. Hooking motion is used to dislodge foreign body and maneuver it into mouth for removal.

Hemodynamic Monitoring

Description

Hemodynamic monitoring refers to measurement of pressure, flow, and oxygenation of blood within the cardiovascular system. Both invasive (internally placed devices) and noninvasive (external devices) measurements are made.

- Values commonly measured include systemic and pulmonary arterial pressures, central venous pressure (CVP), pulmonary capillary wedge pressure (PCWP), cardiac output, and O_2 saturation of the hemoglobin of arterial and mixed venous blood.
- From these measurements the clinician calculates several values, including the resistance of the systemic and pulmonary arterial vasculature and O_2 content, delivery, and consumption.
- When these data are integrated with clinical assessment, the nurse can derive a detailed and accurate picture of the patient's problem and the effect of therapy. It is important that all measures be made with attention to technical aspects. False or inaccurate data are potentially misleading and thus dangerous.

The specific hemodynamic measurements are discussed in Lewis/Collier/Heitkemper, *Medical-Surgical Nursing,* edition 4, pp. 1953-1954.

Nursing Management

Assessment of hemodynamic status requires integration of data from many sources and comparison of the data over time.

- Observations begin with the patient's general appearance. Does the patient appear weak, tired, exhausted? There may be too little cardiac reserve to sustain minimum activity.
- Changing skin color or temperature may indicate diminished cardiac output. If shock is developing, BP and even heart rate might be relatively stable, yet the patient may become increasingly pale and cool because of vasoconstriction of the peripheral circulation.
- Conversely, the patient may remain warm and pink yet develop tachycardia and BP instability. These features are characteristic of septic shock.

The heart rate is often a useful indicator of the hemodynamic state. As tissue perfusion becomes compromised, heart rate increases. Although heart rates of 100 beats/min are common among stressed, compromised, critically ill patients, further increases in heart rate may herald compromised perfusion. In patients in whom heart rate cannot increase, such as with arteriovenous (AV) block, the mixed venous oxygen saturation (SvO_2) can be a useful indicator of impending compromise.

In addition to high-technology measurements available to the ICU nurse, simple observations may provide useful insights into the patient's hemodynamic status.

- Mental clarity reflects cerebral perfusion.
- Urine output reflects renal perfusion.
- The patient with diminished GI perfusion may develop hypoactive or absent bowel sounds and may have nausea and vomiting when GI motility is impaired by a lack of perfusion.

By carefully monitoring the patient, the astute nurse is able to recognize early cues and manage problems before they escalate.

Intraaortic Balloon Pump

Description
The intraaortic balloon pump (IABP) provides temporary circulatory assistance to the compromised heart by reducing afterload (by reduction in systolic pressure) and augmenting the aortic diastolic pressure. Table 57 lists clinical conditions for which the IABP is used.

Procedure
The IABP consists of a sausage-shaped balloon, a pump that inflates and deflates the balloon, control devices for synchronizing the balloon inflation to cardiac contraction, and fail-safe devices. (See Figs. 61-7 and 61-8 in Lewis/Collier/Heitkemper, *Medical-Surgical Nursing,* edition 4, p. 1962.)

- The balloon is inserted percutaneously or surgically into the femoral artery, advanced toward the heart, and positioned in the descending thoracic aorta just below the left subclavian artery but above the renal arteries.
- A pneumatic device cyclically fills the balloon with helium during diastole and deflates it during systole.
- The ECG is used to trigger deflation on the R wave and inflation on the T wave. The arterial wave is used to refine timing so that inflation occurs at the arterial dicrotic notch and deflation occurs just before systole.
- IABP support is referred to as counterpulsation because the timing of balloon inflation is opposite ventricular contraction.

Table 57	Indications and Contraindications for the Intraaortic Balloon Pump

Indications

Preinfarction, accelerating, or crescendo angina (when conventional modes of therapy, such as bed rest, nitrates, β-blockers, and calcium channel blockers have failed)

Severe cardiac disease (when undergoing cardiac catheterization or noncardiac surgery)

Acute myocardial infarction with any of the following*:

Ventricular aneurysm accompanied by ventricular dysrhythmias

Acute ventricular septal defect

Acute mitral valve regurgitation

Cardiogenic shock

Continuing chest pain

Preoperative, intraoperative, and postoperative open heart surgery (e.g., aneurysectomy, revascularization, or valve replacement); often used to wean from cardiopulmonary bypass

Cardiogenic shock

Contraindications

Irreversible brain damage

Terminal or untreatable diseases of any major organ system

Ruptured or dissecting aortic or thoracic aneurysm

Generalized peripheral vascular disease (may prevent placement of balloon)

Insufficient aortic valve (considered an *absolute* contraindication)

*Allows time for emergency angiography and corrective cardiac surgery to be performed.

Complications

Complications are common with the IABP. Patients receiving an IABP are prone to infections. Insertion site infection or sepsis from an unknown source require catheter removal. Vascular injuries such as dislodging of plaque, arterial dissection, and compromised distal extremity circulation are common. Thrombus and embolus formation add to the risk of distal circulation compromise. Peripheral nerve damage can occur, particularly when a cutdown is performed for insertion.

- To reduce these risks, hourly neurovascular assessment is necessary. Because the balloon pumping can cause physical destruction of platelets, thrombocytopenia is common and coagulation status indicators must be monitored.

- Displacement of the balloon can occlude the left subclavian, renal, or mesenteric arteries.
- If the balloon develops a leak, the catheter must be changed immediately to avoid a gas embolus. A malfunction of the balloon or console triggers fail-safe alarms and automatic unit shutdown.

Nursing Management

The patient with an IABP is relatively immobile, limited to side-lying or supine positions with the bed elevated no more than 15 degrees. The leg in which the catheter is inserted must not be flexed at the hip. The patient may be receiving ventilatory support and will likely have multiple invasive lines, which increase the challenge of comfortable positioning. Skin care and comfort measures are required.

As the patient improves, the patient is "weaned" from IABP; that is, circulatory support provided by the IABP is gradually reduced.

- Even if the patient is stable without the IABP, pumping is usually continued every third or fourth beat until the line is removed. This reduces the risk of thrombus formation around the catheter. Detailed frequent hemodynamic assessment continues to be required during the weaning phase.

INTUBATION, ENDOTRACHEAL

Description

Endotracheal intubation is the insertion and placement of a tube into the trachea through the nose (nasal intubation) or mouth (oral intubation) (Fig. 10).

- Indications for endotracheal intubation are to (1) prevent or relieve upper airway obstruction, (2) prevent aspiration, (3) facilitate secretion removal, and (4) provide a closed system for positive pressure ventilation.

If *oral intubation* is selected, the patient is placed in a supine position with the head extended, the neck fully flexed, and the jaw pulled forward. The endotracheal tube is passed through the mouth and vocal cords and into the trachea with the aid of a laryngoscope or bronchoscope.

- Problems with oral intubation include easy dislodgement, poor toleration, difficult oral hygiene, difficulty swallowing, inability to communicate, and lip laceration.

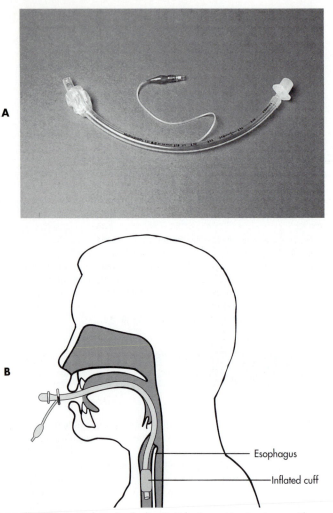

Fig. 10 A, Endotracheal tube. **B,** Tube in position in airway with cuff inflated.

If *nasal intubation* is selected, insertion is performed by manipulating the tube through the nose, nasopharynx, and vocal cords.

- The advantages of nasal intubation compared with oral intubation include better oral hygiene, continued ability to swallow, better communication, and less sedation. However, nasal intubation is associated with complications, including sinusitis, otitis media, and epistaxis after removal.

Nursing Management

Before intubation the nurse should ensure that the patient is properly oxygenated.

- If the patient is conscious, the nurse should explain why endotracheal intubation is necessary, the procedure involved, and sensations (gagging and a feeling of suffocation) that may be experienced during the procedure.
- The nurse should explain that because of the inflated cuff, it will not be possible to talk when the tube is in place but speech will be possible after the tube is removed.

After intubation nursing responsibilities include (1) assessing correct tube placement, (2) inflating the cuff, (3) assessing oxygenation status and acid-base balance and reporting untoward changes, (4) suctioning to remove secretions, (5) providing mouth care, (6) alternating placement of oral tubes to prevent pressure necrosis, (7) preventing accidental disconnection from the ventilator or extubation, and (8) preventing cuff overinflation.

After insertion the nurse should immediately verify correct tube position by observing for symmetric rise and fall of both sides of the chest and auscultation of bilateral breath sounds.

- If correct tube position is not verified, the physician should immediately reposition the tube because this is an emergency. No oxygen will be delivered to the lungs or the entire tidal volume will be delivered to one lung, placing the patient at risk for *pneumothorax.*

See the procedure for suctioning in Table 23-4 in Lewis/Collier/Heitkemper, *Medical-Surgical Nursing,* edition 4, p. 603.

Cuffs are plastic balloons that encircle the endotracheal tube. A cuff is required during endotracheal intubation because the tube passes through the epiglottis, splinting it open. The patient cannot protect the airway from aspiration.

- The nurse should record cuff pressure after intubation and once per shift to confirm that the cuff is properly inflated. (For nursing management with artificial airways, see Table 23-5 in Lewis/Collier/Heitkemper, *Medical-Surgical Nursing,* edition 4, p. 605.)

Meticulous care is required to prevent skin excoriation or pressure sores as a result of pressure from the tube, tube holder, or adhesive tape.

- To prevent this complication, the adhesive tape may be removed once a day and the tube moved to the other side of the mouth.

Table 58   Complications of Endotracheal Tubes and Nursing Management

Complications	Causes	Prevention/treatment
■ Tube obstruction	Patient biting tube; tube kinking during repositioning; cuff herniation; dried secretions, blood, or lubricant; tissue from tumor; trauma; foreign body	**Prevention:** Place bite block. Sedate patient prn. Suction prn. Humidify inspired gases. **Treatment:** Replace tube.
■ Tube displacement	Movement of patient's head; movement of tube by patient's tongue; traction on tube from ventilator tubing; self-extubation	**Prevention:** Secure tube to upper lip. Restrain patient's hands. Sedate patient prn. Ensure that only 2 inches of tube extend beyond lip. Support ventilator tubing. **Treatment:** Replace tube.
■ Sinusitis and nasal injury	Obstruction of paranasal sinus drainage; pressure necrosis of nares	**Prevention:** Avoid nasal intubations. Cushion nares from tube and tape/ties. **Treatment:** Remove all tubes from nasal passages. Administer antibiotics.

■ Tracheoesophageal fistula	Pressure necrosis of posterior tracheal wall resulting from overinflated cuff and rigid nasogastric tube	**Prevention:** Inflate cuff with minimal amount of air necessary. Monitor cuff pressures q8hr. **Treatment:** Position cuff of tube distal to fistula. Place gastrostomy tube for enteral feedings. Place esophageal tube for secretion clearance proximal to fistula.
■ Mucosal lesions	Pressure at tube and mucosal interface	**Prevention:** Inflate cuff with minimal amount of air necessary. **Treatment:** May resolve spontaneously. Perform surgical intervention.
■ Laryngeal or tracheal stenosis	Injury to area from end of tube or cuff, resulting in scar tissue formation and narrowing of airway	**Prevention:** Inflate cuff with minimal amount of air necessary. Monitor cuff pressures q8hr. Suction area above cuff frequently. **Treatment:** Perform tracheostomy. Place laryngeal stent. Perform surgical repair.
■ Cricoid abscess	Mucosal injury with bacterial invasion	**Prevention:** Inflate cuff with minimal amount of air necessary. Monitor cuff pressures q8hr. Suction area above cuff frequently. **Treatment:** Perform incision and drainage of area. Administer antibiotics.

From Thelan LA and others, editors: *Critical care nursing: diagnosis and management*, ed 2, St Louis, 1994, Mosby.

Mouth care should be provided at least once every 8 hours. The presence of an oral endotracheal tube stimulates oral secretions. If not removed, these secretions can dry and crust in the mouth and provide a medium for bacterial growth.

Complications of Endotracheal Intubation

The major complications of endotracheal (ET) intubation result from injury to the hypopharynx, larynx, and trachea and are related to the pressure exerted on upper airway structures by the tube and cuff. Improper tube placement, aspiration, oral and nasal pressure sores, and accidental extubation are also potential problems. Table 58 summarizes complications seen in patients with ET tubes.

MECHANICAL VENTILATION

Description

Mechanical ventilation is the process in which air or O_2-enriched air is moved in and out the lungs mechanically. Mechanical ventilation is not curative. It is a means of supporting patients until they recover the ability to breathe independently. Indications for mechanical ventilation are listed in Table 61-11 in Lewis/Collier/Heitkemper, *Medical-Surgical Nursing,* edition 4, p. 1973.

Types of Mechanical Ventilators

There are two major types of mechanical ventilators: negative-pressure and positive-pressure ventilators.

- Negative-pressure ventilators are composed of chambers that encase the chest or body and surround it with intermittent subatmospheric or negative pressure. Intermittent negative pressure around the chest wall causes the chest to be pulled outward. This reduces intrathoracic pressure. Air rushes in through the upper airway, which is outside the sealed chamber. Expiration is passive. An artificial airway is not required.
- Positive-pressure ventilation is the primary method used with acutely ill patients. During inspiration the ventilator forces air into the lungs under positive pressure. Unlike spontaneous ventilation, intrathoracic pressure is raised rather than lowered during lung inflation. Expiration occurs passively as in normal expiration. Positive pressure may be added during expiration, but expiration remains passive.

A nursing care plan for the patient on mechanical ventilation is presented in Lewis/Collier/Heitkemper, *Medical-Surgical Nursing,* edition 4, p. 1984.

Ostomies

Types of Ostomies

A *stoma* is created when the intestine is brought through the abdominal wall and sutured to the skin. It may be permanent or temporary. Fecal matter is diverted from the colon through the stoma to the outside of the abdominal wall.

- An *ileostomy* is an opening from the ileum through the abdominal wall and is also referred to as a *conventional* or *Brooke* ileostomy. It is most commonly used in surgical treatment of ulcerative colitis, Crohn's disease, and familial polyposis.
- A *cecostomy* is an opening between the cecum and the abdominal wall. Both cecostomies and ascending colostomies are uncommon. They are usually temporary and most often are used for fecal diversion before surgery or for palliation.
- A *colostomy* is an opening between the colon and the abdominal wall. The proximal end of the colon is sutured to the skin. The types of colostomies are shown in Figure 11.
- A *temporary colostomy* is usually performed to protect an end-to-end anastomosis after a bowel resection or as an emergency measure after bowel obstruction (e.g., malignant tumor), abdominal trauma (e.g., gunshot wound), or a perforated diverticulum. Temporary colostomies are usually located in the transverse colon.
- *Loop colostomy* and *double-barrel colostomy* are most commonly performed as temporary colostomies, but they may be permanent. A comparison of colostomies and ileostomy is shown in Table 59.

The actual procedures to perform ostomy surgeries are discussed in Chapter 40 in Lewis/Collier/Heitkemper, *Medical-Surgical Nursing,* edition 4, p. 1244.

Nursing Management

In the preoperative period it is important to review the information the patient has received from the physician. The family and the patient usually have many questions concerning the procedures.

- If available, an enterostomal therapy (ET) nurse or therapist should visit with the patient and the family.
- The nurse or ET nurse must determine the patient's ability to perform self-care, identify support systems, and determine potential adverse factors that could be modified to facilitate learning during rehabilitation.
- In some institutions the ET nurse marks the stoma site before surgery. An improperly placed stoma complicates rehabilita-

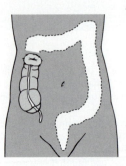
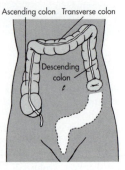

Ascending colon Transverse colon

Descending colon

Ascending colostomy

Descending colostomy

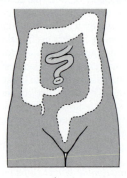

Ileostomy

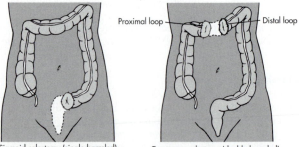

Proximal loop

Distal loop

Sigmoid colostomy (single-barreled)

Transverse colostomy (double-barreled)

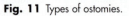

Fig. 11 Types of ostomies.

Table 59 Comparison of Colostomy and Ileostomy

	Colostomy			Ileostomy
	Ascending	Transverse	Sigmoid	
Stool consistency	Semiliquid	Semiformed	Formed	Liquid to semiliquid
Fluid requirement	Increased	Possibly increased	No change	Increased
Bowel regulation	No	Uncommon	Yes (if there is a history of a regular bowel pattern)	No
Appliance and skin barriers	Yes	Yes	Dependent on regulation	Yes
Irrigation	No	No	Possible every 24-48 hr (if patient meets criteria)	No
Indications for surgery	Perforating diverticulitis in lower colon; trauma; inoperable tumors of colon, rectum, or pelvis; rectovaginal fistula	Same as for ascending; birth defect	Cancer of the rectum or rectosigmoidal area; perforating diverticulum; trauma	Ulcerative colitis, Crohn's disease; diseased or injured colon, birth defect, familial polyposis, trauma, cancer

tion by increasing time and expense of pouch change routine. It can also contribute to skin irritation and poor adaptation.

- The patient and the family should understand the extent of surgery and the type of stoma and its care.
- If the patient desires a referral and the physician agrees, a trained ostomy visitor from the United Ostomy Association can provide meaningful psychologic support.

Colostomy Care

Postoperative nursing care should focus on assessing the stoma, protecting the skin, selecting the pouch, and assisting the patient to adapt psychologically to a changed body. See the nursing care plan for the patient with a colostomy or ileostomy in Lewis/Collier/Heitkemper, *Medical-Surgical Nursing,* edition 4, p. 1228.

The stoma should be pink. A dusky-blue stoma indicates ischemia and a brown-black stoma indicates necrosis. The nurse should assess and document stoma color every 8 hours until the stoma remains pink for 3 days. There is mild to moderate swelling of the stoma the first 2 to 3 weeks after surgery. A skin barrier should be applied to protect the peristomal suture line and skin surrounding the stoma. Solid skin barriers include Stomahesive (Convatec), karaya, and Comfeel (Coloplast). The skin should be washed with warm water and dried thoroughly before the barrier is applied.

- With an open-ended, transparent, plastic, odor-proof pouch it is easy to protect the skin and to observe and collect the drainage. The pouch must fit snugly to prevent leakage around the stoma. The size of the stoma is determined with a stoma measuring card. Although the pouch is usually applied after surgery, the colostomy does not function until 2 to 4 days postoperatively, when peristalsis has been adequately restored.
- The volume, color, and consistency of the drainage are recorded. Each time the pouch is changed, the condition of the skin is observed for irritation. A pouch should *never* be placed directly on irritated skin.
- A colostomy in the ascending and transverse colon has semiliquid stools and is more difficult to regulate than a colostomy on the left side of the colon. The patient needs to be instructed to use a drainable pouch. A colostomy in the sigmoid or descending colon has semiformed or formed stools and can be regulated by the irrigation method. The patient may or may not wear a drainage pouch. A nondrainable pouch should have a gas filter.
- For most patients with colostomies, there are few, if any, dietary restrictions. A well-balanced diet and adequate fluid intake is important. The patient's medical and surgical history need to be considered when individualizing dietary instructions. For the effects of various foods on stoma output, see

Table 40-32 in Lewis/Collier/Heitkemper, *Medical-Surgical Nursing,* edition 4, p. 1247.

Colostomy irrigations are intended to regulate bowel function, treat constipation, or prepare the bowel for surgery. If control is achieved, there should be little or no spillage between irrigations. The patient who establishes regularity may need to wear only a pad or cover over the stoma. The patient who cannot or chooses not to establish regularity by irrigations must wear a pouch at all times. The procedure for colostomy irrigation is presented in Table 60.

- The procedure should not be rushed; the patient should feel relaxed. The patient or family member must be instructed in the procedure and must be able to demonstrate the ability to irrigate before being independent. This can be done in the outpatient setting.

Patient Teaching

- The patient should be able to perform skin care, control odor, care for the stoma, and identify signs and symptoms of complications. The patient should know the importance of fluids and food in the diet, have names and addresses of the United Ostomy Association, and know when to seek medical care. Outpatient follow-up by an ET nurse is recommended.
- Patients need to be discharged with written pouch change instructions, teaching literature relevant to the type of stoma they have, a list of equipment they use (including names and phone numbers), a list of equipment retailers, outpatient follow-up appointments with the surgeon and ET nurse, and the phone numbers of the surgeon and nurse.

Ileostomy Care

Care of the ileostomy is presented in the nursing care plan for the patient with a colostomy or ileostomy in Lewis/Collier/Heitkemper, *Medical-Surgical Nursing,* edition 4, p. 1228.

- Immediately after surgery, intake and output must be accurately monitored. The patient should be observed for signs and symptoms of fluid and electrolyte imbalance, particularly potassium, sodium, and fluid deficits.
- In the first 24 to 48 hours after surgery the amount of drainage from the stoma may be negligible. Once peristalsis returns, the patient may experience a period of high volume output of 1000 to 1800 ml per day. Later on the average amount can be 500 to 800 ml daily.

Patient Teaching

The patient should be instructed to drink at least 1 to 2 L of fluid daily; more may be necessary when diarrhea occurs and in the summer, when perspiration is increased. Diarrhea from an ileostomy produces acidosis from the loss of bicarbonate. The physician may instruct the patient to take an electrolyte solution at home (e.g., 1

Table 60	Equipment and Procedure for Colostomy Irrigation

Equipment
　　Lubricant
　　Irrigation set (1000-2000 ml container, tubing with irrigating
　　　　cone, clamp)
　　Irrigating sleeve with adhesive or belt
　　Toilet tissue to clean around stoma
　　Disposal sack for soiled dressing

Procedure
　　1. Place 500-1000 ml of lukewarm water (not to exceed
　　　　105° F) [40.5° C] in container. Volume is titrated for indi-
　　　　vidual; use enough irrigant to distend bowel but not
　　　　enough to cause cramping pain. Most adults use 500-
　　　　1000 ml of water.
　　2. Ensure comfortable position. Patient may sit in chair in
　　　　front of toilet.
　　3. Clear tubing of all air by flushing it with fluid.
　　4. Hang container on hook or IV pole (18-24 in) above
　　　　stoma (about shoulder height).
　　5. Apply irrigating sheath and place bottom end in bed pan
　　　　or toilet bowl.
　　6. Lubricate cone and insert cone tip gently into stoma and
　　　　hold tip securely in place to prevent back flow.
　　7. Allow irrigation solution to flow in steadily for 5-10 min.
　　8. If cramping occurs, stop the flow of solution for few sec-
　　　　onds, leaving cone in place.
　　9. Clamp tubing and remove irrigating cone when desired
　　　　amount of irrigant has been delivered or when patient
　　　　senses colonic distention.
　10. Allow 30-45 min for solution and feces to be expelled.
　　　　Initial evacuation is usually complete in 10-15 min. Close
　　　　off irrigating sheath at bottom to allow ambulation.
　11. Clean, rinse, and dry peristomal skin well.
　12. Replace colostomy drainage pouch or desired stoma
　　　　covering.
　13. Wash and rinse all equipment and hang to dry.

teaspoon of salt and 1 teaspoon of baking soda in 1 quart of water). Fluids rich in electrolytes should be encouraged.

- Usually a low-roughage diet is ordered initially. Fiber-containing foods are reintroduced gradually. Later there are no dietary restrictions except for foods that are troublesome (e.g., high roughage-popcorn) for the patient. Return to a normal, presurgical diet is the goal.
- The ileal stoma often bleeds easily when it is touched because it has a high vascular supply. The patient should be told that minimal oozing of blood is normal.

General Nursing Considerations Related to Ostomies

- The patient should not be forced to learn to care for the ostomy. The nurse should watch for clues that the patient is ready. Teaching at the appropriate time is an important part of the care and can contribute to a smooth adjustment process.
- Supportive measures by nursing include helping the patient acquire knowledge, providing or recommending support services, and identifying coping mechanisms that are effective. The nurse provides support by responding to the physiologic needs of stoma care and the psychosocial needs of self-esteem.
- Discussion of sexuality and sexual function need to be incorporated in the plan of care. The nurse can help the patient understand that sexual function or sexual activity may be affected, but sexual intimacy does not have to be altered.
- The social impact of the stoma is interrelated with the psychologic, physical, and sexual aspects. Concerns of people with stomas include the ability to resume sexual activity, altering clothing styles, the effect on daily activities, sleeping while wearing a pouch, passing gas, the presence of odor, cleanliness, and deciding when or if to tell others about the ostomy.

OXYGEN THERAPY

Description

The goal of O_2 therapy is to supply the patient with adequate O_2 to maximize the O_2-carrying ability of blood. O_2 is usually administered to treat hypoxemia caused by (1) respiratory disorders such as chronic obstructive pulmonary disease (COPD), cor pulmonale, pneumonia, atelectasis, lung cancer, and pulmonary emboli; (2) cardiovascular disorders such as myocardial infarction, dysrhythmias, angina pectoris, and cardiogenic shock; and (3) central nervous system (CNS) disorders such as overdose of narcotics, head injury, and disordered sleep (sleep apnea).

Methods of Administration

There are various methods of O_2 administration (see Table 24-13 in Lewis/Collier/Heitkemper, *Medical-Surgical Nursing,* edition 4, p. 648). The method of administration selected depends on factors such as fraction of inspiratory O_2 (FIO_2) and humidification required, patient cooperation, and comfort. Various methods include nasal cannula, face mask, nasal catheter, rebreathing and nonrebreathing masks, transtracheal catheter, and Venturi mask.

- Oxygen obtained from cylinders or wall systems is dry. Dry O_2 has an irritating effect on mucous membranes and dries secretions. Therefore it is important that O_2 be humidified when administered, either by humidification or nebulization.

Complications

O_2 supports combustion and increases the rate of burning. This is why it is important that smoking be prohibited in the area in which O_2 is being used. A "No Smoking" sign should be prominently displayed on the patient's door. The patient should also be cautioned against smoking with O_2 prongs or a catheter in place.

- In some cases of respiratory distress, such as long-standing COPD, increasing O_2 flow rate may be quite harmful. When O_2 is administered in high concentrations, the hypoxic stimulus is eliminated and the rate and depth of ventilation decreases. The patient will subsequently develop hypercapnia and eventually *CO_2 narcosis.* The patient's mental status and vital signs should be assessed before starting O_2 therapy and frequently thereafter.

Infection can be a major hazard of O_2 administration. Heated nebulizers present the highest risk. Constant use of humidity supports bacterial growth with the most common infecting organism *Pseudomonas aeruginosa.* Disposable equipment that operates as a closed system should be used and changed every 48 hours to prevent infection. There should be a hospital policy stating the required frequency of equipment changes based on the type of equipment. Both equipment and respiratory secretions should be gram-stained and cultured frequently.

Chronic Oxygen Therapy at Home

An improved prognosis has been noted in patients with COPD who receive nocturnal or continuous O_2 to treat hypoxemia. The longer continuous daily use of O_2 is maintained, the greater the improvement.

- Periodic reevaluations are necessary for the patient who is using chronic supplemental O_2. Generally the patient should be reevaluated every 6 months during the first year of therapy and annually after that, as long as patient remains stable.

Nursing Management
Goals
The patient receiving O_2 will have no skin breakdown from the breathing device, no complaints of mucosal discomfort, no evidence of respiratory infection, and no evidence of fire due to the presence of O_2.

See the nursing care plan for the patient receiving oxygen in Lewis/Collier/Heitkemper, *Medical-Surgical Nursing,* edition 4, p. 651.

Nursing Diagnoses/Collaborative Problems
- Risk for impaired skin integrity related to the O_2 administration device and humidity
- Risk for injury related to fire hazard secondary to O_2-enriched environment
- Risk for infection related to presence of environmental pathogens and bacterial contamination of equipment
- Altered oral and nasal mucous membranes related to O_2 therapy
- Potential complication: CO_2 narcosis in patient with COPD related to excessive O_2 administration in a person with hypercapnia
- Potential complication: O_2 toxicity related to enriched O_2 environment

Patient Teaching
- Teach patient and family not to increase O_2 flow rate unless directed to do so by a physician or nurse to prevent problems related to removing the patient's hypoxic drive.
- Teach patient about precautions related to home O_2 therapy to eliminate the risk of fire at home.

PACEMAKERS

Description
The artificial cardiac pacemaker is an electronic device used in place of the sinoatrial (SA) node, the natural cardiac pacemaker of the heart. The artificial cardiac pacemaker is an electrical circuit in which the battery provides electricity that travels through a conducting wire to the myocardium, and the myocardium stimulates the heart to beat (i.e., it "captures" the heart).
- Recent advances in technology have been applied extensively to pacemakers. This has resulted in sophisticated, noninvasive,

programmable single- and dual-chambered pacemakers with specialized circuits that weigh only 40 to 50 g. Pacemakers have been developed that are more physiologically accurate, pacing both atrium and ventricle, and increasing the heart rate when appropriate

Types of Pacemakers

Permanent pacemakers are those that are implanted totally within the body and *temporary pacemakers* are those with the power source outside the body.

- The permanent pacemaker power source is implanted subcutaneously in the chest or abdomen and is attached to pacer electrodes, which are threaded transvenously to right ventricle or right atrium. Indications for insertion of a permanent pacemaker are listed in Table 61.
- Temporary pacemakers are used with a lead or wire threaded transvenously to the right ventricle and with a wire attached to a power source externally. Indications for temporary pacing are listed in Table 62.

Complications

Pacemaker malfunction is manifested by failure to sense or failure to capture. *Failure to sense* occurs when the pacemaker fails to recognize spontaneous atrial or ventricular activity, and it fires inappropriately. Failure to sense may be caused by pacer lead fracture, battery failure, or displacement of electrode. *Failure to capture* occurs when electrical charge to myocardium is insufficient to produce atrial or ventricular contraction. Failure to capture may be caused by pacer lead fracture, battery failure, electrode displacement, or fibrosis at the electrode tip.

Table 61	Indications for Permanent Pacemaker Therapy

Sinus node dysfunction
Third-degree AV block
Fibrosis or sclerotic changes of cardiac conduction system
Sick sinus syndrome
Mobitz II second-degree AV block
Hypersensitive carotid sinus syndrome
Chronic atrial fibrillation with slow ventricular response

AV, Atrioventricular.

Table 62	**Indications for Temporary Pacing**

- Maintenance of adequate HR and rhythm during special circumstances such as surgery and postoperative recovery, cardiac catheterization or coronary angioplasty, during drug therapy that may cause bradycardia, and before implantation of a permanent pacemaker
- As prophylaxis after open heart surgery
- Acute anterior MI with second-degree or third-degree AV block or bundle branch block
- Acute inferior MI with symptomatic bradycardia and AV block
- Termination of AV nodal reentry or reciprocating tachycardia associated with WPW syndrome, atrial flutter, or ventricular tachycardia
- Suppression of ectopic atrial or ventricular rhythm
- Electrophysiologic studies to evaluate patient with bradydysrhythmias and tachydysrhythmias

AV, Atrioventricular; *HR*, heart rate; *MI*, myocardial infarction; *WPW*, Wolff-Parkinson-White.

Complications of invasive temporary or permanent pacemaker insertion include infection and hematoma formation at the site of insertion of pacemaker power source, pneumothorax, failure to sense or capture with possible bradycardia and significant symptoms, perforation of atrial or ventricular septum by pacing wire, and appearance of "end-of-life" battery parameters on testing the pacemaker.

- Measures taken to prevent and assess complications include prophylactic IV antibiotic therapy before and after insertion, assessment of chest x-ray after insertion to check lead placement and to rule out the presence of pneumothorax, careful observation of insertion site, and continuous ECG monitoring of patient's rhythm.
- After pacemaker insertion the patient is maintained on bed rest for 24 hours, and minimal arm and shoulder activity is allowed to prevent dislodgement of newly implanted pacemaker leads.

Nursing Management

Nursing interventions include observation for signs of infection by assessing the incision for redness, swelling or discharge; temperature elevation should also be noted. Careful monitoring of patient's rhythm is used to detect problems with sensing or capturing.

- The patient with a newly implanted pacemaker may frequently have many questions about activity restrictions and fears concerning body image and becoming a "cardiac cripple" after the procedure.
- The goal of pacemaker therapy should be to enhance physiologic functioning and quality of life. This should be emphasized to the patient, and the nurse should give concrete advice on activity restrictions. Basic information for the patient with a pacemaker is outlined in Table 63.

Table 63	Educational Information for Patients with Pacemakers

- Maintain follow-up care with a physician because it is important to check pacemaker site and to begin regular pacemaker function checks with magnet and ECG evaluation.
- Watch for signs of infection at incision site (e.g., redness, swelling, drainage).
- Keep incision dry for 1 wk after discharge.
- For activity restriction, avoid direct blows to generator site. (Avoid contact sports such as football or use of rifle.)
- Avoid close proximity to high-output electrical generators or to large magnets such as MRI scanner. These devices can reprogram pacemaker.
- Microwave ovens are perfectly safe to use and do not threaten pacemaker function.
- Travel without restrictions is allowed. Metal case of small implanted pacemaker rarely sets off an airport security alarm.
- Learn how to take pulse rate.
- Carry pacemaker information card at all times, preferably in an easily accessible place such as wallet or purse.

RADIATION THERAPY

Description

Radiation therapy is a local treatment modality for cancer. An estimated 60% of all persons with cancer will receive radiation therapy in treating their disease.

- Radiation is the emission and distribution of energy through space or a material medium. The target of radiation is deoxyribonucleic acid (DNA) damage, resulting in an irreversible loss of proliferative capacity. Cancer cells that are more likely to be dividing are at increased risk for permanent damage with cumulative radiation doses. Normal cells usually recover from radiation damage if therapy is kept within certain doses.
- Cellular sensitivity to radiation varies throughout the cell cycle with cells being most sensitive to lethal damage in the M and G_2 phases and least sensitive to damage during the S or synthesis phase. Damage to DNA in cells that are not in the M phase will be expressed when division occurs.
- Table 64 describes the radiosensitivity of various cancerous tumors.

Types of Radiation Therapy

- *External radiation* therapy (telepathy) is given by external beam and is the most common form of treatment.
- *Internal radiation* (brachytherapy) means "close" treatment and consists of implantation or insertion of radioactive materials directly into the tumor or in close proximity to the tumor. This method is commonly used for tumors of the head and neck and gynecologic malignancies. Implants, such as prostate implants, may also be permanent with insertion of radioactive seeds into tumors.

Side Effects of Therapy

Possible side effects from radiation therapy may be divided into phases: *acute effects* occur during treatment and for up to 6 months after completion of therapy, *subacute effects* occur in the next 6 months after completion of therapy, and *late effects* occur 1 year and beyond.

- Actively proliferating tissue, such as GI mucosa, esophageal and oropharyngeal mucosa, and bone marrow, exhibit early, acute responses to radiation therapy. Cartilage, bone, kidney, and central and peripheral nervous tissue manifest subacute or late responses.

Table 64 ·· **Tumor Radiosensitivity**

High	Moderate	Mild	Poor
Ovarian dysgerminoma	Skin carcinoma	Soft tissue sarcomas (e.g., chondrosarcoma)	Osteosarcoma
Testicular seminoma	Oropharyngeal carcinoma	Gastric adenocarcinoma	Malignant melanoma
Hodgkin's disease	Esophageal carcinoma	Renal adenocarcinoma	Malignant gliomas
Non-Hodgkin's lymphoma	Breast adenocarcinoma	Colon adenocarcinoma	Testicular nonseminoma
Wilms' tumor	Uterine and cervical carcinoma		
Neuroblastoma	Prostate carcinoma		
	Bladder carcinoma		

- Common radiation therapy side effects are fatigue, anorexia, bone marrow suppression, erythema, mucositis, nausea, vomiting, diarrhea, cough, fever, night sweats, and changes in functioning of the ovaries and testes.

Nursing Management

Caring for the person with an implant requires that the nurse be aware that the patient is radioactive. If a patient has a temporary implant, the patient is radioactive during the time the source is in place. If the patient has a permanent implant, radioactive exposure to the outside and others is low, and the patient may be discharged with precautions.

- Helping the patient to cope with the anxiety of receiving radiation is an essential component of the nursing role. The necessity of coming for treatment five times per week forces the individual to confront the cancer on an almost daily basis.
- Demands on the patient and family and the disruption of normal activities created by the treatment schedule are difficult to handle. In conjunction with the social worker, the nurse needs to assist with planning for transportation with available resources such as the American Cancer Society, churches, and community resources.
- The impact of radiation on the quality of life of the patient undergoing therapy may be minimized with information and support.

For nursing management of anorexia, skin and oral reactions, GI reactions, pulmonary effects, and reproductive effects associated with radiation therapy, see Lewis/Collier/Heitkemper, *Medical-Surgical Nursing,* edition 4, pp. 282-288.

SURGICAL PROCEDURES INVOLVING THE FEMALE REPRODUCTIVE SYSTEM

Types of Surgical Procedures

A variety of surgical procedures are carried out when either benign or malignant tumors of the female reproductive system are found.

Hysterectomy. A hysterectomy may be done either vaginally or abdominally. A vaginal route is often used when vaginal repair is to be done in addition to removal of the uterus. The abdominal route is used when large tumors are present and the pelvic cavity is to be explored or when the tubes and ovaries are to be removed at the same time. The abdominal route can present more postoperative problems because it involves an incision and the opening of the abdominal cavity. In both vaginal and abdominal hysterectomies the ligaments that support the uterus are attached to the vaginal cuff so that the normal depth of the vagina is maintained.

Salpingectomy and oophorectomy. Postoperative care of the woman who has undergone removal of a fallopian tube *(salpingectomy)* or an ovary *(oophorectomy)* is similar to that for any patient having abdominal surgery. One exception is that if a large ovarian cyst is removed, there may be abdominal distention because of the sudden release of pressure in the intestines.

- When both ovaries are removed *(bilateral oophorectomy),* surgical menopause results. The symptoms are similar to those of regular menopause but may be more severe because of the sudden withdrawal of hormones. Attempts are made to leave at least a portion of an ovary.
- Replacement therapy with estrogen is given to most patients to preserve secondary sex characteristics, avoid symptoms of menopause, and to prevent bone loss and the development of osteoporosis.

Vulvectomy. Although cancer of the vulva is relatively uncommon, the extent of the required surgery and the psychologic implications for the patient demand the best in nursing management.

- It is important that the nurse recognize the extent of the vulvectomy and the impact it will have on the patient's life. An honest, open attitude with the patient and her partner preoperatively can be most helpful in the postoperative period.

Pelvic exenteration. When other forms of therapy are ineffective in the treatment of cancer and no metastases have been found outside of the pelvis, pelvic exenteration may be performed.

- Although different types are done, this radical surgery usually involves removal of the uterus, ovaries, fallopian tubes, vagina, bladder, urethra, and pelvic lymph nodes. In some situations the descending colon, rectum, and anal canal may also be removed. Candidates for this procedure are selected on the basis of their likelihood of surviving the surgery and their ability to adjust to and accept the resulting limitations.

Nursing Management of Gynecologic Tumors
Goals
The patient with a gynecologic tumor will actively participate in treatment decisions, achieve satisfactory pain and symptom management, recognize and report problems promptly, maintain preferred lifestyle as long as possible, and continue to practice cancer detection strategies.

See the nursing care plan for the patient with total abdominal hysterectomy in Lewis/Collier/Heitkemper, *Medical-Surgical Nursing,* edition 4, p. 1609.

Nursing Diagnoses
- Anxiety related to threats of a malignancy and lack of knowledge related to disease process and prognosis
- Pain related to pressure secondary to enlarging tumor
- Body image disturbance related to loss of body part
- Altered sexuality patterns related to physiologic limitations and fatigue
- Anticipatory grieving related to poor prognosis of the disease

Nursing Interventions

Although early diagnosis and treatment of tumors of the female reproductive tract have improved, a relatively high associated death rate remains. The chief reason may be that women do not sufficiently participate in good preventive care.

- In their many contacts with women, nurses can play a major role in advocating preventive care. Nurses have to be well informed about reproductive tract screening schedules and malignancies, especially the early signs and symptoms, and the various diagnostic studies and treatment measures available.

A detailed description of postoperative nursing care for each of these surgical procedures, and internal and external radiation therapy for cervical and uterine cancer is provided in Lewis/Collier/Heitkemper, *Medical-Surgical Nursing,* edition 4, pp. 1616-1620.

TOTAL PARENTERAL NUTRITION

Description

Total parenteral nutrition (TPN) (also called hyperalimentation) is a relatively safe and practical method for delivering total nutritional needs by an IV route. TPN is used when the GI tract cannot be used for the ingestion, digestion, and/or absorption of essential nutrients.

- The goal of TPN is to keep the patient in positive nitrogen balance and to allow for growth of new body tissue, which can be drastically depleted by prolonged inability to eat normally.
- Indications for TPN include patients with severe injury, surgery, or burns and those who are malnourished as a result of medical treatment or disease processes. Regular IV glucose solutions contain no protein and have 170 cal/L, whereas TPN contains protein, dextrose (20%-50%), electrolytes, trace elements, vitamins, and possibly fat emulsion.
- All TPN solutions should be prepared by a pharmacist or trained technician using strict aseptic techniques under a laminar flow hood. Nothing should be added to hyperalimentation solutions after they are prepared by the pharmacy.

Administration of TPN

TPN may be administered via a central line into the superior vena cava (most common route) or through a peripherally inserted central (PIC) catheter usually placed into the basilic or cephalic vein.

- Central hyperalimentation is indicated when long-term nutritional support is necessary, when the patient has high protein and caloric requirements, and when suitable peripheral veins are not available.
- Peripheral parenteral nutrition (PPN) is administered through a large peripheral vein when (1) nutritional support is needed for only a short time (up to 2 weeks), (2) protein and caloric requirements are not excessively high, (3) the risk of a central catheter is too great, or (4) nutritional support is used to supplement inadequate oral intake.
- Once established for TPN, a single-lumen central catheter should not be used for the administration of blood or antibiotics, the drawing of blood samples, or central venous pressure monitoring.

Nursing Management

Infection is one of the major concerns with TPN solutions. It is essential that proper aseptic techniques be followed.

- Millipore filters should be placed on all parenteral lines. When the filter is used, it should be placed proximal to the catheter hub. Filters are changed every 24 hours.
- New IV tubing is changed with each new bottle of TPN. Tubing and the filter should be clearly labeled with the date and the time they are put into use.

A metabolic complication of parenteral nutrition is hyperglycemia. At the beginning of TPN therapy the solution is infused at a gradually increasing rate over a 24- to 48-hour period. In this way the pancreas can adapt to the increased amount of glucose in the circulation by producing more insulin.

- Blood glucose levels should be checked at the bedside every 4 to 6 hours with a glucose-testing meter. A sliding scale of insulin may be ordered to keep the level below 180 to 200 mg/dl.

Nurses must be aware that speeding or slowing the infusion rate is contraindicated. Speeding up the rate results in a large amount of glucose entering the circulation. Conversely, slowing the rate may result in a hypoglycemic state because it takes time for the pancreatic islet cells to adjust to a reduced glucose level.

- Checking the amount infused and the rate every ½ to 1 hour is recommended. An infusion pump should be used during administration of TPN so that the infusion rate can be maintained and an alarm will sound if the tubing becomes obstructed.

Solutions must also be examined for signs of contamination, such as a cloudy appearance. If contamination is suspected, the solution should be promptly returned to the pharmacy for replacement. It is the nurse's responsibility to ensure that the TPN solution is discontinued and replaced with a new solution if it is still infusing at the end of 24 hours.

Vital signs should be monitored every 4 hours. Daily weights give an indication of the patient's nutritional status as therapy progresses. Blood levels of glucose, electrolytes, and protein; a complete blood cell count; and enzyme studies are followed daily or every other day.

Dressings covering the catheter site are changed according to institutional protocol, from every other day to once a week. Frequently, specially trained nurses from the IV team or the nutritional support team are responsible for these dressing changes. Some institutions allow the staff nurses to do the dressing changes after special instruction.

- The procedure for changing the dressing is similar to that followed after catheter insertion. The institutional routine should be followed.
- The site is carefully observed for signs of inflammation and infection. Phlebitis can readily occur in the vein as a result of the hypertonic infusion and can become infected. In immunosuppressed patients signs of inflammation or infection can be subtle, if present at all.
- If an infection is suspected during a dressing change, a culture specimen of the site and drainage should be sent for analysis and the physician should be notified immediately.
- If the patient exhibits signs and symptoms of a systemic infection, the catheter tip is usually suspect unless another cause can be found. Cultures of blood, sputum, urine, wound drainage, and the catheter tip, if it has been removed, are done at once. A chest x-ray is taken to detect changes in pulmonary status.
- The current bottle of TPN solution with tubing and filter should also be cultured and replaced with an entirely new setup.
- A new central line may be immediately established or replaced by a peripheral route. It is important that a glucose source be maintained to prevent rebound hypoglycemia.

Additional information related to nursing management of TPN is presented in the the nursing care plan for the patient receiving total parenteral nutrition in Lewis/Collier/Heitkemper, *Medical-Surgical Nursing,* edition 4, p. 1121.

Tracheostomy

Description

A *tracheotomy* is a surgical incision into the trachea for the purpose of establishing an airway. A *tracheostomy* is the tracheal stoma or opening that results from a tracheotomy. Correct placement of the tube requires careful dissection; for this reason a tracheotomy is not performed as an emergency unless required to relieve upper airway obstruction. A tracheotomy can be performed in the ICU with the patient under local anesthesia, but it is performed most frequently in the operating room.

Indications for tracheostomy are to bypass an upper airway obstruction, facilitate removal of secretions, facilitate weaning from a respirator by reducing anatomic dead space and lowering airway resistance, permit long-term mechanical ventilation, and improve patient comfort. Patient comfort may be increased because no tube is present in the mouth.

- The patient can eat and speak if the tracheostomy cuff can be deflated or a speaking tube is used. Because the tube is more secure, patient mobility is increased.
- Most clinicians believe a tracheostomy should be performed after 7 to 10 days of mechanical ventilation if extubation is not possible, or earlier if it appears likely that an extended period of mechanical ventilation will be required.
- When the patient can expectorate secretions and maintain adequate gas exchange without mechanical ventilation, the tracheostomy tube can be removed. The stoma is covered with dressing and tape. Epithelial tissue begins to form in 24 to 48 hours, and the opening will close in several days.

Nursing Management

Goals

The patient with a tracheostomy will communicate needs, maintain a patent airway, have a normal white blood cell (WBC) count and temperature, have usual appetite with normal body weight maintained, and have normal swallowing function.

See the nursing care plan for the patient with a tracheostomy in Lewis/Collier/Heitkemper *Medical-Surgical Nursing,* edition 4, p. 608.

Nursing Diagnoses/Collaborative Problems

- Ineffective airway clearance related to difficulty expectorating sputum
- Altered nutrition: less than body requirements related to decreased oral intake, altered taste sensation, and swallowing difficulty

- Impaired verbal communication related to use of artificial airway and cuff
- Impaired swallowing related to tracheostomy tube
- Ineffective management of therapeutic regimen related to lack of knowledge about care of tracheostomy at home
- Risk for infection related to bypass of airway defense mechanisms and impaired skin integrity
- Potential complication: hypoxemia related to misplaced or improperly functioning tube

Nursing Interventions

- Before the tracheotomy the nurse should explain to the patient and family the purpose of the procedure and inform them that the patient will not be able to speak if an inflated cuff is used. Patient and family should be told that normal speech will be possible as soon as the cuff can be deflated.

Care should be taken not to dislodge the tracheostomy tube during the first few days when the stoma is not mature or healed.

- Because tube replacement can be difficult, several precautions are required: (1) a replacement tube of equal or smaller size is kept at the bedside, readily available for emergency reinsertion, (2) the first tube change is performed by a physician usually no sooner than 7 days after tracheotomy, and (3) tracheostomy tapes are not changed for at least 24 hours after the insertion procedure.
- Retention sutures are often placed in the tracheal cartilage when the tracheostomy is performed. The free ends should be taped to the skin in a place and manner that leaves them accessible if the tube is dislodged.
- The cleaning procedure removes mucus that has accumulated on the inside of the tube. If humidification is adequate, this accumulation of mucus should not occur and a tube without an inner cannula can be used. See Table 65 for a listing of tracheostomy care.

Patient Teaching

- Assess ability of patient and family to provide care at home, including airway care and ability to respond appropriately to emergencies to determine if home care is feasible.
- Teach clean suction technique, good hand washing, home preparation of sterile saline solution, use of one catheter for 24 hours, methods of cleaning and reusing catheters, and clean technique for tracheostomy care.
- Make referral for visiting nurse or home care to provide ongoing assistance and support.
- Provide opportunities for patient to discuss care and concerns about caring for tracheostomy at home to alleviate anxiety.

Table 65	**Tracheostomy Care**

1. Explain procedure to patient.
2. Collect necessary sterile equipment such as suction catheter, gloves, water, basin, drape, tracheostomy ties, tube brush or pipe cleaners (usually in a disposable set), 4 × 4s, hydrogen peroxide (3%), and tracheostomy dressing (optional).
3. Position patient in semi-Fowler's position.
4. Assemble needed materials on bedside table next to patient.
5. Suction and oxygenate patient.
6. Wash hands. Put on goggles and gloves.
7. Unlock and remove inner cannula.*
8. If disposable inner cannula is used, replace with new cannula. If nondisposable cannula is used:

    Immerse inner cannula in 3% hydrogen peroxide and clean inside and outside of cannula with tube brush or pipe cleaners.

    Drain hydrogen peroxide from cannula. Immerse cannula in sterile water. Remove from sterile water and shake dry.

    Insert inner cannula into outer cannula with curved part downward; lock in place.
9. Remove dried secretions from stoma with 4 × 4 pad soaked in hydrogen peroxide. Rinse with sterile water and another 4 × 4 pad. Gently pat dry area around stoma.
10. Change tracheostomy ties.† *To prevent accidental tube removal,* secure tracheostomy tube by gently applying pressure to flange of tube.
11. As alternative, patient may prefer tracheostomy ties made of Velcro, which are easier to adjust. Plastic intravenous tubing may also be preferred because it is easily cleaned and dries without need to replace ties.
12. Unless excessive amounts of exudate, avoid using tracheostomy dressing. If drainage is excessive, place dressing around tube. Change dressing frequently.

---

*Many tracheostomy tubes do not have inner cannulas. Care for these tubes includes all steps except those for inner cannula care.
†Do not change tracheostomy ties for 24 hours after tracheotomy procedure.

TUBE FEEDING

Indications for tube feeding as a supplemental form of nutrition include:

- The patient who has a functioning GI tract but cannot take oral nourishment
- Persons with anorexia, orofacial fractures, head and neck cancer, neurologic or psychiatric conditions that prevent oral intake, extensive burns, and those who are receiving chemotherapy or radiation therapy

Tube feedings are easily administered, safer, more physiologically efficient, and less expensive than parenteral nutrition. They are used to provide nutrients by way of the GI tract (alone or as a supplement to oral or parenteral nutrition) or as a treatment for malnutrition.

Types of feeding tubes include:

- Nastrogastric (NG) tube, which is most commonly used for short-term problems
- Esophagostomy, gastrostomy, or jejunostomy tubes for extended feeding
- Transpyloric tube placement for feeding below the pyloric spinchter

The procedure for tube feeding includes (1) having the patient sitting or lying with the head of bed elevated 30 to 45 degrees, (2) maintaining tube patency by irrigating after feeding; if feedings are continuous, monitor built-in alarm on feeding pump, and (3) checking proper tube placement before each feeding and with continuous feedings every 4 hours.

Nursing considerations include the following:

- The patient should be weighed daily or several times a week.
- Accurate intake and output records should be maintained
- Frequent blood glucose checks must be done if the patient is prone to the development of nonketotic-hyperosmolar hyperglycemia from high-glucose formula feedings.
- Feedings that have been opened and not refrigerated or feedings that have been infusing longer than 8 hours should be discarded to minimize bacterial growth.
- If a pump is being used, the tubing should be changed every 24 hours.

Additional information on tube feeding is discussed in Lewis/Collier/Heitkemper, *Medical-Surgical Nursing,* edition 4, p. 1115.

PART THREE

REFERENCE APPENDIX

BLOOD GASES
Normal Values

	Arterial (sea level)	**Venous**
pH	7.35-7.45	7.34-7.37
pO_2*	80-100 mm Hg	30-40 mm Hg
pCO_2	35-45 mm Hg	41-51 mm Hg
HCO_3^-	22-26 mEq/L	24-30 mEq/L
O_2 sat	95%-99%	60%-80%
Base excess	-2 to $+2$	0 to $+4$

*In a patient >60 years old, PaO_2 is equal to 80 mm Hg minus 1 mm Hg for every year over 60. Expected $PaO_2 = FIO_2 \times 5$.

Interpreting ABGs

1. Check pH $\uparrow$ = Alkalosis; $\downarrow$ = acidosis
2. Check pCO_2 $\uparrow$ = CO_2 retention (hypoventilation); respiratory acidosis or compensating for metabolic alkalosis
   $\downarrow$ = CO_2 blown off (hyperventilation); respiratory alkalosis or compensating for metabolic acidosis
3. Check HCO_3^- $\uparrow$ = Nonvolatile acid is lost; HCO_3^- gained (metabolic alkalosis or compensating for respiratory acidosis)
   $\downarrow$ = Nonvolatile acid is added; HCO_3^- is lost (metabolic acidosis or compensating for respiratory alkalosis)
4. Determine imbalance
5. Determine if compensation exists

Determining the Imbalance in ABGs

If: pH $\uparrow$ and pCO_2 $\downarrow$
or
pH $\downarrow$ and pCO_2 $\uparrow$ **Then** respiratory disorder

If: pH $\uparrow$ and HCO_3^- $\uparrow$
or
pH $\downarrow$ and HCO_3^- $\downarrow$ **Then** metabolic disorder

If: pCO_2 $\uparrow$ and HCO_3^- $\uparrow$
or
pCO_2 $\downarrow$ and HCO_3^- $\downarrow$ **Then** compensation is occurring

If: pCO_2 $\uparrow$ and HCO_3^- $\downarrow$
or
pCO_2 $\downarrow$ and HCO_3^- $\uparrow$ **Then** mixed imbalance

BLOOD LABORATORY VALUES

Test	Conventional Units	SI Units
Complete Blood Count		
RBC	$4.5\text{-}6.0 \times 10^6/\mu L$ (males)	$4.5\text{-}6.0 \times 10^{12}/L$
	$4.0\text{-}5.0 \times 10^6/\mu L$ (females)	$4.0\text{-}5.0 \times 10^{12}/L$
WBC	$4.0\text{-}11.0 \times 10^3/\mu L$	$4.0\text{-}11.0 \times 10^9/L$
Hb	13.5-18 g/dl (males)	135-180 g/L
	12-16 g/dl (females)	120-160 g/L
Hct	40%-51% (males)	0.40-0.51
	38%-44% (females)	0.38-0.44
Chemistry		
Albumin	3.5-5 g/dl	507-725 μmol/L
Alkaline phosphatase	30-120 U/L	0.5-2.0 μkat/L
Alanine aminotransferase (ALT/SGPT)	5-36 U/L	0.08-0.6 μkat/L
Ammonia	30-70 μg/dl	17.6-41.1 μmol/L
Amylase	0-130 U/L	0-2.17 μkat/L
Aspartate aminotransferase (AST/SGOT)	7-40 U/L	0.12-0.67 μkat/L
Bilirubin		
Total	0.2-1.3 mg/dl	3.4-22.0 μmol/L
Direct	0.1-0.3 mg/dl	1.7-5.1 μmol/L
Indirect	0.1-1.0 mg/dl	1.7-17 μmol/L
BUN	10-30 mg/dl	1.8-7.1 mmol/L
BUN:Cr ratio	10:1-15:1	
Calcium	9-11 mg/dl	2.25-2.74 mmol/L
Cholesterol	140-200 mg/dl (age dependent)	3.6-5.2 mmol/L
HDL	>45 mg/dl (males)	>1.2 mmol/L
	>55 mg/dl (females)	>1.4 mmol/L
LDL	<130 mg/dl	<3.4 mmol/L

Test	Conventional Units	SI Units
Chloride	95-105 mEq/L	95-105 mmol/L
CO_2	20-30 mEq/L	20-30 mmol/L
Creatinine	0.5-1.5 mg/dl	44-133 μmol/L
Glucose	70-120 mg/dl	3.89-6.66 mmol/L
Iron	50-150 μg/dl	9.0-26.9 μmol/L
Lactic dehydrogenase (LDH)	50-150 U/L	0.83-2.5 μkat/L
Lipase	0-160 U/L	0-2.66 μkat/L
Magnesium	1.5-2.5 mEq/L	0.75-1.25 mmol/L
Osmolality	285-295 mOsm/kg	285-295 mmol/kg
Phosphorus	2.8-4.5 mg/dl	0.90-1.45 mmol/L
Potassium	3.5-5.5 mEq/L	3.5-5.5 mmol/L
Protein	6-8 g/dl	60-80 g/L
Sedimentation rate	<15 mm/hr (males) <20 mm/hr (females)	
Sodium	135-145 mEq/L	135-145 mmol/L
T_3	110-230 ng/dl	1.7-3.5 nmol/L
T_4	5-12 μg/dl	64-154 nmol/L
Triglyceride	40-150 mg/dl	0.45-1.69 mmol/L
Uric acid	2.5-6.5 mg/dl	149-387 μmol/L
Coagulation		
Platelets	150-400 × 10^3/μL	150-400 × 10^9/L
PT	10-14 sec	Same as conventional unit
APTT	30-45 sec	Same as conventional unit
FSP	<10 mg/L	Same as conventional unit

BLOOD PRODUCTS*

Description	Special considerations	Indications for use
Packed RBCs Packed RBCs are prepared from whole blood by sedimentation or centrifugation. One unit contains 250-350 ml.	Use of RBCs for treatment allows remaining components of blood (e.g., platelets, albumin, plasma) to be used for other purposes. There is less danger of fluid overload. Packed RBCs are preferred RBC source because they are more component specific.	Severe or symptomatic anemia, acute blood loss.
Frozen RBCs Frozen RBCs are prepared from RBCs using glycerol for protection and frozen. They can be stored for 3 yr at −188.6°F (−87°C).	They must be used within 24 hr of thawing. Successive washings with saline solution remove majority of WBCs and plasma proteins.	Autotransfusion, patient with previous febrile reactions to transfusions. Infrequently used because filters remove most WBCs.
Platelets Platelets are prepared from fresh whole blood within 4 hr after collection. One unit contains 30-60 ml of platelet concentrate.	Multiple units of platelets can be obtained from one donor by plateletpheresis. They can be kept at room temperature for 1-5 days, depending on type of collection and storage bag used. Expected increase is 10,000/μL/U.	Bleeding caused by thrombocytopenia, platelet levels <10,000-20,000/μL (10-20 × 10⁹/L).

Fresh Frozen Plasma

Liquid portion of whole blood is separated from cells and frozen. One unit contains 200-250 ml. Plasma is rich in clotting factors but contains no platelets. It may be stored for 1 yr. It must be used within 2 hr after thawing.

Use of plasma in treating hypovolemic shock is being replaced by pure plasma preparations such as albumin plasma expanders.

Bleeding caused by deficiency in clotting factors (e.g., DIC, hemorrhage, massive transfusion).

Albumin

Albumin is prepared from plasma. It can be stored for 5 yr. It is available in 5% or 25% solution.

Albumin 25 g/100 ml is osmotically equal to 500 ml of plasma. Hyperosmolar solution acts by moving water from extravascular to intravascular space.

Hypovolemic shock, hypoalbuminemia.

Cryoprecipitates and Commercial Concentrates

Cryoprecipitate is prepared from fresh frozen plasma, with 10-20 ml/bag. It can be stored for 1 yr. Once thawed, must be used.

See Table 28-19 in Lewis/Collier/Heitkemper, *Medical-Surgical Nursing*, edition 4, p. 801.

Replacement of clotting factors, especially factor VIII and fibrinogen.

*Component therapy has replaced use of whole blood, which accounts for <10% of all transfusions.

DIC, Disseminated intravascular coagulation; *Hct*, hematocrit; *RBC*, red blood cell; *WBC*, white blood cell.

BREATH SOUNDS
Normal Sounds

Type	Normal site	Duration	Characteristics
Vesicular	Peripheral lung	I > E	Soft and swishing sounds; abnormal when heard over the large airways
Bronchial	Trachea and bronchi	E > I	Louder, coarser, and of longer duration than vesicular; abnormal if heard over peripheral lung
Bronchovesicular	Sternal border of the major bronchi	E = I	Moderate in pitch and intensity; abnormal if heard over peripheral lung

E, Expiration; *I,* inspiration.

Adventitious Sounds

Type	Waveform	Characteristics	Possible clinical condition
Coarse crackle		Discontinuous, explosive, interrupted; loud; low in pitch	Pulmonary edema; pneumonia in resolution stage
Fine crackle		Discontinuous, explosive, interrupted; less loud than coarse crackles, lower in pitch, and of shorter duration	Interstitial lung disease; heart failure; atelectasis
Wheeze		Continuous, of long duration, high-pitched, musical, hissing	Narrowing of airway; bronchial asthma; chronic obstructive pulmonary disease
Rhonchus		Continuous, of long duration, low-pitched, snoring	Production of sputum (usually cleared or lessened by coughing)
Pleural friction rub		Grating, rasping noise	Rubbing together of inflamed parietal linings; loss of normal pleural lubrication

CANCER SCREENING GUIDELINES: SPECIFIC CANCER SITES

Screening	High-risk profile	Medium and low-risk profile
Lung Cancer Early detection method not available; annual chest x-ray (advised by some physicians); observation by patient for change in respiratory status; increased frequency of infections and change in cough, sputum, breathing, voice	History of more than 20 pack-years of smoking (1 pack a day for 20 years); exposure to airborne carcinogens, especially asbestos, uranium, hydrocarbons; age range 40-80 yr; chronic lung disease	History of less than 20 pack-years of smoking; nonsmokers; former smokers after 10 yr
Colon and Rectal Cancer Blood test on stools every year after age 50 and digital rectal examination annually after age 40; sigmoidoscopic examination (preferably flexible) every 3-5 yr after age 50; observation by patient for changes in bowel pattern: diarrhea, constipation, pain, flatus, black tarry stools, bleeding	History of familial polyposis, ulcerative colitis, Crohn's disease; personal or family history of colon or rectal cancer; diet high in fat and low in fiber; age range 40-75 yr	Persons with no known risk factors

Prostatic Cancer

Digital rectal examination at age 40 and annually thereafter; prostate specific antigen blood test every year for men aged 50 and older; observation by patient for dysuria, blood in urine, difficulty in producing stream of urine

Presence of prostatic hyperplasia; presence of prostatic infection; African-American; increased risk with age

Presence of one risk factor, excluding age

Cervical Cancer

Pap test and pelvic examination every year for those who are or have been sexually active or who have reached age 18; colposcopy if suspicious area is noted; observation by patient for abnormal vaginal bleeding or discharge, pain or bleeding with sexual intercourse

Early intercourse (before age 20) with multiple partners; poor personal hygiene; history of herpesvirus type II infection, cervical dysplasia

No known risk factors

Based on the *American Cancer Society 1995 Recommendations.*

Continued.

CANCER SCREENING GUIDELINES: SPECIFIC CANCER SITES—cont'd

Screening	High-risk profile	Medium and low-risk profile
Endometrial Cancer		
Pap test every year; pelvic examination every year; endometrial biopsy every year for women at menopause and at risk; observation by patient for abnormal uterine bleeding, pain, change in menstrual pattern	Infertility; ovarian dysfunction; obesity; uterine bleeding; estrogen therapy over long period of time; diabetes; age range 30-80 yr	Presence of one risk factor, excluding estrogen therapy, over long period of time
Skin Cancer		
Self-examination monthly with suspicious lesions evaluated promptly; physical examination every year; observation by patient for sore that does not heal, change in wart or mole	Prolonged exposure to sun; previous radiation exposure; fair, thin skin; positive family history of dysplastic nevus syndrome (DNS)	Presence of one risk factor, excluding prolonged exposure to sun

Breast Cancer

Monthly breast self-examination; breast examination by health professional every 3 yr for women age 20-40 yr and every year after age 40; baseline mammogram at age 40, every 1-2 yr between ages 40 and 49, and every year after age 50; observation by patient for lump or thickening; discharge from nipple, pain in breast

Caucasian; early menarche, late menopause; fibrocystic breast disease; infertility; more than age 30 for first pregnancy; personal history of breast cancer; mother or sister with history of breast cancer; obesity; age range 35-65 yr

Excluding family history of breast cancer, fewer than two risk factors

COMMONLY USED FORMULAS

Parameter	Formula	Normal range
Alveolar-arterial oxygen gradient ($AaDO_2$)	$PAO_2 - PaO_2$	<15 mm Hg
Alveolar partial pressure of oxygen (PAO_2)	$FIO_2 (713) - PaCO_2/0.8$	
Anion gap	$Na - (HCO_3^- + Cl)$	8-16 mEq/L
Cardiac index (CI)	CO/Body surface area (BSA)	2.2-4.0 L/min/m^2
Cardiac output (CO)	$HR \times SV$	4-8 L/min
Cerebral perfusion pressure (CPP)	$MAP - ICP$	80-100 mm Hg
Ejection fraction (EF)	$\dfrac{SV}{\text{End diastolic volume}} \times 100$	60% or greater
Mean arterial pressure (MAP)	$\dfrac{2(DPB) + SBP}{3}$	70-105 mm Hg

Pulmonary vascular resistance (PVR)

$$\frac{PAM - PCWP}{CO} \times 80$$

<250 dyne sec/cm^5

Pulmonary vascular resistance index (PVRI)

$$\frac{PAM - PCWP}{CI} \times 80$$

160-380 dyne sec m^2/cm^5

Stroke volume (SV)

$$\frac{CO \times 1000}{HR}$$

60-180 ml/beat

Stroke volume index (SVI)

$$\frac{SV}{BSA} \quad \text{or} \quad \frac{CI}{HR} \times 1000$$

30-65 ml/m^2/beat

Systemic vascular resistance (SVR)

$$\frac{MAP - CVP}{CO} \times 80$$

800-1200 dyne sec/cm^5

Systemic vascular resistance index (SVRI)

$$\frac{MAP - CVP}{CI} \times 80$$

1970-2390 dyne sec m^2/cm^5

DBP, Diastolic blood pressure; *FIO$_2$*, fraction of inspired oxygen; *ICP*, intracranial pressure; *PAM*, mean pulmonary artery pressure; *PCWP*, pulmonary capillary wedge pressure; *SBP*, systolic blood pressure.

CONVERSION FACTORS

1 kg	= 1 L fluid	1/150 gr	= 0.4 mg
1 mg	= 1000 µg	1 tsp	= 5 ml
1 kg	= 2.2 lb	1 tbsp	= 15 ml
1 gr	= 60 or 65 mg	1 oz	= 30 ml
1/100 gr	= 0.6 mg	1 mm Hg	= 1.36 cm H_2O

DYSRHYTHMIA CHARACTERISTICS

Pattern	Rate and rhythm
NSR	60-100 bpm and regular
Sinus bradycardia	<60 bpm and regular
Sinus tachycardia	>100 bpm and regular
PAC	Usually 60-100 bpm and irregular
Atrial flutter	*Atrial:* 250-350 bpm and regular
	Ventricular: >100 bpm and irregular
Atrial fibrillation	*Atrial:* 350-600 bpm and irregular
	Ventricular: >100 bpm and irregular or possibly any rate
Junctional rhythms	40-140 bpm and regular
First-degree heart block	Normal and regular
Second-degree heart block	
Type I (Mobitz I, Wenckebach)	*Atrial:* Normal and regular
	Ventricular: Slower and irregular
Type II (Mobitz II)	*Atrial:* Usually normal and regular or irregular
	Ventricular: Slower and regular or irregular
Third-degree heart block	Ventricular rate 20-40 bpm and regular
PVC	60-100 bpm and irregular
Ventricular tachycardia	100-250 bpm and regular or irregular
Ventricular fibrillation	Not measurable and irregular

bpm, Beats per minute; *NSR,* normal sinus rhythm; *PAC,* premature atrial contraction; *PSVT,* paroxysmal supraventricular tachycardia; *PVC,* premature ventricular contraction.

P wave	PR interval	QRS complex
Normal	Normal	Normal
Normal	Normal	Normal
Normal	Normal	Normal
Abnormal shape	Normal or variable	Normal (usually)
Sawtooth	Variable	Normal (usually)
Chaotic	Not measurable	Normal (usually)
Abnormal (may be hidden)	Variable	Normal (usually)
Normal	>0.20 sec	Normal
Normal	Progressively lengthened	Normal width, with pattern of one non-conducted QRS
P wave occurs in multiples	Normal or prolonged	Widened, preceded by two or more P waves
Normal, but no connection with QRS complex	Variable	Normal or widened, no connection with P waves
Not usually present	Not measurable	Wide and distorted
Not usually present	Not measurable	Wide and distorted
Absent	Not measurable	Not measurable

ELECTROCARDIOGRAM (ECG) MONITORING: WAVEFORM

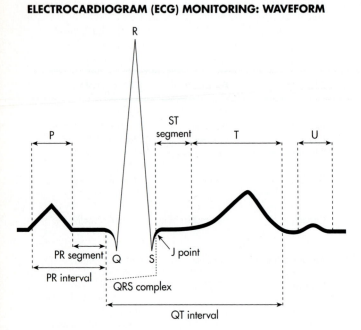

P wave	Represents atrial depolarization.
PR segment	Represents time required for impulse to travel through atrioventricular (AV) node, where it is delayed, and through bundle of His, bundle branches, and Purkinje fiber network, just before ventricular depolarization.
PR interval	Represents time required for atrial depolarization and impulse to travel through conduction system and Purkinje fiber network, inclusive of P wave and PR segment. It is measured from beginning of P wave to end of PR segment. Normally measures 0.12 to 0.20 sec in duration.
QRS complex	Represents depolarization of both ventricles and is measured from beginning of Q (or R) wave to end of S wave. Also measured from end of PR interval to J point. Normally measures from 0.04 to 0.10 sec.
J point	Represents junction where QRS complex ends and ST segment begins.
ST segment	Represents early ventricular repolarization. Measured from J point to beginning of T wave.
T wave	Represents ventricular repolarization.
U wave	Represents late ventricular repolarization. Not normally seen in all leads.
QT interval	Represents total time required for ventricular depolarization and repolarization and is measured from beginning of QRS complex to end of T wave.

GLASGOW COMA SCALE

Category of response*	Appropriate stimulus
Eyes open	Approach to bedside Verbal command Pain
Best verbal response	Verbal questioning with maximum arousal
Best motor response	Verbal command (e.g., "raise your arm, hold up two fingers") Pain (pressure on prox- imal nail bed)

*Specific behaviors that are seen as responses to testing stimulus in each of these three areas are given a numerical value and can be plotted on a graph. Graph visually plots a place on consciousness continuum to determine whether patient is stable, improving, or deteriorating.

Response	Score†
Spontaneous response	4
Opening of eyes to name or command	3
Lack of opening of eyes to previous stimuli but opening to pain	2
Lack of opening of eyes to any stimulus	1
Untestable	U
Appropriate orientation, conversant, correct identification of self, place, year, and month	5
Confusion, conversant, but disorientation in one or more spheres	4
Inappropriate or disorganized use of words (e.g., cursing), lack of sustained conversation	3
Incomprehensible words, sounds (e.g., moaning)	2
Lack of sound, even with painful stimuli	1
Untestable	U
Obedience of command	6
Localization of pain, lack of obedience but presence of attempts to remove offending stimulus	5
Flexion withdrawal,* flexion of arm in response to pain without abnormal flexion posture	4
Abnormal flexion, flexing of arm at elbow and pronation, making a fist	3
Abnormal extension, extension of arm at elbow usually with adduction and internal rotation of arm at shoulder	2
Lack of response	1
Untestable	U

†The sum can be interpreted by comparing it to the highest score of 15 for a fully alert person and the lowest possible score of 3. A score of 8 or less is generally indicative of coma.

HEART SOUNDS
Normal Sounds

Sound	Auscultation site	Timing	Pitch
S_1 (M_1 T_1)	Apex	Beginning of systole	High
S_1 split	Apex	Beginning of systole	High
S_2 (A_2 P_2)	A_2 at 2nd ICS, RSB; P_2 at 2nd ICS, LSB	End of systole	High
S_2 physiologic split	2nd ICS, LSB	End of systole	High
S_2 persistent (wide) split	2nd ICS, LSB	End of systole	High
S_2 paradoxic (reversed) split (P_2 A_2)	2nd ICS, LSB	End of systole	High
S_2 fixed split	2nd ICS, LSB	End of systole	High
S_3 (ventricular gallop)	Apex	Early in diastole just after S_2	Dull, low
S_4 (atrial gallop)	Apex	Late in diastole just before S_1	Low

CAD, Coronary artery disease; *CHF,* congestive heart failure; *ICS,* intercostal

Clinical occurrence	End-piece/ pt. position
Closing of mitral and tricuspid valves; normal sound	Diaphragm/ pt. supine
Ventricles contracting at different times due to electrical or mechanical problems (e.g., longer time span between $M_1 T_1$ caused by right bundle-branch heart block, or reversal $[T_1 M_1]$ caused by mitral stenosis)	Same as S_1
Closing of aortic and pulmonic valves; normal sound	Diaphragm/ pt. supine
Accentuated by inspiration; disappears on expiration; sound that corresponds with respiratory cycle due to normal delay in closure of pulmonic valve during inspiration; accentuated during exercise or in individuals with thin chest walls; heard most often in children and young adults	Same as S_2
Heard throughout respiratory cycle; caused by late closure of pulmonic valve or early closure of aortic valve; occurs in atrial septal defect, right ventricular failure, pulmonic stenosis, hypertension, or right bundle-branch heart block	Same as S_2
Because of delayed left ventricular systole, aortic valve closes after pulmonic valve rather than before it (normally during expiration the two sounds merge); causes may include left bundle-branch heart block, aortic stenosis, severe left ventricular failure, MI, and severe hypertension	Same as S_2
Heard with equal intensity during inspiration and expiration due to split of pulmonic and aortic components, which are unaffected by blood volume or respiratory changes; may be heard in pulmonary stenosis or atrial septal defect	Same as S_2
Early and rapid filling of ventricle, as in early ventricular failure, CHF; common in children, during last trimester of pregnancy and possibly in healthy adults over age 50 yr	Bell/patient in left lateral or supine position
Atrium filling against increased resistance of stiff ventricle, as in CHF, CAD, cardiomyopathy, pulmonary artery hypertension, ventricular failure; may be normal in infants, children, and athletes	Same as S_3

space; *LSB,* left sternal border; *MI,* myocardial infarction; *RSB,* right sternal border.

Murmurs

Type	Timing	Pitch	Quality	Auscultation site	Radiation
Pulmonic stenosis	Systolic ejection	Medium-high	Harsh	2nd ICS, LSB	Toward left shoulder, back
Aortic stenosis	Mid-systolic	Medium-high	Harsh	2nd ICS, RSB	Toward carotid arteries
Ventricular septal defect	Late systolic	High	Blowing	4th ICS, LSB	Toward right sternal border
Mitral insufficiency	Holosystolic	High	Blowing	5th-6th ICS, left MCL	Toward left axilla
Tricuspid insufficiency	Holosystolic	High	Blowing	4th ICS, LSB	Toward apex
Aortic insufficiency	Early diastolic	High	Blowing	2nd ICS, RSB	Toward sternum
Pulmonary insufficiency	Early diastolic	High	Blowing	2nd ICS, LSB	Toward sternum
Mitral stenosis	Mid-late diastolic	Low	Rumbling	5th ICS, left MCL	Toward axilla
Tricuspid stenosis	Mid-late diastolic	Low	Rumbling	4th ICS, LSB	Usually none

ICS, intercostal space; *LSB,* left sternal border; *MCL,* midclavicular line; *RSB,* right sternal border.

Internet Introduction

The Internet can be an excellent resource on nursing, health care, and particularly on current health care and medical research. The Internet's power to the nursing student or the practitioner comes from its diversity of current and archived information sources that can support one's data needs, including the latest clinical trial protocols for AIDS drugs, a list of the latest drugs and treatments for AIDS/HIV, the latest medical or nursing journal research abstracts, national and international conferences on women's health issues, alternative healing resources, the latest information on the *Ebola* virus hemorrhagic fever, and much more.

Getting onto the Internet

Universities and colleges normally provide a campus-wide local area network (LAN) and Internet access through student computer center accounts. If access is provided by your institution, you need to do the following:

1. Establish a student account with the computer center. The center will provide phone numbers, a password, and technical information on how to access the campus and Internet resources (E-mail, FTP, Telnet, World Wide Web, etc.).

2. Configure your modem to access your institution's computer network if you are using a computer at home. Dialing into the institution's computer network requires access software, a phone line, and a high-speed modem installed on your computer. If you do not have a home computer, computers at your institution should be configured for direct or remote access to the campus-wide local area network and the Internet.

3. Last, take Internet "how-to" courses given by the computer center or library staff. These courses will reduce your learning time and get you on-line and active in a shorter period of time.

Where to Look by Using Internet Information-Browsing Tools

Your aim is to spend as little time as possible on the highway and as much time as possible accessing and retrieving information at your destination. Knowing where to look and by what means to access and then retrieve information once there is very important. The following sections discuss the major tools used to search the Internet for information.

E-Mail as a Search Tool

E-mail, or electronic mail, is based on Internet TCP/IP protocols for sending and receiving messages worldwide. E-mail is the most heavily used network application. When you sign up for a computer account to use your institution's computer system, you will be provided with an E-mail address. Your institution's computer system will have a computer software program that allows you to send and receive E-mail.

Mailing Lists to Browse for Information

E-mail bulk mailings, called Usenet Newsgroups and Listservers, give people the chance to transmit comments, questions, answers, and opinions to a large group of people who share a similar interest. Newsgroups and Listservers are ongoing on-line moderated or unmoderated discussion groups devoted to specific topics. Both share, via E-mail messages, information to those who have subscribed to receive messages. The information shared can be of great interest to nursing students and professionals. It may include the latest research findings in nursing, literature reviews of current research or books, or discussions of current issues in health care and case management.

Usenet Newsgroups are based on a worldwide-distributed electronic bulletin board system (BBS) with over 40,000 postings (messages) daily. Messages come from hundreds of thousands of computer users worldwide who post to "newsgroups" on this electronic bulletin board. Topics and discussions range from the serious to the lighthearted.

A Listserver is an automated bulk E-mail list computer system for discussion groups. Similar to bulk mailings from the post office placed in your home mailbox, this computer program adds or removes subscribers to discussion groups; it also posts E-mail messages daily. If you subscribe to a group, your E-mail address is added to the group's mailing list, and you then receive all of its postings.

For the student nurse there is a Listserver that lets you "talk" with nursing students from around the world. It is called SNURSE-L. To subscribe, send an E-mail to "LISTSERV@UBVM.CC.BUFFALO.EDU" with no subject line. In the body of the message, put SUB SNURSE-L <your full name>.

How do you find other newsgroups or listservers? The easiest way is to go to your local bookstore and look for a copy of the "Internet Yellow Pages" or a similar book that provides a comprehensive list and description of newsgroups and listservers and how to subscribe to them via E-mail. Once you have become comfortable with the Internet, you can surf to various World Wide Web or Gopher sites and download a "list of lists" of such groups to join.

Anonymous FTP and Archie as Information-Browsing Tools

Many computer systems on the Internet have set aside specific areas on their networks for archived files that you can download to your own computer. These sites are called "anonymous FTP" because anyone can log on using the password "anonymous." Files at anonymous sites can be anything from software programs to complete text such as the King James Bible and files such as pictures and sound bytes.

FTP is based on Internet TCP/IP file transfer protocols. It is a means for anyone on the Internet to transfer files from one network site to their own computer. FTP is a resident software program on your institution's computer system that provides a standardized text-based method of transferring files over a telephone line.

What does that mean? By typing in a command, such as GET File "X" you are able to transfer files from a network to your computer. If you have used DOS or UNIX computer commands (GET, SEND, etc.), the procedure will seem rather straightforward; if not, you will require some help to learn the commands at first.

With hundreds of anonymous FTP sites on the Internet, how do you find, browse and retrieve a specific file? A software program called Archie was designed to help you locate and retrieve files from anonymous FTP sites. Using Archie is similar to using your library's electronic card catalog, where you search the library's holdings by title, author, or subject and then go to the shelf to select the book or journal. Archie searches by keywords and then creates a list of "hits" showing where these "hits" are located. You then use FTP commands to retrieve and download the desired files to your own computer. To get into Archie, you type the word Archie at your computer system prompt and follow the directions for conducting a search.

Gopher and Veronica as Information-Browsing Tools

Not all information is located in FTP sites or can be searched via Archie. A vast amount of information is located and maintained on networks that can be located and retrieved by using a menu-driven system called "Gopher." Gopher "to go for" is a software program that is a menu-based server designed to identify, locate, maintain, and retrieve information that is held in text format throughout the Internet.

Networks had to have some way to organize the information they maintained so that anyone could log on to the system and locate and retrieve information efficiently. Since a network can be made of many computers and information could be located anywhere on the system, the Gopher software provides both the means to locate and to retrieve information throughout a network and the Internet.

If you look at your library's electronic catalog, the first screen you will see is the system's main "menu." By selecting each menu item, you use the various features of the electronic catalog. Similarly, Gopher menus let you navigate throughout the Internet to various computer network systems to locate and retrieve stored information by using the various menu items found on the Gopher.

Information can be stored anywhere on the Internet. It can be retrieved in two ways. First, a Gopher menu can point to where the information is stored; by keying on that menu item, you are transported to where the information is maintained. Second, the menu item can actually be the information you want; it is then retrieved by simply keying on the item. Gopher menu design is straightforward. By keying on a menu item, you receive information or are directed to where information is maintained.

With more than 1,000 Gophers existing on the Internet, a means to search, browse, and retrieve Gopher information needed to be developed. Veronica is the browser software designed to locate information stored at various gopher sites. The software searches all Gopher menus throughout the Internet by key terms found either in Gopher directories or menu titles, records the number of "hits" that match, and then creates a separate menu of the "hits" for you to use to retrieve the information. Keep in mind that no universal standard for terms used in Gopher directories or menu titles exists, so when doing a Veronica search, you will need to be "creative."

Since Veronica is a Gopher information browser, it is normally a menu item on nearly all Gophers. Select it as a menu item, choose the search method (directory or titles), and press the "Enter" key. A small box will appear in the middle of your computer screen; in it, type in your search term(s) and hit the "Enter" key. As in Archie, a list of "hits" matched will be created. You simply choose from the menu of "hits" and browse and retrieve the information.

WAIS as an Information-Browsing Tool

Unlike Gophers, Wide Area Information Servers (WAIS) are information servers located on various networks that have *fully indexed databases*. WAIS is very similar to your library's electronic catalog database. It includes fully searchable databases by keywords found in text documents maintained in the databases. WAIS has achieved limited success because of the vast amount of technical expertise needed to create and maintain such a database.

WAIS is a Gopher menu item similar to Veronica. Locate it on your institution's Gopher and select it. Once it is selected, you will find a list of WAIS that can be searched. Since WAIS includes subject area databases such as AIDS/HIV, select the one that fits your data needs. As in Veronica, a small box appears and you key in searchable terms in the selected WAIS database. As with Veronica, a menu of "hits" is generated to locate and retrieve information held in the particular database.

World Wide Web and Lynx as Information-Browsing Tools

FTP, Gopher, Archie, Veronica, and WAIS offer ways to locate, identify, and retrieve information held through the various networks that make up the Internet. Another server that allows you to surf the net for information is the World Wide Web. The Web incorporates many of the various tools, protocols, and utilities found elsewhere on the Internet. The Web software takes the Gopher server one step further by using what is called "hypertext" documents.

Hypertext documents contain not only information but also links to other documents that contain information and more links. Hypertext linking is the chief feature of the World Wide Web. Another characteristic is that it is highly graphic. By tabbing onto highlighted words found in a document and pressing the "Enter" key, you are transported to other documents, to other Web sites, and other linkages throughout the Internet.

Web documents can often be highly "graphic," with media types such as PostScript or GIF graphics, sound bytes, and QuickTime movies. Being highly pictorial, your computer (or the institution's computer) requires software browsers such as Mosaic or Netscape to display these features. Your computer will also need a color monitor, a high-speed video graphics board, a sound board, and a high-speed modem, with a direct link to the Internet to make full use of these features.

Lacking any of these aids, you can still access the Web via a text-based information browser called Lynx. Lynx accesses the Web's hypertext documents and its linkages only. As in Gopher and other TCP/IP Internet features, to see if Lynx is available to you, type the word <lynx> at your institution's computer system prompt and press the "Enter" key. A hypertext document should appear on your computer screen. Tab to the highlighted text and press the "Enter" key, and you will be linked to other hypertext documents throughout the Web. Like Gophers, the World Wide Web has various information browsers located as hypertext items available for searching the Web by key words and phrases.

Putting Your Information Search All Together

The following is an example of how one can do a search for information to be used in an undergraduate medical-surgical or pharmacology course. The topic selected is AIDS/HIV drugs and treatments. The World Wide Web and the Netscape software were used to conduct the search. The same search can be done using Veronica or Lynx, and it would have similar results.

I want to locate a current and comprehensive list of the AIDS/HIV drugs and treatments, a brief description of their use and side effects, and at least one example of an AIDS drug being used in clinical research trials. I use Netscape's netsearch feature and type in the word <health> and press the "Enter" key. A list of World Wide Web site "hits" matching the term is produced. I then look over the "hit" list and choose what I consider to be the best place to start, which is a comprehensive list of health-related resources on the Internet (http://wwww.yahoo.com/health/).

Once I choose this "hit" and press the "Enter" key, a list of 34 health-related World Wide Web resources appear. When I select "Diseases and Conditions," a hypertext document titled "Health: Diseases and Conditions: AIDS/HIV" appears with 36 AIDS/HIV resources listed on it. I choose the first item on the list: "AIDS and HIV—Information and Resources." This selection then opens up to another hypertext document titled "AIDS Treatment Data Network." Within this document is a hypertext link to "Clinical Trials" and a "Glossary of Brief Descriptions of Drugs and Treatments." Other hypertext link documents include "Treatment Review," an on-line newsletter about current and proposed treatments and drugs, and "Alternative Treatments," which discusses the use of herbs and other forms of therapy that have not undergone extensive clinical trials.

When I choose "Clinical Trials," a published directory of clinical trials for the New York area, Connecticut, New Jersey, Philadelphia, and the National Institutes of Health in Bethesda, Maryland, appears. Under "Clinical Trials" is a separate item about a protease inhibitor called saquinavir and its expanded access program. I open this hypertext document and find that this drug is discussed in some detail. Then I print the information. Next, I go to the glossary and open this hypertext document. It contains nearly 14 pages of drugs and treatments and their side effects. I print these pages.

This search is completed in less than 30 minutes, and I have obtained nearly 20 pages of printed materials. To go to this site if using Netscape, type <http://www.yahoo.com/health/> to obtain the resource list. Choose "Diseases and Conditions," and this will take you into the AIDS/HIV hypertext. Using Lynx and Veronica will produce Web and Gopher sites with similar information.

Bibliography

Pitter, Keiko et al: *Every student's guide to the Internet,* New York, 1995, McGraw-Hill.

Acknowledgment

The Internet Introduction was contributed by Douglas A. Coffin, RN, PhD, Assistant Professor, Florida International University, Miami, Florida.

MEDICATION ADMINISTRATION
Equivalent Weights and Measures

Metric	Apothecary	Household
Weight		
1 kg	2.2 pounds	
1000 mg = 1 gram	gr xv	
60 or 65 mg	gr i	
30 mg	gr ss (one half)	
1 μg (mcg) = 0.001 mg		
Volume		
	4 quarts	1 gallon
1000 ml = 1 liter = 1000 cc	Approx. 1 quart	1 quart
500 ml	Approx. 1 pint (½ qt)	16 ounces
240 or 250 ml	℥viii (8 fluidounces)	1 cup or 1 glass
30 ml = approx. 30 cc	℥i (1 fluidounce)	2 tbsp
16 ml = approx. 16 cc	℥iv (4 fluidrams)	1 tbsp
8 ml	℥ (2 fluidrams)	2 tsp
4 to 5 ml	℥ (1 fluidram)	1 tsp
1 ml = approx. 1 cc	Minims xv or xvi	

Drug Calculations

Ratio and proportion:

1. To set up a ratio and proportion, put on the right-hand side what you already have or what you already know (e.g., 1000 mg:1 ml).
2. On the left-hand side put X, or what you want to know (e.g., 750 mg:X).
3. The equation should look like this:
   750 mg:X = 1000 mg:1 ml
4. Multiply the two inside numbers. Multiply the two outside numbers.
   1000X = 750
5. Solve for X:
   $$X = \frac{750}{1000} = 0.75 \text{ ml}$$

IV Drip Rate

$$\frac{\text{Total number of milliliters to be infused}}{\text{Total number of minutes infusion is to run}} \times \text{Drop factor}$$
$$= \text{Rate (drops per minute)}$$

Abbreviations for Medication Administration

	Unabbrev. form	Meaning
a	ante	before
ac	ante cibum	before meals
ad lib	ad libitum	freely
AM	ante meridiem	morning
bid	bis in die	twice each day
$\bar{c}$	cum	with
cap	capsule	capsule
cc, cm^3	cubic centimeter	cubic centimeter (ml)
D/C or DC	discontinue	terminate
elix	elixir	elixir
g, gm	gram	1000 milligrams
gr	grain	60 milligrams
gtt	gutta	drop
h, hr	hora	hour
hs	hora somni	at bedtime
IM	intramuscular	into a muscle
IV	intravenous	into a vein
IVPB	IV piggyback	secondary IV line
kg	kilogram	2.2 lb (1000 g)
KVO	keep vein open	very slow infusion rate
Ⓛ	left	left
L	liter	liter
μg, mcg	microgram	one millionth of a gram
mg	milligram	one thousandth of a gram
mEq	milliequivalent	the number of grams of solute dissolved in 1 milliliter of a normal solution
min or m	minim	minim ($\frac{1}{15}$ or $\frac{1}{16}$ ml)
ml, mL	milliliter	one thousandth of a liter
ng	nanogram	one billionth of a gram
$\bar{o}$	no or none	no or none
OD	oculus dexter	right eye
OS	oculus sinister	left eye
os	os	mouth
OTC	over-the-counter	nonprescription drug
OU	oculus uterque	each eye
pc	post cibum	after meals
PM	post meridiem	after noon
PO	per os	by mouth, orally
prn	pro re nata	according to necessity

	Unabbrev. form	Meaning
pt	patient	patient
q	quaque	every
qd	quaque die	every day
qh	quaque hora	every hour
q4h, q4°	every 4 hours	every 4 hours around the clock
qid	quater in die	four times each day
qod	quaque aliem die	every other day
qs	quantum satis	sufficient quantity
Ⓡ	right	right
℞	receipt	take
s̄	sine	without
SL	sub linguam	under the tongue
SOS	si opus sit	if necessary
ss	semis	a half
stat	statim	at once
SC,SQ	subcutaneous	into subcutaneous tissue
tbsp	tablespoon	tablespoon (15 ml)
tid	ter in die	three times a day
TO	telephone order	order received over the telephone
tsp	teaspoon	teaspoon (4 or 5 ml)
U	unit	a dosage measure for insulin, penicillin, heparin
VO	verbal order	order received verbally
t, tt	one, two	one, two (as in "gr t," "gr tt")
ʒ	dram	4 or 5 ml
℥	ounce or fluid-ounce	ounce (30 milliliters)
×	times	as in two times a week
>	greater than	greater than
<	less than	less than
=	equal to	equal to

Techniques of Administration
Angles of Injection

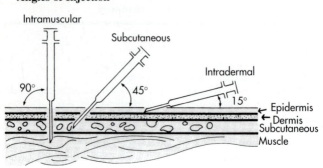

Injection Sites
Subcutaneous

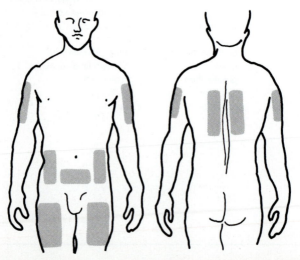

Intramuscular: deltoid muscle

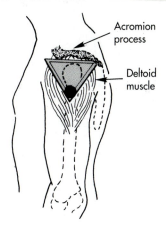

Acromion process

Deltoid muscle

Intramuscular: dorsogluteal muscle

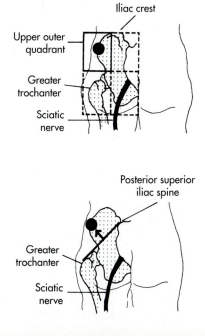

Iliac crest

Upper outer quadrant

Greater trochanter

Sciatic nerve

Posterior superior iliac spine

Greater trochanter

Sciatic nerve

Intramuscular: vastus lateralis muscle

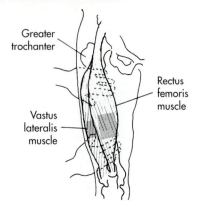

Greater trochanter

Rectus femoris muscle

Vastus lateralis muscle

Intramuscular: ventrogluteal muscle

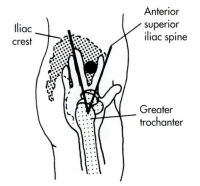

Iliac crest

Anterior superior iliac spine

Greater trochanter

Z-Track Technique

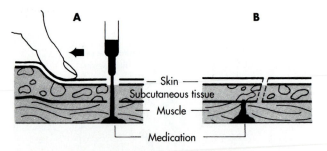

A

B

Skin

Subcutaneous tissue

Muscle

Medication

A, In Z-track intramuscular injection, skin is pulled laterally, then injection is administered. **B,** After needle is withdrawn, skin is released. This technique helps prevent medication from leaking.

Intermittent IV
Peripheral vein intermittent infusion device
1. Irrigate device with 1 ml of normal saline.
2. Administer prescribed medication.
3. Irrigate device with 1 ml of normal saline after medication administration is completed.
4. If policy, perform a final irrigation with 1 ml of heparin solution (100 units of heparin per ml of normal saline).

Central vein intermittent infusion device
1. Irrigate device with 2 to 5 ml of normal saline (volume depends on type of infusion catheter and agency policy).
2. Administer prescribed medication.
3. Irrigate device with 2 to 5 ml of normal saline when medication administration is completed.
4. Irrigate device with 2 to 5 ml of heparin solution (100 units of heparin per ml of normal saline).

Heparin Flush
Peripheral vein intermittent infusion device
1. Irrigate device with 1 ml of normal saline.
2. Administer prescribed medication.
3. Irrigate device with 1 ml of normal saline after medication administration is completed.
4. If policy, perform a final irrigation with 1 ml of heparin solution (100 units of heparin per ml of normal saline).

Central vein intermittent infusion device
1. Irrigate device with 2 to 5 ml of normal saline (volume depends on type of infusion catheter and agency policy).
2. Administer prescribed medication.
3. Irrigate device with 2 to 5 ml of normal saline when medication administration is completed.
4. Irrigate device with 2 to 5 ml of heparin solution (100 units of heparin per ml of normal saline).

Intravenous Needle Site Complications

	Infiltration	Phlebitis
Assessment		
Color	Pale	Red
Temperature	Cool to cold	Warm to hot
Swelling	Rounded	Cordlike vein path
Pain	Yes, usually	Yes
Flow	Slowed or stopped	No change or may be slowed
Nursing Actions	Tourniquet proximally (flow continues—infiltration)	Discontinue IV; usually call IV team
	Lower bottle (blood in tubing—no infiltration)	Note irritating solution (Valium, Keflin, KCl running too fast)
	Discontinue IV	Warm compresses; elevate and immobilize part
	Call IV team	
	Get order for warm compresses and elevate part	

NURSING DIAGNOSES*

Health Perception–Health Management Pattern
Altered Health Maintenance
Altered Protection
Effective Management of Therapeutic Regimen: Individual
Energy Field Disturbance
Health-Seeking Behaviors (Specify)
Ineffective Management of Therapeutic Regimen: Individuals
Ineffective Management of Therapeutic Regimen: Community
Ineffective Management of Therapeutic Regimen: Families
Noncompliance (Specify)
Risk for Infection
Risk for Injury
Risk for Perioperative Positioning Injury
Risk for Poisoning
Risk for Suffocation
Risk for Trauma

Nutritional-Metabolic Pattern
Altered Nutrition: Less than Body Requirements
Altered Nutrition: More than Body Requirements
Altered Nutrition: Potential for More than Body Requirements
Altered Oral Mucous Membrane
Effective Breastfeeding
Fluid Volume Deficit
Fluid Volume Excess
Hyperthermia
Hypothermia
Impaired Skin Integrity
Impaired Swallowing
Impaired Tissue Integrity
Ineffective Breastfeeding
Ineffective Infant Feeding Pattern
Ineffective Thermoregulation
Interrupted Breastfeeding
Risk for Altered Body Temperature
Risk for Aspiration
Risk for Fluid Volume Deficit
Risk for Impaired Skin Integrity

Modified from *NANDA nursing diagnoses: definitions and classifications 1995-1996,* North American Nursing Diagnosis Association; and Gordon M: *Manual of nursing diagnoses,* St Louis, 1995, Mosby.
*Grouped by functional health patterns.

Elimination Pattern

Altered Urinary Elimination
Bowel Incontinence
Colonic Constipation
Constipation
Diarrhea
Functional Incontinence
Perceived Constipation
Reflex Incontinence
Stress Incontinence
Total Incontinence
Urge Incontinence
Urinary Retention

Activity-Exercise Pattern

Activity Intolerance
Altered Growth and Development
Altered Tissue Perfusion (Specify Type) (Renal, cerebral, cardiopulmonary, gastrointestinal, peripheral)
Bathing/Hygiene Self-Care Deficit
Decreased Cardiac Output
Disorganized Infant Behavior
Diversional Activity Deficit
Dressing Self-Care Deficit
Dysfunctional Ventilatory Weaning Response
Dysreflexia
Fatigue
Feeding Self-Care Deficit
Impaired Gas Exchange
Impaired Home Maintenance Management
Impaired Physical Mobility
Inability to Sustain Spontaneous Ventilation
Ineffective Airway Clearance
Ineffective Breathing Pattern
Potential for Enhanced Organized Infant Behavior
Risk for Activity Intolerance
Risk for Disorganized Infant Behavior
Risk for Disuse Syndrome
Risk for Peripheral Neurovascular Dysfunction
Toileting Self-Care Deficit

Sleep-Rest Pattern

Sleep Pattern Disturbance

Cognitive-Perceptual Pattern

Acute Confusion
Altered Thought Processes
Chronic Confusion
Chronic Pain
Decisional Conflict (Specify)
Decreased Adaptive Capacity: Intracranial
Impaired Environmental Interpretation Syndrome
Impaired Memory
Knowledge Deficit (Specify)
Pain
Sensory-Perceptual Alterations
Unilateral Neglect

Self-Perception–Self-Concept Pattern

Anxiety
Body Image Disturbance
Chronic Low Self-Esteem
Fear (Specify Focus)
Hopelessness
Personal Identity Disturbance
Powerlessness
Risk for Loneliness
Risk for Self-Mutilation
Self-Esteem Disturbance
Situational Low Self-Esteem

Role-Relationship Pattern

Altered Family Processes
Altered Family Process: Alcoholism
Altered Parenting
Altered Role Performance
Anticipatory Grieving
Caregiver Role Strain
Dysfunctional Grieving
Impaired Social Interaction
Impaired Verbal Communication
Parental Role Conflict
Relocation Stress Syndrome
Risk for Altered Parent/Infant/Child Attachment
Risk for Altered Parenting
Risk for Caregiver Role Strain
Risk for Violence: Self-Directed or Directed at Others
Social Isolation

Sexuality-Reproductive Pattern

Altered Sexuality Patterns
Rape-Trauma Syndrome
Rape-Trauma Syndrome: Compound Reaction
Rape-Trauma Syndrome: Silent Reaction
Sexual Dysfunction

Coping–Stress Tolerance Pattern

Defensive Coping
Family Coping: Potential for Growth
Impaired Adjustment
Ineffective Community Coping
Ineffective Individual Coping
Ineffective Denial
Ineffective Family Coping: Compromised
Ineffective Family Coping: Disabling
Posttrauma Response
Potential for Enhanced Community Coping

Value-Belief Pattern

Potential for Enhanced Spiritual Well-Being
Spiritual Distress

TEMPERATURE CONVERSION FACTORS

°C	°F	°C	°F	°C	°F	°C	°F
34.0	93.2	36.4	97.5	38.8	101.8	41.2	106.1
34.2	93.6	36.6	97.9	39.0	102.2	41.4	106.5
34.4	93.9	36.8	98.2	39.2	102.6	41.6	106.8
34.6	94.3	37.0	98.6	39.4	102.9	41.8	107.2
34.8	94.6	37.2	99.0	39.6	103.3	42.0	107.6
35.0	95.0	37.4	99.3	39.8	103.6	42.2	108.0
35.2	95.4	37.6	99.7	40.0	104.0	42.4	108.3
35.4	95.7	37.8	100.0	40.2	104.4	42.6	108.7
35.6	96.1	38.0	100.4	40.4	104.7	42.8	109.0
35.8	96.4	38.2	100.8	40.6	105.2	43.0	109.4
36.0	96.8	38.4	101.1	40.8	105.4		
36.2	97.2	38.6	101.5	41.0	105.9		

°C = Temperature in Celsius (centigrade) degrees. (°C × 9/5) + 32 = °F.
°F = Temperature in Fahrenheit degrees. (°F − 32) × 5/9 = °C.

URINE LABORATORY VALUES

Test	Normal	Abnormal finding and significance
■ Color	Amber yellow	Dark, smoky color suggests hematuria. Yellow brown to olive green indicates excessive bilirubin. Orange red or orange brown is caused by phenazopyridine (Pyridium) or urobilin in excess. Cloudiness of freshly voided urine indicates infection. Colorless urine indicates excessive fluid intake, renal disease, or diabetes insipidus.
■ Smell	Aromatic	On standing, urine becomes more ammonia-like in smell. In urinary tract infections, urine smells unpleasant.
■ Protein	0-150 mg/24 hr 0-18 mg/dl	Persistent proteinuria is characteristic of acute and chronic renal disease, especially involving glomeruli. In absence of disease, positive finding may be caused by high-protein diet, strenuous exercise, dehydration, fever, or emotional stress. Vaginal secretions may contaminate urine specimen and give positive finding.
■ Glucose	None	Glycosuria indicates diabetes mellitus or low renal threshold for glucose reabsorption (if blood glucose level is normal). Small amounts may be found after glucose loading (e.g., glucose tolerance test).
■ Ketones	None	Altered carbohydrate and fat metabolisms indicate diabetes mellitus and starvation. Findings can also be seen in dehydration, vomiting, and severe diarrhea.
■ Bilirubin	None	Presence of bilirubinuria is as significant as jaundice in detection of liver disorders. Bilirubin may appear in urine before jaundice becomes visible or may be present in persons with hepatic disorders who do not have recognizable jaundice.

■ Specific gravity	1.003-1.030	Specific gravity of morning urine specimen reflects maximum concentrating ability of kidney and is 1.025 to 1.030. Low specific gravity indicates dilute urine and possibly excessive diuresis. High specific gravity indicates dehydration. If it becomes fixed at about 1.010, this indicates renal inability to concentrate urine, suggesting that kidney is progressing to end-stage renal disease.
■ Osmolality	300-1300 mOsm/kg	Measurement is a more accurate method than specific gravity for determining diluting and concentrating ability of kidneys. Deviations from normal indicate tubular dysfunction. Findings indicate if kidney has lost ability to concentrate or dilute urine. (Not part of routine urinalysis.)
■ pH	4.0-8.0 (average 6.0)	If more than 8.0, finding may be the result of standing of urine or urinary tract infections because bacteria decompose urea to form ammonia. If less than 4.0, may indicate respiratory and metabolic acidosis.
■ RBC	0-4/hpf	Bleeding in urinary tract is caused by calculi, cystitis, neoplasm, glomerulonephritis, tuberculosis, kidney biopsy, or trauma.
■ WBC	0-5/hpf	Increased number of WBCs in urine (pyuria) indicates urinary tract infection or inflammation.
■ Casts	None-occasional hyaline	Casts are molds of the renal tubules and may contain protein, WBCs, RBCs, or bacteria. Noncellular casts are hyaline in appearance, and a few may be found in normal urine. Casts indicate renal dysfunction or urinary tract infections.
■ Culture for organisms	No organisms in bladder, <10⁴ organisms/ml result of normal urethral flora	Bacteria counts >10^5/ml indicate urinary tract infection. Organisms most commonly found in urinary tract infections are *Escherichia coli*, enterococci, *Klebsiella*, *Proteus*, and streptococci.

hpf, High-powered field; *RBC*, red blood cell; *WBC*, white blood cell.

INDEX